SCOLIOSIS AND SPINAL PAIN SYNDROME

New understanding of their origin
and ways of successful treatment

VALENTYN SERDYUK
Professor, Doctor of Medical Sciences
(Honoured Inventor of Ukraine)
Department Traumatology and Orthopaedic Surgery
Odessa National Medical University
Ukraine

BYWORD BOOKS™

First Edition 2014

ISBN 978-81-8193-116-0

Cover Design: Netra Shyam
Typesetter: Jacob Thomas

Published by
Byword Books Private Limited
GF-15, Virat Bhavan
Mukherjee Nagar Commercial Complex
Delhi 110009, India
email: bywordbooks@gmail.com
website: www.bywordbooks.in

Printed in India at Manipal Technologies Ltd., Manipal, India

'Everything is simple when it has already been discovered
and is incredibly difficult if one does not yet know
where to look for it!'

—Hans Selye

Dedicated to my family,
in particular, to Lilia Serdyuk-Savishcheva,
my wife and best friend, whose moral support and assistance
helped me to write this book

Contents

Introduction

HAVING WORKED AS A PRACTITIONER SINCE 1966, I have managed to accumulate considerable experience and expertise in the field of orthopaedics and traumatology. During the past two decades, I focused on in-depth case studies of spinal pain and associated spinal deformities, including scoliosis, degenerative disc disease, osteoarthritis and spondylosis deformans.

The seeds of my interest in this subject were sown by Professor Ivan Gerzen, the eminent Ukranian scientist and founder of the Department of Traumatology and Orthopaedics at the Odessa National Medical University, during his consultations at the beginning of my medical work as a graduate student. Subsequently, as I went on to practise as an orthopaedic surgeon–traumatologist, seeing and helping several patients every day, I always tried to find an answer to the question that was uppermost in my mind: what are the causes of these diseases? Knowing the causes could help us eliminate the effects, enabling us to commence not with symptomatic but aetiology-based treatment, which would be much more effective.

It is widely accepted that osteochondrosis is a major cause of back pain and that it is related to age. While I agree with this, I am still trying to discover the origin of other diseases, and whether there is a connection between the pathology of the skeleton and internal diseases. It is said that the modern way of life, which is characterized by physical and emotional overload, environmental degradation and, often, the consumption of low-quality water and food, is the source of all the trouble. But then how do we explain the occurrence of spinal pain and the same diseases thousands of years ago, when the earth's ecology was undisturbed and people paid much more attention to the welfare of their bodies? Does this mean that the same causes existed back then as well as today?

The problem of spinal pain is multifaceted, i.e. such pain can be associated with an extremely wide range of factors, such as traumatological, oncological, helminthological and haematological. I have not analysed these areas in this book. My goal is to establish the initial causes of spinal deformities, spinal pain, and the diseases of the central and peripheral nervous systems and internal organs that arise from such deformities. I am particularly interested in analysing the existence of deformities during the first few years of life, before they result in osteochondrosis, spondylosis and other pathological conditions typically seen in an adult.

There are a considerable number of publications on spinal pain, spinal diseases (osteochondrosis, spondylosis) and, particularly, scoliosis. In addition, hundreds of excellent handbooks, manuals and guidelines for practitioners, and a large number of monographs, dissertations and articles in journals and newspapers have been published on the subject.

One gets the impression that the number of such patients is continuously increasing, and the establishment of new centres of spinal pathology, manual therapy, etc. seems to prove this. Perhaps the main reason for the rise in the number of patients is that, over the years, increasing pressure is being placed on the spine, especially in the case of children and adolescents. Youngsters spend many hours sitting at a desk and in front of a computer. Many have weak muscles and do not always have a healthy diet.

Thousands of people suffering from spinal pain have turned not only to medical professionals, but traditional healers as well. As the patients are generally satisfied, one could have let the situation remain as it is. But this problem is the subject of extensive research, and has been so for centuries. Many generations of physicians have taken a keen interest in the origin of human diseases, including spinal pain. Physicians of all times have been engaged in the treatment of such patients. Notably, there is the ancient Egyptian papyrus entitled 'The Secret Book of a Doctor', which is written by Ebers and dates back to 2500 BC. Attempts were made to unlock this secret. The famous ancient Indian texts expounding the ayurvedic system of medicine were written around 700 BC. According to this system, human diseases are the result of an imbalance between the different substances of the body. Doctors used drugs to eliminate harmful substances from the body and replace them with beneficial ones.

The research was continued by the ancient Greek poet and doctor, Homer (900 BC); the philosopher, mathematician and doctor, Pythagoras (580 BC); and finally, Hippocrates (460–377 BC), who was held in high esteem by his colleagues and called the 'father of medicine'. His followers believed that all diseases including spinal problems are associated with an imbalance of four fluids: blood, black bile, yellow bile and phlegm (mucus), as well as four related properties: heat, cold, dryness and humidity. Among the other prominent representatives of Greek medicine who explored this area were Democritus (460–370 BC), Plato (427–347 BC), Aristotle (384–322 BC) and Celsus (25 BC–AD 50).

The most outstanding scholar of antiquity, second to Hippocrates, was the Roman physician, Claudius Galen (c. BC 130–210). He was a doctor of the imperial family and his authority over the physicians of the Middle Ages was indisputable. His works completed the era of ancient medicine. Incidentally, it was Galen who suggested the term 'scoliosis', which means 'curve'. He was also the originator of the terms 'lordosis' and 'kyphosis'. Galen's impact was so great that his scientific works remained the basis for the study of medicine and, in particular, human anatomy for the next 13 centuries. However, he still could not find the answer to the question regarding the origin of human diseases. Centuries have passed since then, but the problem is viewed with the same sense of urgency, as evidenced by the growing number of publications.

Spinal neurosurgery is developing at a rapid pace today, having reached a very high technical level. Everyone knows about myelocele, which can be confirmed by a CT scan. Unfortunately, medical decisions mostly consider surgical options and not those which focus on allowing a patient to help himself. Are herniated discs as dangerous as claimed, or are they perhaps yet another excuse for the excessive activity of neurosurgeons? There is no consensus on how the herniated disc is formed in various regions of the spine. The most important aspect is that neither patients nor physicians have ever been fully satisfied with the results of surgical treatment for spinal pain.

What about the problem of scoliosis? Ask any physician whether it is possible to cure scoliosis and he will say 'no'. Is that really so?

In this book, I draw upon my long, personal experience with many thousands of observations to explain the seemingly 'entirely clear' and old problem of spinal pain and spinal deformity. For over 20 years, almost every day I have seen and continue to see patients suffering from pain in different regions of the spine. In many cases, the problem had started decades earlier and the patient had already received treatment from physicians of different specialties (neurologists, psychiatrists, cardiologists, urologists, oncologists, internists, etc.). The choice of the specialist usually depended on the prevalent clinical symptoms. Very often, the effect of the treatment was short-lived, which left the patient disappointed.

While seeing patients, I tried to combine all their statements to form a single picture of the disease. Eventually, I began to get an idea of the recurring symptoms. These belonged to a standard set of symptoms that occurred with slight variations in each child or adult patient. Having defined one of the symptoms, I was able to predict the occurrence of all the others. This was confirmed in hundreds and even thousands of cases. I gradually gained a large amount of practical knowledge that enabled me to arrive at some very important conclusions.

Eventually, I became firmly convinced that I had no right to remain silent any longer and should share all the knowledge I had accumulated together with my fellow physicians and patients. Apart from a dozen articles on this issue and several appearances on radio and local television, I had done nothing to make my findings and conclusions known. This book was first published in Russian in 2010. I am sure that the material presented in this English edition will help a large number of physicians to improve their efficiency and ease the suffering of many people.

Every time a patient from a different city or country comes to consult me, I ask him and myself a question: why has he not found the necessary help at home? I doubt that the physicians there lack professionalism. Probably the explanation is that the literature available to them does not contain a simple and clear explanation of the mechanism of spinal pain in its various manifestations. Perhaps the textbooks available on anatomy lack information on the comparative anatomy, for example, of the cervical vertebrae.

A roentgenologist generally describes in a barren medical style the observed signs of pathology, but the clinician can hardly understand them. Everybody agrees that spinal pathology lies at the heart of all diseases, but what conclusions can be drawn from this? There are no practical recommendations for patients on what to do in everyday life and at work, and what measures to take to prevent spinal pain.

In this book, I attempt to analyse the problems mentioned above and share my understanding of the origin of diseases and the factors responsible for their progression. In addition, I discuss the existing methods of diagnosis and treatment, besides explaining the essence of my proposals. The book is intended as a source of information not only for healthcare professionals and medical students, but also for a wider audience. That is why the extremely complicated material is presented in a semi-scientific style.

Probably it is time to reconsider some of the established views on the causes of spinal pain and spinal deformities. Indeed, like nature, our knowledge is all about dynamic development. It is continuously updated, and more and more facts are absorbed into our store of knowledge with the passage of time. I am fully aware that the orthodox medical fraternity will deny much of what is presented in this book. It is always very hard to abandon common practice or view things from a new angle. I am prepared to accept this. What you find in the following pages is not a figment of my imagination, but a presentation of facts meant for individual analysis by the reader.

And finally, when I started on this book, I did not possess much expertise in the area of scoliosis and other spinal deformities, and did not have any great knowledge of the pathogenesis of spinal pain. We started out by making an analysis of the clinical material we had collected. I did not have even a shadow of doubt about the correctness of the conclusions of my predecessors. The validity of the main guidelines and indicators for surgical and conservative treatment of spinal deformities seemed to be indisputable. However, our examination of many thousands of patients and analysis of the results of the treatment we prescribed provided us with an enormous amount of factual material which made it possible to see the problem of scoliosis and spinal pain in a way that departs from the standard view.

On the basis of our experience, we were able to reveal the mechanism of progression of lateral spinal curvature, the nature of osteochondrosis and deforming spondylosis, persistent pelvic pain syndrome and fibromyalgia, as well as the connection of human diseases with spinal deformities. The knowledge we had gathered allowed us to make useful recommendations not only for children with initial presentations of various diseases, but also for adults with existing chronic medical problems.

Nowadays, there are no doubts about the benefits of physiotherapy, therapeutic physical training and spa treatment, which together constitute the entire scheme of rehabilitation of patients with spinal diseases. Also, if indicated, timely surgical treatment can be the right choice for some patients. The purpose of this book is not to make the reader question the value of the accumulated knowledge of other professionals. Instead, the aim is to encourage professionals to provide care to patients as soon as possible, starting with the maternity ward, then in a children's clinic, a sanatorium, etc. The active prevention of spinal diseases must be the main focus of the experts.

And now, allow me to take you through the pages of this book, which might help you consider old problems from a new perspective. I hope you find the experience a useful and enjoyable one.

Valentyn Serdyuk
(www.orthopedics.com.ua)

Ukraine
September 2013

1 Evolution of medical thinking on the causes of spinal deformities and pain

I HAVE BEEN WORKING AS AN ORTHOPAEDIST-TRAUMATOLOGIST for over four decades. I graduated from Odessa Medical Institute in 1966 and thereafter completed primary training at Kyiv Institute of Orthopaedics in 1971. For my PhD thesis on plastic surgery for Achilles tendon defects, I initially focused on reconstructive orthopaedics and later worked on the treatment of severe injuries of major joints, including injuries complicated by purulent infection. In my doctoral dissertation, I described, for the first time, the application of magnetic therapy in the treatment and prevention of complications of open limb injuries.

In 1990, I began studying the problems of spinal pain and spinal deformities systematically. Around the same time, similar work was being done by other members of the Department of Traumatology and Orthopaedics of Odessa National Medical University and the city trauma centre, where I have been working as a professor for nearly 20 years now. Among those working in this area were Professor V.F. Wenger, Professor E.V. Kulazhenko, and Honoured Inventor of Ukraine V.I. Gruntovskiy. Docent V.S. Esipenko, who has greatly influenced my work, and physiotherapist V.A. Domrachev were my first teachers and mentors in vertebrology. They exposed me to the basic techniques of manual therapy. Since these physicians had specialized experience in vertebrology, I directed patients with spinal pain to them. This continued until I found that they were receiving repeated visits from patients with recurrent pain, as well as patients seeking help following unsuccessful attempts at repositioning of their vertebrae under anaesthesia. These cases raised doubts about the accuracy of applied treatment.

Soon, A.A. Unanov, a manual therapist and doctor of therapeutic exercises, who later became a doctor of pedagogical sciences and a professor, gained distinction in our city. He had achieved great success in one of the district clinics, as was evidenced by the large flow of patients to the clinic. However, as it turned out, his patients, too, kept visiting him repeatedly (sometimes 10 times or more) because of recurring pain. It was then that I began to explore the degree of success attained by other vertebrologists. I found that they, too, had failed to provide their patients with effective treatment, as demonstrated by the numerous cases of re-treatment. As a result of their failure, many

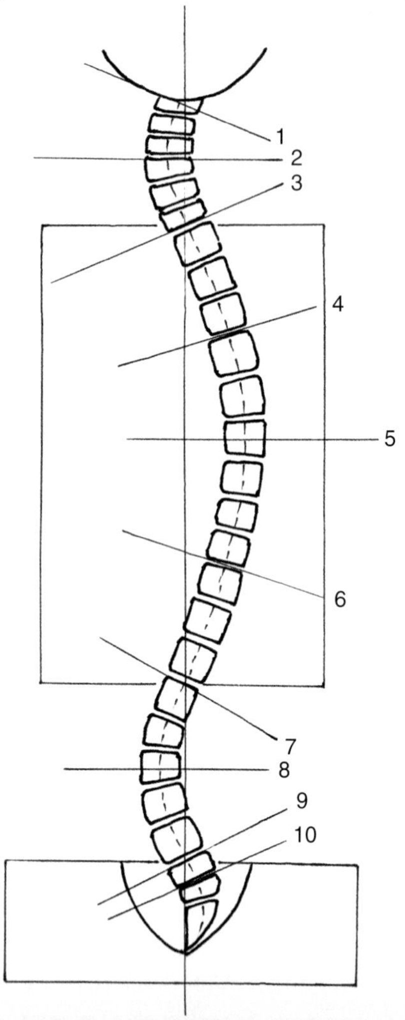

Fig. 1.1. Localization of rotational displacements of vertebrae in cervical, thoracic, lumbar and sacral regions of the spine in shortening of the left leg. 1–10 — areas of their typical location

manual therapists gave up on treating patients with spinal pain.

That was when I started to ask myself what was really going on. What was the explanation for this situation? Was it a situation when the vertebrologists were making deliberate mistakes in their work in order to retain patients for as long as possible for the sake of money or was it something beyond their knowledge or understanding?

On observing how each of the specialists functioned, I concluded that they were honest and conscientious people. I, therefore, felt that their failure had to be attributed to a lack of knowledge of something which was apparently common. This something led to the exacerbation of pain and caused patients to seek retreatment.

I took it upon myself to examine patients with the complaint of spinal pain. I found that the pain was located in areas where rotational displacement of vertebrae could be detected by the finger. In all patients, without exception, the location of the rotations was similar, as if typical (the cervical, thoracic, lumbar and sacral regions of the spine), although the pain might have been localized to only one or two sites (Fig. 1.1).

I also observed the following two types of chest deformity in all the patients I examined:

First type: This type was characterized by anteposition of the right collarbone (clavicle) and marked asymmetry of the left half of the chest, as well as anteposition of the left costal arch. There was a rib hump at the back on the same side of the chest that had a clavicle deformation (Figs 1.2 and 1.3).

Second type: In the case of anteposition of the left clavicle, all the features of the first type of deformity of the chest were mirrored on the opposite side (Fig. 1.4).

Once I was sent to examine a patient diagnosed with dislocated right clavicle at the sternoclavicular junction. Careful examination revealed that it was a case of the clavicle deformity described above, caused by chest torsion and scoliosis of a curvature of 3–4 degrees.

My most interesting finding was that every single patient I examined, regardless

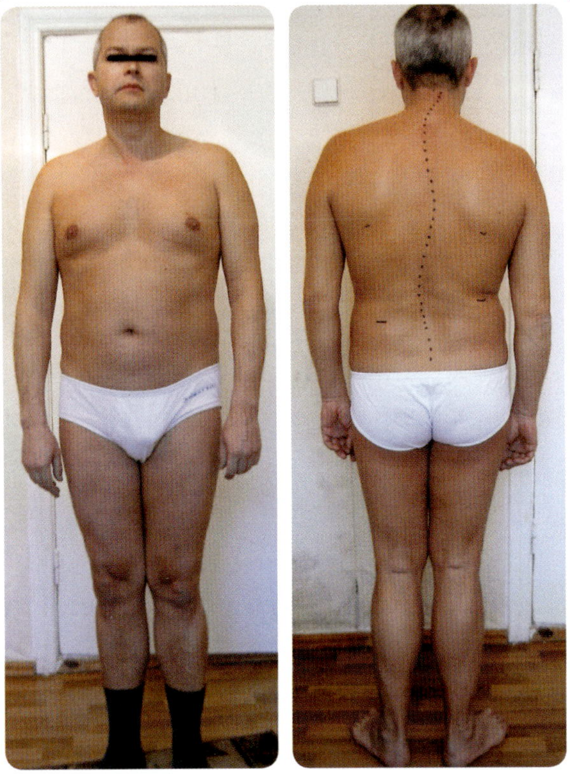

A B

Fig. 1.2.
A - Displacement of the right clavicle (collarbone) and left half of the chest anteriorly
B - The same patient: thorax deformation—right-sided rib hump; left-sided pelvic tilt

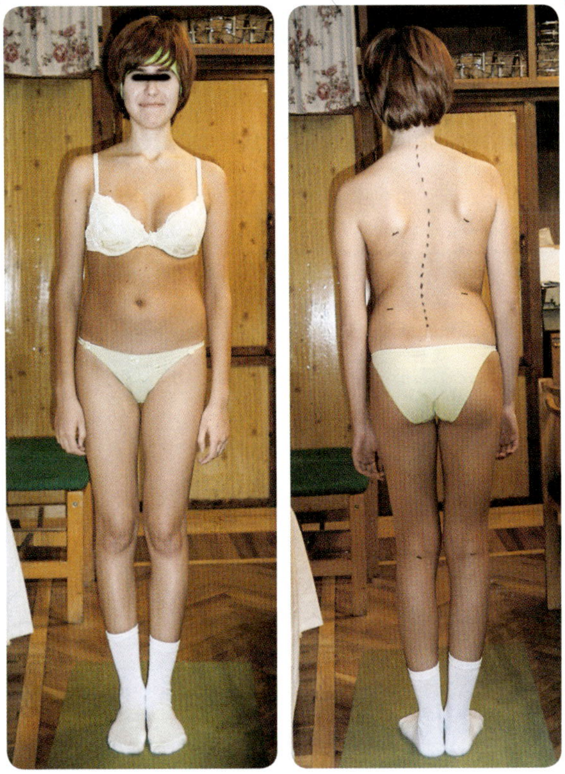

A B

Fig. 1.3.
A - Asymmetry of the left part of thorax with left-sided anterior displacement of costal arch
B - The same patient: thorax deformation—right-sided rib hump; left-sided pelvic tilt

of the age group, suffered from either the first or second type of deformity. *Thus, the development of chest deformity was a regular feature.* Over the next few years, I examined hundreds of other patients, which allowed me to establish the existence of a number of other regularly recurrent symptoms. For example, on the side of the chest where the arc of the ribs came forward, there was a clearly visible shortening of the lower limb (Fig. 1.5).

In our early work on vertebrological issues, we tried to determine the extent of the shortening of the lower limb with a measuring tape. The measurement was carried out by standard methods: from the front upper iliac spine to the bottom of the inner ankle. Since we had determined the position of the lower limb in relation to the pelvis, we measured what is known as relative shortening. It is considered more precise to determine the length of the lower limb by measuring its two segments separately. The first segment runs from the lower edge of the greater trochanter to the knee joint (thigh length), while the second is from the knee joint to the bottom of the outer ankle, which is the length of the tibia. This method of measurement is called absolute or anatomical.

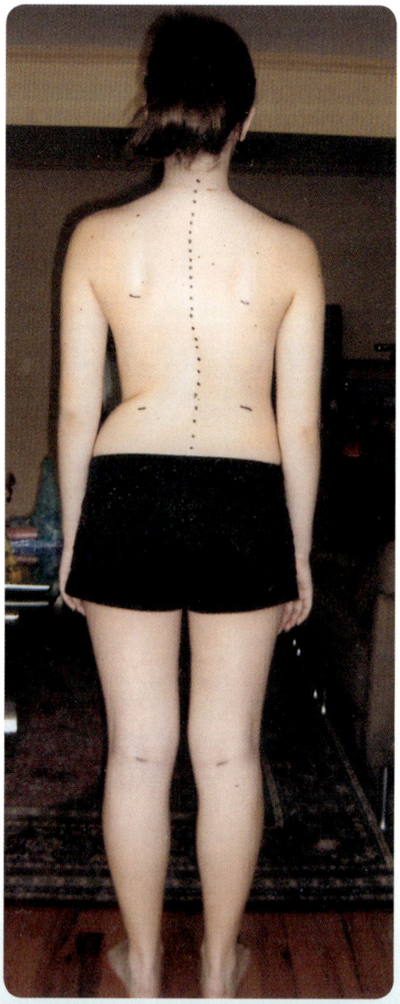

Fig. 1.4. Development of left-sided hump in right-sided body tilt due to shortening of the right leg

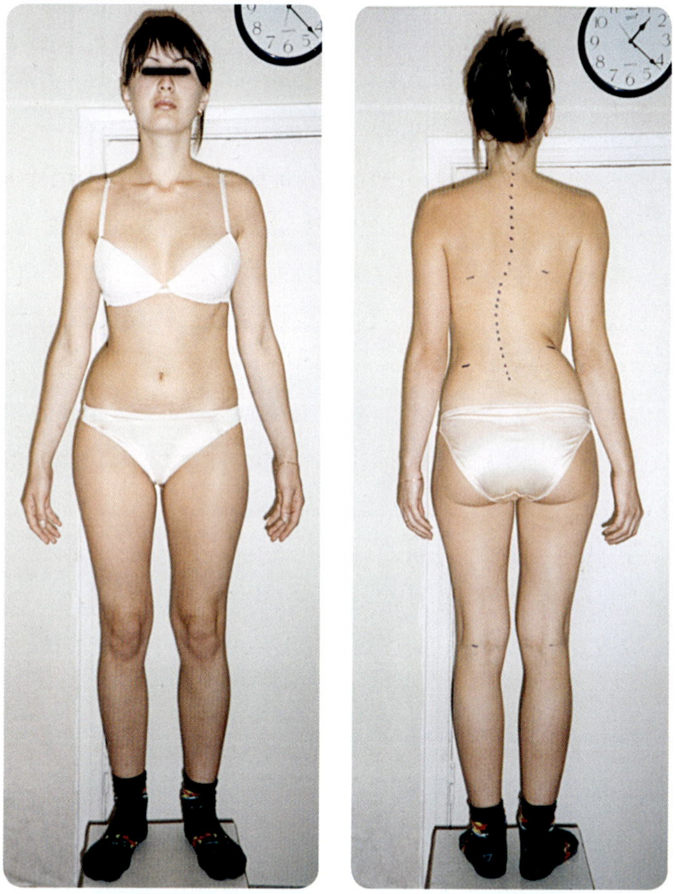

A B

Fig. 1.5. Patient S., 20 years.
A - The left half of the thorax protrudes anteriorly
B - Shortening of the left leg 30 mm; severe hypotrophy of left gluteal muscles, hypoplasia of pelvic bones on the left side; varus deformity of the left tibia

I must say that tape measurements do not yield accurate data because the skin may give rise to a bias, especially among obese people. The literature contained very little information on attempts to measure the length of the legs through radiography or the use of special devices. An interesting study, conducted at the Moscow Scientific Research Institute of Medical Instrumentation, calculated the extent of shortening of the lower limbs by measuring the difference between the pressure of the feet as the patient stood on a special platform connected to a computer. Such methods were not used in everyday orthopaedic practice due to lack of proper equipment.

When examining patients in our clinic, we inserted special orthopaedic insoles under the heel that was shorter. The insoles, which were of different thickness, eliminated shortening and helped to determine the extent of shortening. The data that we gathered led us to the conclusion that the leading symptom was not an absolute shortening, i.e. an anatomical reduction of the length of the thigh and/or shinbone, but relative shortening of a compensatory nature. The relative shortening of the limb was always accompanied by varying degrees of muscle tension in the spinal extensors on both sides. However, during the initial stages of our work, the mechanism and causes of the development of muscular asymmetry were not clear to us.

The extent of shortening of the limb varied widely from 3 mm to 50 mm and above. Age made no difference. In an adult male of 55–60 years of age, the shortening could be of 3 mm, and in a child of 5–6 years of age it could be of 15–20 mm. The sex also made no difference—the extent of shortening could be 40–55 mm irrespective of whether it was a boy or a girl. Thus, the degree of shortening seemed to bear no relation to gender, age and the physical development of the body. However, it clearly seemed to be of a hereditary nature.

Another regularly recurring symptom I observed was that on the side on which the lower limb was relatively shortened, the lower third of the thigh and tibia had a marked varus deformity (curvature with the angle open medially). This could be of varying degrees. The valgus deformity (curvature with the angle open outwards) of the lower limbs was encountered much less frequently. The first time I noticed the varus deformity was during a visit to Arlington Cemetery near Washington (USA). During the guard of honour at the Tomb of the Unknown Soldier, a tall athletic guard was standing with his back to me. He wore pants that were tight-fitting at the thighs and cruses. The left lower limb had an obvious varus deformity of the knee. However, this young man was certainly healthy and without any complaints, otherwise he could not have served in the army and even less so, in the honour guard, for which the best are likely to be recruited.

Considering the frequency with which this varus deformity occurred, I began to take a closer look at the people I saw around me, as well as our patients. We found that the varus deformity of the lower limbs occurred mainly on the left (according to our observations, in 83%–85% of cases) and less frequently on the right. The deformity was negligible among young people (Figs 1.5 and 1.6), whereas it was often perceptible even from a distance among older people (Fig. 1.7). This led me to draw certain conclusions on unilateral varus or valgus deformity of the thigh and tibia in people of all ages, especially in those who had suffered no injury of the corresponding lower limb in the past. If in youth the deformity was not accompanied by pain; in adulthood, constant pressure from the internal or external thigh condyle on the meniscus and cartilage surface of the tibia and other elements of the knee led to the development of deforming arthrosis with severe pain. It is quite possible that these varus (or valgus) deformities of the thigh and tibia, which distort the limb by causing shortening, could be important aetiological factors in the development of Perthes disease, aseptic necrosis of the femoral head and, eventually, deforming coxarthrosis. If the mechanism of deformation becomes clear, we can perhaps stop this process somehow and even reverse it.

For the moment, however, let us keep to the main point without venturing too far ahead. Another regularly recurring symptom was that on the side of the varus (or valgus) deformity of the tibia (i.e. on the side of the relatively shorter lower limb), the volume of the buttocks was significantly smaller than on the opposite side (Fig. 1.8). Most of the patients with severe scoliosis, apart from showing such a decrease in the volume of one buttock, suffered from hypoplasia of the pelvic bones (Figs 1.9–1.12). A possible explanation for this situation is that shortening of the leg since early childhood had caused a gradual increase of working hypotrophy in all soft or bone tissues.

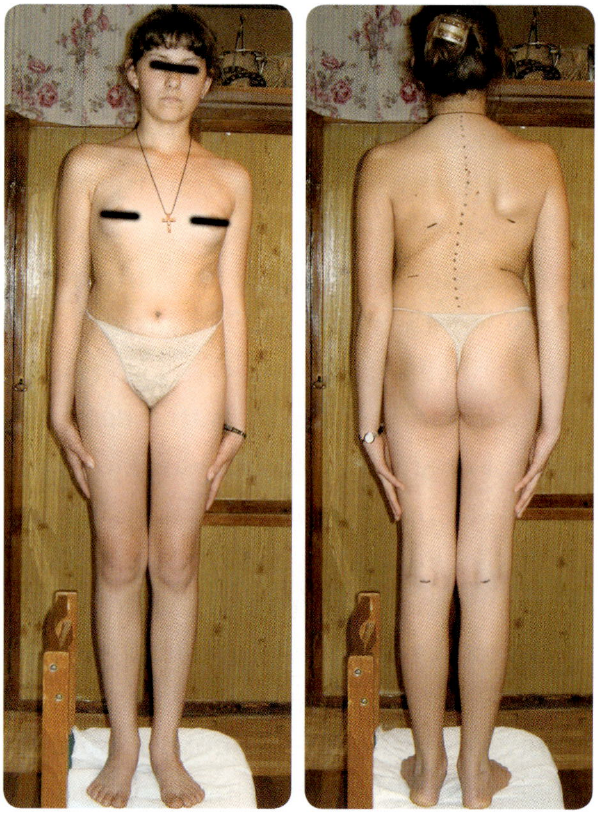

A B

Fig. 1.6. Patient B., 14 years.
A - Anterior protrusion of the right collarbone and left side of the thorax
B - Shortening of the left leg 7 mm; right-sided rib hump; wasting the left gluteal region; varus deformity of the left tibia; plano-valgus foot

The readers may confirm my observations themselves, in all people without exception, whether children or adults. The deformities described are most noticeable in summer or when a person is dressed in tight pants. For some reason, most of these people (in my experience, up to 83%–85%) have their head tilted to the right when seen from the front, the right clavicle protruding more than the left and the left rib arch protruding forward as well. In addition, in *most women*, the left breast protrudes forward. Viewed from the back, the right side of the thorax is deformed due to the formation of the rib hump (the shoulder blade sticks out in lean people and the volume of the left leg and left buttock are less than that of their right counterparts. The left leg has a varus deformity. Of course, the severity of the symptoms varies, but they are always present.

Later we discovered two other symptoms. One was a limitation in the rotation of the head in the direction of the leg that was relatively shortened. The other was related to the volume of the back muscles. The muscles that straighten the body (M. erector spinae and M. latissimus dorsi) are attached together to the sacrum. Hypothetically, having the same leg length and equal muscle force, their contours on the right and left should be identical. However, in the case of relative shortening of the left leg, the volume of both muscles becomes much larger on the right than that on the left (Figs 1.13 and 1.14). Similarly, in the case of relative shortening of the right leg, the volume of both these muscles on the left is significantly larger than that on the opposite side.

While searching for the causes of the development of the deformities mentioned above, we noted that 100% of the patients, regardless of age, had lateral (scoliotic) curvature of the spine. The curvature was of varying degrees of severity. We illustrate this with a few photographs of patients of different ages (from 4 to 84 years of age). Almost all the patients examined had shortening of the left leg and, accordingly, right-sided scoliosis. Shortening of the right leg, and accordingly, left-sided scoliosis were present only in rare cases (Figs 1.13–1.15).

I was shocked by the finding regarding scoliosis and naturally, decided to scan the existing literature and to learn the findings of other orthopaedic surgeons. The results were quite contradictory. In different

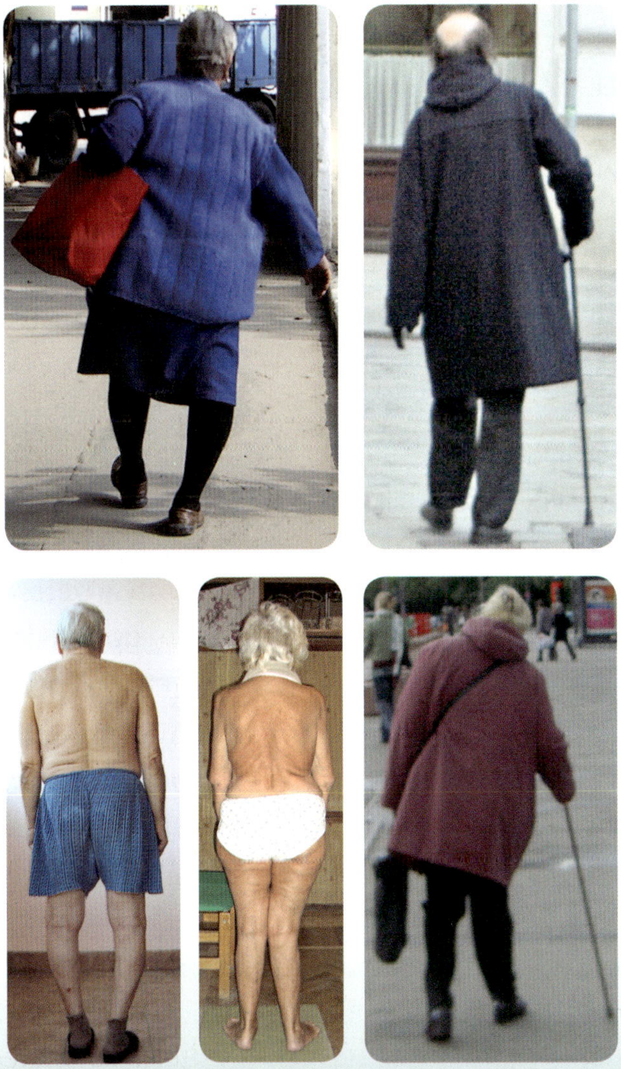

Fig. 1.7. Types of varus and valgus deformities of the lower extremities in the elderly

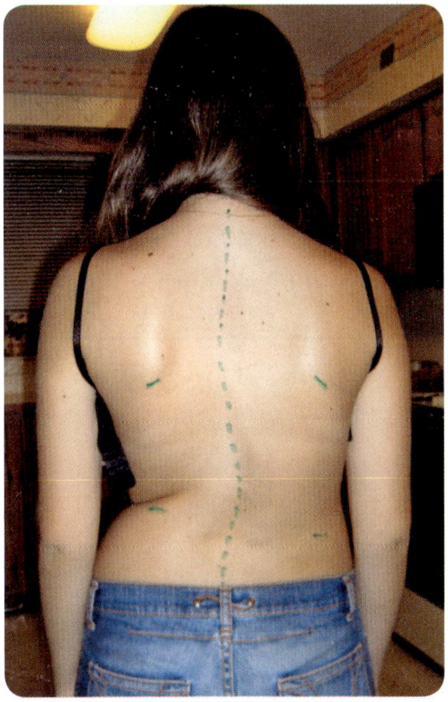

Fig. 1.8.
Volume of the gluteal muscles is more on the left than on the right due to the relative shortening of the right leg

studies, the frequency of scoliosis ranged from 10% to 90%. This variation was probably due to differences in the methods of assessment of children, adolescents and adults. In particular, the initial extent of the disease was evaluated differently. However, even if one left room for possible biases, the frequency of scoliosis was still very high. The traditional explanations for the occurrence of scoliosis were weakness of the back muscles, postural disturbance due to uncomfortable school desks, carrying bags full of books, etc. Hereditary factors and hormonal disorders were also said to play an important role.

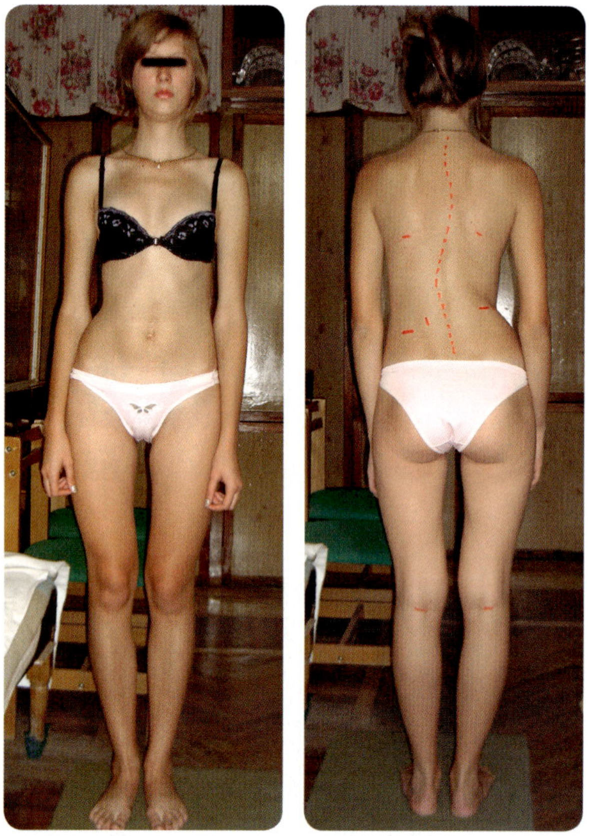

A B

Fig. 1.9. Patient G., 14 years.
A - Displacement of the right collarbone and left side of the thorax with the breast protruding anteriorly; relative shortening of the left leg 48 mm
B - Right-sided rib hump; substantial wasting of gluteal muscles on the left side; hypoplasia of pelvic bones on the left side; varus deformity of the left tibia; plano-valgus deformity of the left tibia; plano-valgus foot

I then decided to examine various groups of healthy people and draw my own conclusions. I started by seeing some children in kindergarten, located in my neighbourhood. This idea had occurred to me after meeting a group of kids on the street. Since it was summer, the children were in T-shirts and it was easy to make out that some of them clearly had a chest deformity. So, I introduced myself to the school management as an orthopaedic surgeon and, together with a nurse, examined 40 children about 6 years of age. I found that all of them had scoliotic spinal deformity of varying severity. At that time, I was not paying much attention to the length of the legs, since my first and foremost concern was whether or not they had scoliosis. Then I examined a group of toddlers of up to 3 years of age. All of them too had a spinal deformity, though it was barely noticeable. I would like to draw attention to the fact that the children I examined were only in kindergarten and did not have to carry the kinds of loads that older children have to carry.

Some days later, an Olympics champion in rhythmic gymnastics needed my consultation as she was suffering from severe pain in the legs. Upon examining her, I found several subluxations in the lumbar spine. The pain was brought under control with the help of treatment. It was extraordinary that even such a well-trained athlete

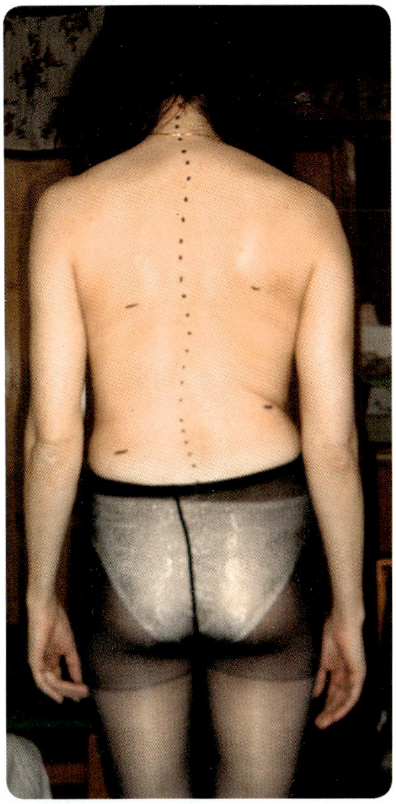

Fig. 1.10.
Patient S., 36 years.
Shortening of the left leg 23 mm; wasting of gluteal muscles on the left side, hypoplasia of pelvic bones; right-sided scoliosis

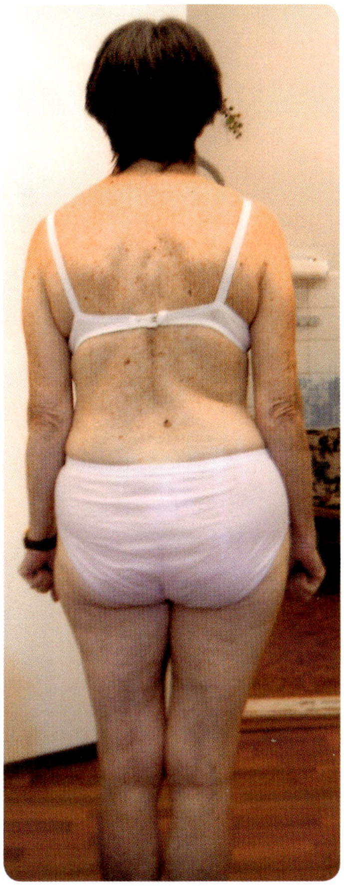

Fig. 1.11.
Patient S., 36 years.
Shortening of the left leg 33 mm; wasting of muscles of left gluteal region; hypoplasia of pelvic bones on the left side; right-sided scoliosis

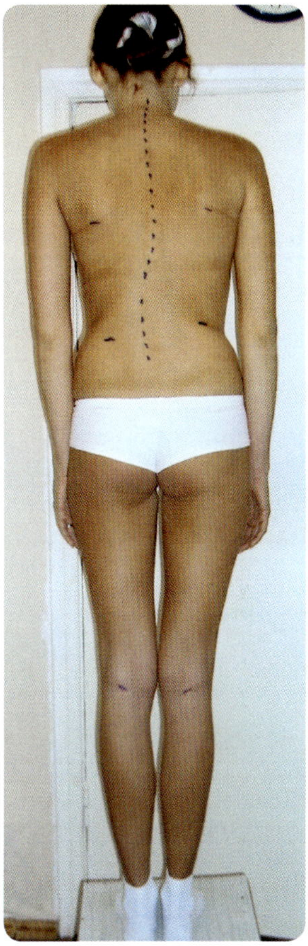

Fig. 1.12.
Patient L., 23 years.
Relative shortening of the left log 10 mm; hypotrophy of gluteal muscles on the left side, hypoplasia of pelvic bones on the left side; right-sided scoliosis

had a highly visible deformity of the spine, consistent with scoliosis of a curvature of 2nd degree. In addition, there was a deformity of one of the collarbones, which protruded forward. I sought permission to examine all the gymnasts who were present in the gym at that time and all the girls lined up in a row. Since they all wore swimsuits, both their clavicles were clearly visible. I was amazed by what I saw. Every girl had a clavicle asymmetry either on the left or right side. This made it obvious that weakness of the spinal muscles or lack of fitness was not the cause. So, what was it?

In search of an answer I examined a group of athletes. These were people with a high level of physical fitness, and powerful muscles of the corpus and limbs. You might have probably guessed by now that all the athletes I examined had a clavicle asymmetry, deformity of the chest with a rib hump on the side concerned, and rotary subluxation of vertebrae in the same places—cervical, upper-chest and middle-chest, lower thoracic and lumbar. All of them had scoliosis of a greater or lesser degree

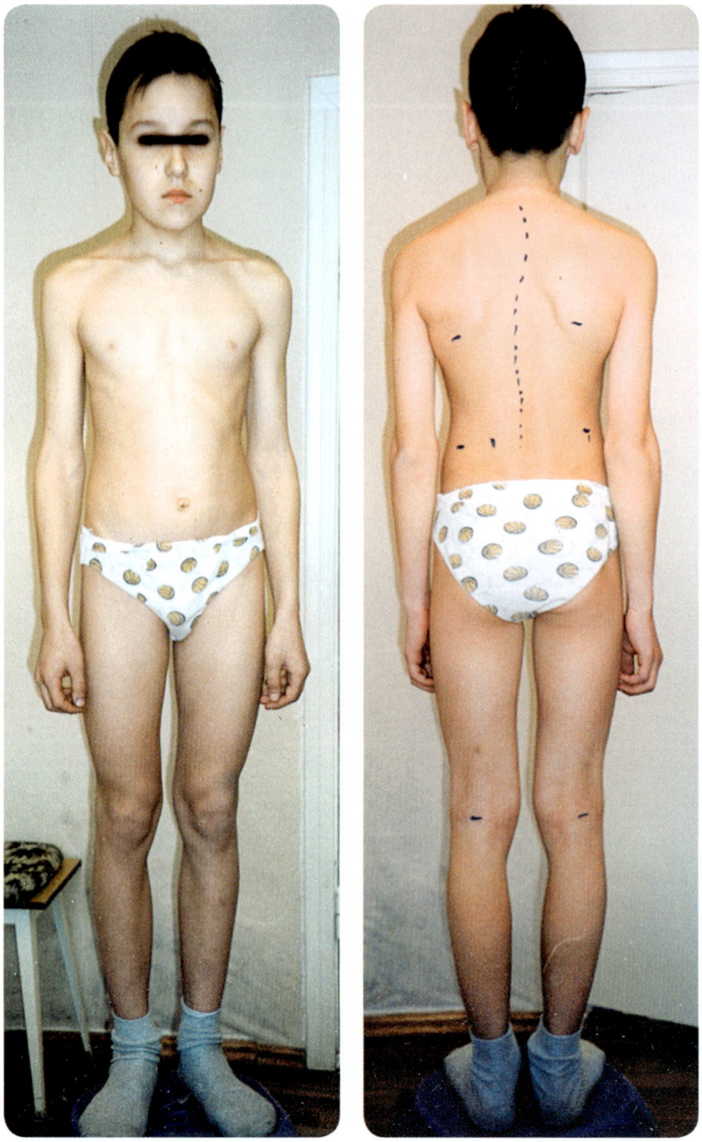

A **B**

Fig. 1.13. Patient S., 12 years.
A - Relative shortening of the left leg 10 mm; head is tilted to the right; the right clavicle and left costal arch are protruding
B - Right half of the thorax posteriorly and forms a rib hump; slightly marked varus deformity of the left tibia; volume of spine extensors on the right is bigger than on the left; plano-valgus foot

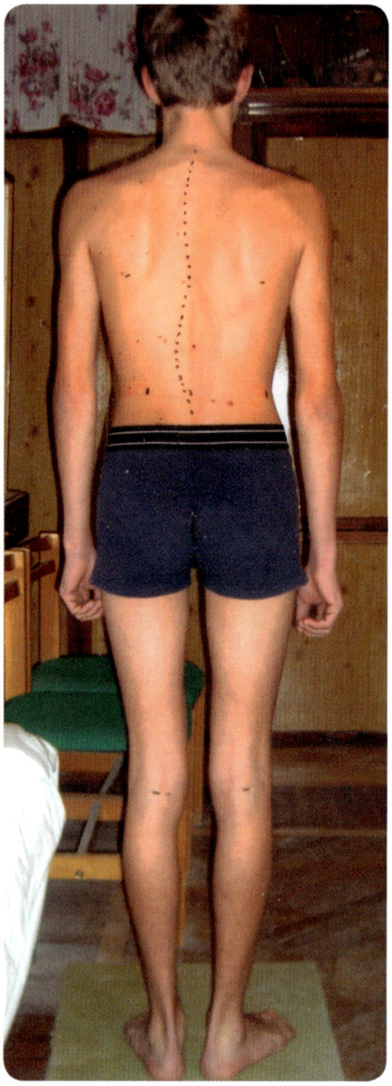

Fig. 1.14. Patient Y., 15 years. Relative shortening of the left leg 15 mm; the right scapula protrudes posteriorly forming the rib hump; pelvis is tilted to the left; volume of gluteal muscles on the left is smaller than on the right side; slightly marked varus deformity of the left tibia; volume of the back extensors on the right is much larger than on the left

(Fig. 1.16). And all this in spite of the massive amount of muscles! In those parts of the spine where there were subluxations, applying pressure with the finger caused pain.

Next, we decided to examine a large group of children from a prestigious school in Odessa. The arguments in favour of this decision included the fact that since education here was rather expensive, these children's parents would be wealthy and capable of giving them a good diet. Further, practically all the children had good physical training and could swim or ride a horse. Finally, children in this school were under

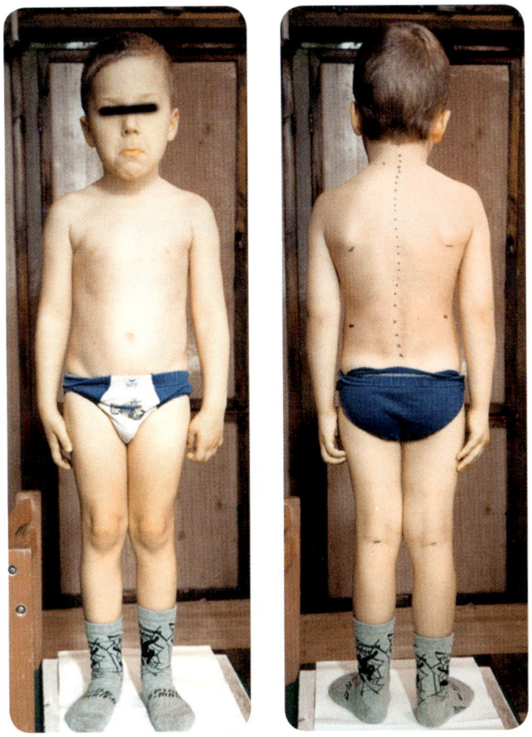

A B

Fig. 1.15-1. Patient G., 4 years.
A - Relative shortening of the left leg 7 mm; head is tilted to the right; facial asymmetry; slightly pronounced anteversion of the left costal arch
B - Right-sided scoliosis with initial signs of the rib hump formation on the right; slight hypotrophy of left gluteal muscles; weakly pronounced left-sided pelvic tilt; left-sided flat-valgus foot deformity

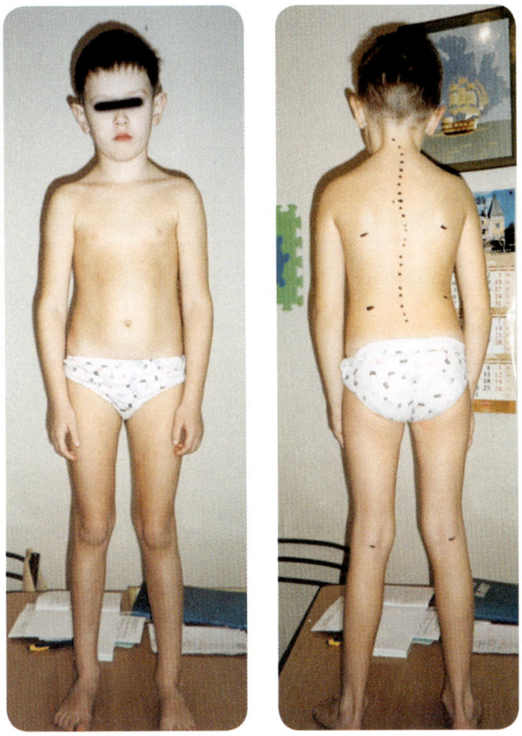

A B

Fig. 1.15-2. Patient K., 6 years.
A - Relative shortening of the left leg 7 mm; facial asymmetry; head is tilted to the right; slightly marked deformity of the chest
B - Right-sided scoliosis with initial signs of the rib hump formation on the right; tilt of the pelvis to the left; wasting of gluteal muscles on the left, hypoplasia of pelvic bones on the left; left-sided flat-valgus foot deformity

constant medical care, so one would expect them to be healthy. Where else, indeed, could one find healthy children? I sought the director's permission to examine 100 children of 8–10 years of age. Since the children were being examined free of charge, by a professor of orthopaedics, there were no problems with attendance. I examined the children only in the presence of their parents. Of the 100 children examined, 100 cases of scoliotic deformity were detected, as a rule, barely noticeable. In all cases, there was a visible deformity of the collarbone and protrusion of the costal arch on the opposite side. In some cases, the rib hump was hidden by adipose tissue, although it was present without a doubt. I discussed my findings with the parents and made the relevant recommendations. However, I still had not found an answer to the question: Why did all these examined children have a scoliotic posture?

My daily work and the visits of patients with complaints of spinal pain eventually forced me to give up my mass examinations of people. Moreover, I did not see the

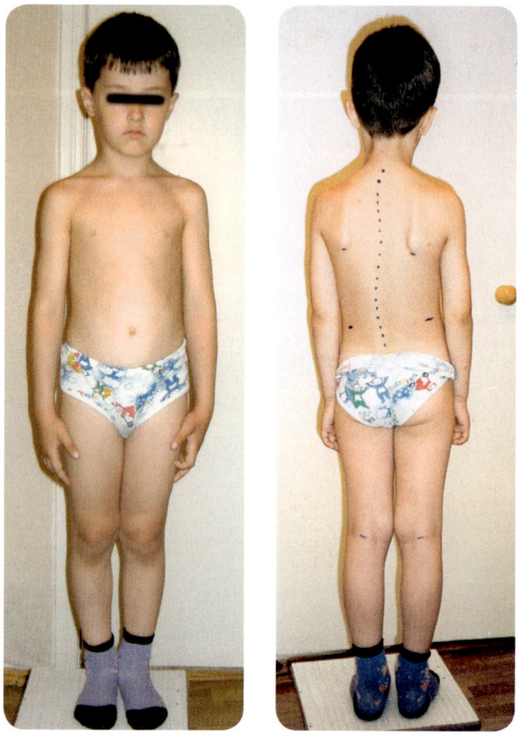

A B

Fig. 1.15-3. Patient S., 6 years.
A - Relative shortening of the left leg 15 mm; slightly marked deformity of the chest — anteversion of the right collarbone and left costal arch
B - Right-sided scoliosis with formation of the rib hump on the right; pelvis is tilted to the left; wasting of gluteal muscles on the left, slightly marked hypoplasia of pelvic bones on the left; slight varus deformity of the left tibia; plano-valgus foot

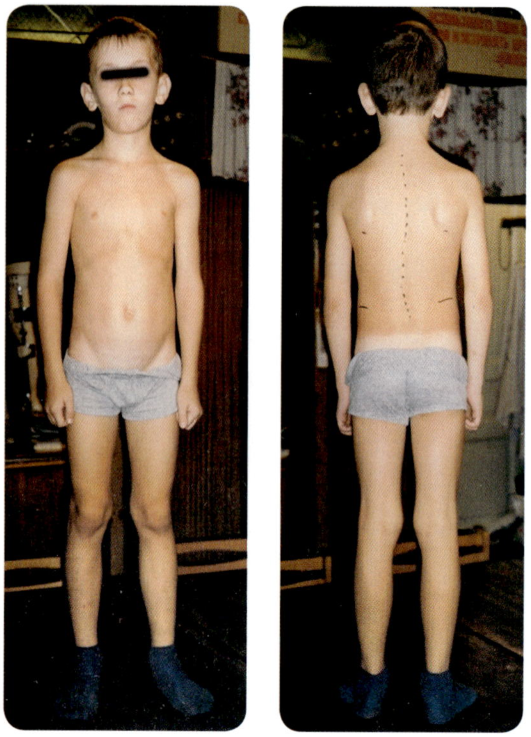

A B

Fig. 1.15-4. Patient A., 8 years.
A - Relative shortening of the left leg 7 mm; head is tilted to the right; facial asymmetry, divergent strabismus; anteversion of the right clavicle; left rib arc protrudes anteriorly
B - Right-sided scoliosis with initial signs of the rib hump formation on the right; slight hypotrophy of gluteal muscles on the left; weakly pronounced pelvic tilt to the left; plano-valgus foot

point in continuing with them. After all, everyone I had examined had a scoliotic deformity of a greater or lesser degree. The question which seemed more relevant now pertained to the nature of spinal pain. The traditional explanation implicated osteochondrosis, both among adults and children. I must say that in the first stage of my research, I fully seconded this hypothesis. Indeed, the reduction in disc height and the consequent decrease in the intervertebral space led to a decrease in the diameter of the intervertebral foramen formed by the arch of the vertebral body and the articular processes. As a result, compression of the spinal rootlets occurred. This was compounded by the presence of osteophytes in spondylosis deformans. Other than scoliosis, the spinal pain could be precipitated by osteochondrosis and spondylosis deformans, as well as other pathological conditions that caused injury to the spinal roots. These included primary and metastatic tumours, tuberculosis, leishmaniasis, multiple myeloma, syphilis, osteomyelitis and spondylolisthesis. According to the

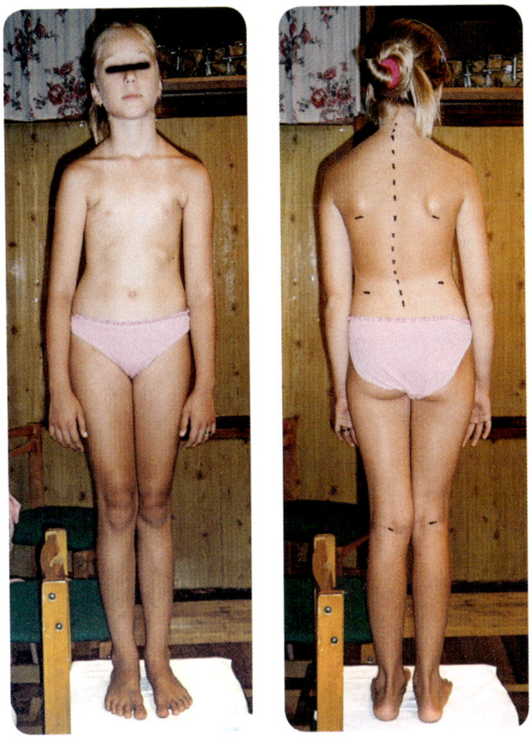

A B

Fig. 1.15-5. Patient B., 9 years.
A - Relative shortening of the left leg 18 mm; head is tilted to the right, facial asymmetry; slightly marked chest deformity — the right clavicle and left rib arc are protruding anteriorly
B - Right-sided scoliosis with formation of the rib hump on the same side; pelvis is tilted to the left; wasting of gluteal muscles on the left; hypoplasia of pelvic bones on the left; slight varus deformity of the left tibia; plano-valgus feet, more marked on the left side

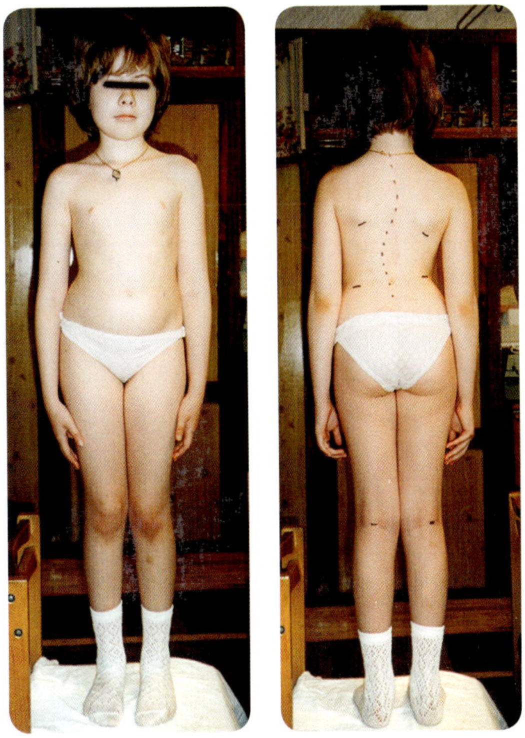

A B

Fig. 1.15-6. Patient K., 10 years.
A - Relative shortening of the left leg 20 mm; head is tilted to the right, facial asymmetry; deformation of the chest, anteversion of the right clavicle and left costal arch
B - Right-sided scoliosis with formation of the rib hump on the right; pelvis is tilted to the left; wasting of gluteal muscles on the left; hypoplasia of pelvic bones on the left; slight varus deformity of the left tibia; plano-valgus foot

statistics, the leading cause of spinal pain is a neurosurgical pathological process, most often arising from the destruction of the (vertebral) body or the vertebral arches and intervertebral disc or nucleus, or both of them, together with the formation of disc herniation.

There is another cause of spinal pain. Some vertebrologists believe that cartilaginous rings located in the facet joints, or the so-called meniscoids, can shift towards the intervertebral foramina, resulting in the compression of nerve roots.

A comparison of the frequency of the occurrence of neurosurgical and orthopaedic conditions among patients suffering from spinal pain showed that those with neurosurgical conditions accounted for only 10%–15% of patients. Those with orthopaedic conditions, such as scoliosis, osteochondrosis, deforming spondylosis and spondylolisthesis, accounted for 80% or more.

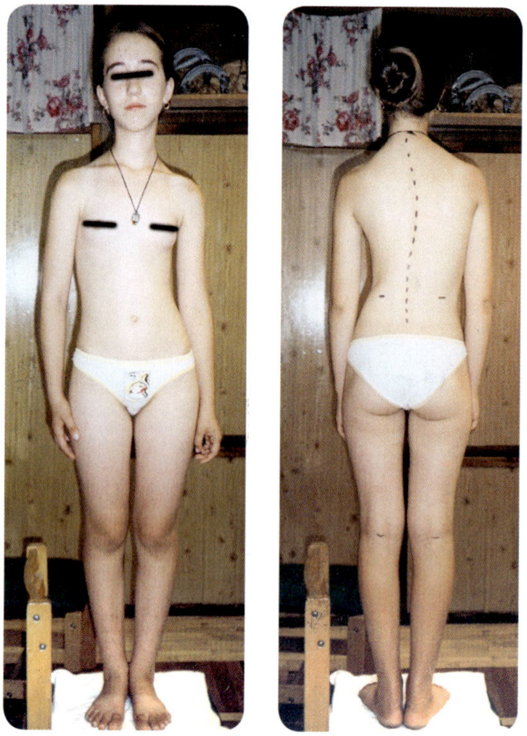

A B

Fig. 1.15-7. Patient B., 13 years.
A - Relative shortening of the left leg 10 mm; slight tilt of the head to the right, facial asymmetry; divergent strabismus; slight deformation of the chest — left breast is protruding
B - Right-sided scoliosis with formation of rib hump on the right

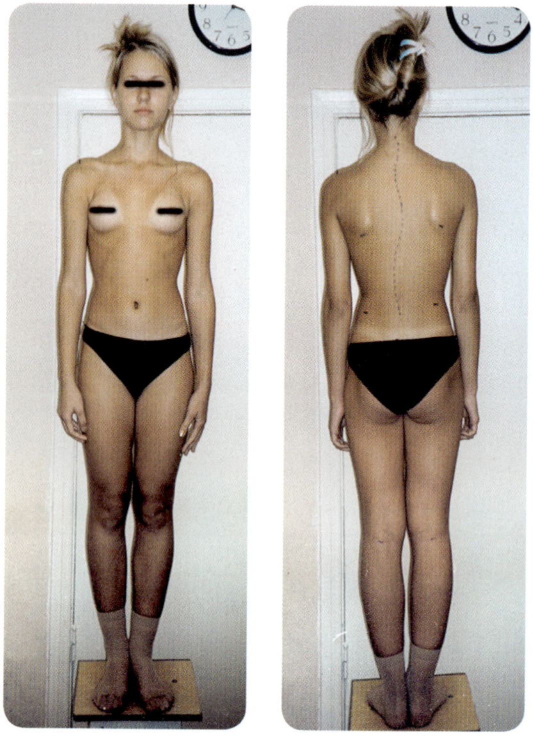

A B

Fig. 1.15-8. Patient B., 13 years.
A - Relative shortening of the left leg 20 mm; head is tilted to the right, facial asymmetry; deformation of the thorax with noticeable anteversion of the right clavicle and left costal arch
B - Right-sided scoliosis with formation of noticeable rib hump on the right; wasting of gluteal muscles on the left; slight varus deformity of the left tibia

In 1997–98, I learnt from numerous articles in the local newspapers about the achievements of A.I. Bobyr, a Russian orthopaedist with a PhD in Medical Sciences. Dr Bobyr reported that he had been successful in relieving pain as well as in treating osteochondrosis. I attended one of his lectures, which was also attended by many of my colleagues. During the lecture, we were shown a colour film dealing with several interesting facts. However, in my view, their interpretation was incorrect. Dr Bobyr often expressed the idea that osteochondrosis, which causes spinal pain, was a major disease of the century, affecting millions of people. According to him, this disease was caused by a sedentary lifestyle, lack of faith in God, malnutrition, poor quality of water and several other factors. His recommendations for the treatment of the problem included wearing magnetic insoles, performing physiotherapeutic exercises, taking a nutritious diet, maintaining a healthy lifestyle, attending church regularly and, most importantly, undergoing manual therapy, for which he used his own technique. In contrast to Dr Kasian, who set spondyles with arm-kick, Dr Bobyr approached the

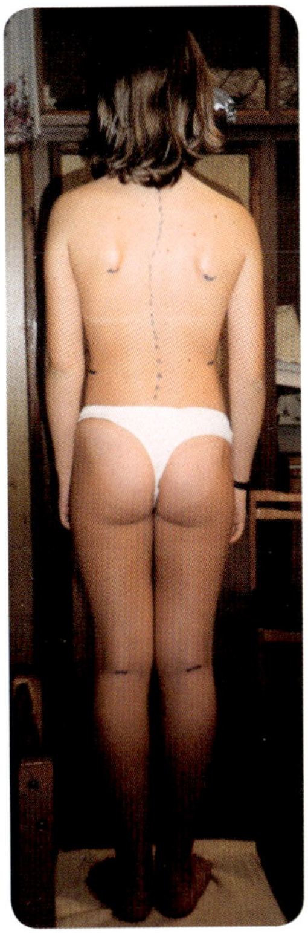

Fig. 1.15-9.
Patient D., 10 years. Relative shortening of the right leg 45 mm; wasting of right gluteal area; tilt of the body to the right; left-sided scoliosis; protrusion of the left scapula

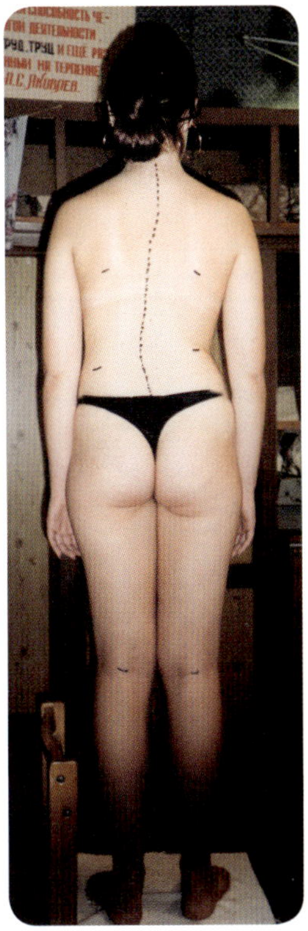

Fig. 1.15-10.
Patient I., 16 years. Relative shortening of the left leg 23 mm; right-sided scoliosis with formation of the rib hump; pelvis is tilted to the left; hypoplasia of gluteal muscles and pelvic bones on the left

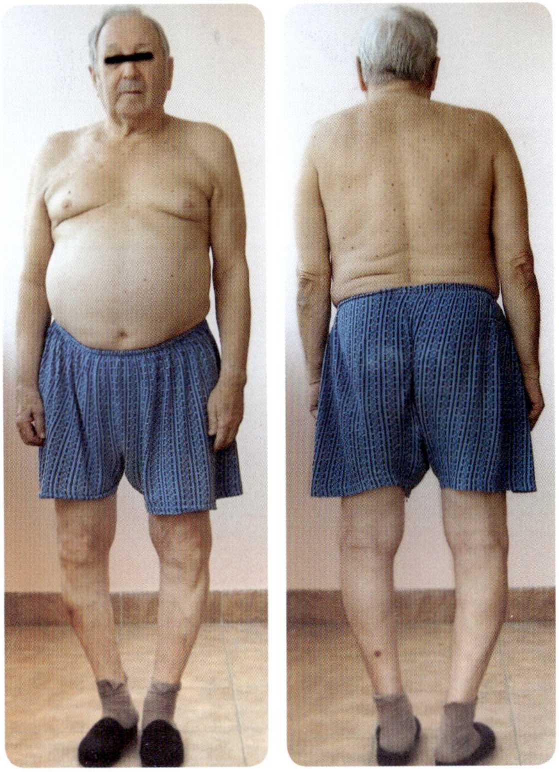

A B

Fig. 1.15-11. Patient L., 84 years.
A - Relative shortening of the left leg 10 mm; head is tilted to the right, facial asymmetry; left side of the thorax is protruding; deformity is barely visible due to fat deposits
B - Right-sided scoliosis with formation of rib hump on the right; body is tilted to the left; hypotrophy of gluteal muscles and hypoplasia of pelvic bones on the left; varus deformity of both lower limbs more pronounced on the left side; plano-valgus deformity of the left foot

patient from the back and lifted him from under his arms with a good shake. This was followed by a session of back massage.

I left this lecture feeling depressed by all that I had seen and heard. I also felt a sense of shame because despite knowing that there was a need to find the real reasons for the occurrence of deformities of the human body, I had given up my search for these reasons. Thus, as before, it was of primary importance to me now to find out the truth sooner or later and reveal it to the people.

Soon, I had the opportunity to visit Syria at the invitation of our university graduates to select patients with various orthopaedic diseases for surgical treatment in the trauma centre of Odessa. During my stay in this country, I examined at least 150 people. As expected, in addition to various pathologies of the limbs, I found that all the patients had deformities of the thorax, scoliosis, rotational vertebral subluxations with local pain, and

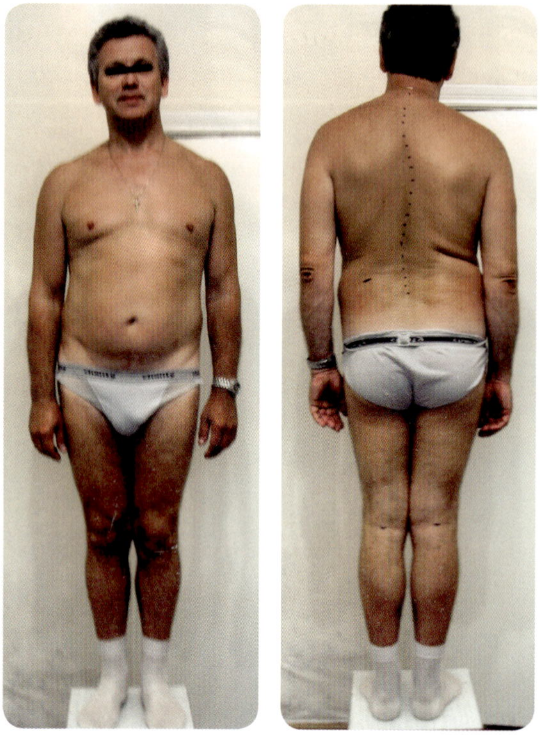

A B

Fig. 1.15-12. Patient N., 53 years.
A - Relative shortening of the left leg 25 mm; head is slightly tilted to the right, facial asymmetry; left side of the thorax is protruding, deformity is barely visible due to fat deposits
B - Right-sided scoliosis with formation of rib hump on the right; pronounced tilt of the body to the left; hypotrophy of gluteal muscles and hypoplasia of pelvic bones on the left; slight varus deformity of the left tibia; plano-valgus foot

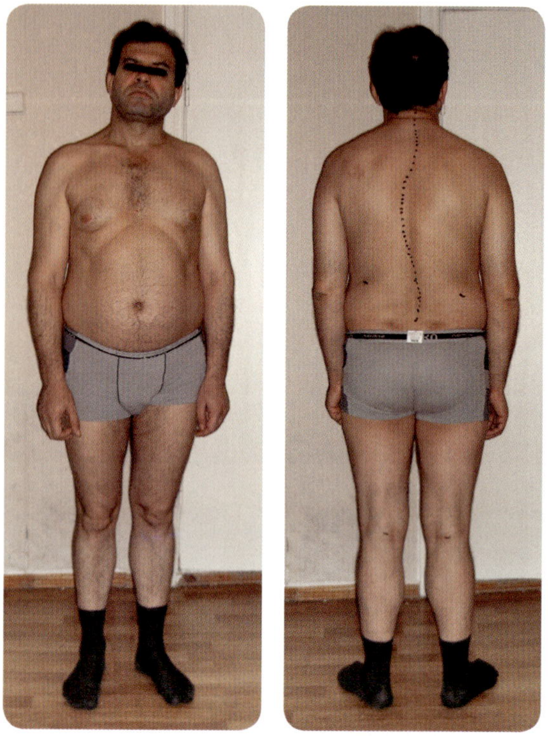

A B

Fig. 1.15-13. Patient R., 45 years.

A - Relative shortening of the right leg 38 mm; head is slightly tilted to the left, facial asymmetry; the right side of the thorax is protruding

B - Left-sided scoliosis with formation of rib hump on the left; marked tilt of the body to the right; hypotrophy of gluteal muscles and hypoplasia of pelvic bones on the right

shortening of one leg that was not associated with a positive history of poliomyelitis. I would like to emphasize that my patients were deeply religious Muslims, who worked on their fields day and night, drank clean water from mountain springs and ate organic food. If one were to believe Dr Bobyr's theory, these people simply could not have had osteochondrosis. What then caused the intense pain in their spine?

Next summer, I took my wife and younger son on a cruise. For some reason the ship was detained and we had to stay in Venice for about a week. Having nothing better to do, I turned my attention to the tourists. Standing at the footbridge, which the tourists had to cross as they walked from the port to the city, I had the opportunity to observe large groups of tourists from England, Germany, France, the USA, Japan and other countries. They were scantily dressed because of the heat and as they were walking in my direction, I got a front view of them. I was extremely surprised by what I saw. All

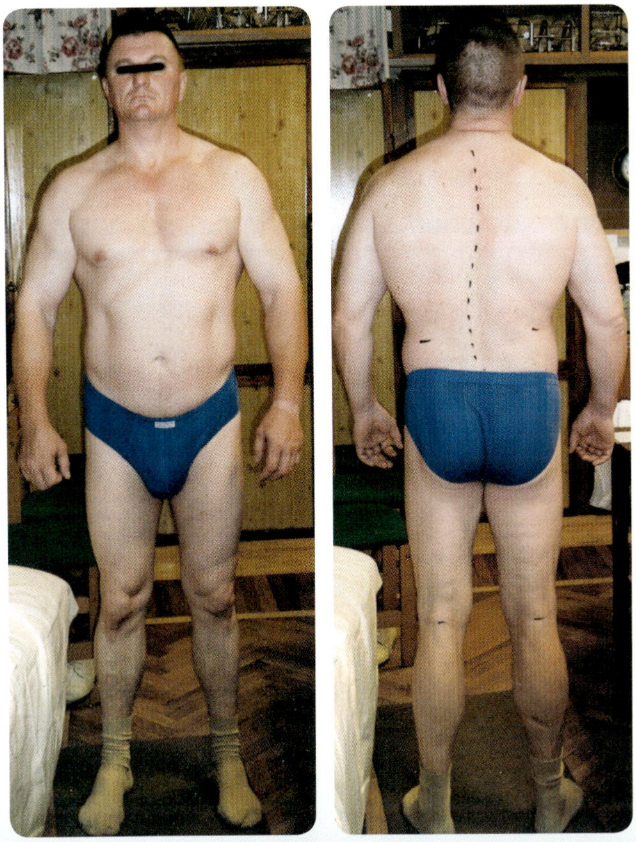

Fig. 1.16. Patient M., 44 years.
Relative shortening of the left leg 18 mm; right-sided scoliosis; spinal pain

these people had asymmetry of the shoulder girdle (with one shoulder drooping lower than the other and one collarbone protruding more than the other. This meant that they all had a scoliotic posture. It should be noted that these were people from different countries, and that these countries afforded their populations with a high standard of living, good food and a clean environment, besides being culturally enlightened. Hence, it was once again apparent that the causes of scoliosis were something other than those put forward by Dr Bobyr. I speculated that perhaps the condition was due to the structural features of the skeleton of modern man. Feeling calmer temporarily, I continued to explore the city of Venice. One day, we visited the Museum of the Academy of Painting. On display were a large number of originals of famous artists of the Renaissance era—Michelangelo, Leonardo da Vinci, Giorgione, Titian, Veronese, Tintoretto, Raphael, Caravaggio, Rubens, Dürer and others. In one of the halls, I saw a full-length depiction of Jesus Christ facing me. I saw that his right collarbone protruded more than the left. Also, his body was skewed to the left and the left rib arch protruded forward. I have since noticed these features of the body structure of Jesus Christ in several other paintings and wooden crucifixes. A similar pattern of chest deformity could be seen on another canvas depicting St Mark. The most amazing thing is that the paintings date back to the 16th and 17th centuries. Therefore, this deformity cannot be explained by any factors that are unique to modern man.

With the aim of exploring this further, I visited many museums and, after returning from Venice, I looked at several sculptures and portraits in which the shoulder girdle was exposed. Each time, I found what I wanted, i.e. clear asymmetry of the chest was evident even in a bronze figure from the ancient Greek period, a figure found by Jacques-Yves Cousteau underwater at the site of a shipwreck. I came across similar deformities while studying ancient frescoes displayed in the Kiev Museum of Art. One of them had a close-up view of a centaur, a man with the body of a horse; his powerful chest was deformed and asymmetrical. Later, there were other observations.

In the summer of 1999, I visited the Metropolitan Museum of Art in New York. There, in the hall displaying the arts of ancient Greece and Rome, I saw plenty of marble figures, including the torsos of warriors and noblemen. The nude figures, which had been made with great care by the ancient sculptors, all had the same features: one collarbone protruded forward, as did the costal angle on the opposite side. There were also figures with a costal humpback. As a rule, the sculptures of people in a standing posture were such that one leg was bent at the knee joint (Figs 1.17 and 1.18). As it became clear many years later, this was due to the shortening of one leg. A shorter leg was usually bent at the knee because that position was comfortable.

During a visit to the Historical Museum of Ulm (Germany) in January 2000, I came across the figure of a child, carved out of wood. According to the inscription, the statue of a child, in three-quarters of natural growth, had been made in the 17th century. It was the child Jesus. The sculptor had carved every part of the child's body very meticulously. It did not require more than one look to find the various elements of the skeleton pathology we have been discussing. Other than the presence of chest

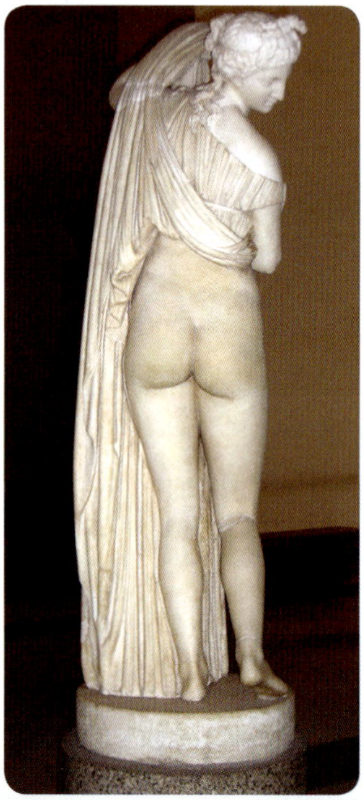

Fig. 1.17. Figure of a woman, Rome, 500 AD. Pelvic tilt to the right, towards shortening

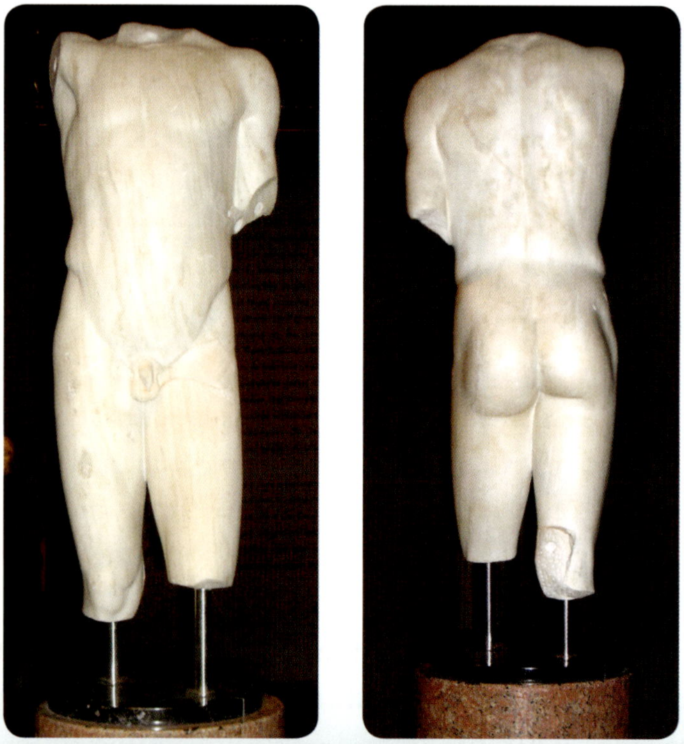

Fig. 1.18. Figure of a man, Rome, about 450 AD. Tilt of the body to the left, towards shortening

asymmetry and the marked rib hump typical of scoliosis of a curvature of 3–4 degrees, the left leg was shorter than the right and there was severe hypotrophy of the left gluteal region.

Later, while observing various television presenters, I noticed that each of them, too, had an asymmetry of the body, which was inclined either to the right or the left. One day, they were showing a former US president, his wife and daughter on television, and again, in each of their cases, one shoulder was higher than the other. I made a similar observation while viewing a large group portrait of a monarch of one of the Nordic countries, his wife and children. Both the former US president and the Nordic monarch, of course, must have had a healthy lifestyle and diet, supervised by physicians, but this did not prevent the occurrence of deformity of the body, and hence, the spinal deformity.

As we continued to examine more and more patients, we began to notice that the asymmetry of the body included the face as well (Fig. 1.19). In most cases, the left ear, eyebrow, eye, nostril, mouth angle and angle of the labial fold were located lower than the right. This was invariably accompanied by a prolapse of the left shoulder and a right-sided scoliotic posture. As in other cases of asymmetry, I thought at first that these changes occurred only among modern human beings (Figs 1.20 and 1.21). Gradually, however, my views began to change. While at an exhibition on the life of Peter I at the Historical Museum in Moscow, I came across a life-size depiction of his face, commissioned by the emperor (Fig. 1.22). I noticed a marked facial asymmetry.

Later, during a visit to a Protestant church in Copenhagen (Denmark), designed by Bertel Thorvaldsen (1770–1844), I saw a bust of the architect, whose right eyebrow was higher than the left (Fig. 1.23). There was also a beautiful sculpture of St James, whose left eyebrow was clearly lower than the right (Fig. 1.24).

In the Pergamon Museum, which has the famous bust of Nefertiti (Fig. 1.25), the Bode Museum and the Historical Museum in Berlin, I noticed the same thing—the busts of Napoleon, Hitler, Charlemagne, two brothers from Rome (Nicolo and Filippo Strozzi, 1454–1493) and others had similar signs of asymmetry.

The same could be noticed on the great portraits of the Zimmerman family, in which the parents and children had clearly visible signs of facial asymmetry (Figs 1.26–1.28).

In 2005, during another visit to New York, I went to the Brooklyn Museum of Fine Arts. There I found that a figure of the Buddha, carved out of wood and dating back to the 12th–13th centuries AD, also bore evidence of asymmetry of the body and face (Fig. 1.29). In addition, facial asymmetry was noticeable in the sculptures and pictorial depictions of persons belonging to the ancient Persian, Egyptian and Roman periods (Figs 1.30–1.32). When I took a look at the marble and terracotta busts, as

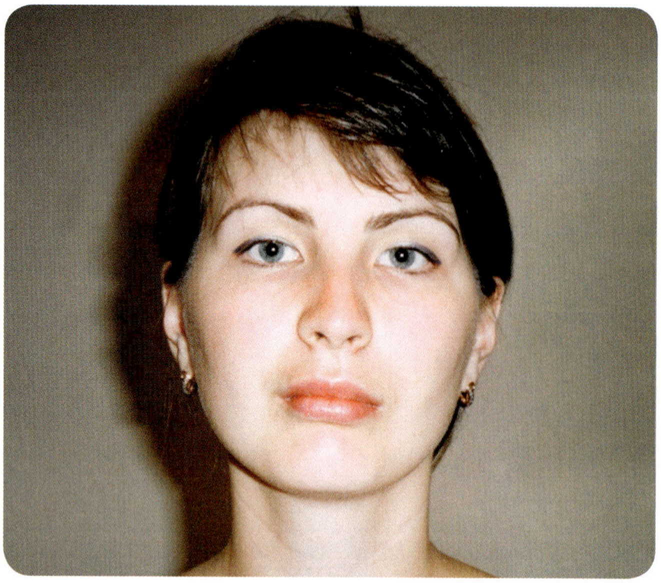

A

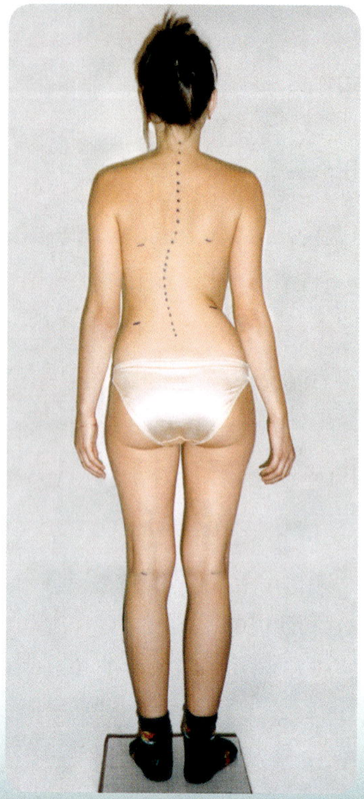

B

Fig. 1.19. Patient S., 20 years.
A - Facial asymmetry; left palpebral fissure is narrower that the right; shortening of the left leg 30 mm
B - Dropping of the left shoulder with formation of right-sided scoliotic posture; severe hypotrophy of gluteal muscles and pelvic bones on the left; varus deformity of the left tibia

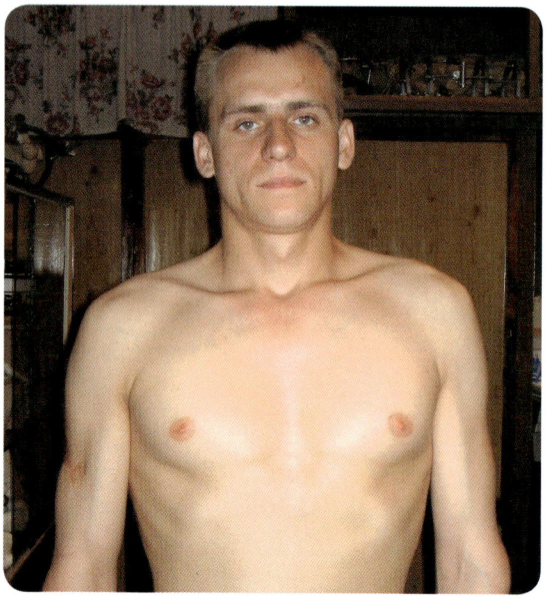

A

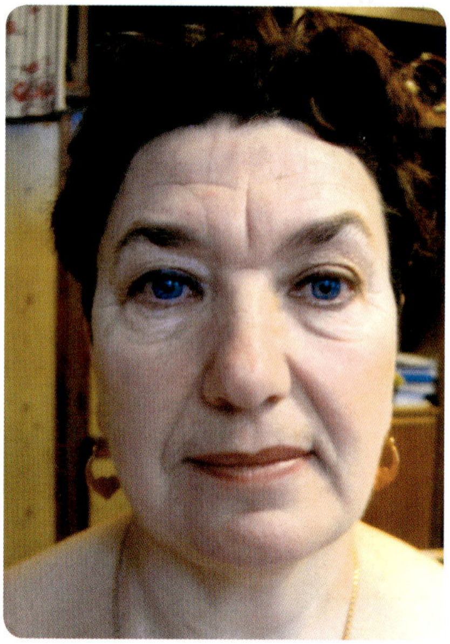

B

Fig. 1.20.
A - Asymmetry of the body; right eyebrow and right ear are located lower than those of the left half; right half of the chest is protruded more than the left half
B - Facial asymmetry; right eyebrow and right ear are located lower than those of the left half; right palpebral fissure is narrower than the left

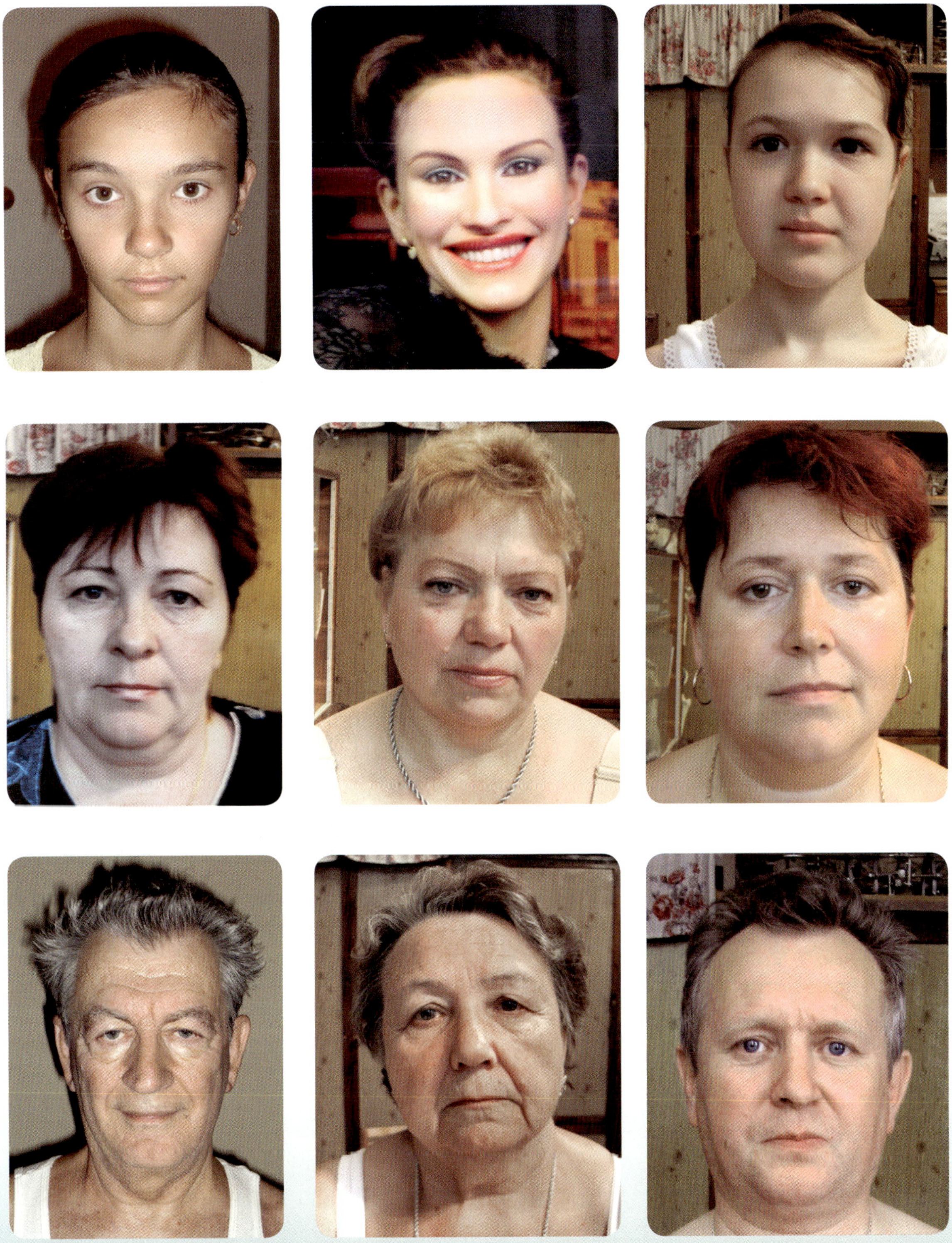

Fig. 1.21.
Asymmetry of the modern human face

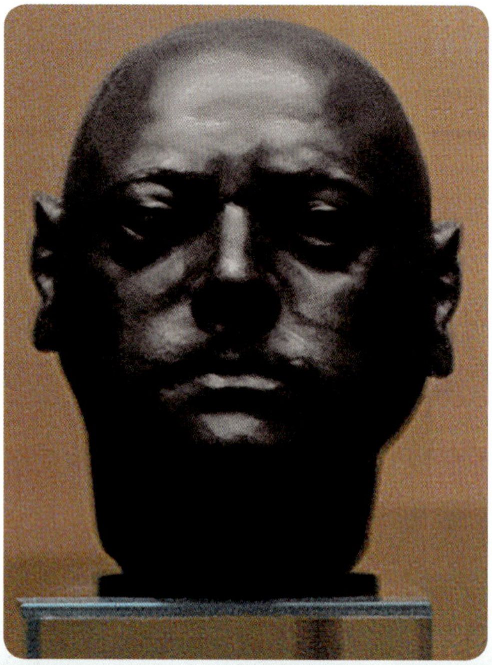

Fig. 1.22.
Intravital copy of the head of Emperor of Russia Peter the First

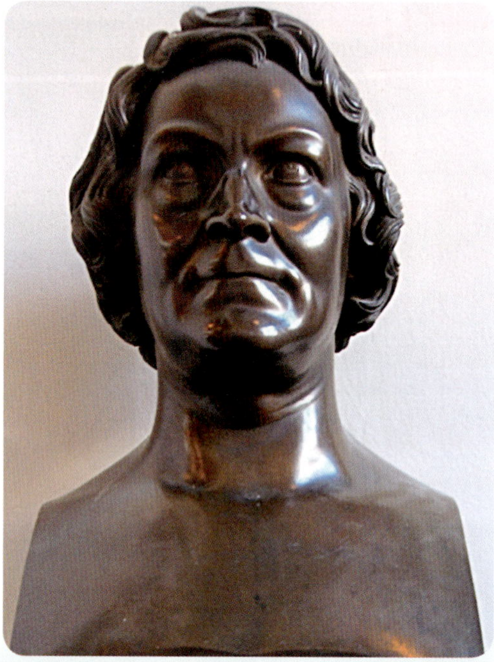

Fig. 1.23.
Bust of Bertel Thorvaldsen with signs of facial asymmetry

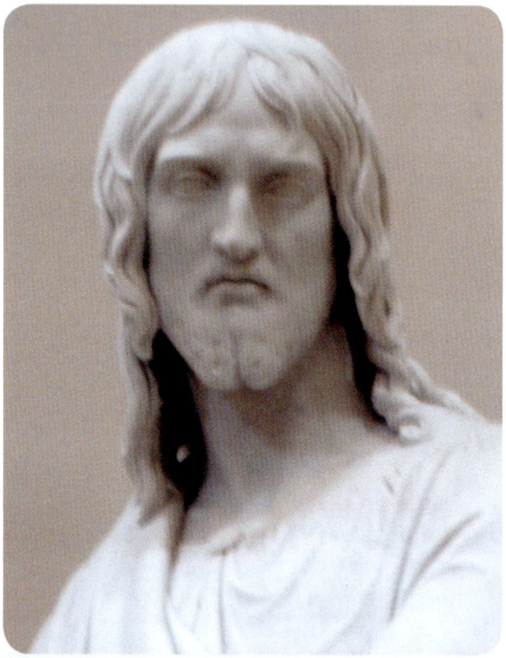

Fig. 1.24.
Marble statue of St. Jacob with signs of facial asymmetry

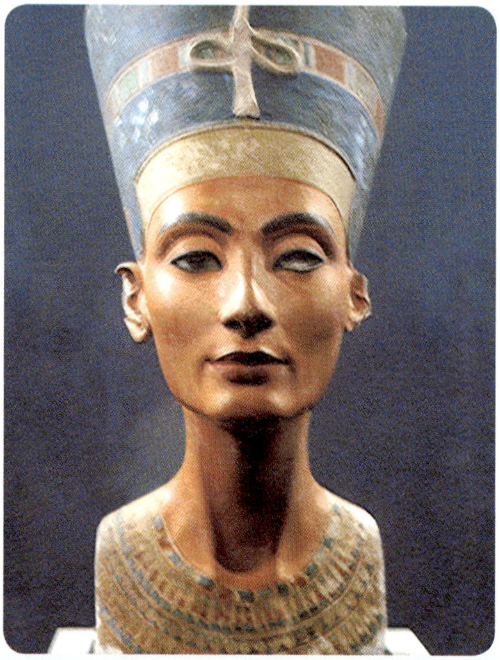

Fig. 1.25. Bust of Nefertiti with signs of facial asymmetry (slight hypotrophy of the right zygomatic area, right eyebrow is lower than the left)

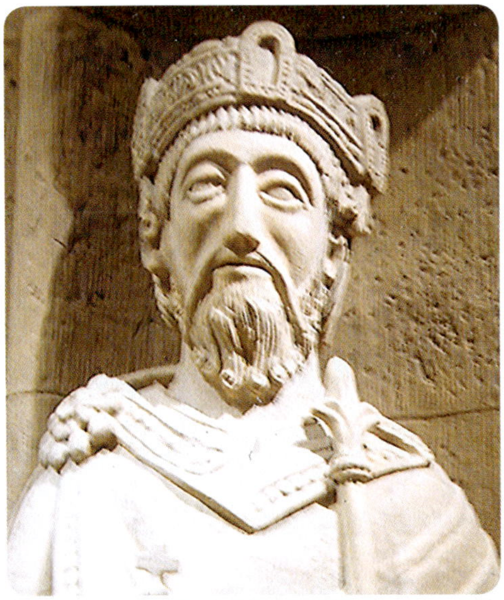

Fig. 1.26.
Marble sculpture of Charles the Great with signs of facial asymmetry

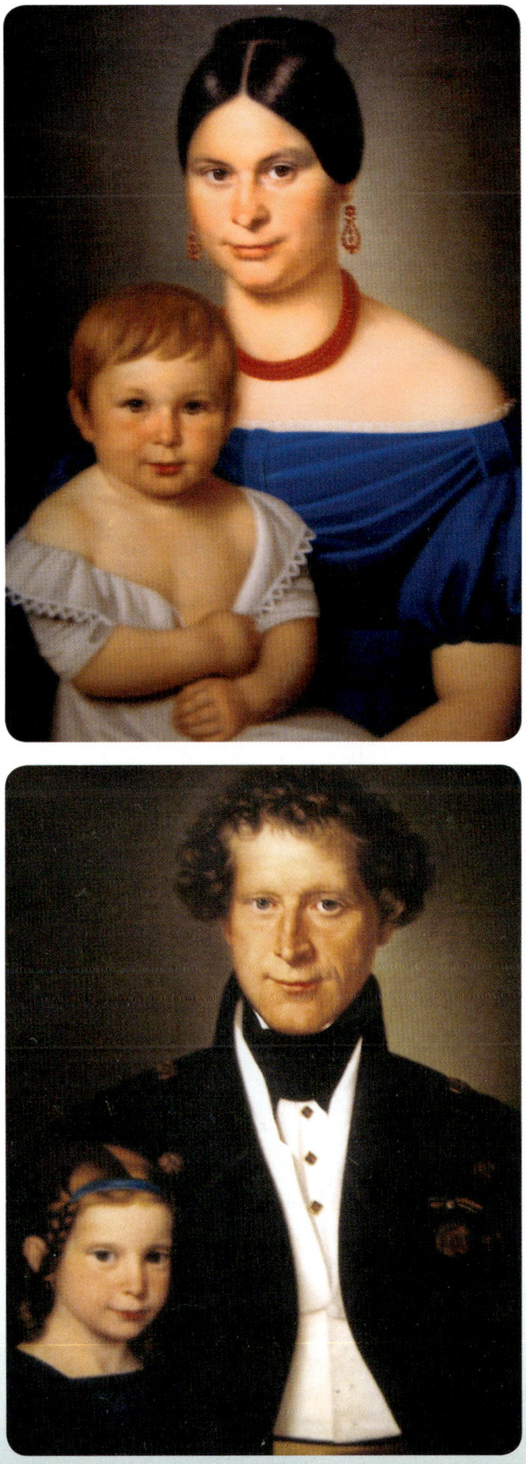

Fig. 1.27.
Portraits of historical figures with facial asymmetry

well as portraits on canvas and wood from different periods, I immediately noticed signs of asymmetry of the face and body (Figs 1.33–1.37).

One day we made a visit to the Louvre in Paris to examine the portrait of Mona Lisa (La Giaconda) by Leonardo da Vinci, as well as the statue of the goddess of beauty, Venus de Milo. And we saw exactly what we had expected to see. Mona Lisa had facial asymmetry, while Venus had all kinds of body deformities.

In 2008, the popular Ukranian weekly, *Arguments and Facts*, published an article entitled 'Slaves of black colonizers. Were they aliens?' by Savely Kashnitsky (No. 34, page 36), which gave a fascinating cultural heritage of an ancient civilization of Latin America. This civilization, called the Olmec, flourished in the third millennium BC and left a heritage consisting of several enormous heads (up to 3 metres long and weighing tens of tons), carved out of stone (Fig. 1.38). As can be seen in the photograph of the head, there is a clearly visible facial asymmetry—the left cheek and nostril protrude

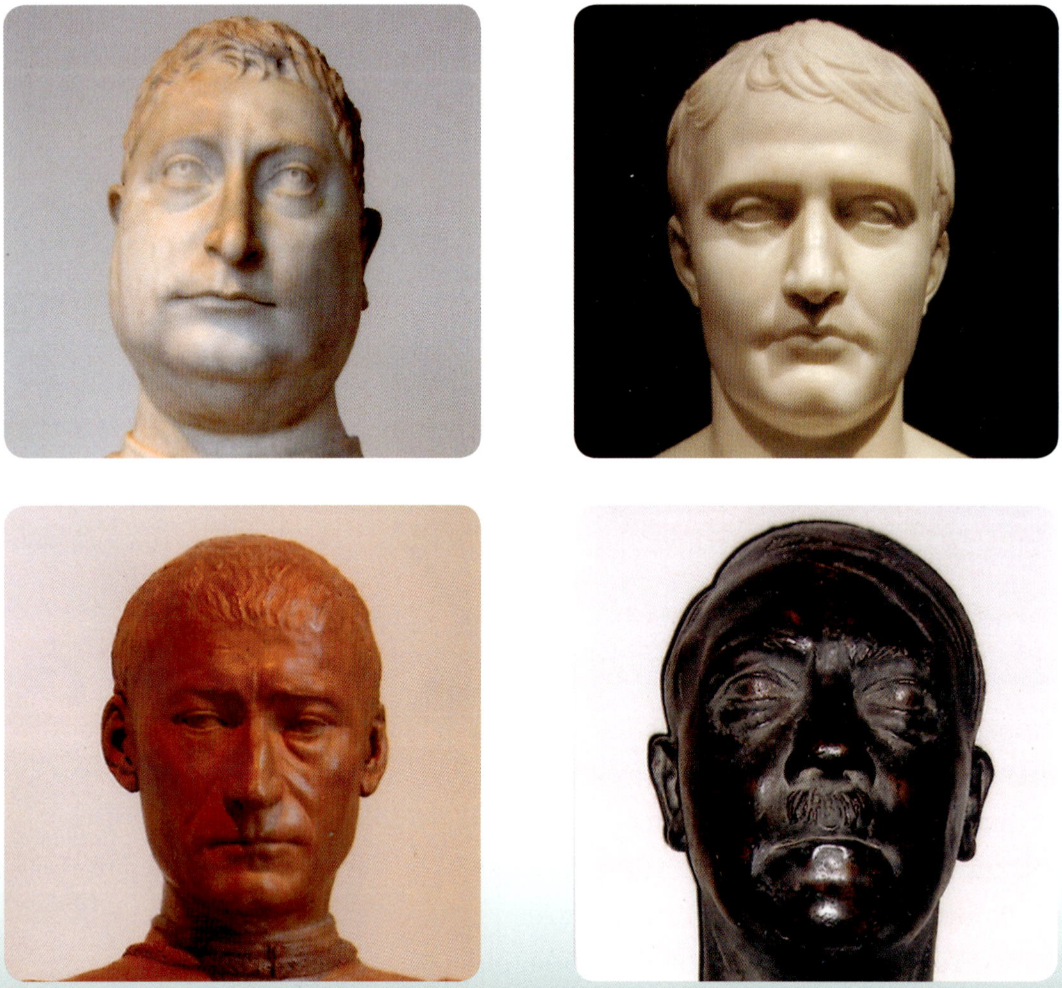

Fig. 1.28. Sculptures of historical figures with facial asymmetry

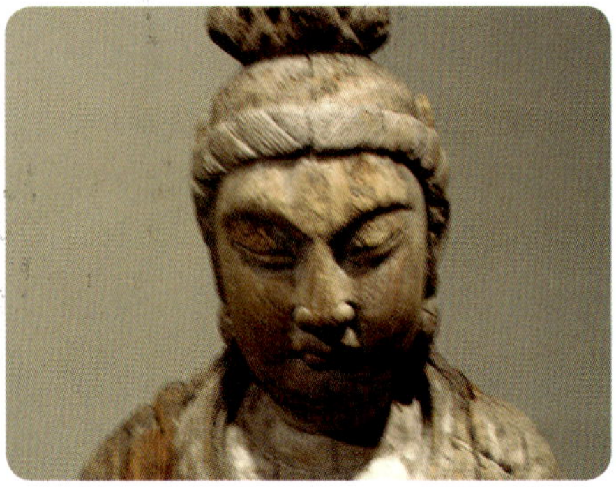

Fig. 1.29.
Figure of Buddha carved out of wood; executed in China during the Ching Dynasty (1115–1234).
Right eyebrow, nostril and angle of the mouth are located lower than on the left side and the right half of the face is poorly developed in comparison with the left

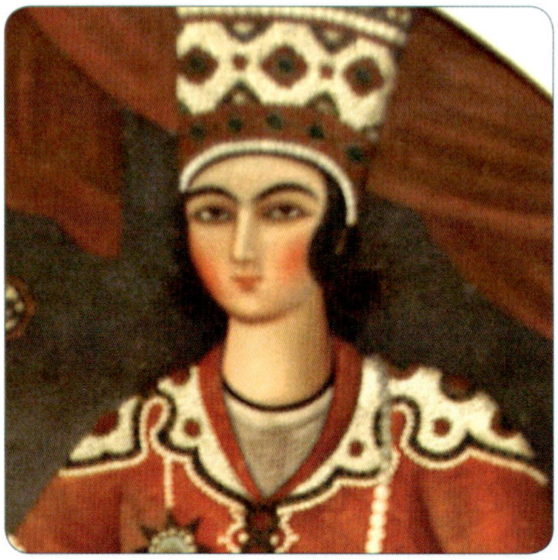

Fig. 1.30.
Picturesque depiction of inhabitant of ancient Persia with facial asymmetry

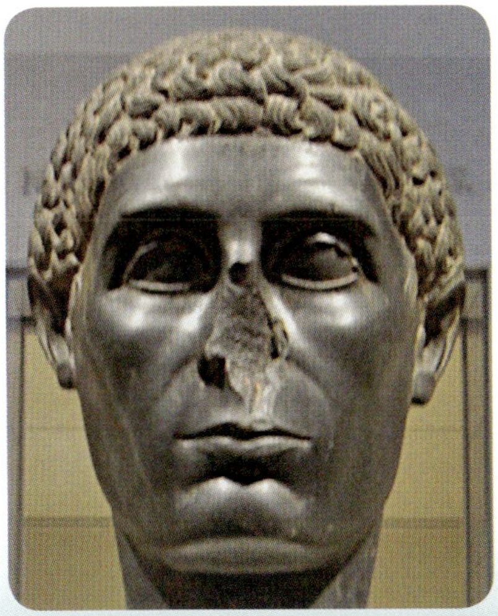

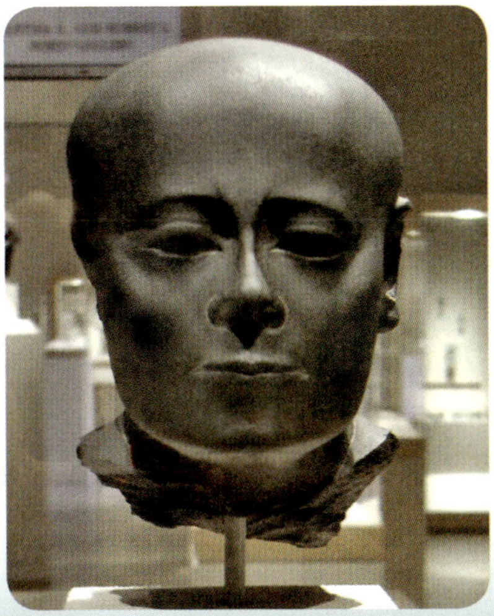

Fig. 1.31. Sculptures of persons with signs of asymmetry related to the period of ancient Egypt and Rome

forward more than the right. The same goes for the left half of the lip and the left eye.

The following conclusions can be drawn from these findings:

- Asymmetry of the body, in particular the face and chest, is not unique to modern human beings. It is noticeable also in people who lived a few centuries or even millennia ago.
- Asymmetry of the body is accompanied by the formation of a rib hump, which is a manifestation of scoliotic deformity.
- Asymmetry of the chest is always accompanied by a difference in the length of the lower limbs. This, in most cases, is of a compensatory nature.
- Asymmetry of the body is characteristic of all human beings, regardless of social status, nationality, religion, age, physical fitness, sex, etc.

Thus, we realized that asymmetry in the structure of the human body is essential and always present. After that, I stopped observing people walking towards me on the streets. However, I started looking at them from the back and eventually became aware of another characteristic feature which I have mentioned earlier. The volume of the buttocks was smaller on the side of the relatively shorter leg. In some people (adults) with severe scoliosis, along with the decrease in the volume of one buttock, there was also hypoplasia of the pelvic bones on the same side. This situation could be explained by the fact that due to the decrease in the length of the leg (since early childhood), there was a gradual increase of working hypotrophy in all tissues, whether soft or bone tissues.

Although some points had been clarified, many new questions had emerged. These included the following.

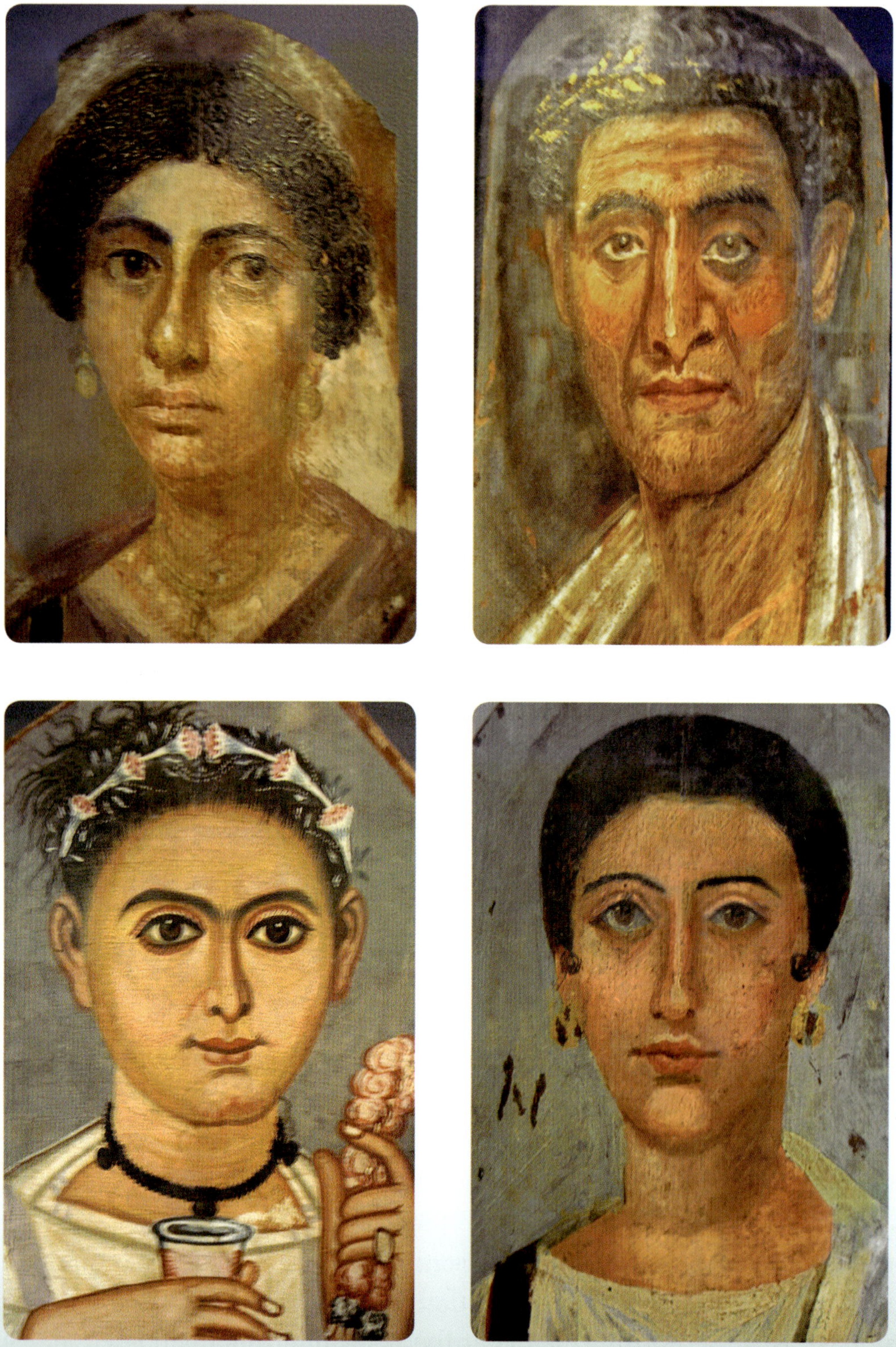

Fig. 1.32.
Picturesque depictions of persons with signs of asymmetry related to the period of ancient Egypt and Rome

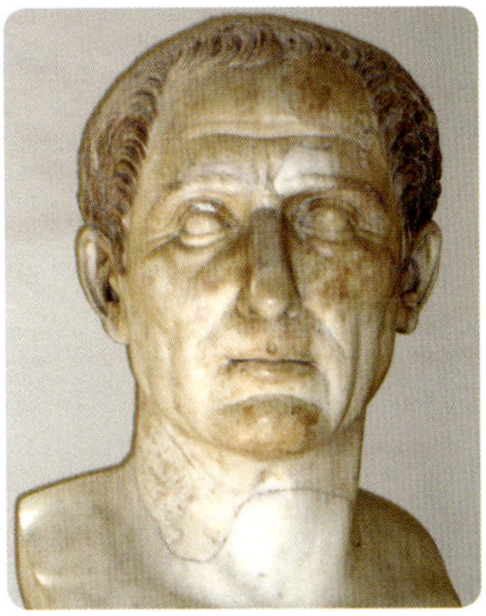

Fig. 1.33.
Marble bust of Roman Emperor Caesar (Archaeological Museum of Naples, Italy) Facial asymmetry: its right half is less developed than the left, right eyebrow and right ear are located lower than the left; right palpebral fissure is narrower than the left, right nostril is less developed

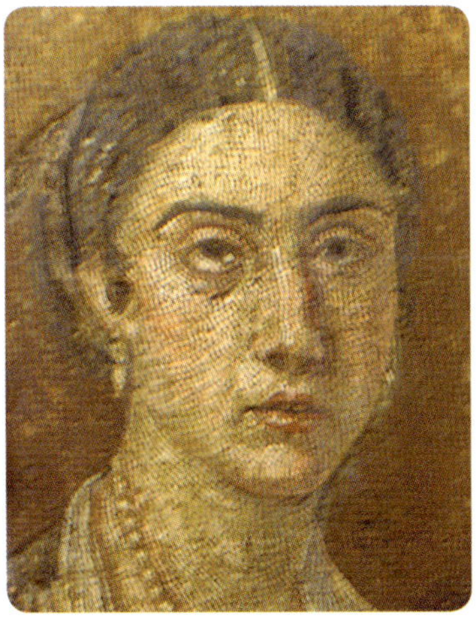

Fig. 1.34.
Mosaic panel from the Archaeological Museum of Naples (Italy), found during excavations of Pompeii. Young woman's face is slightly tilted to the right; left eyebrow is located lower than the right, left palpebral fissure is narrower

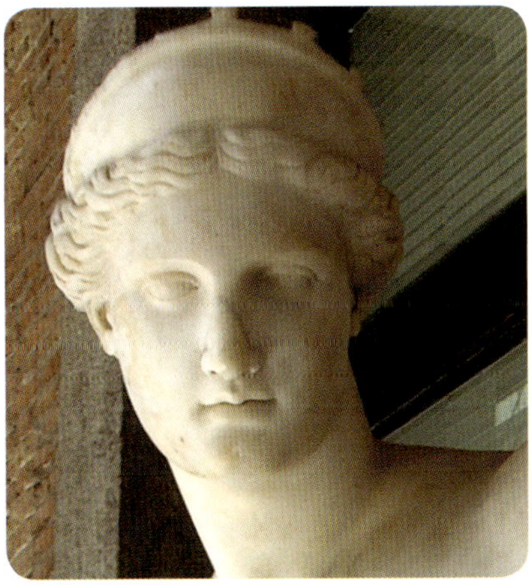

Fig. 1.35.
Marble figure of Aphrodite, 400 AD (Archaeological Museum of Naples, Italy).
Facial asymmetry: the left eyebrow, nostril and ear are located below the right ones; the left eye is narrower than the right

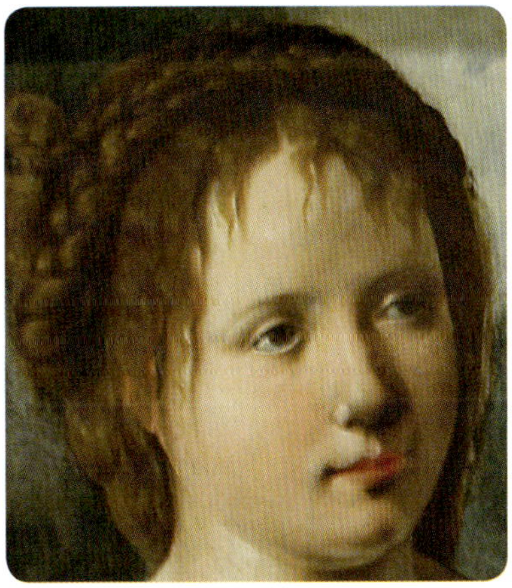

Fig. 1.36.
The head of Bacchus. A painting by Maerten van Heemskerck (1498–1574) from the Museum of Fine Arts in Vienna (Austria).
The head is tilted to the right, left eyebrow is lower than the right, left orbital fissure is narrower than the right

- What is the cause of asymmetry of the body? Is asymmetry a sign of pathology? Moreover, if it is characteristic of each human being whether living in the present or the past, is it the norm? What is at the bottom of this phenomenon, especially considering that the creations of nature are usually so efficient? Is this, perhaps, one of those occasional defects of nature, such as dwarf trees?
- Is asymmetry characteristic only of human beings?

Is there any connection between asymmetry of the body and the development of the initial forms of disease among children? How do we explain the fact that a huge number of relatively healthy children grow up to become adult patients? Incidentally, this pattern is not confined only to the former Soviet countries which had low standards of living, but is just as prevalent in developed countries, including the USA, Germany, Japan and France.

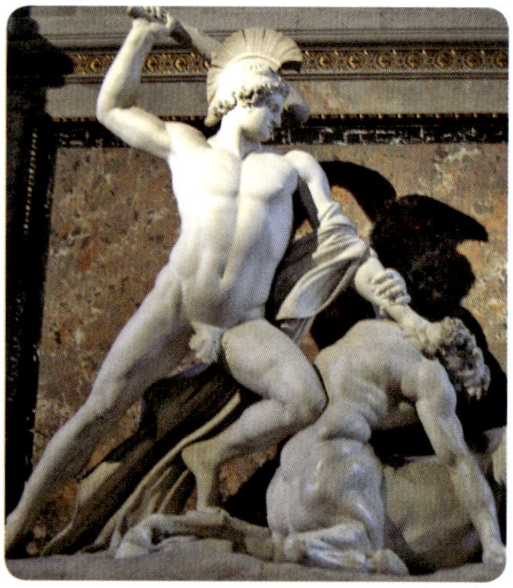

Fig. 1.37.
Marble sculpture 'Tesnus killing Centaur' by Antonio Canova (Rome, 1805) from the Museum of Fine Arts in Vienna (Austria). The left side of the warrior's chest is more anterior than the right

Throughout the history of humankind, the origin of diseases has been a major concern. The reasons that have been considered are numerous: constant stress, environmental issues, nutritional problems, poor quality of water, etc. All these factors cause diseases today and probably did earlier as well. But what about ancient times, when the environment was clean and nature pristine? The food was organic, the water was not contaminated by garbage and there were no chemical industries, nuclear power plants, fertilizers, etc. There was a marked culture of cultivating the body with a strong emphasis on physical development and great attention to physical health and fitness. The ancient Olympic games bear testimony to this. Nevertheless, there were sick people. Diseases occurred even in ancient times, as is evident from the manuscripts of ancient civilizations. Why did diseases emerge at that time? And why do they still emerge?

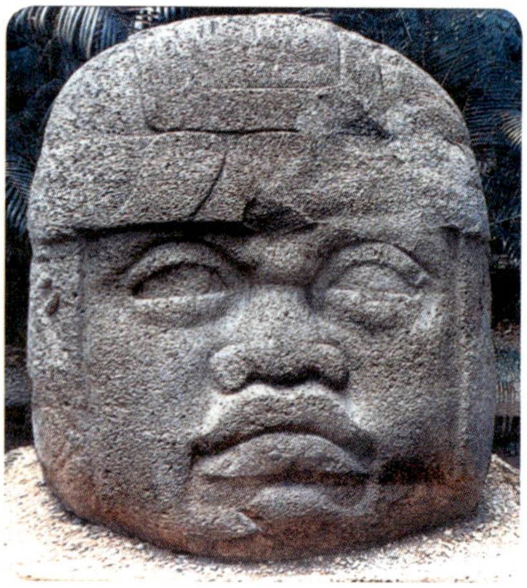

Fig. 1.38.
Marble sculpture of ancient Olmec with signs of facial asymmetry

This means that some reasons existed in days long gone and continue to exist even today. The fact that they have persisted through the millennia shows that there is a certain pattern in the development of body deformities. But what pattern? I had to find it out. This became the key goal of my research.

- Why are people born with limbs of different lengths? What happens in the body? There is a view that this is due to a difference between the velocity of the circulation of bio-impulses in the right and left hemispheres of the brain. Is this true?

- We connect the deformities of the body, and thus human diseases, with the upright posture. There is even a view that human diseases can be attributed to the quick transition from walking on four limbs (as the ancient humanoid did) to two. This argument will not hold because animals walk on four limbs but suffer from the same diseases as human beings. Any veterinarian can confirm this. What, then, is the answer?
- Why does rotation of the vertebrae or so-called rotary subluxation take place? The only explanation that has occurred to us is that it is due to the difference in the length of the lower limbs. However, tetrapods, and even sprawlers, have rotary subluxation, although shortening of four or more legs will probably not have the same impact as shortening of one leg in a human being.
- The literature suggests that in nature, there are two types of limb shortening: (i) relative, which is due to asymmetry of the muscles and (ii) absolute, which is associated with the presence of bones of different length. What we need to ascertain is the most important cause of the formation of skeleton deformities.
- Is there a connection between spinal deformities among children and the development of various diseases among adults?
- What is the cause of spinal pain among children? When we speak of spinal pain in adults, osteochondrosis or spondylosis deformans could be cited as reasons. But what about a child of the age of 1.5–2 years, who shows the signs both of bilateral plexitis and bilateral sciatica (lumboischialgia), i.e. when his whole body aches, including his head, feet and hands? He has a severe allergy, stomach ulcers and constipation. Can we still blame it on osteochondrosis or spondylosis deformans? There must be some other reasons, a knowledge of which would help us to cure children and, therefore, reduce the number of adult patients. When I made this list of questions, I was somewhat fearful that I might be misunderstood during my search for the answers. As a result, over the next several months, I stopped dealing with the problem of spinal pain and decided not to reveal my findings on the development of spinal deformities.

It was a stalemate situation

But it would be wrong to say that the literature did not contain any data on body asymmetry. Moreover, some time after I started my own research, I discovered another useful source of information. This was the outstanding Renaissance artist Leonardo da Vinci (1452–1519). He diligently studied anatomy, and had set himself the task of illustrating the anatomical studies of Claudius Galen, who coined the word 'scoliosis'.

Another prominent painter, sculptor and architect of the Renaissance period who had meticulously represented the proportions of the human body was Michelangelo.

He adorned the Sistine Chapel in Rome with a myriad paintings that clearly depicted the human body, besides making dozens of sculptures which are considered masterpieces. The painter Albrecht Durer lived and worked in Germany in the same period. He was the author of a four-volume work on the proportions of the human body.

In the beginning of the 19th century (1825), Dr Parri made a statement on asymmetry of the human skeleton, while Bergson described asymmetry of the face in 1837. Finally, I want to share what I learnt from an excellent article written by Professor G.M. Ter-Egiazarov and his colleagues in 1977. Published in the *Journal of Orthopaedics, Traumatology and Prosthetics (Russia)* and entitled 'Hemihypoplasia', the article pointed out that the human skeleton is asymmetrical, with 40%–80% of people showing shortening of the left lower limb. In the authors' view, this feature is not limited to human beings and apes, but is characteristic also of several other mammals, including foxes and wolves.

The authors had examined 122 children with asymmetry of the body, which they termed hemihypoplasia. Among the features of facial asymmetry were a difference in the height of the eyebrows, uneven contraction of the palpebral fissure, difference in smoothing of the contours of the upper and lower jaws, reduced volume of the soft tissue of one cheek, and asymmetry of the mouth angles, nose wings, tongue and ears. The authors had also observed deformity of the chest, anterior protrusion of the costal arch on the affected side and asymmetry of the breast. Children's posture varied considerably. In addition, they had observed asymmetry of the shoulder girdles, configuration of the shoulder blades and waist triangles, as well as tilting of the pelvis and static scoliosis. Asymmetry of the upper limbs was also found to occur, though less commonly than asymmetry of the lower ones. The difference in length of the legs ranged from 10 mm to 40 mm, and of the arms, up to 30 mm.

The irregular length of the lower limbs led to significant changes in static, pace and curvature of the spine. This necessitated accurate measurement of the length of the legs to ensure that they could be properly aligned. Owing to the fact that using a measuring tape could result in errors of up to 1 cm, the authors measured the bones of the lower limbs using the method proposed by Merilli (cited from G.M. Ter-Egiazarov in co-authorship, 1977).

The children with hemihypoplasia were observed over a 6-year period. It was found that the difference between the length of the legs increased during the period of most intensive growth. Considering the dramatic progression of shortening (more than 4 cm) of the lower limb, surgical lengthening was recommended. A very important conclusion of the authors was that asymmetry of the length of the lower limbs can lead not only to the development of scoliosis, but also deformities of the hips, legs, feet, etc.

I was very happy with the information provided in the article, as the authors' conclusions were almost similar to ours. We had reached these conclusions on our own, without even knowing about the long-term observations made by Professor G.M. Ter-Egiazarov *et al*. However, the authors' conclusions left me disappointed at the same time because the main questions, i.e. those relating to the origin of asymmetry and the causes of the natural development of spinal deformity in everyone, whether a child or an adult, remained unanswered. A separate point to be noted is that while Professor G.M. Ter-Egiazarov and his colleagues conducted bone measurements, i.e. estimated the absolute length of the limb, we measured relative shortening, for which radiological studies were not required. Having familiarized ourselves with whatever could be gleaned from this article, we saw a clear need for further research.

The world-renowned Russian orthopaedist and trauma surgeon Professor G.A. Ilizarov also drew attention to the important role of the difference between the length of the legs in scoliosis. Professor Ilizarov pioneered the compression–distraction osteosynthesis method and designed an apparatus for lengthening of the limbs. One of his students wrote a dissertation on surgical elimination of scoliotic deformity through lengthening of the shortened limb using the Ilizarov apparatus.

After a long time, one cool autumn day when it was pouring outside, I felt that someone was pushing me to leave my warm and cosy office and go to the Medical University Library. The last time I had been there was several months ago. Thus I had no idea what to look for. Shortly after I reached the library, the lights went out. I was not sure about what to do next and went to the second floor. Again I got the same feeling, as if someone was leading me to a dark corner on the far side, where, as it turned out, there was a stand on which some of the books of the library funds were exhibited. There, under the glass, I saw a little book that revolutionized my mind and showed me the path to follow. The book, *Symmetry of Nature and the Nature of Symmetry*, was written by A. Urmantsev and published in Moscow in 1974.

The information this book contains on symmetry and asymmetry in general and in nature, in particular, is so vital for an understanding of what is to follow that I feel it appropriate to briefly outline the main points which might be interesting for the reader. The concepts of 'symmetry' and 'asymmetry' were suggested by a famous mathematician, sculptor, monk and healer, Pythagoras of Regiuma (Southern Italy, the Great Greece back then), who lived at the turn of the 6th century BC. He proposed the 'pillars' theory, according to which the slope of the foundation leads to the distortion of the whole structure that is based on the foundation. Although this theory makes more sense to architects and builders, it is also applicable to the assessment of the pelvis and spine.

Louis Pasteur, the world-renowned microbiologist (1822–1895), discovered the chemical asymmetry of protoplasm and said that asymmetry was the basic property of life, transmitted persistently by inheritance.

An outstanding Russian scholar, Vladimir Vernadsky (1863–1945), made a significant contribution in the area of symmetry and asymmetry in nature, to which he dedicated 30 years of his life. He made the following points, which have been defended and accepted unconditionally by scientists around the world.

- 'In nature there is a fundamental asymmetry of the universe. Thus, the globe itself is asymmetrical—the Southern hemisphere is more elongated than the Northern. Also, the rotating forces of the earth are asymmetrical.'
- 'Every living material has a "dissymmetry (asymmetry)"—the feature through which all life-related forms lack equality of the right and left sides.'

At present, we have pinpointed three basic types of asymmetry—structural or crystallographic, geometrical and dynamic. In biology, the use of the methods of crystallography and the ideas underlying it in research facilitated the birth of the new sciences of molecular biology and bio-symmetry. These sciences led to several discoveries, including the discovery of the fine structure of the most important biopolymers, DNA and RNA.

The explorations, both of theoreticians and those conducting experiments in the area of geometrical and dynamic asymmetry of nature, led to numerous findings in various fields of knowledge, including physics, crystallography, chemistry, biology, mathematics and philosophy. The results of these studies were contained in seminal works both by Russian and foreign scientists. In the field of biology, these included *Biogeochemical Essays* by V.I. Vernadsky (1940), *The Asymmetry of Protoplasm* by G.F. Gause (1940), *Fundamentals of the Comparative Anatomy of Invertebrates* by V.N. Beklemishev (1952), W. Arnold, R. Steel, H. Mueller 'On the magnetic asymmetry of muscle fibers', *Proc Natl Acad Sci* (USA) 1958:44:1–11, *Symmetry in Nature* by I.I. Shafranovsky (1968), *Origin of Life* by J. Bernal (1969), and *Bio-symmetrical and Biorhythmic Phenomena and Signs in Agricultural Plants* by G. Sulima (1970). A collection of papers entitled *Symmetry in Nature* (1971) occupies a special place among the works on symmetry due to its fascinating contents. These papers discuss symmetry with physics, crystallography, chemistry, geology, geography, astronomy, biology, medicine, mathematics and philosophy. There is another interesting monograph *Symmetry in Nature* (1971) by A.G. Volokhonsky.

Discussing the nature of asymmetry, the physicists T.S. Tikhoplav and V.Y. Tikhoplav (2002), stated, '...the surface of every cell, tissue or organ, regardless of its functions, is always negatively charged, while its internal layers are positively charged. The presence of a potential difference between the surface and inner layers, the so-called bio-potential, testifies to the vital processes.' As I shall discuss the various aspects of symmetry and asymmetry in greater detail in a subsequent chapter, I shall, for the moment, confine myself to a brief enumeration of the main conclusions I reached after reading Y.A. Urmantsev's book. These points are necessary for understanding the origins of the deformities of the spine.

- Organisms in the lower stages of evolution display various features of symmetry. However, fewer such features are encountered as we go higher up the evolutionary tree, including the human body.
- In engineering, mechanics, crystallography and mathematics, one comes across the isomorphism of symmetry or, more simply, true symmetry.
- On the other hand, in biology, agriculture and medicine one observes a polymorphism of symmetry, i.e. all living matter is characterized by asymmetry, and there is no life beyond it.

It is probably due to the magnetic asymmetry of muscle fibres that cardiac muscles work throughout life, sometimes even despite a tremendous overload. An example of asymmetry is the simultaneous presence of positive and negative charges in the tissues, including in a single cell, which leads to the existence of bio-potentials. Different polarities ensure the movement of bio-currents from the central nervous system to the periphery and back. There are numerous examples of asymmetry in nature. These include asymmetry of the two halves of a leaf, asymmetry of the arrangement of leaves on a branch, and asymmetrical eyes, ears and eyebrows. The two halves of the face are asymmetrical, as are the left and right halves of the nose and lips The law of unity and the struggle of opposites are also manifestations of asymmetry. The variety of asymmetries is infinite when one considers paired opposites such as man–woman, positive–negative, hot–cold, right–left, up–down, sunrise–sunset, short–long, wide–narrow, thick–thin, good–bad and alive–dead. *Thus, the asymmetrical structure of a living organism perhaps constitutes the foundation of its life.*

So far, we have come to the conclusion that there is no symmetry in living organisms, in general, and the human body, in particular. While the apparent asymmetry of the eyes, hands, eyebrows, etc. does not entail serious consequences, the asymmetry of the body muscles and of the legs, in terms of different lengths, lead to an imbalance of the pelvis. The greater the difference in length, the greater the severity of inclination. The laws of mechanics and, more precisely, biomechanics come into play here. The bias of the base, in our case the base of the pelvis, leads to the development of skeletal deformities.

At this stage, it is necessary to describe the features of the stages in the process of the development of skeletal deformities. The following information has been gathered by us and the conclusions are based on our personal views.

An examination of the trees outside would make it easier for the reader to understand the mechanism of spinal deformity. The first time I paid attention to them in this context was through the window of a train, while I was travelling to Kiev on some work. The matter became even clearer when on a winter day, while looking out of the car window on my way to Munich, I saw the spruce, pine and other trees lining the slopes, their branches bare. All the trees, regardless of the angle of inclination of the slope, rose vertically relative to the horizontal plane of the Earth (Fig. 1.39). The extension axis of a tree was perpendicular to it. When a tree began to grow not strictly vertically but was inclined somewhat sideways, it became vertical nonetheless as it grew later (Fig. 1.40).

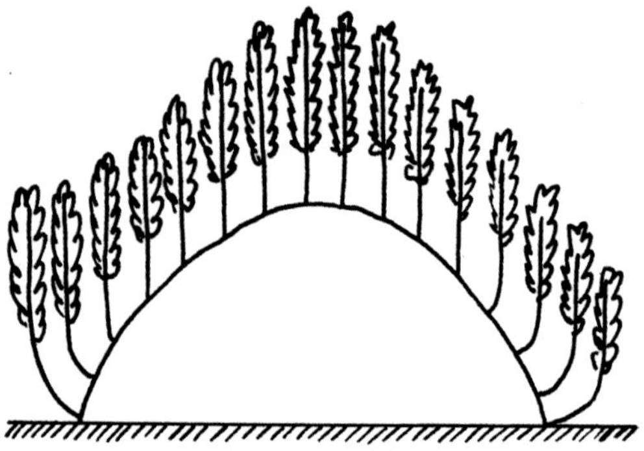

Fig. 1.39.
Trees located on the slopes of hills and mountains are growing straight vertically

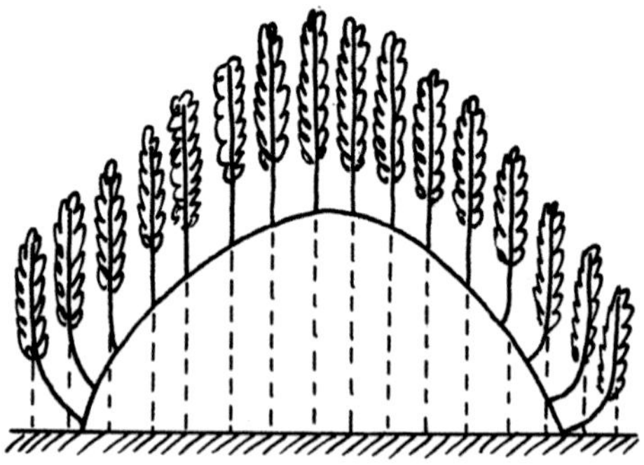

Fig. 1.40.
Axes of the trees are perpendicular to the Earth's surface

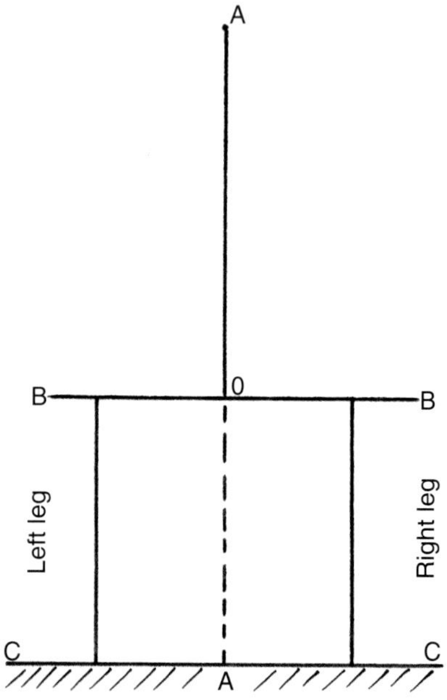

Fig. 1.41.
In the case of equal leg length, the axis of the spine is perpendicular to the Earth's surface

As to why this happens, the answer is that this is how the law of gravity works. Since this is a universal law, the phenomenon can be observed anytime and anywhere—in Europe, Asia, Africa and America, in every city, every mountain and even on a small hill.

Let us now get back to the skeleton, or rather, the human body when viewed from the back. If the lower limbs were of the same length, then the A–A axis of the spine would have been perpendicular to the axis of the pelvis, B–B, and the horizontal surface of the earth, C–C (Fig. 1.41). However, we already know that this does not happen in nature and one leg is necessarily shorter than the other, resulting in a change in the A–A spinal axis. If we take the case of shortening of the left leg (Fig. 1.42), it will initially be perpendicular to the new plane—the B_1–B_1 axis

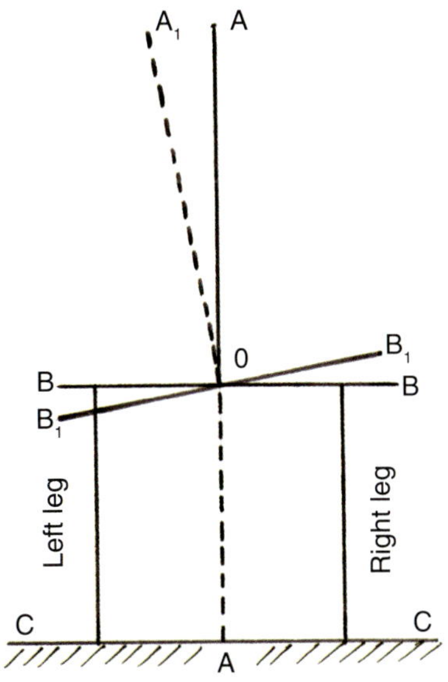

Fig. 1.42.
In shortening of the left leg, the axis of the spine turns into a broken curve

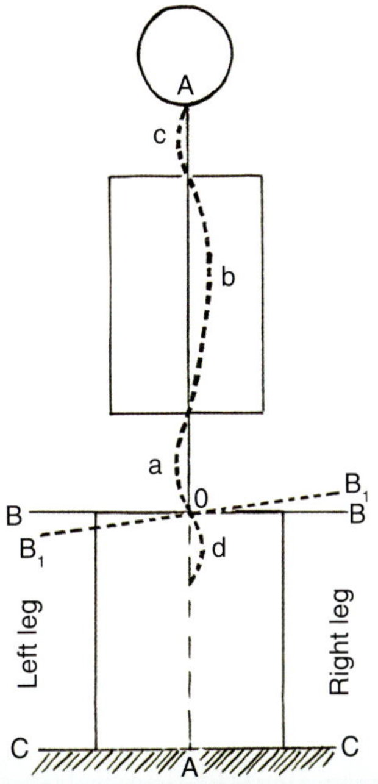

Fig. 1. 43.
Formation of right-sided scoliosis in shortened left leg

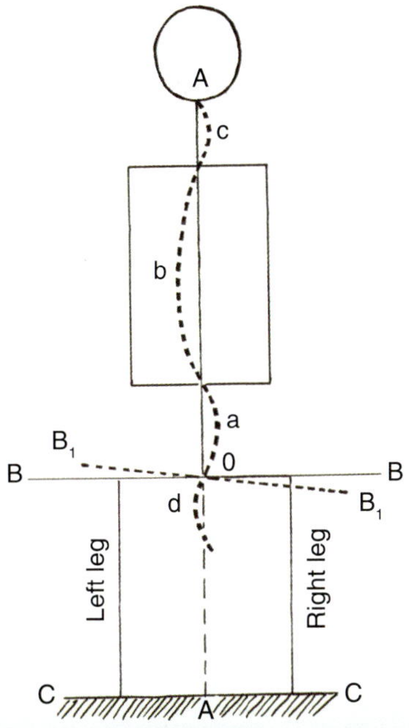

Fig. 1.44.
Formation of left-sided scoliosis in shortened right leg

of the pelvis, and become the broken curve A_0–A_1. Then, however, obeying the laws of gravity, as is the case with a tree, the O–A_1 axis will tend to become perpendicular to the horizontal axis of the earth, C–C.

Eventually, the first arc («a») of the S-shaped scoliosis deformity is formed. Subsequently, following the same rules, the second arc («b») is formed and then the third («c»). The «a» arc appears in the lumbar spine, the «b» arc in the thoracic spine and the «c» arc in the cervical spine. Shortening of the left leg leads to right-sided scoliosis (Fig. 1.43) and shortening of the right to left-sided scoliosis (Fig. 1.44). A fourth arc («d») may also be formed in the area of the sacrum that has non-united sacral vertebrae, as well as other evidence of dysplasia of this part of the spine. Later on, I found support for my conclusion in the textbooks on anatomy by V.P. Vorobiev (1932) and G.P. Ivanov (1949), who described the pattern of spinal deformity in the case of uneven legs. I acknowledge that the authors found this information in earlier sources of literature.

Conclusions

1. The main conclusion is that everyone has a scoliotic deformity of the spine. In early childhood, it is functional, i.e. it is a physiological norm. However, as a person gets older, the scoliotic curvature develops into an actual or structural deformity. Its severity depends on the extent of shortening of one of the lower limbs. This

shortening can be absolute, i.e. when there is a decrease in the length of the thigh and/or crus or relative, as in muscle asymmetry. While absolute shortening occurs only among some people, relative shortening is typical of all human beings.

Functional hypotrophy of the gluteal muscles on the side of the shortened leg can be clearly observed even among children of 4–5 years of age. Two more features become noticeable among children of 10–12 years of age: (i) there is a delay in the development of bones in the corresponding half of the pelvis and (ii) there is a marked decrease in the volume of soft tissues of the thigh and crus on the side of the shortened leg.

2. If the spinal deformity has been caused by true shortening of the growing thigh or crus or both, surgical treatment is advisable. If the key aetiological factor for the deformity is muscle asymmetry, the treatment must be conservative and should be aimed at the recovery of muscular balance.
3. It is extremely important to understand the fact that correction of muscle imbalance in childhood will not only eliminate the leading aetiological factor for scoliosis, but will also help to prevent absolute shortening of the limbs. Stimulation of the growing zones by increasing load on the underdeveloped bone will promote its active development, and the sooner this is done, the greater is the benefit.

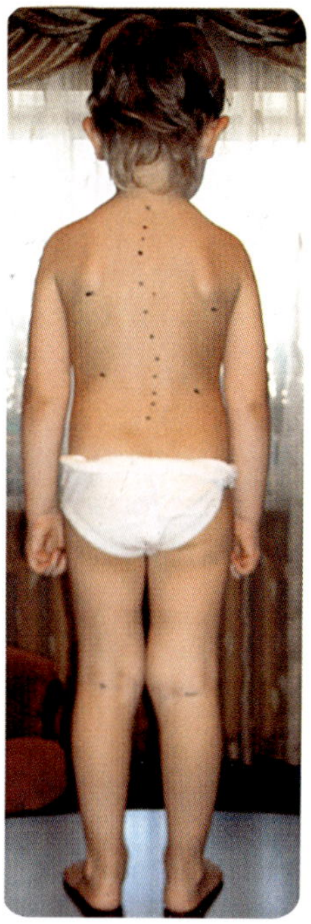

Fig. 1.45.
Visible signs of body asymmetry in a 2-year child; relative shortening of the right leg 3 mm

We have yet to deal with the question of the origin of the rib hump. How does the rib hump develop? While functional scoliosis is associated only with lateral curvature of the spine, actual or structural scoliosis consists not merely of a distortion, but also a rotation of the spine about its axis of wedge-modified vertebrae. This rotation is localized in the thoracic region of above deformity. And as the thoracic vertebrae are the site of attachment of the ribs, turning of the vertebrae causes deformity of the chest and protrusion of the ribs in one direction. It is to be noted that this deformity begins to form among children as early as the time they take their first steps, before they start going to school and sitting at desks. Figure 1.45 provides an example of a 2-year-old child with relative shortening (3 mm) of the right leg. There are clear signs of chest deformity and protrusion of the left shoulder, indicating the beginning of the formation of the rib hump. In addition, there are signs of hypotrophy of the gluteal area.

We would like to draw the reader's attention to the fact that the child in question has already developed a plano-valgus foot. In our view, such foot deformities are a compensatory mechanism, aimed at giving the body upright stability. The greater the inclination of the body, the more the foot will turn outwards. Something similar happens in nature. The lower extremities (fins) of seals, which have a huge body and short hind legs, also have a pronounced valgus formation. This can be easily verified by watching a seal at a circus or in a zoo.

It would seem that everything is now clear and understandable, but it is only seemingly clear and many questions remain unanswered. For example, why does torsion (rotation) of vertebrae take place? Is this process random or regular? What is the role of muscle asymmetry? In which regions or levels of the spine does torsion occur? Why are there three or four arcs, and not more or less? Why is it that the left leg is shortened in the majority of people (according to statistics, up to 80% or more) and the right in much fewer (20%). Is this true?

We understand the role of the asymmetry of body muscles in the formation of spinal deformity. Perhaps there are other reasons associated with skeletal abnormalities.

We say that one leg is shorter than the other. The question is the extent to which it is shorter. Are there any standards of shortening? And why are all people born with legs of different lengths as well as other evidence of asymmetry?

Is it possible to correct scoliosis if we proceed according to the thesis that the main cause of spinal deformity lies in muscle asymmetry? Of course, such an approach is unacceptable in cases of bone abnormalities, but such cases have been very rare among thousands of patients that I have examined personally. The large number of unanswered questions compelled us to study specific literature. The following chapters present the results of these studies, and also describe the path that resulted in our scientific discovery: 'Regularity of development of scoliotic deformation of the spinal column in all its sections on the ground of zones of instability. They appear as a consequence of one-sided hypertonus of spinal muscles, linked with asymmetry of function of the brain's hemispheres.'

2 Anatomical aspects of the problem

CONTINUOUS AND LONG-STANDING CONTACTS with patients allowed us to identify a complex of complaints, which were, to some extent, similar among children of different ages and adults. The older the patient was, the more pronounced were his disease symptoms. The other important factors included the duration of the pathological process, as well as the localization of vertebral rotational subluxation.

It was also found that the above-mentioned abnormalities of patients' general condition, proper functioning of the musculoskeletal system and of various organs were associated with dysfunctions of the spinal cord, brain, spinal nerves and their plexuses (cervical, brachial, lumbar, sacral and coccygeal), etc. While trying to discover the origin of these pathological conditions, we realized that it was necessary to study carefully the human anatomy and the anatomy of the spine in particular. It was particularly important to identify anomalies, developmental variations and even malformations associated with abnormal spine structure. We had to find answers regarding the association between muscular asymmetry, the anatomical structure of the spine and its various deformities, on the one hand, and the various types of pain and dysfunctions in a single organ or even an organ system, on the other.

We had a great deal of difficulty putting together this chapter. As we wanted to avoid presenting a huge amount of data on human anatomy, we set ourselves the task of providing only those data which would be sufficient for the reader to understand the origin of pain, other symptoms and specific dysfunctions. Thus, the chapter contains only minimal, basic information. Readers who are interested in an in-depth study of the anatomy of the skeletal, peripheral, central and autonomic nervous systems will need to explore further on their own.

This chapter first provides information on the normal anatomy of the spine, and then goes on to describe the structure of the central and peripheral nervous systems, as well as the role of the autonomic nervous system in the functioning of the body. Variations among different people, anomalies and malformations, as well as signs of body asymmetry, are described in separate sections.

2.1 Normal anatomy of the spine and peripheral and autonomic nervous systems

Vertebral column: The vertebral column (VC) (Fig. 2.1.1) consists of separate vertebrae, which are interconnected by intervertebral discs, joints and ligaments. The number of vertebrae varies between 32 and 35, and in rare cases, reaches 37 due to a larger number of sacral and coccygeal vertebrae. The VC includes 7 cervical vertebrae (vertebrae cervicales), 12 thoracic vertebrae (vertebrae thoracicae) and 5 lumbar

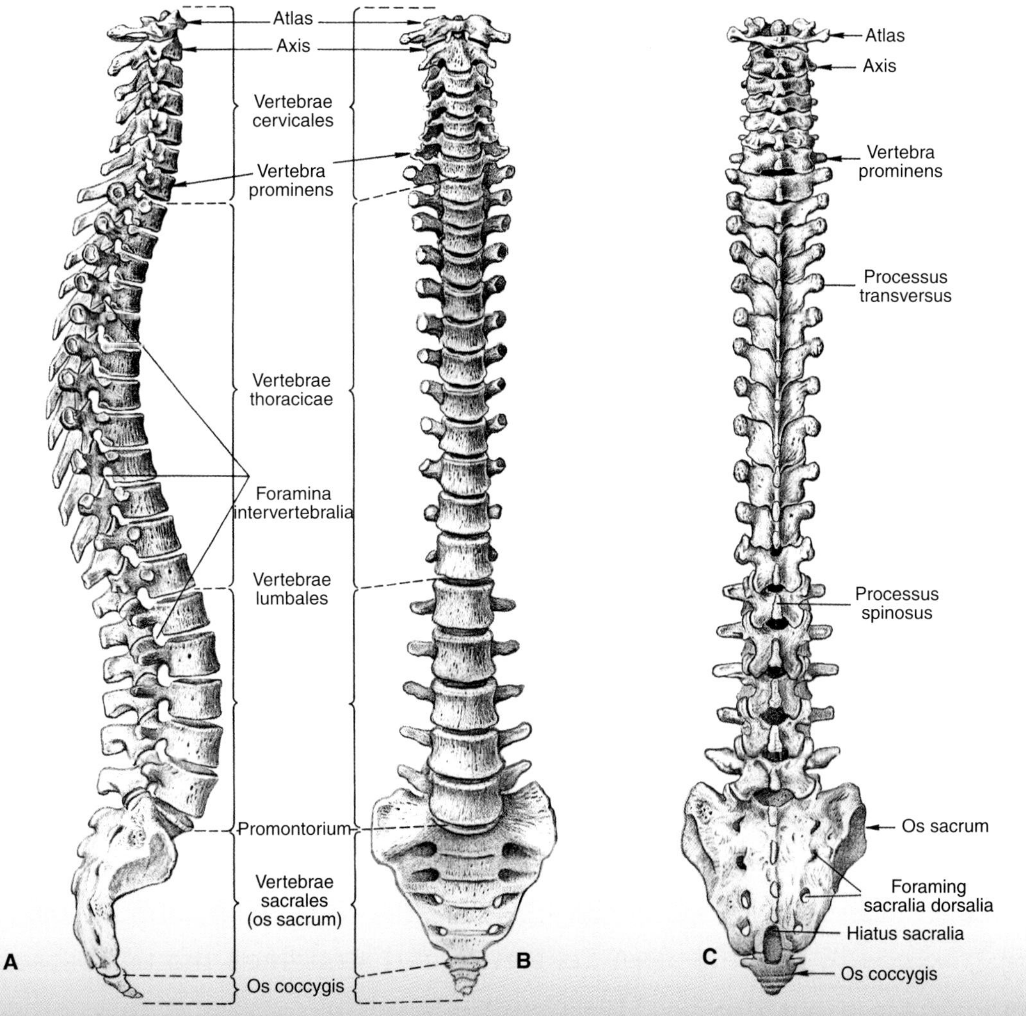

Fig. 2.1.1. Vertebral column, *columna vertebralis:* **A** - view from the right side, **B** - front view, **C** - rear view

vertebrae (vertebrae lumbales). The sacral region has 4–6 vertebrae (vertebrae sacrales), which are fused to form the sacrum (os sacrum), while the coccygeal region has 4–5 rudimentary vertebrae (vertebrae coccygeae), which form the coccyx (os coccygis).

The length of the spine can vary significantly and determines the length of the trunk. In males, the average length of the spine is 73–75 cm and in females, 69–71 cm. Thirty centimeters account for the thoracic region, 17 cm for the lumbar region, and 11–12 cm for the cervical and sacrococcygeal regions. In the elderly, the spine is usually shortened to some extent due to the formation of more or less marked kyphosis (gibbus), compression and ossification of the intervertebral cartilages, and involution of vertebral bodies.

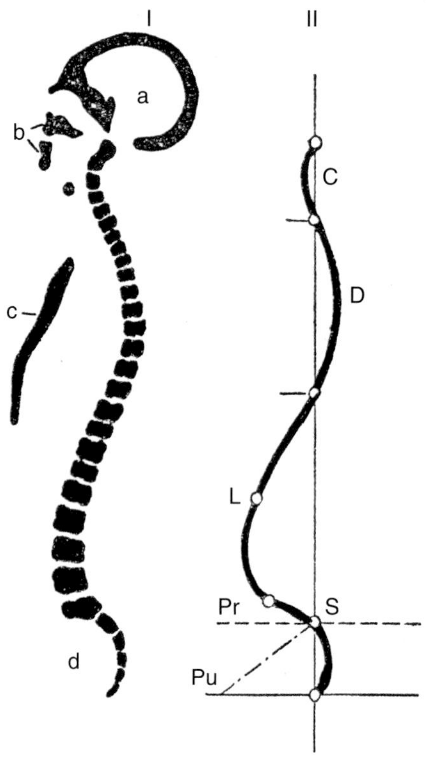

Fig. 2.1.2.
Scheme of curvatures of the spine in the sagittal plane:
I - anteroposterior curvatures of the spine: a - cranial cavity, b - the upper and lower jaw, c - sternum, d - pubis; II - intersection of vertical line of gravity with the curvature of spine (three upper and two lower circles); C - cervical region; D - thoracic; L - lumbar; S - sacral; Pr - promontorium; Pu - pubis

The VC of an adult male has four curves (Fig. 2.1.2). The upper cervical curve, which is convex in the forward direction (lordosis, from the Greek *lordoo*, or curving forward or bending), is formed by all the cervical and upper thoracic vertebrae. The peak of the curve is located at the level of the 5th and 6th cervical vertebrae. The peak of the second thoracic curve, which is concave in the backward direction (kyphosis, from the Greek *kyphos*, or hump), is located at the level of the 6th and 7th thoracic vertebrae. The lower thoracic and all lumbar vertebrae form the third lumbar curve (lordosis). Anteriorly, the most prominent lumbar vertebrae, the 4th and 5th, and the most prominent sacral vertebra, the 1st, form the promontorium. The sacrum and coccyx form the fourth curve, which is concave in the backward direction (kyphosis).

The majority of investigators consider the VC curves to be a result of the distribution of the forces of gravity and of muscle tension during growth and development in childhood (Fig. 2.1.3). The VC curves are not pronounced in newborns. Cervical lordosis first develops among children after they attempt to sit up and hold their heads straight. The child's gradual attempts to rise and straighten the head result in the development of certain muscles. This, in turn, curves the cervical region of the VC and simultaneously gives rise to thoracic kyphosis. Sacral curvature may be observed as early as the fifth month of embryonic development.

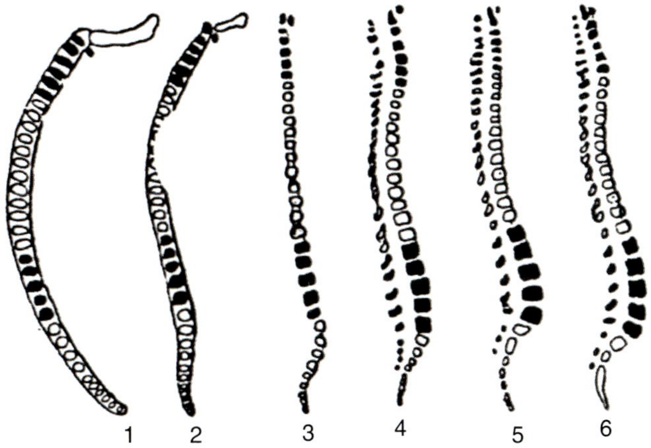

Fig. 2.1.3.
Development of spine curvatures in humans:
1 - 2nd month of embryonic development, 2 - 6th month of embryonic development, and 3 - the newborn; 4 - 4 years, 5 - 13 years old, 6 - spine of an adult man

The final formation of cervical lordosis and thoracic kyphosis occurs at the age of 7 years. Lumbar lordosis develops during the pubertal period. With increasing age, the shape of the VC changes. At an average age of 50 years, the physiological curves of the VC flatten. Among healthy individuals, the changes in the shape of the VC do not affect the normal physiological processes. Some elderly people may develop thoracic kyphosis, commonly known as senile kyphosis.

The appearance of other natural VC curvatures may be explained by the presence of different muscle tractions on the right and left sides of the body. When taking a posterior view of the spine, it is evident that there is a slight curvature to the side (to the left or the right), between the scapulae in the frontal plane—a so-called 'scoliotic deformity' or scoliosis (from the Greek *scolios*, or crooked). Right-sided scoliosis is usually more frequently observed among right-handed persons and left-sided scoliosis among left-handed persons. According to S.F. Mamoiko (cited from G.F. Ivanov, 1949), lateral (scoliotic) curvature is an acquired pathological condition of the spine and is not found among healthy individuals. G.F. Ivanov (1949) himself thought that this condition was a result of normal asymmetry (Fig. 2.1.4).

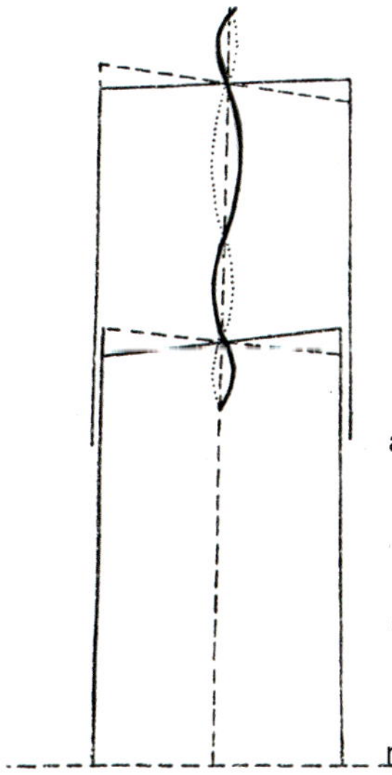
Fig. 2.1.4.
Scheme of frontal curvatures of the spine (scoliosis) — normal asymmetry; rear view. Dashed line denotes scoliosis and tilt of pelvis and shoulders of a man with normal leg length; solid line denotes the same in a man having leg shortening; inclined horizontal line denotes the position of transverse axis of the body relative to shoulders and pelvis

A spinal motion segment (SMS), also known as a 'functional spinal unit', is a structural unit of the spine. This conventional unit consists of two adjacent vertebrae, the intervertebral disc and all the ligaments and muscles between them. A thoracic SMS also includes the costovertebral and costotransverse joints.

Generally, all vertebrae have a similar structure, but they acquire certain features depending on the region of the spine. Thus, all vertebrae (except the 1st cervical vertebra) have a vertebral body (corpus vertebra), which is located anteriorly, and a vertebral arch (arcus vertebralis), which is located posteriorly. These are interconnected by the pediculus arcus (pedunculi arcus). The vertebral corpora and arches enclose the vertebral foramina, which collectively form the spinal canal (canalis vertebralis). A vertebral arch has a few processes: the spinous process (processus spinosus), located posteriorly in the midline, and the articular processes, some of which are directed downwards and some upwards (processus articulares superiores et inferiores). The latter posteriorly enclose superior and inferior vertebral incisures, which form the intervertebral foramina (foramina intervertebralia).

Cervical vertebrae: The transverse processes of these have foramina (*foramina transversalia*) through which passes the neurovascular bundle containing the vertebral artery. The top two cervical vertebrae, i.e. the atlas (Fig. 2.1.5) and the epistropheus or axis (Fig. 2.1.6), have a special shape because of the role they play in the formation of the rotating junction with the skull. The shape of the next five vertebrae differs significantly from that of the first two. Their bodies are smaller, and their superior and inferior surfaces are concave (Fig. 2.1.7). The length of the spinous processes, which lie horizontally, increases from the upper to the lower vertebrae. Thus, the long process of the 7th cervical vertebra protrudes dorsally and can be palpated easily. For this reason, this vertebra is described as prominent (vertebra prominens) (Fig. 2.1.8).

Thoracic vertebrae: The thoracic vertebrae (Fig. 2.1.9) are connected with the ribs. Thus, the upper and lower surfaces of their body (fovea costalis superior et inferior) have areas for articulation with the costal heads. The foveae of adjacent vertebrae form one complete fossa, into which the costal head comes. The spinous processes of the thoracic vertebrae overlie each other like the tiles on a roof, especially in the lower thoracic region. From the 8th

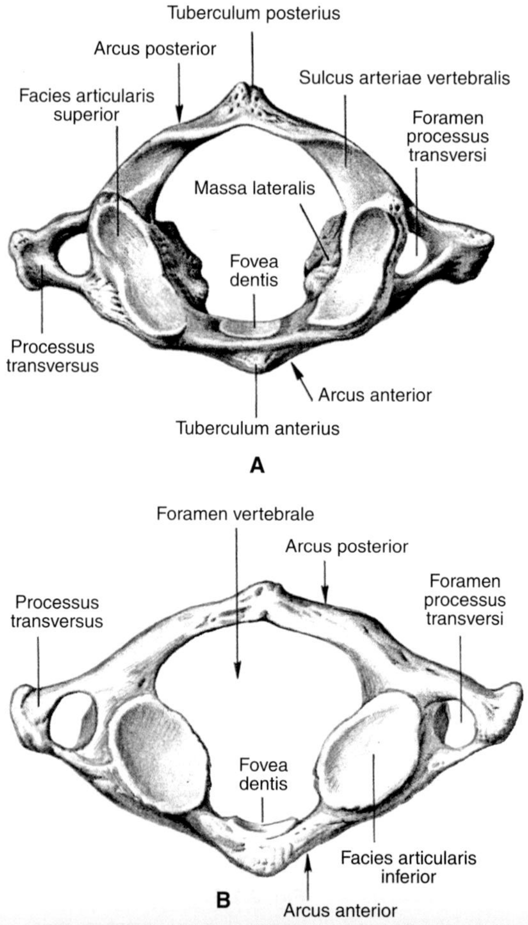

Fig. 2.1.5.
A - the first (I) cervical vertebra, *atlant*, atlas, (top view); **B** - the first (I) cervical vertebra, *atlant*, atlas (bottom view)

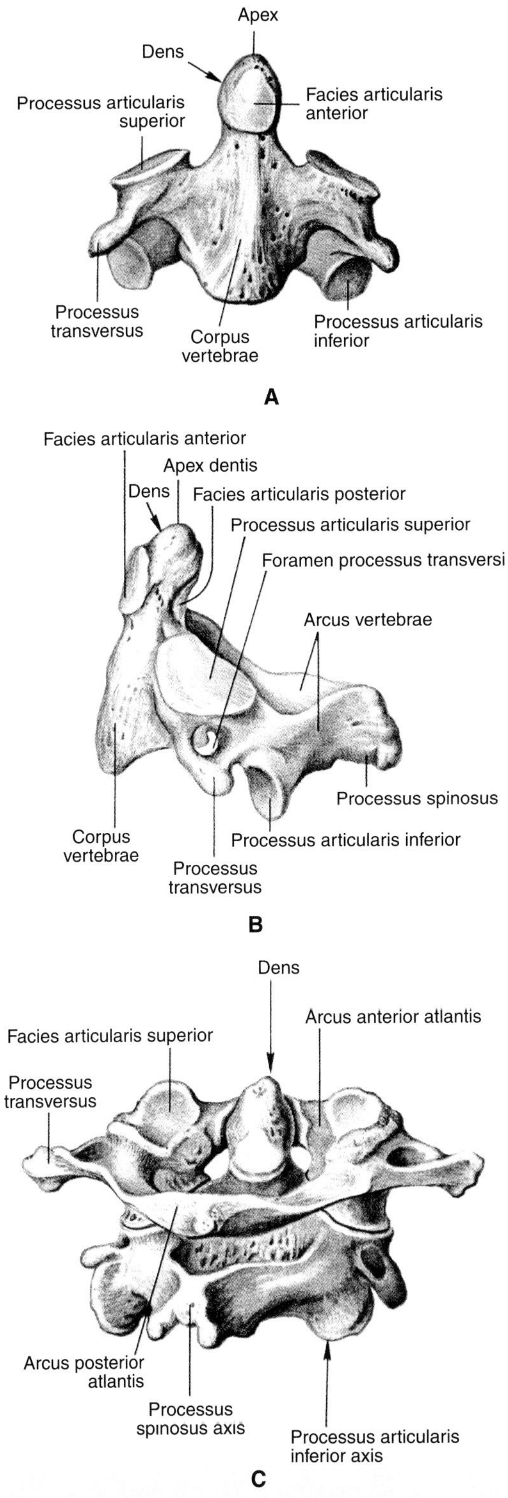

Fig. 2.1.6.
A - the second (II) cervical, axial vertebra, axis; front view; **B** - the second (II) cervical, axial vertebra, axis; view from the left side; **C** - the first (I) and second (II) cervical vertebrae, rear and lateral (right) view

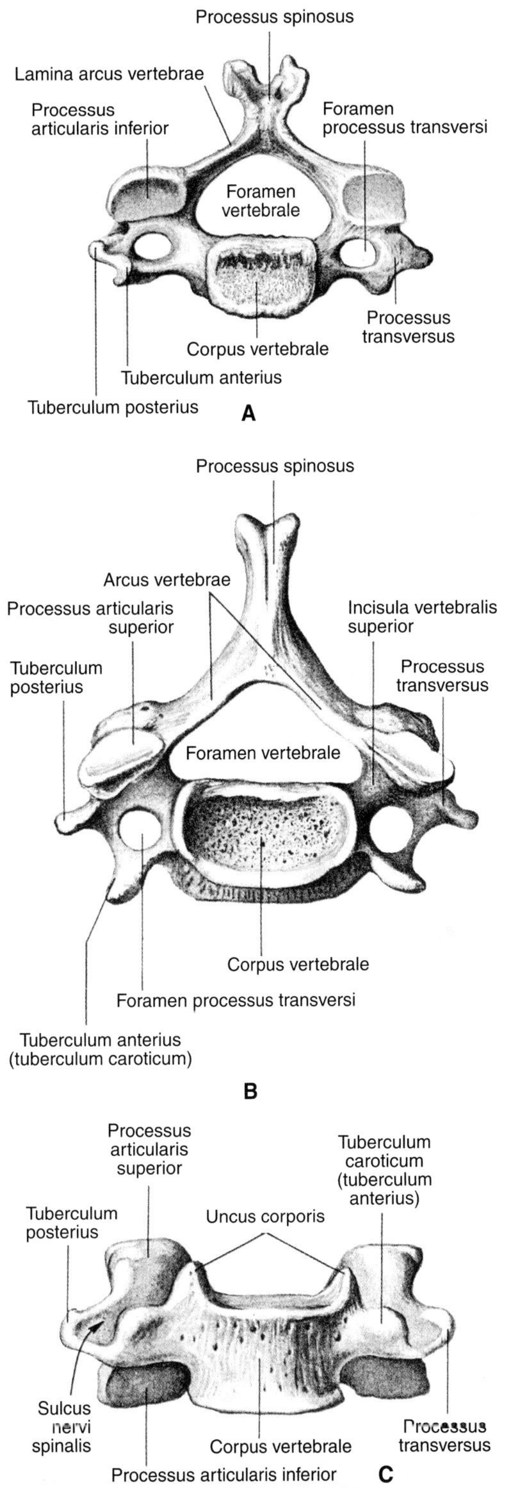

Fig. 2.1.7.
A - The sixth (VI) cervical vertebra, *vertebra cervicalis VI*; front view; **B** - the sixth (VI) cervical vertebra, *vertebra cervicalis VI*; top view; **C** - the fourth (IV) cervical vertebra, *vertebra cervicalis IV*; bottom view

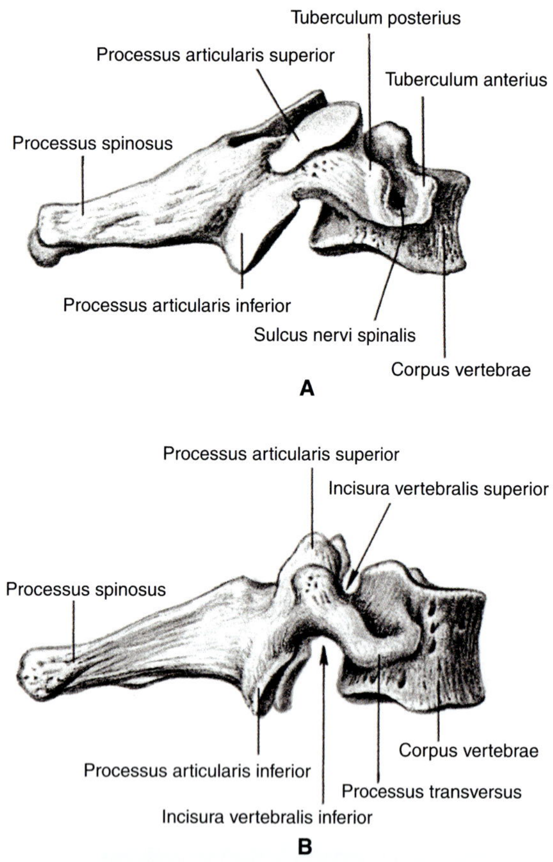

Fig. 2.1.8.
A - the sixth (VI) cervical vertebra, *vertebra cervicalis VI* (view from the right); **B** - the seventh (VII) cervical, prominent vertebra, *vertebra prominens VII* (view from the right)

vertebra downwards, the inclination of the spinous processes decreases, and the process of the 12th vertebra lies horizontally.

Lumbar vertebrae: The lumbar vertebrae (Fig. 2.1.10) are much larger than the thoracic vertebrae. The vertebral foramina is also bigger. The inferior articular processes are very large and their articular surfaces are turned outward. These features of the lumbar intervertebral joints allow for forward and backward movements of the lumbar spine. On each superior articular process, there is a small mamillary process (processus mamillaris),

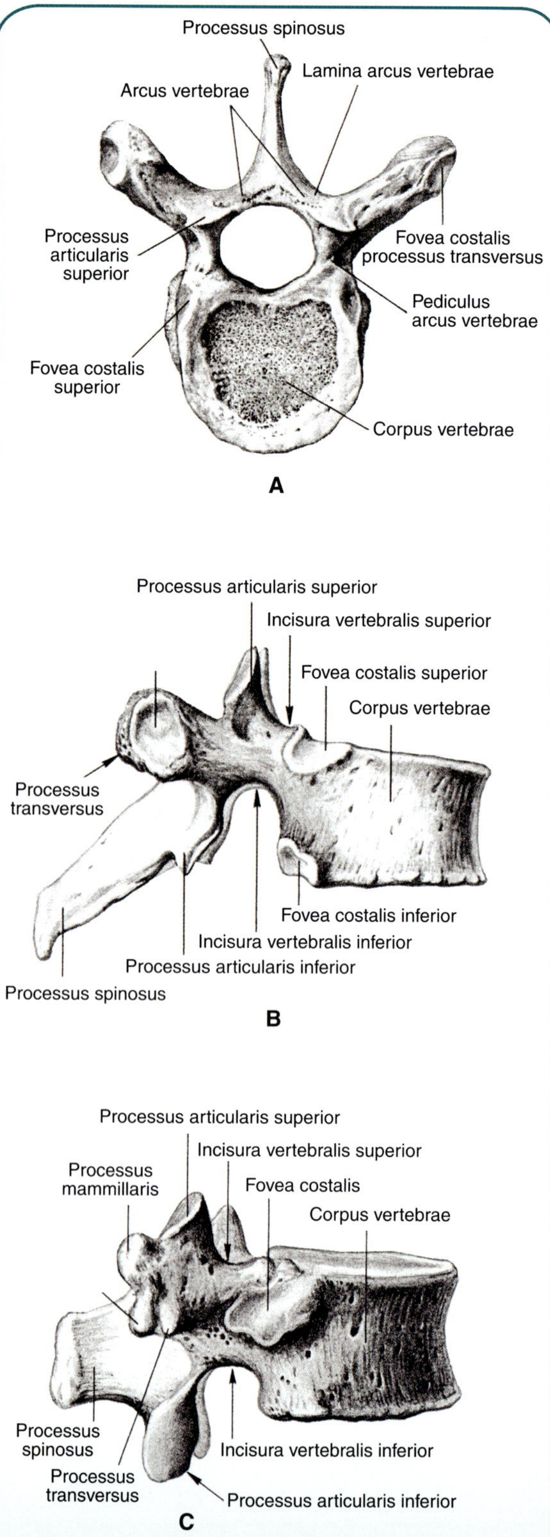

Fig. 2.1.9.
A - the eighth (VIII) thoracic vertebra, *vertebra thoracica VIII* (top view); **B** - the eighth (VIII) thoracic vertebra, *vertebra thoracica VIII* (view from the right); **C** - the twelfth (XII) thoracic vertebra, *vertebra thoracica XII* (view from the right)

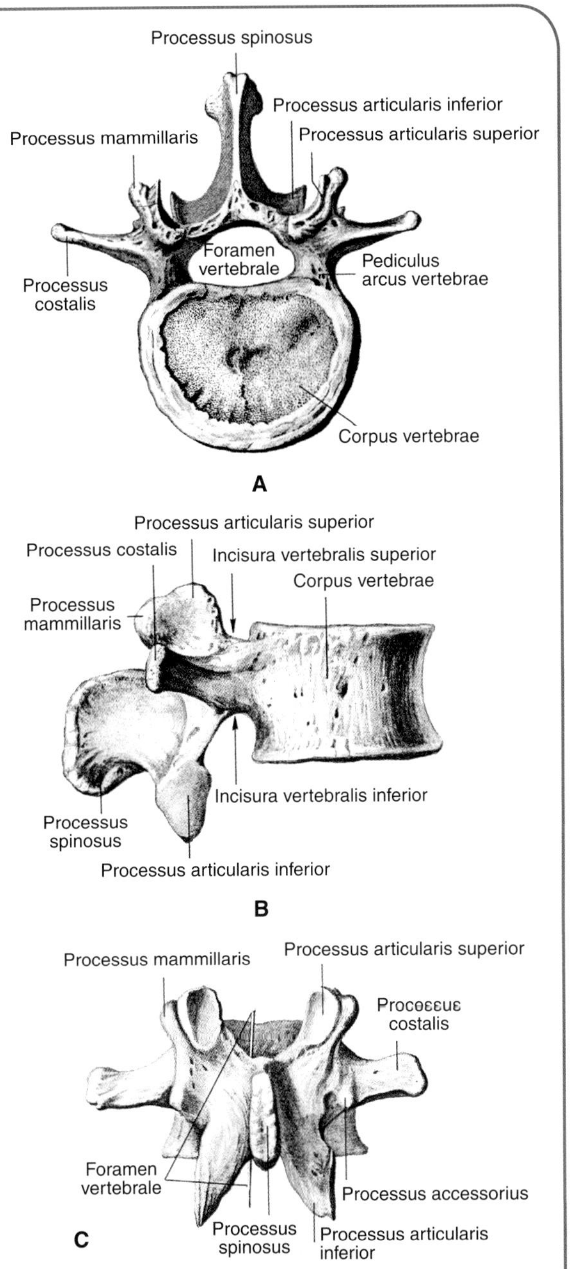

Fig. 2.1.10.
A - the third (III) lumbar vertebra, *vertebra lumbalis III* (top view); **B** - the third (III) lumbar vertebra, *vertebra lumbalis III* (view from the right); **C** - the third (III) lumbar vertebra, *vertebra lumbalis III* (rear view)

and behind the base of the transverse process is an additional process (processus accessorius).

Sacrum: The sacrum (Fig. 2.1.11) is a region of the spine that forms the posterior wall of the pelvic cavity. The position of

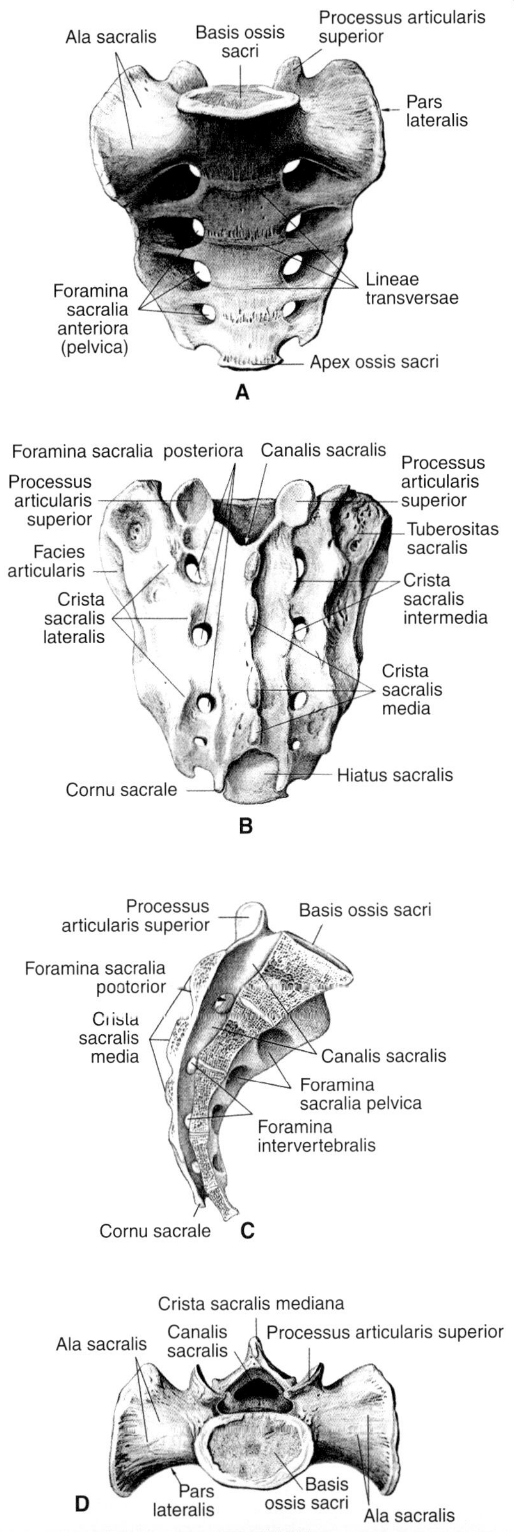

Fig. 2.1.11.
A - sacrum, *os sacrum*; front view (pelvic surface, *facies pelvica*); **B** - sacrum, *os sacrum*; rear view (dorsal surface, *facies dorsalis*); **C** - sacrum, *os sacrum*; right side (mid-longitudinal cutting); **D** - sacrum, *os sacrum*; top view

the sacrum allows it to play a unique role in body mechanics. The sacrum consists of five vertebrae, which fuse during different periods of life. By the age of 16 years, the lower caudal vertebrae begin to fuse to form a single structure. The upper sacral vertebrae fuse completely only by the age of 25 years. Thus, it is quite late by the time the sacrum forms as a single bone. The anatomical variations of this region include fusion of the 5th lumbar vertebra with the sacrum (sacralization of L_5). In some cases, S_1 is observed to be a part of the lumbar region of the spine (lumbarization of S_1). In such cases, the sacrum consists of four vertebrae.

The anterior surface of the sacrum (facies pelvina) is concave and is crossed by four transverse ridges. These are traces of vertebral fusion. Moreover, there are four foramina on either side of the median line, the lower ones being smaller than the upper ones. The nerves of the sacral plexus leave the pelvic cavity through the anterior sacral foramina. The dorsal surface of the sacrum (facies dorsalis) is convex and tuberous. Between the lateral and medial crests, there are posterior sacral foramina, through which posterior branches of the sacral nerves and vessels go out. An intervertebral joint is formed by the base of the sacrum together with the 5th lumbar vertebra. An orifice of the sacral canal is also located here. The 1st sacral vertebra protrudes anteriorly to form the promontorium. Intervertebral ganglia are located in the intersacral canals, which correspond to the intervertebral foramina. The inferior opening of the sacral canal (hiatus sacralis) varies in size and shape. At the apex of the sacrum there is an oval facet for articulation with the coccyx. The sacrum is connected to the bones of the pelvis through a number of ligaments, apart from articular surfaces.

The terminal part of a cavity or a bag formed by the dura mater is located in the sacral canal. This cavity contains the rootlets of the segments of the caudal spinal cord, which are a part of the cauda equina. The membrane-covered nerves forming the sacral plexus are also located here.

Coccyx: The coccyx (tailbone or os coccygis) (Fig. 2.1.12) looks like a flat, slightly concave, rough wedge. The anterior surface of the coccyx is slightly concave, while the posterior one is slightly convex. The coccyx consists of four, or less frequently five or six, fused vestigial tail vertebrae. The sacrum and coccyx are interconnected by articular processes, which are also called coccygeal horns (cornua coccygea), and also through ligamentous connections.

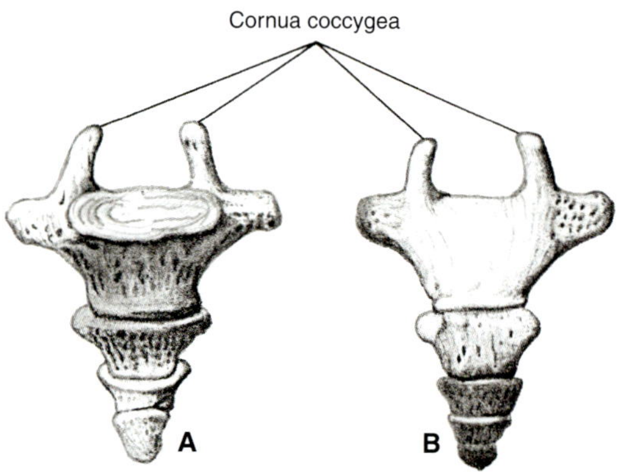

Fig. 2.1.12.
Coccyx, *os coccygis*; **A** - front view; **B** - rear view

Spinal muscles (Figs 2.1.13–2.1.15)

Extension of the spine: This is performed by muscles located on the posterior surface of the trunk and the neck. These muscles are: the trapezius muscle (m. trapezius), superior and inferior serratus muscles (mm. serrati post. sup. et inf.), splenius cervicis and capitis muscles (m. splenius cervicis et capitis), extensor spinae (m. erector spinae), transversospinal muscle (m. transverso-spinalis) and short muscles of the back.

Flexion of the spine: This is performed by the anterior cervical muscles, i.e. the sternocleidomastoid or sternomastoid muscle, the scalene muscles and the longus capitis and colli muscles (m. sterno-cleido-mastoideus, mm. scaleni ant., med. et post., m. longus capitis et m. longus colli); the abdominal muscles (transverse and rectus); and the iliopsoas muscle (m. ilio-psoas).

Lateral flexion of the spine is performed according to the rule of the parallelogram of forces, i.e. the simultaneous contraction of flexors and extensors leads to the flexion of the spine in a direction given by the resultant of the two forces.

Rotation of the spine: The unilateral contraction of the following muscles allows for the rotation of the spine about its longitudinal axis: the sternocleidomastoid muscle, the superior part of the trapezius muscle, the scalene muscles and the abdominal external oblique muscle, together with the internal oblique muscle of the opposite side. Circular movements of the spine are performed due to sequential contraction of all muscle groups.

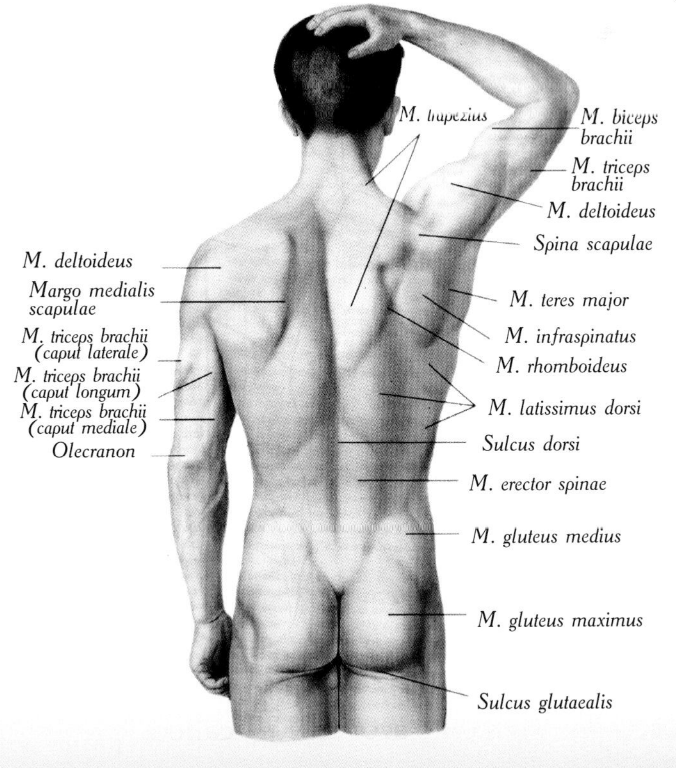

Fig. 2.1.13.
The relief of muscles of the trunk; rear view

Ligamentous apparatus of the spine

The vertebrae are interconnected by fibrous cartilaginous plates or discs (disci intervertebrales), with intervertebral joints and ligaments. The ligaments play a variety of roles, such as strengthening the spine by limiting its mobility. Intervertebral discs are located between the bodies of all the vertebrae, except C_I–C_{II}. The discs have the functions of providing support, fixation, and shock-absorption. They also provide some mobility to

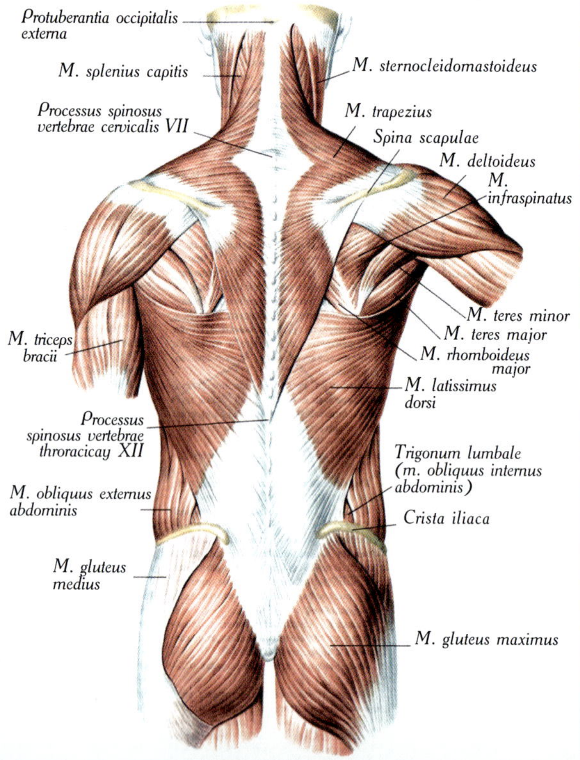

Fig. 2.1.14.
Back muscles, *mm. dorsi*
(superficial muscles)

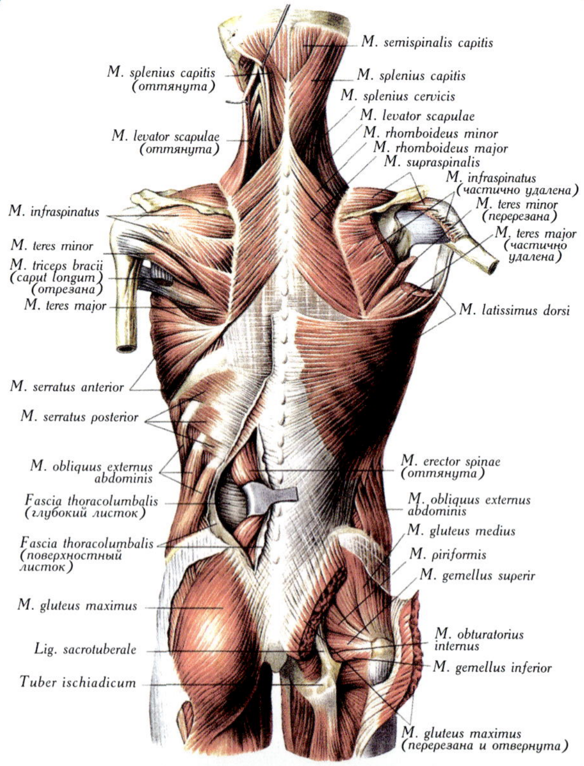

Fig. 2.1.15.
Back muscles and posterior muscles of the neck (superficial muscles: the first, second and third layers; trapezius and left latissimus dorsi muscles are removed)

the SMS (Fig. 2.1.16). The outer side of the disc, called the annulus (annulus fibrosus), consists of densely interwoven collagen fibres that grow into the periosteum. These fibres protect the horizontal surfaces of the vertebral bodies from traumatization by providing a strong interconnection between the disc and the bodies of the adjacent vertebrae. Fibres become completely calcified by the end of the second decade of life.

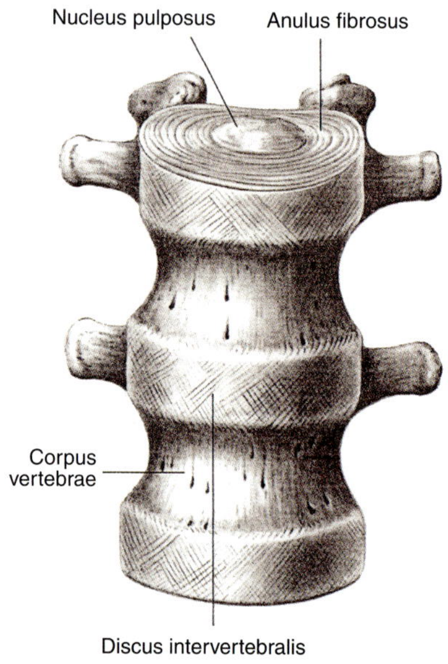

Fig. 2.1.16.
Intervertebral discs, *disci intervertebrales*; front view

There are no fibres in the centre of the disc which, instead, contains a jelly-like substance called the nucleus pulposus (Fig. 2.1.17). It is soft, glassy in appearance and has the tendency to protrude. The nucleus pulposus is composed of cartilaginous cells, collagen fibres and intercellular substance. The latter contains proteins, glycosaminoglycans, etc. Polar pH-groups provide nutrition to the nucleus pulposus via diffusion, a process facilitated by the high ability of the nucleus to retain water. This ability enables the VC to absorb shocks and bumps during movements such as jumping and running. The discs of the cervical SMS are more or less of the same height. Those in the thoracic region are very thin. The height of the lumbar discs is greater than that of the others, and reach the maximum in the L_{IV}–L_{V} segment.

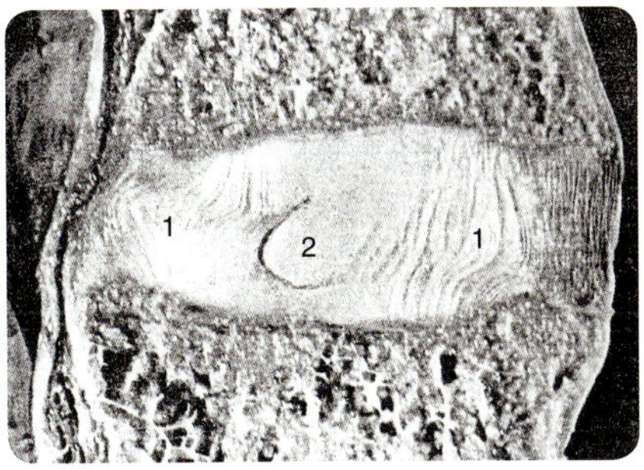

Fig. 2.1.17.
Sagittal cutting of lumbar vertebrae (L_{IV}–L_{V}) and the intervertebral disc:
1 - annulus fibrosus; **2** - nucleus pulposus

There are anterior and posterior longitudinal ligaments on the corresponding surfaces of the vertebral bodies (Fig. 2.1.18). An anterior longitudinal ligament (lig. longitudinale anterius) passes across the front of the vertebral body. It is well expressed in the lumbar region and only slightly in the cervical. These ligaments prevent overextension of the spine, and are firmly connected with the vertebrae and loosely connected with the intervertebral discs. A posterior longitudinal ligament (lig. longitudinale posterius) runs across the back of the vertebral body and prevents the spine from bending. It is firmly connected with the disc and loosely connected with the vertebral body. This ligament is well expressed in the cervical region and hardly expressed in the lower lumbar region, which gives rise to the possibility of the occurrence of certain conditions, such as herniation and protrusion of the nucleus pulposus.

There are tight, dense membranes located along all the spaces down the spine, between the arcs of the adjacent vertebrae (except for the intervertebral foramina). Known as the yellow ligaments (ligamenta flava) (Fig. 2.1.19), these are very thick

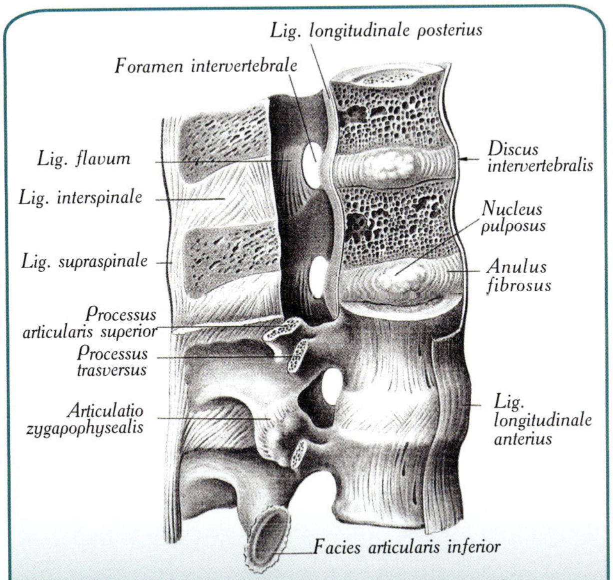

Fig. 2.1.18. Ligaments and joints of the spine

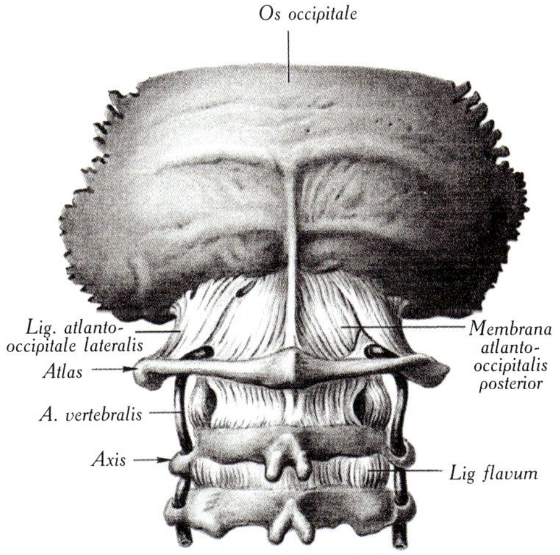

Fig. 2.1.19.
Ligaments of cervical vertebrae and the occipital bone (rear view)

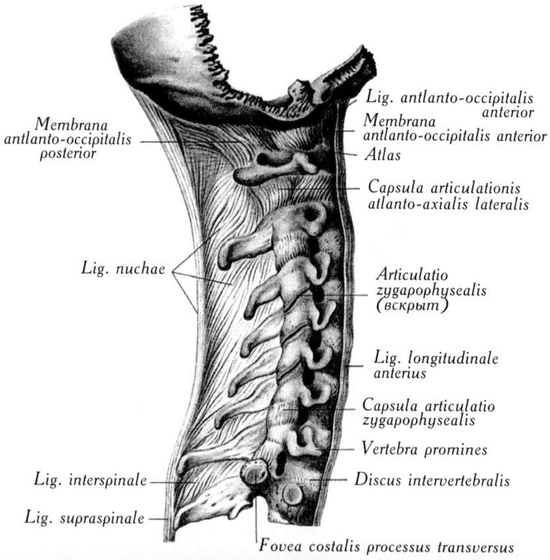

Fig. 2.1.20.
Ligaments and joints of the cervical spine

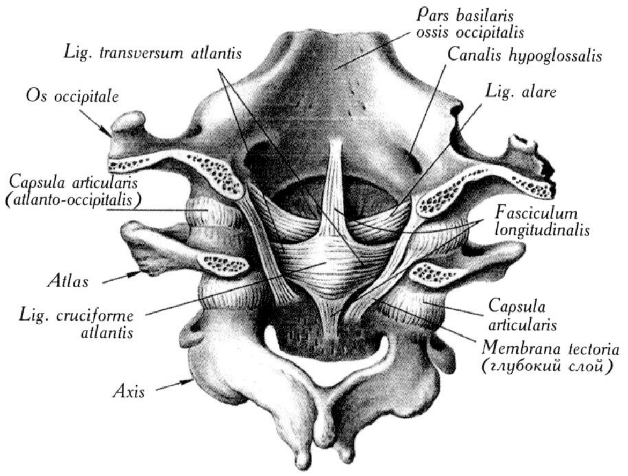

Fig. 2.1.21.
Ligaments and joints of cervical vertebrae and occipital bone (view from inside)

(2–7 mm in the lumbar region) and thus strong. The gaps between the spinous processes are packed with interspinous ligaments (lig. interspinalia). In contrast to the yellow ligaments, these are very weak and do not perform a mechanical role. A strong supraspinal ligament (lig. supraspinale) is located above the spinous processes. This extends throughout the VC (Figs 2.1.20 and 2.1.21).

In the cervical part of the VC, interspinous and supraspinal ligaments extend beyond the spinous processes and form a thick and strong nuchal ligament (lig. nuchae) which, together with the neck muscles, holds the head in equilibrium.

Vascular supply to the spine

The cervical region of the VC is supplied mainly by the vertebral artery (a. vertebralis). Arising from the subclavian artery (a. subclavia), it passes through holes in the transverse processes of six cervical vertebrae, sending out branches to the spinal cord and medulla oblongata (Fig. 2.1.22).

In the thoracic region of the VC, arterial trunks arise from the intercostal arteries (a. intercostales). At the level of the costal heads, each of these arteries divides into anterior and posterior branches. The anterior branches run forward between the internal and external intercostal muscles, supplying these muscles and the skin. The posterior branches run backward, supplying the muscles and skin of the back.

There are four pairs of lumbar arteries (aa. lumbales), which correspond to the intercostal arteries. These, too, are divided into anterior and posterior branches. They send branches to the vertebral canal. The middle sacral artery (a. sacralis media), running down to the coccyx, sends out branches to the sacral and coccygeal vertebrae.

There are numerous veins in the VC and these are arranged in plexuses (plexus

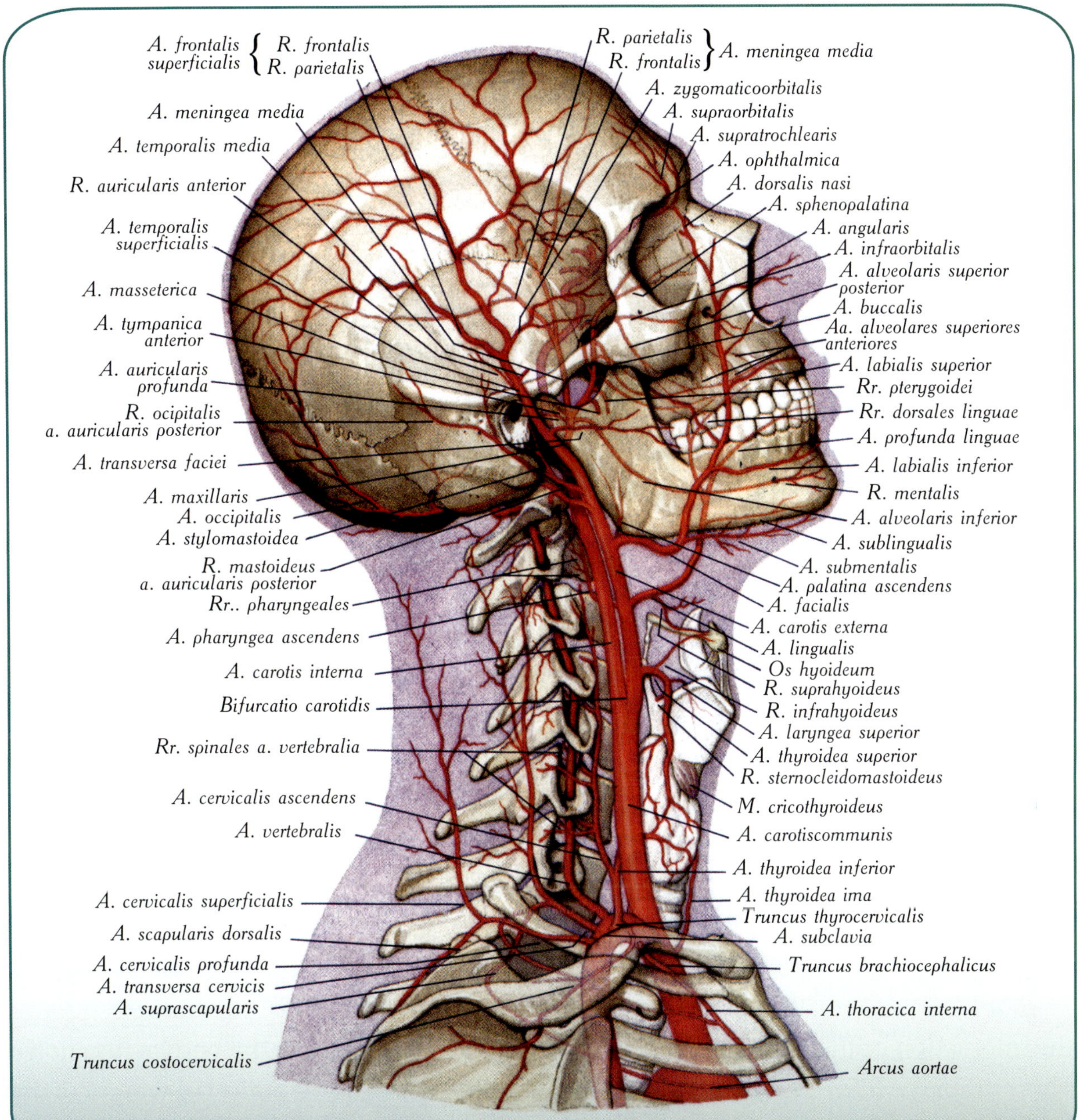

Fig. 2.1.22. Arteries of the head and neck (view from the right side [semi-schematic])

venosus) that lie along the spine, on its outer and inner surfaces. There are both anterior and posterior veins. These plexuses are interconnected throughout the spine to the superior and inferior vena cava via posterior branches (rami posteriores). Vertebral veins (vv. intervertebrales), together with the spinal nerves, run through the intervertebral foramina (Fig. 2.1.23).

Central nervous system

The central nervous system (CNS) consists of parts that are located within the cranium and the VC.

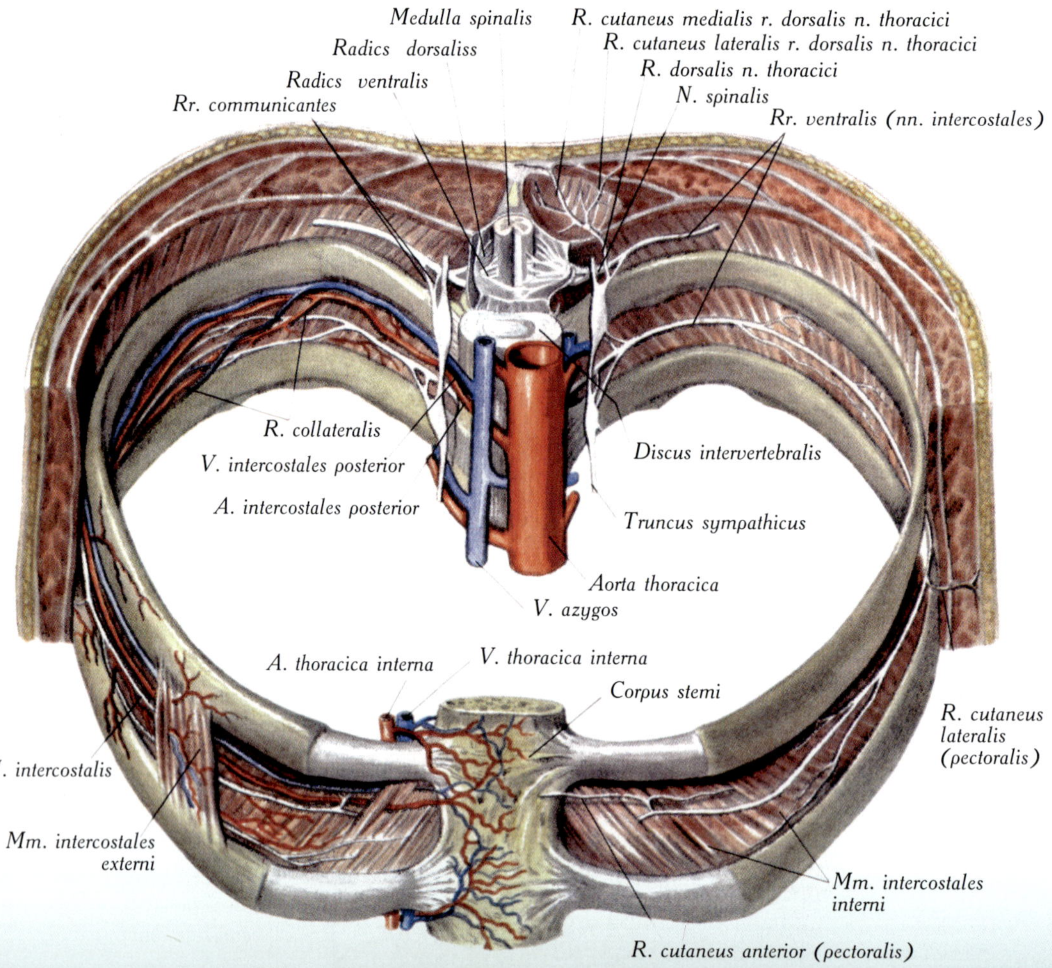

Fig. 2.1.23.
Intercostal nerves, arteries and veins (view from the top and slightly anteriorly)

Brain (encephalon): The supreme organ of the nervous system, the brain, regulates the interaction of the organism with the environment, as well as the body's functions. This part of the CNS is enclosed in the cranial cavity. In an adult male, the weight of the brain (without the dura mater) is approximately 1375 g. Its weight varies according to age, sex and individual characteristics. The brain consists of the brainstem, cerebellum and cerebrum. The areas where the 12 cranial nerves originate are located on the inferior surface of the brain (Fig. 2.1.24).

Spinal cord: The spinal cord (SC), or medulla spinalis (Figs 2.1.25–2.1.27), and brain are genetically, morphologically and functionally interconnected. There is no sharply defined border between the two, with one running into the other.

The SC is located within the spinal canal, from the 1st cervical vertebra to the 1st lumbar vertebra or the upper margin of the 2nd lumbar vertebra. To some extent, it curves together with the parts of the VC that it passes through. At the level of the lower margin of the foramen magnum and the upper margin of the 1st cervical vertebra, the

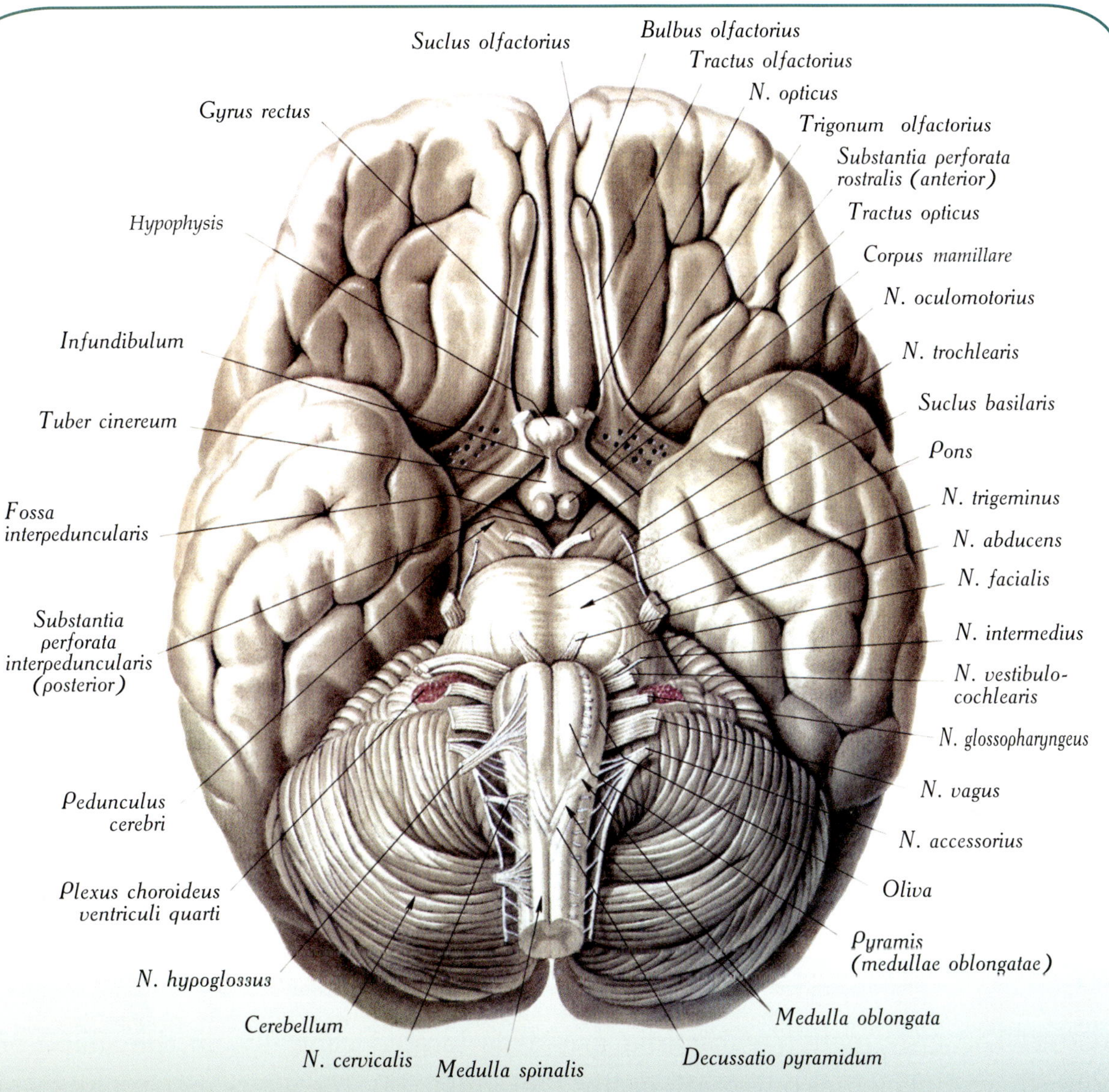

Fig. 2.1.24. Brain, *encephalon*; bottom view (inferior surface)

SC runs into the medulla without any sharply defined borders. The SC only partially fills the cavity of the vertebral canal. The space remaining within the walls of the canal is filled with adipose tissue, vessels, meninges and cerebrospinal fluid.

In an adult, the length of the SC varies between 40 cm and 45 cm, and its width, between 1.0 cm and 1.5 cm. It weighs approximately 35 g. The diameter of the SC is the same along its entire length. There are, however, two intumescences. One is the cervical intumescence, which is located at the level of the 3rd to 4th cervical vertebrae and is the site of origin of the spinal nerves that supply the upper extremities. The other is the lumbosacral intumescence, which is located at the level of the 9th to 10th thoracic to 1st lumbar vertebrae. This is the site of origin of the nerves supplying the lower extremities.

A transverse section of the SC (Fig. 2.1.28) shows the presence of white and grey

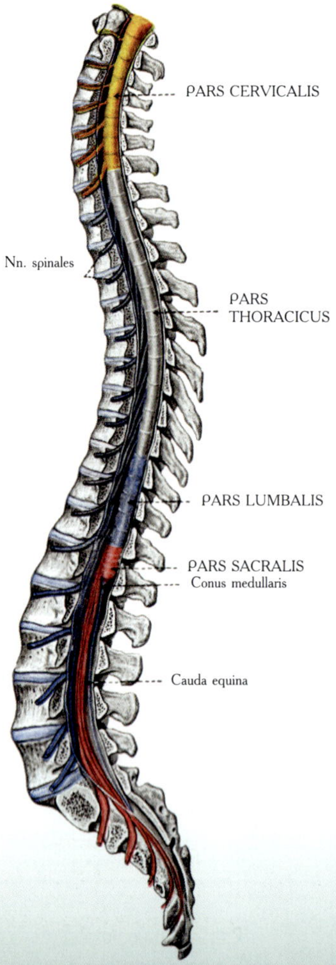

Fig. 2.1.25. Medulla spinalis *in situ*

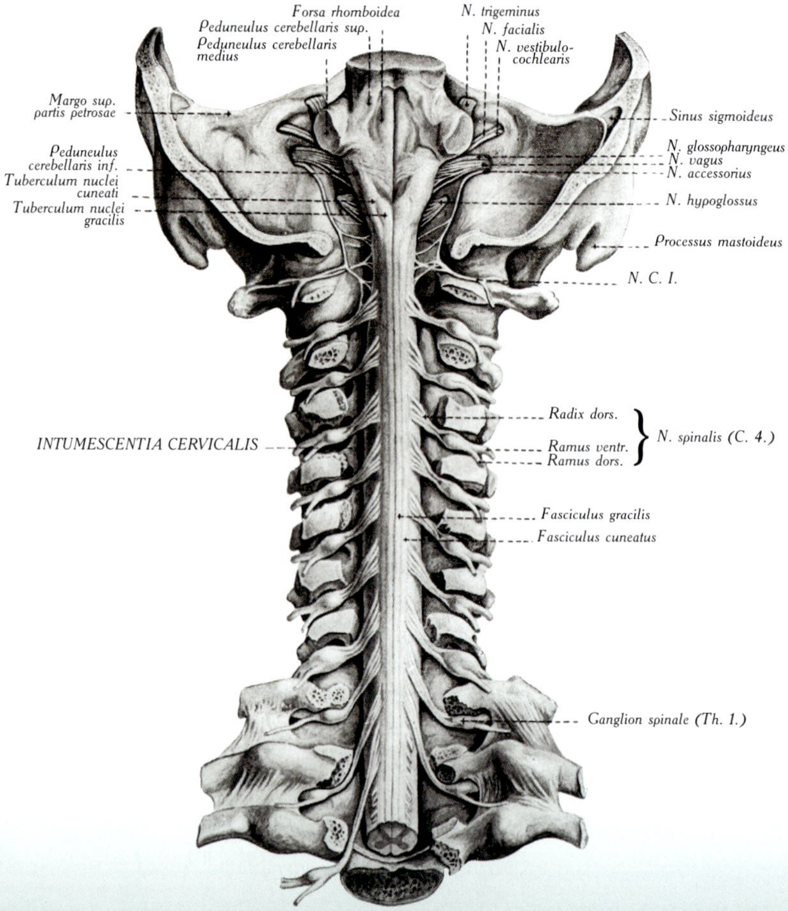

Fig. 2.1.26.
Pars cervicalis medullae spinalis

matter. The grey matter (substantia grisea) is located centrally, in the shape of a butterfly with its wings outspread or like the capital 'H'. The white matter (substantia alba) lies at the periphery of the SC, around the grey matter. It consists of a complex of myelinated and non-myelinated nerve fibres of varying length and diameter, as well as supportive tissue, i.e. neuroglia and vessels, which are surrounded by a small amount of connective tissue. The nerve fibres of the white matter are bundled together.

The grey matter of the SC consists mainly of nerve cell bodies and their non-myelinated processes. Moreover, it includes the processes of nerve cells that are located in other parts of the SC and brain, as well as neuroglia, vessels and associated connective tissue. The nerve cells of the grey matter form discrete masses, i.e. nuclei or centres of the SC, which have constant topography.

Meninges of the brain and spinal cord

The brain and SC are enclosed in three membranes (meninges) each (Figs 2.1.29 and 2.1.30). These are the dura mater, the outermost membrane; the arachnoid mater, which is located inwards from the dura; and the pia mater, the innermost layer. Each meninx of the SC continues to form a similarly named cerebral meninx.

There is a space, called epidural space, between the dura mater of the SC and the vertebrae. This space is filled with adipose and loose connective tissue, it contains an extensive network of venous vessels. Between the dura and arachnoid maters is a space called the subdural space. This space contains cerebral and spinal nerves (nerve roots arising from the brain and the SC. The dura and pia maters are supplied with nerves and vessels. The arachnoid mater has no vessels.

Nerve roots, ganglia and nerves arising from the SC are covered with dural sheaths. These sheaths, which play a role in meninx fixation, lie facing the intervertebral foramina.

Nerves enter and leave the CNS. Those located towards the skull or spine form a part of the peripheral nervous system (PNS).

Peripheral nervous system

A living organism is a unique system that is capable of controlling

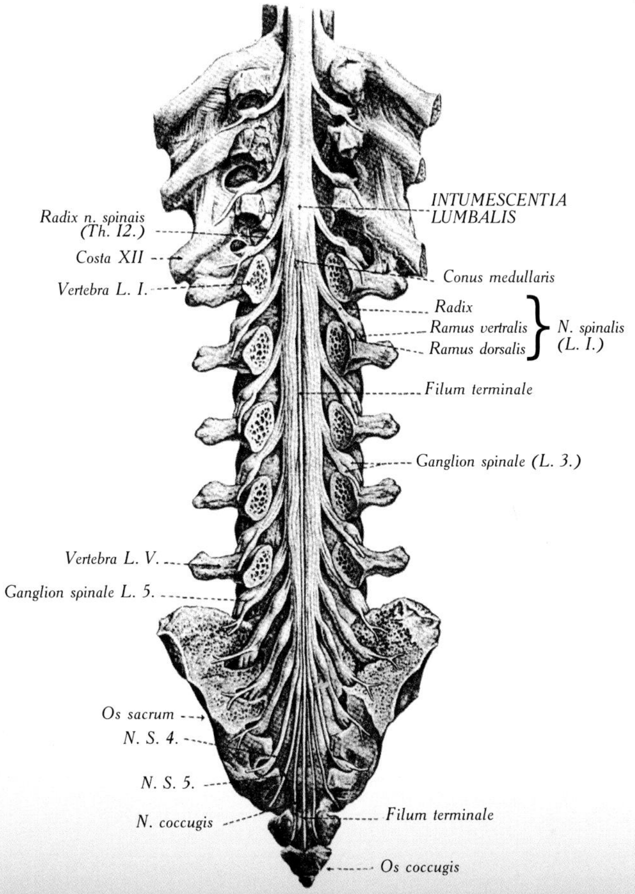

Fig. 2.1.27. Pars lumbalis medulae spinalis et cauda equina

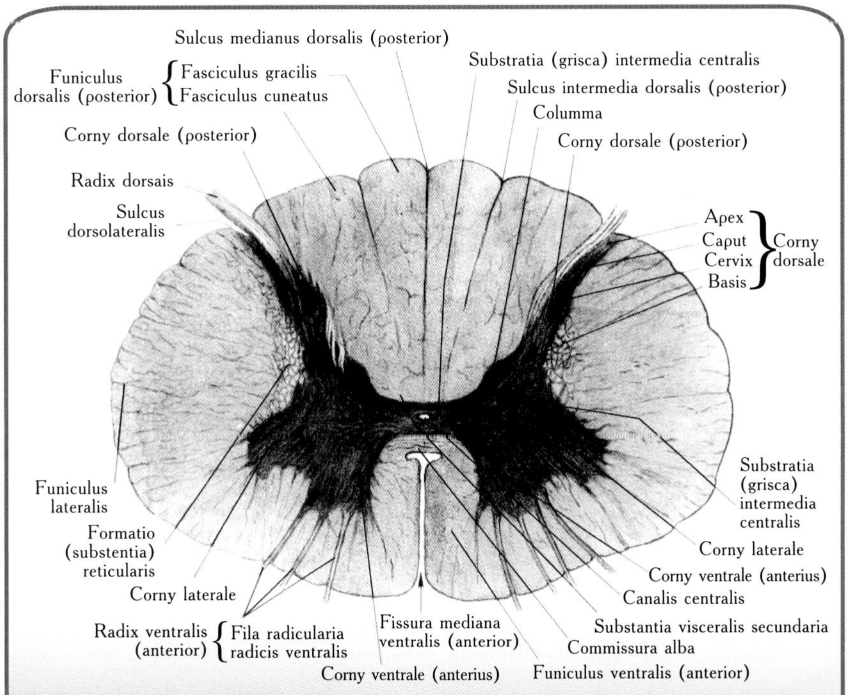

Fig. 2.1.28. Spinal cord, *medulla spinalis*

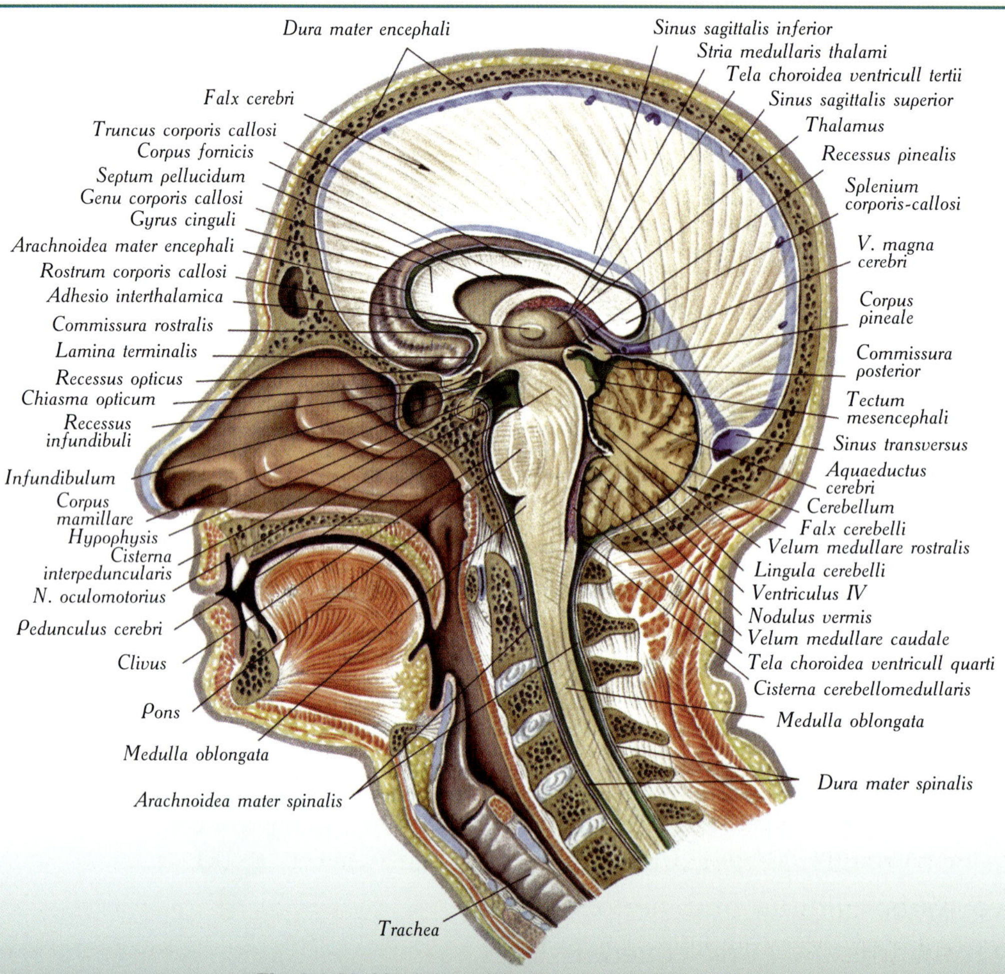

Fig. 2.1.29. Meninges of the brain and spinal cord

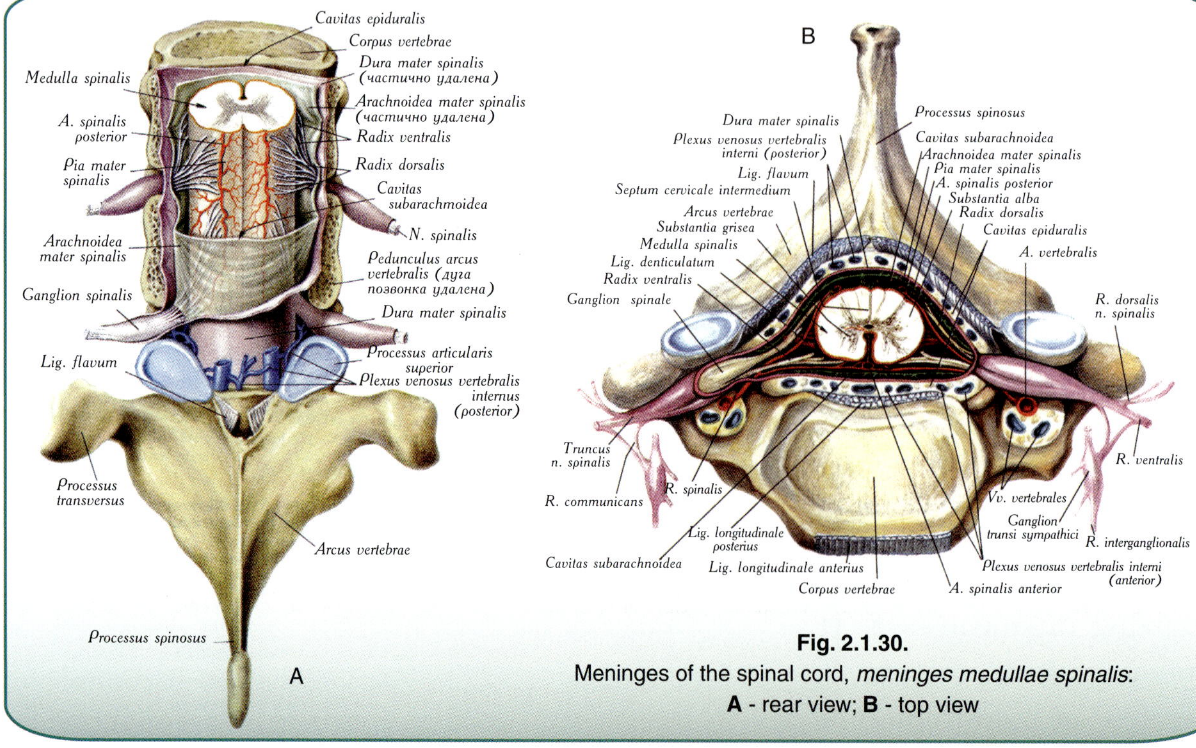

Fig. 2.1.30.
Meninges of the spinal cord, *meninges medullae spinalis*:
A - rear view; **B** - top view

itself. This is achieved through the input of information by neural receptors, followed by central processing of the information and the transfer of signals to the periphery. The PNS is the structural basis for the input and transfer of information. The afferent or sensory nerves (nn. sensorii) transfer information from the periphery to the spinal and cerebral centres, while the efferent or motor nerves (nn. motorii) transfer signals from the centre to the periphery (Fig. 2.1.31).

Specialized neural structures called receptors (receptores) perceive stimuli and convert them into signals, which are then transduced through ascending pathways. The nerves that emerge directly from the brain are called cranial nerves (nn. craniales), while those emerging from the spinal cord are called nn. spinales.

Each nerve consists of a bundle of nerve cell processes. Separate groups of nerve fibres are surrounded by a sheath, called the perineurium, which is composed of connective tissue. The latter penetrates between separate nerve fibres to form an internal sheath, the endoneurium. The outermost layer of connective tissue surrounding a peripheral nerve is called the epineurium. Nerve fibres innervate the skeletal muscles, where they end in motor terminals. Motor nerve fibres directly reach the innervated organ. Sensory nerve fibres originate in various receptors in all organs and tissues of the body, from which they carry signals to the CNS.

Distally from the cranial or spinal ganglia, sensory and motor fibres form mixed nerves. Peripherally, they are interwoven with each other, thus exchanging fibres. Such a network of intersecting nerves is called a neural plexus (plexus nervorum).

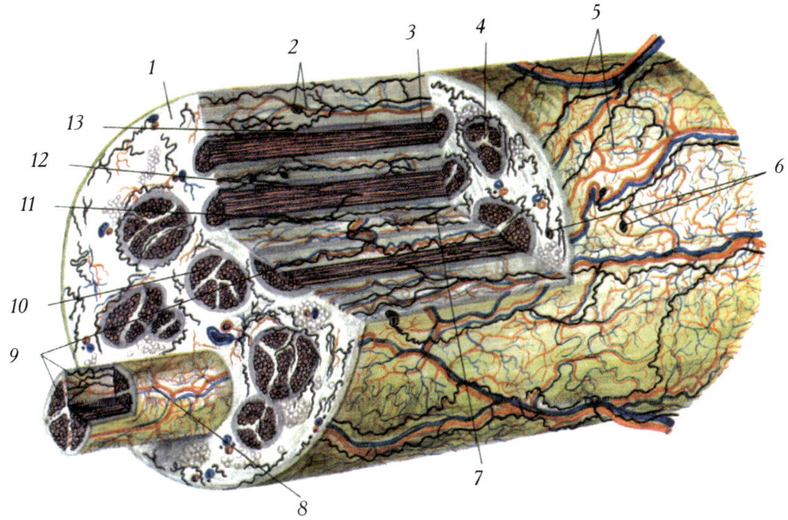

Fig. 2.1.31. The structure of peripheral nerve—innervation and blood supply to the nerve trunk (scheme): 1 - outer epineurium, 2 - inner epineurium (interfascicular tissue); 3 - perineurium 4 - endoneurium 5 - external epineural vascular plexus, 6 - internal epineural vascular plexus; 7 - paraneural vascular plexus, 8 - perineural vascular plexus, 9 - endoneural vascular plexus, 10 - plate-shaped bodies in the epineurium, 11 - plate-shaped bodies in the perineurium, 12 - branch of the nerve trunk supplying its membranes; 13 - blood vessels and nerves penetrating the epineurium

On the basis of their topographical features, the peripheral nerves are divided into cranial nerves (12 pairs), spinal nerves (31 pairs), and vegetative (autonomic) nerves. Cranial nerves are anatomically linked mainly with the brainstem, in which their nuclei are located. These nerves originate from the base of the brain (Fig. 2.1.24). Spinal nerves (Fig. 2.1.32) are paired into symmetrical nerve trunks. They consist of the following:

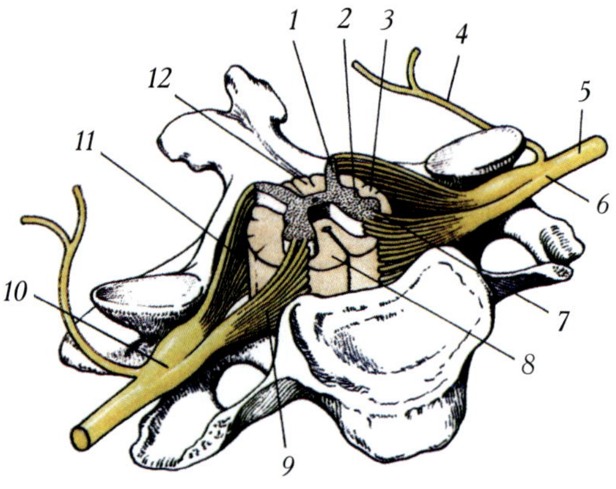

Fig. 2.1.32. Segment of the spinal cord (semi-schematic): 1 - columna posterior; 2 - columna lateralis; 3 - funiculus lateralis; 4 - r. dorsalis; 5 - r. ventralis; 6 - n. spinalis; 7 - columna anterior; 8 - funiculus anterior; 9 - radix ventralis; 10 - ganglion spinale; 11 - radix dorsalis; 12 - funiculus posterior

- Cervical nerves, or nn. cervicales (C_1-C_7) – 8 pairs
- Thoracic nerves, or nn. thoracici (Th_1-Th_{12}) – 12 pairs
- Lumbar nerves, or nn. lumbales (L_1-L_5) – 5 pairs
- Sacral nerves, or nn. sacrales (S_1-S_5) – 5 pairs
- Coccygeal nerve, or n. coccygeus (Co_1-Co_2) – 1 pair

The spinal nerves are mixed, i.e. they contain sensory as well as motor fibres. As each nerve leaves the spinal canal, it almost immediately divides into a branch that contains motor and sensory fibres. The trunk of a spinal nerve is connected with the corresponding ganglion of the sympathetic chain through the rr. communicantes.

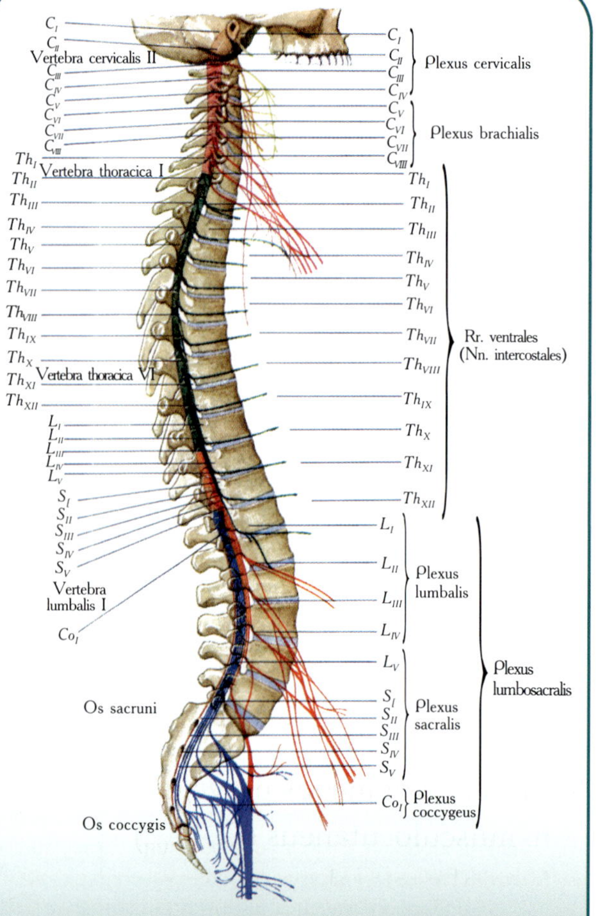

Fig. 2.1.33. Projection of the spinal roots and nerves on the spine (scheme)

Adjacent anterior and posterior branches of the spinal nerves merge to form nerve plexi at different levels: cervical, brachial, lumbosacral and coccygeal (Fig. 2.1.33).

Cervical plexus: The cervical plexus (plexus cervicalis) innervates all the tissues and organs of the neck at the level of the upper four cervical vertebrae (C_1–C_4) (Fig. 2.1.34). It consists of the following branches:

- Lesser occipital nerve, or n. occipitalis minor (C_{II}–C_{III})
- Great auricular nerve, or n. auricularis magnus (C_{III}–C_{IV})
- Transverse cervical nerve, or n. transversus colli (C_{II}–C_{III})
- Supraclavicular nerves or nn. supraclavicularis (C_{III}–C_{IV})
- Phrenic nerve or n. phrenicus (C_{III}–C_{IV}–C_V)

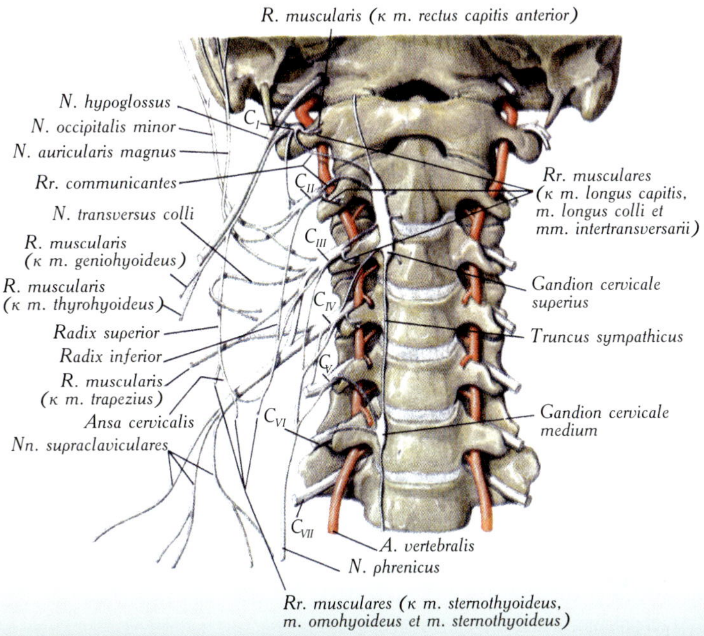

Fig. 2.1.34. Cervical plexus, *plexus cervicalis* (semi-schematic)

Brachial plexus: The brachial plexus (plexus brachialis, referred to as BP here; Fig. 2.1.35) innervates all the tissues and organs of the neck at the level of the lower cervical vertebrae and of the upper limbs. It is formed by anterior branches of the 5th, 6th, 7th and 8th cervical spinal nerves. The BP is divided into supra- and infra-clavicular parts, and consists of the following:

- Muscular branches
- Dorsal scapular nerve, or n. dorsalis scapulae (C_V)
- Long thoracic nerve, or n. thoracicus longus (C_V–C_{VII})
- Subclavian nerve, or n. subclavius (C_{IV}–C_{VI})
- Suprascapular nerve, or n. suprascapularis (C_V–C_{VI})
- Musculocutaneous nerve, or n. musculocutaneus (C_V–C_{VII})
- Lateral pectoral nerve, or n. pectoralis lateralis (C_V–C_{VIII}, Th_I)

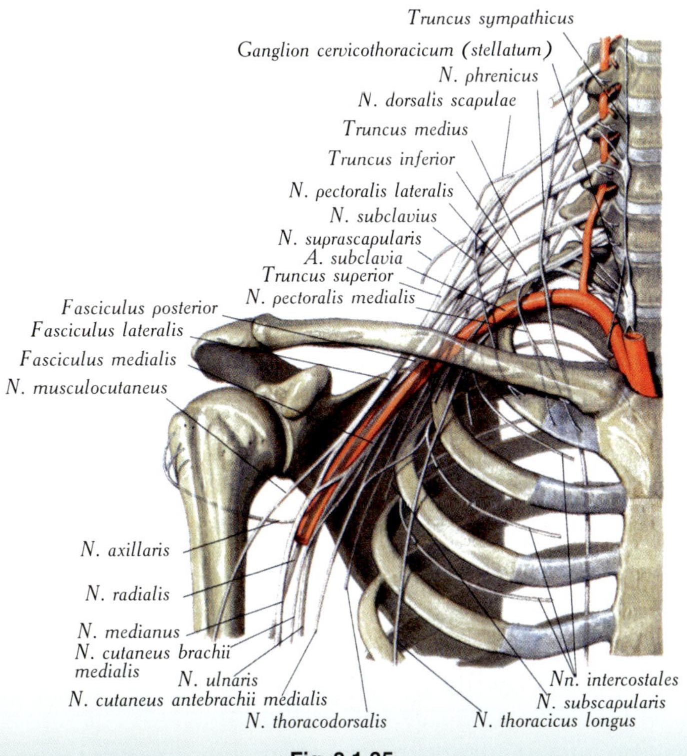

Fig. 2.1.35.
Brachial plexus, *plexus brachialis* (semi-schematic)

- Medial pectoral nerve, or n. pectoralis medialis (C_V–C_{VIII})
- Ulnar nerve, or n. ulnaris (C_{VII}–C_{VIII})
- Medial antebrachial cutaneous nerve or n. cutaneus antebrachii medialis (C_{VIII}, Th_I)
- Medial brachial cutaneous nerve or n. cutaneus brachii medialis (C_{VIII}, Th_I, Th_{II}, Th_{III})
- Median nerve or n. medianus (C_{VI}–Th_I)
- Radial nerve or n. radialis (C_V–C_{VIII}, Th_I)

Thoracic nerves: These nerves (nn. thoracici) innervate the organs of the thoracic cavity.The anterior branches of the lumbar, sacral and coccygeal spinal nerves (L_I–L_V, S_I–S_V, Co_I–Co_{II}) merge to form a single lumbosacral plexus (plexus lumbosacralis). Topographically, this plexus is divided into lumbar (Th_{XII}, L_I–L_{IV}) and sacral plexi (L_{IV}–L_V–Co_I). These innervate the lower extremities, the organs of the small and large pelvis, and the lumbar part of the trunk.

Lumbar plexus: The lumbar plexus (plexus lumbalis, Fig. 2.1.36) consists of the following:

- Muscular branches
- Iliohypogastric nerve or n. iliohypogastricus (Th_{XII}–L_I)
- Ilioinguinal nerve, or n.ilioinguinalis (L_I)
- Genitofemoral nerve or n. genitofemoralis (L_I, L_{II})
- Lateral cutaneous femoral nerve or n. cutaneus femoris lateralis (L_{II}–L_{III})
- Obturator nerve or n. obturatorius (L_I–L_V)
- Accessory obturator nerve or n. obturatorius accessorius (L_{II}–L_{IV})
- Femoral nerve or n. femoralis (L_I–L_{IV})

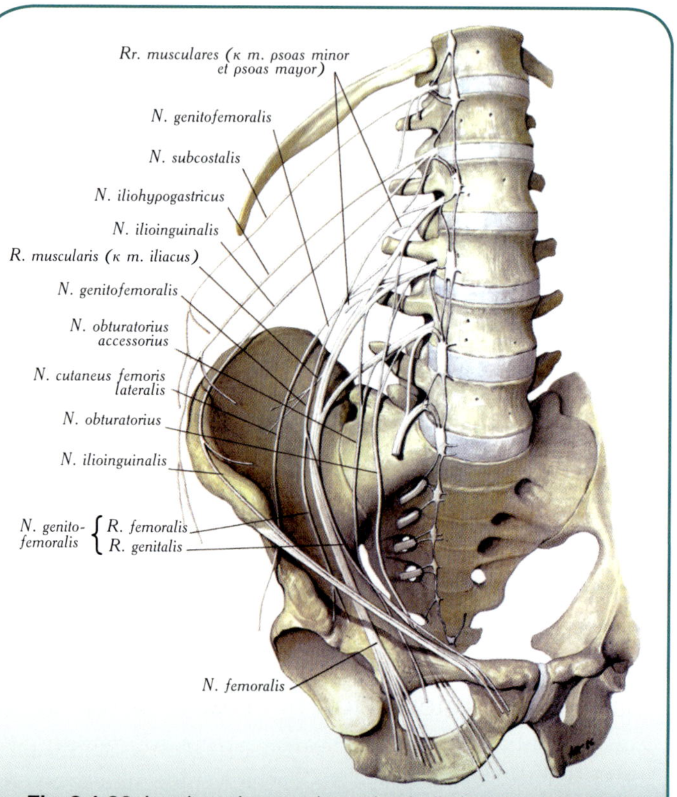

Fig. 2.1.36. Lumbar plexus, *plexus lumbalis* (semi-schematic)

Sacral and coccygeal plexi: These plexi (plexus sacralis et coccygeus) innervate the organs of the small and large pelvis, as well as the sacrum. They include sacral nerves, or nn. sacrales (S_I–S_V, L_{IV}–L_V: S_I–S_{III}) (Fig. 2.1.37).

The sacral plexus consists of the following:

- Internal obturator nerve, or n. obturatorius internus (S_I)
- Nerve to piriformis, or n. piriformis (S_I–S_{II})
- Nerve to quadratus femoris, or n. quadratus femoris (S_I–S_{II})
- Superior gluteal nerve, or n. gluteus superior (L_{IV}–L_V, S_I)
- Inferior gluteal nerve, or n. gluteus inferior (L_V, S_I, S_{II})
- Posterior cutaneous femoral nerve, or n. cutaneus femoris posterior (S_I–S_{II})
- Sciatic nerve, or n. ischiadicus (L_{IV}, L_V, S_I–S_{III})

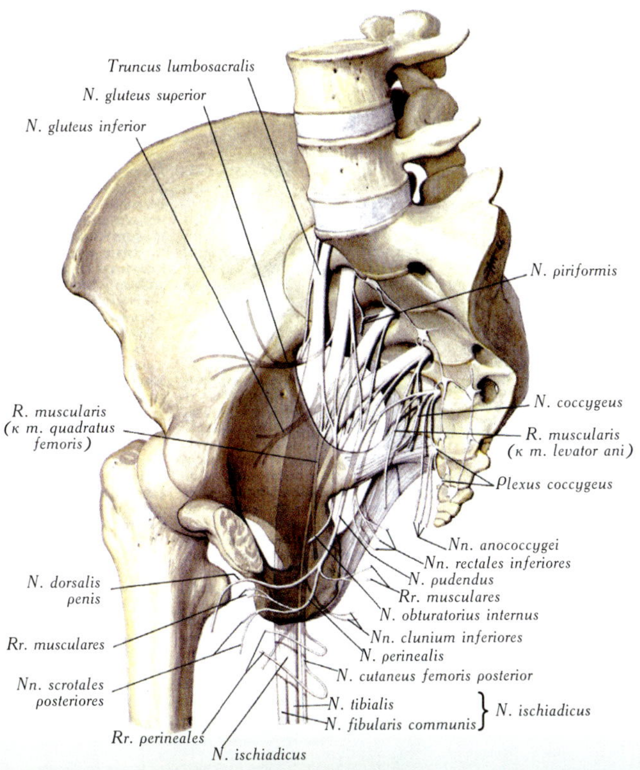

Fig. 2.1.37. Sacral plexus, *plexus sacralis*, and coccygeal plexus, plexus coccygeus

Coccygeal plexus: The coccygeal plexus (plexus coccygeus) innervates the organs of the small pelvis, the coccyx and the sacrum, and consists of the following branches:

1. Coccygeal nerve, or n. coccygeus
2. Anococcygeal nerves, or nn. anococcygei

Vegetative (autonomic) nervous system

Certain components of the PNS have quite a devious connection with the CNS and can function under limited central control, i.e. independently. These components form the vegetative (autonomic) nervous system (systema nervorum autonomicum, referred to as VANS here; Fig. 2.1.38). An example of the autonomous functioning of the VANS is how the body functions during coma. Though the person is not conscious, all the vital functions of the body (breathing, circulation, excretion, digestion, etc.) are performed independently, irrespective of whether or not the brain is functioning.

The VANS innervates the viscera, heart and vessels, organs that have smooth muscle tissue and glandular epithelium, and controls their functioning. It also plays a part in the innervation of cross-striated muscles. The VANS is known to have two parts: an intra-cerebral part, which is a part of the brain and spinal cord, and an extra-cerebral or peripheral part.

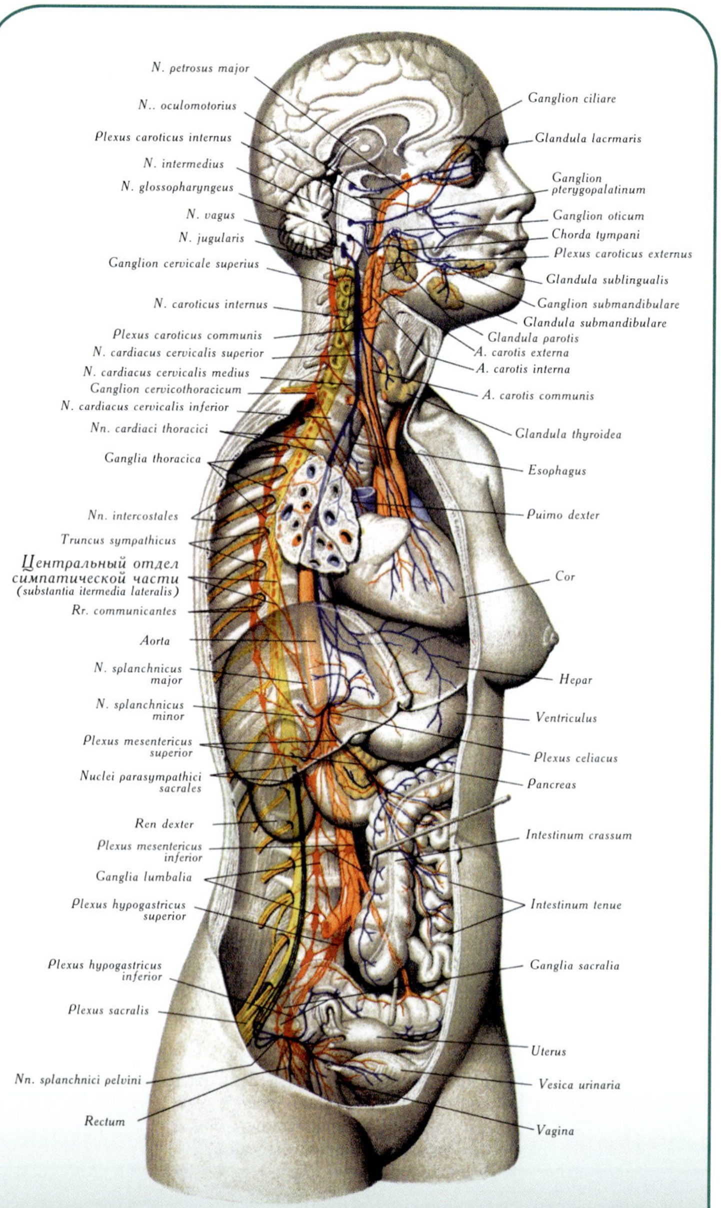

Fig. 2.1.38. Autonomous (vegetative) nervous system (scheme) (red - the sympathetic part, blue - the parasympathetic part)

On the basis of physiological characteristics, the VANS is divided into two systems: sympathetic and parasympathetic. However, there is also a third important division— the diffuse intestinal nervous system. This system is responsible for the innervation and functional coordination of the digestive organs. Its functioning is independent of the sympathetic and parasympathetic systems, but can change under their influence. The ganglia of this system control peristaltic activity, i.e. the movement of food inside the intestine. Acetylcholine is a mediator that excites intestinal smooth muscles.

Sympathetic division of the VANS

The central part of the sympathetic division of the VANS (Fig. 2.1.39) consists of numerous multipolar cells. These are located in the grey matter of the spinal cord, extending from the 8th cervical to the 2nd–3rd lumbar segments. Collectively, these form the sympathetic centre. The peripheral part of the sympathetic VANS consists of the right and left sympathetic trunks (chains) and the nerves originating from these trunks, as well as nerves and ganglia of the plexi situated adjacent to organs or within them.

The vegetative neurons of the spinal cord gather visceral sensory information and transfer it to the CNS, which decides on the body's response to a new situation.

When there is a need for self-defence or in moments of danger and other critical situations, the sympathetic nervous system activates all the vital functions. It causes an increase in lung ventilation, the heart rate, the strength of contraction of the myocardium, blood supply to the muscles, myocardium and brain, muscle contraction, the serum glucose level, etc. (Fig. 2.1.40). The question is how it is possible for the sympathetic nervous system to influence organs located so distantly. The answer is as follows. Increased activity of a sympathetic nerve induces the adrenal medulla to secrete catecholamines. These substances, including the main mediator, noradrenaline, are transported with the blood and affect the activity of various target tissues, causing coordinated and simultaneous changes in their functions. Thus, the efferent pathways of the sympathetic system transmit signals to the organs that directly regulate the internal environment.

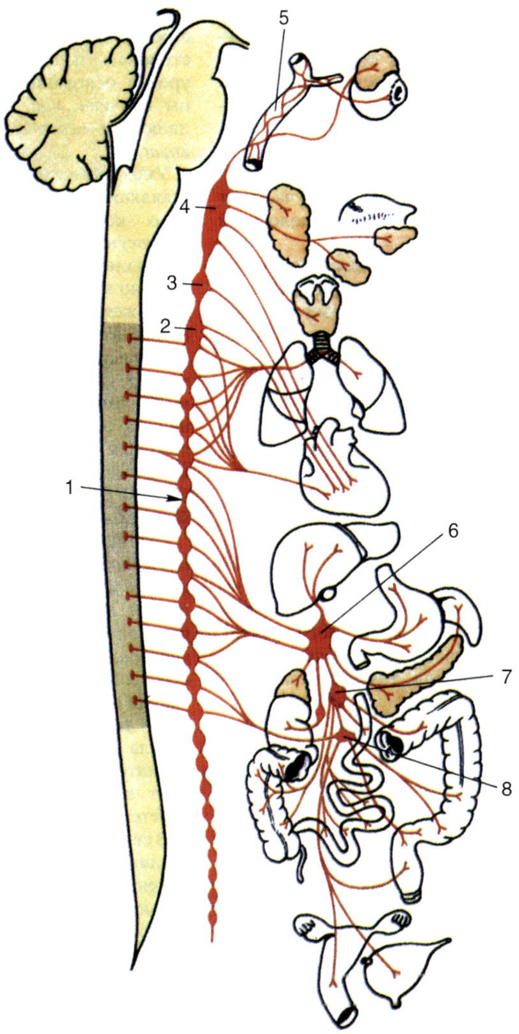

Fig. 2.1.39. The sympathetic part of the autonomic nervous system (scheme): 1 - truncus sympathicus; 2 - ganglion cervicothoracicum (stellatum); 3 - ganglion cervicale medium; 4 - ganglion cervicale superius; 5 - a. carotis interna; 6 - plexus celiacus; 7 - plexus mesentericus superior; 8 - plexus mesentericus inferior

The number of ganglia of a sympathetic trunk, except in the cervical region, basically corresponds to the number of spinal nerves. Thus, there are 3 cervical, 10–12 thoracic, 4–5 lumbar and 4 sacral ganglia, and 1 unpaired ganglion.

Three cervical ganglia were formed as a result of the emergence of eight segmentary sympathetic ganglia. These are the upper, middle and lower ganglia. The latter often merges with the first thoracic ganglion, thus forming the cervicothoracic (stellate) ganglion.

The majority of ganglia are a part of various nervous plexi. The branches of the upper cervical ganglion are the jugular and internal carotid nerves, external carotid and laryngopharyngeal nerves, and the superior cervical cardiac nerve. From the middle cervical ganglion arises the middle cervical cardiac nerve. The branches of the cervicothoracic ganglion are the inferior cervical cardiac nerve, subclavian loop, vertebral nerve and subclavian plexus.

The thoracic part of the sympathetic trunk is located on both sides of the spine, from the 1st to the 12th thoracic vertebrae, approximately in the area of the heads of the

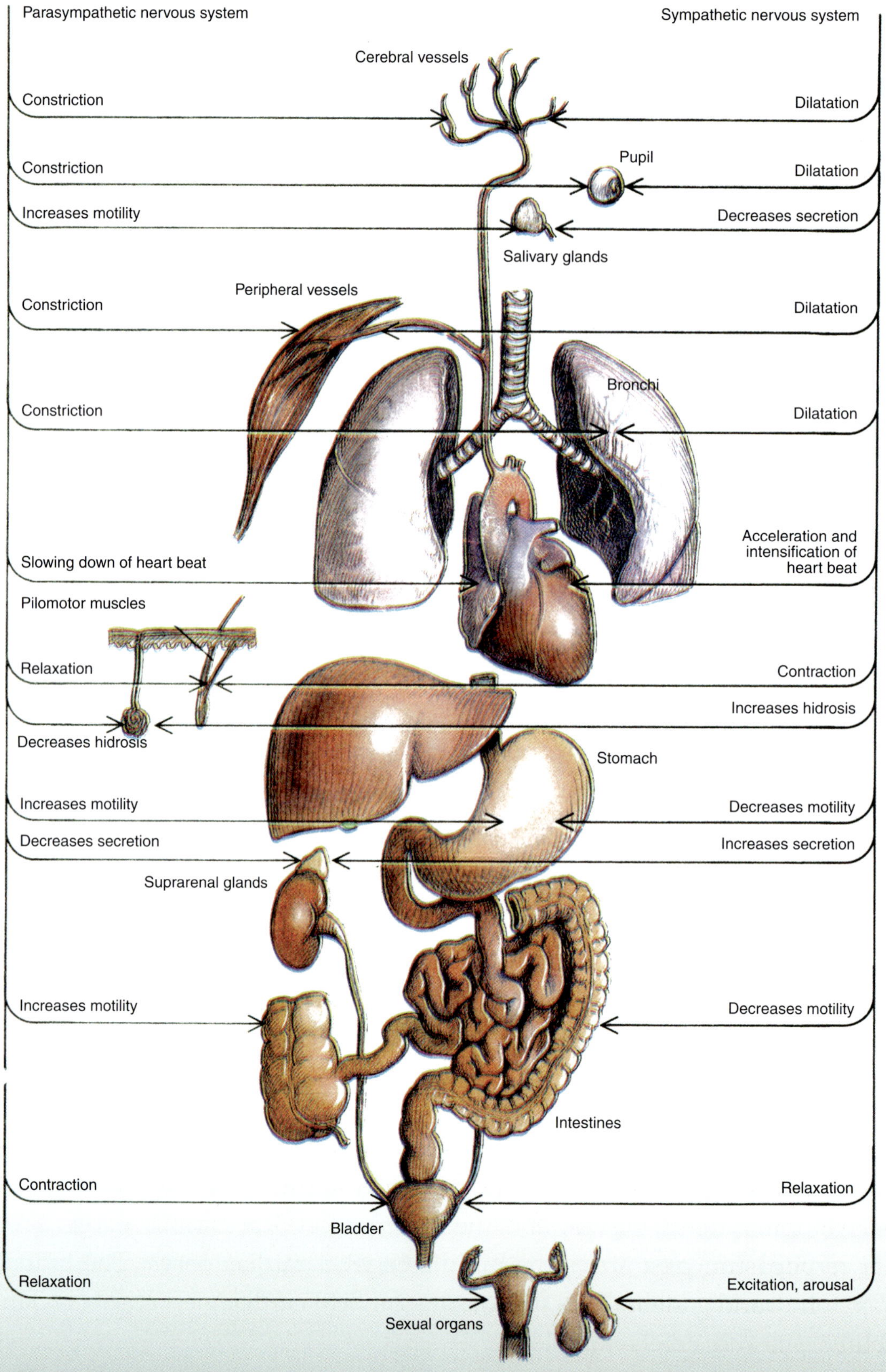

Fig. 2.1.40. Sympathetic and parasympathetic divisions of autonomic nervous systems, organs that they innervate and their impact on every organ

ribs. From each ganglion arise connecting branches to the spinal and intercostal nerves, as well as to the organs of the chest cavity.

The lumbar (celiac) part of the sympathetic trunk passes through the abdominal cavity, between the fascicles of the lumbar part of the diaphragm, and goes on to rest on the anterolateral surface of the bodies of the 1st–5th lumbar vertebrae. Nerves and plexi of the abdominal and pelvic cavities arise from the lumbar part of the sympathetic trunk. These are the nerves of the stomach, liver and gallbladder—the abdominal vegetative, celiac and diaphragmatic nerves, the upper and lower mesenteric nerves, and the aortic and superior hypogastric plexi.

The sacral part of the sympathetic trunk (Figs 2.1.41 and 2.1.42) is located on the pelvic surface of the sacrum, medially from the sacral foramina. The inferior hypogastric plexus and pelvic and sacral splanchnic nerves arise here. In addition, there are smaller vegetative plexi:

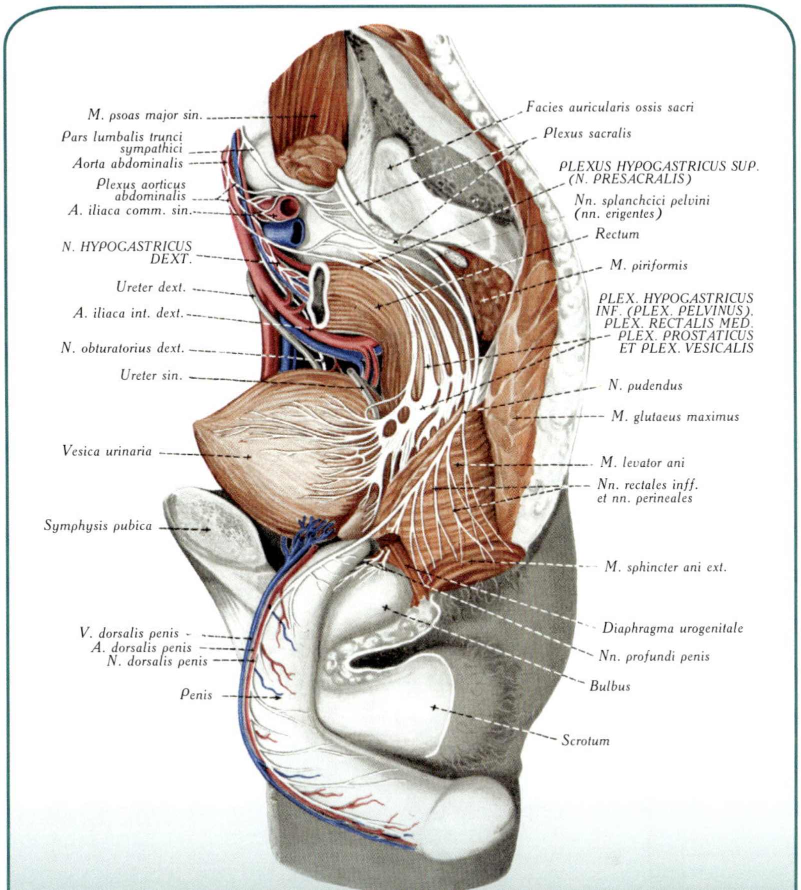

Fig. 2.1.41. Sacral plexus of VANS (male pelvis)

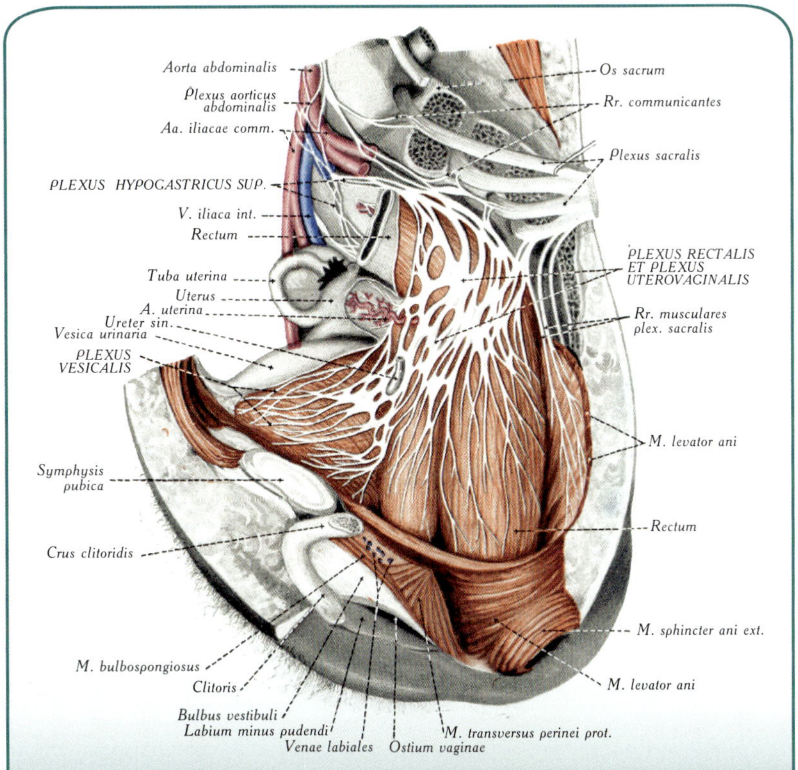

Fig. 2.1.42. Sacral plexus of VANS (female pelvis)

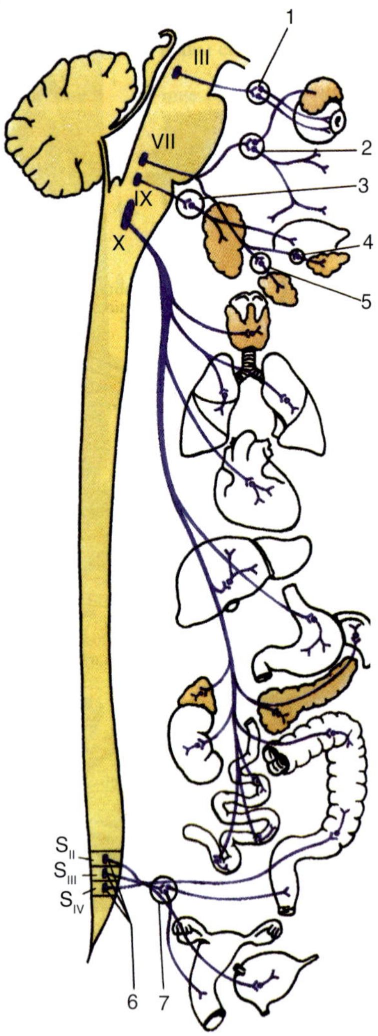

Fig. 2.1.43.
The parasympathetic part of autonomic nervous system (scheme): III - n. oculomotorius; VII - n. facialis; IX - n. glossopharyngeus; X - n. vagus; 1 - ganglion ciliare; 2 - ganglion pterygopalatinum; 3 - ganglion oticum; 4 - ganglion submandibulare; 5 - ganglion sublinguale; 6 - nuclei parasympathici sacrales; 7 - ganglia pelvica

the middle rectal, vesical, prostatic and uterovaginal plexi, the nerves of the cavernous bodies of the penis and the plexus ductus deferentis.

Parasympathetic division of the VANS

The parasympathetic division of the VANS (Fig. 2.1.43), like the sympathetic division, consists of two parts—central (intracerebral) and peripheral (extra-cerebral). Preganglionic fibres extending from both parts form a very important nervous trunk, the vagus nerve (n. vagus), the numerous branches of which innervate the entire parasympathetic system in the heart, lungs and gastrointestinal tract. This nerve also carries sensory information from these organs back to the CNS.

Parasympathetic fibres participate in the formation of the extramural ganglia of the head and neck, i.e. the ciliary, pterygopalatine, oticum, submandibular and hypoglossal ganglia. They are also involved in the formation of some of the ganglia of the vegetative plexi of the thoracic and pelvic cavities. In addition, the parasympathetic division includes the splenic plexus, pancreatic and duodenal nerves, and sigmoid plexus. It also consists of nerves of the salivary glands, heart, trachea, lungs, oesophagus, stomach, intestines, liver, gallbladder, pancreas, spleen, kidneys, bladder, testicles, uterus, vagina, etc.

The terminals of parasympathetic fibres release acetylcholine. Domination of the parasympathetic activity creates conditions that are conducive to rest and restoration of the organism.

2.2 VARIATIONS OF THE HUMAN BODY, ITS ANOMALIES AND MALFORMATIONS

In optimal conditions, an organism and its organs develop without any abnormalities. However, the normal path of embryonic development could be disrupted and the evolving organism could become abnormal, with certain organs or even the whole body becoming anomalous. The causes of such deviations may be external or internal.

External causes: These include concussions and contusions of the embryo through the wall of the maternal body, constriction by the umbilical cord, and occasionally, the occurrence of amniotic strands in the amniotic fluid. As a result, death of foetus or various types of deformities of the face, trunk or limbs may occur. Such types of injuries are known as deformities. Thus, malformation refers to any violation of the integrity of an organism or of its individual parts, the violation usually being visible and accompanied by pathological changes in the organism's function.

Internal causes: The internal factors that disrupt normal foetal development are hereditary factors and impaired function of the endocrine glands (thymus, thyroid, pituitary, etc.). These factors may affect development both in the earliest and later stages. This may result in what is known as anomalies. In some cases, the earlier the factor responsible begins to exercise its influence, the more serious the anomaly becomes. However, the very same factor may cause a less pronounced anomaly, i.e. only weaken the functioning of the body and/or the organ. It is difficult to make a clear distinction between malformations and anomalies, and this division is rather arbitrary. For example, the absence of a hand is considered to be a malformation but the absence of a bone, an anomaly. Some authors describe polydactyly, or fusion of the fingers, as a malformation while others describe it as an anomaly. On the whole, compared to malformations, anomalies are less pronounced and less drastic deviations from normal development, just barely affecting the functions of the body or its parts.

Abnormalities of organs can be manifested as follows:

1. The organ may be positioned wrongly.
2. The organ may be absent (aplasia).
3. The organ may merge with adjacent organs.

4. There may be an additional organ.
5. The shape of the organ may be altered.

All the above anomalies can be diagnosed with absolute certainty. For example, a person who is familiar with the normal structure can easily identify aplasia of an organ, its displacement or splitting, etc. However, in many cases, it is difficult to diagnose a deviation because it may be too mild to be classified. However, it is necessary to remember that various deviations could be explained by observing differences among individuals.

There are always some individual variations in the shape of the nose, mouth, ears and eyes, in hair colour, voice, height, and so on, and there are innumerable combinations of these variants. Thus, one person is never absolutely identical to another. This is true even of the bones and internal organs. For example, there are a number of minor deviations in the positioning of various organs in the thoracic and abdominal cavities, in their shape, as well as their vascular and muscular anatomy. Similarly, there are variations in the structure and size of different bones.

Such variations have been observed even among immediate relatives, such as between parents and their children, between siblings and even between twins. Genes do not guarantee an accurate reproduction of parental traits in the children. Individual differences among organisms are, on the one hand, an expression of the creative power that accounts for evolutionary development and, on the other, a reaction to external stimuli.

The causes of the most marked variations in bone structure are deviations from the normal course of development of the bones at the time of their aniage, or during the ossification period, and the disruption of normal interactions between different parts of a bone or between two adjacent bones. All bony anomalies can be divided into two groups. These are ontogenetic abnormalities, which are distortions of normal development that subsequently result in the formation of bony defects; and phylogenetic abnormalities, which reflect developmental processes and changes experienced by human beings during the transition from the lower animal forms through the course of evolution.

The following discussion addresses only anomalies of the skeleton, and particularly the bones involved in the formation of the spine. It does not deal with the skull, limbs and pelvis. V.A. Dyachenko's classification (1954) of the anomalies of the spine is the most complete one.

Ontogenetic anomalies

1. Developmental anomalies of the vertebral bodies:

   a. Clefts and defects of the vertebral body
   b. Wedge-shaped vertebrae (lateral and posterior)
   c. Aplasia of the vertebral body
   d. Other malformations of the vertebral body, platyspondylia and microspondylia
2. Malformations of the vertebral arches:
   a. Clefts
   b. Partial hypoplasia of the vertebral arch
   c. Abnormal development of the vertebral processes
   d. Anomalies in the interarticular space of the arch (spondylolysis)
3. Mixed anomalies:
   a. Anomalies of segmentation
   b. Hypoplasia of entire regions of the spine
   c. Hypoplasia of certain vertebrae

Phylogenetic anomalies

1. Anomalies of the craniocervical region:
   a. Assimilation of the atlas
   b. Manifestation of the atlas
2. Anomalies of the cervicothoracic region:
   a. Dorsalization of the lower cervical vertebrae (cervical ribs)
   b. Cervicalization of the 1st thoracic vertebra
3. Anomalies of the lumbosacral region:
   a. Sacralization
   b. Lumbarization
4. Anomalies of the sacrococcygeal region

The information given above on the anomalies of the spine covers only those which are observed most commonly and are, therefore, of the greatest interest both to clinicians and radiologists.

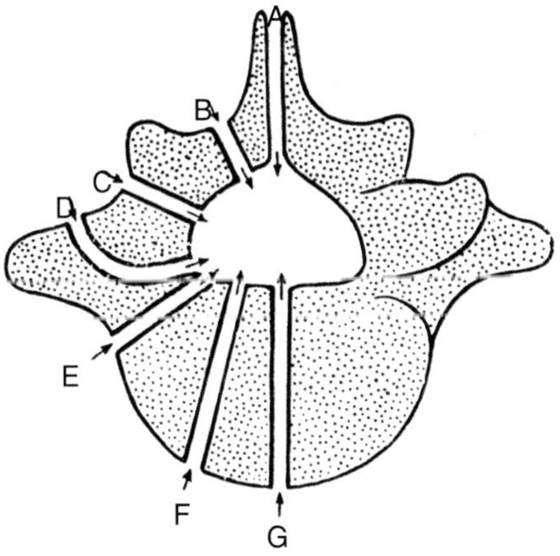

Fig. 2.2.1. Congenital clefts of the spine—*spina bifida*.
Schematic drawing of different types of vertebral clefts; A–D - rear cleft; E–G - front cleft

1. Clefts and defects of vertebral bodies

Congenital clefts or the condition in which the vertebrae remain unfused and open are known as 'spina bifida'. In the majority of cases, these defects are caused by disorders in the development of the vertebral bodies during the foetal stages. The location of the clefts varies (Fig. 2.2.1).

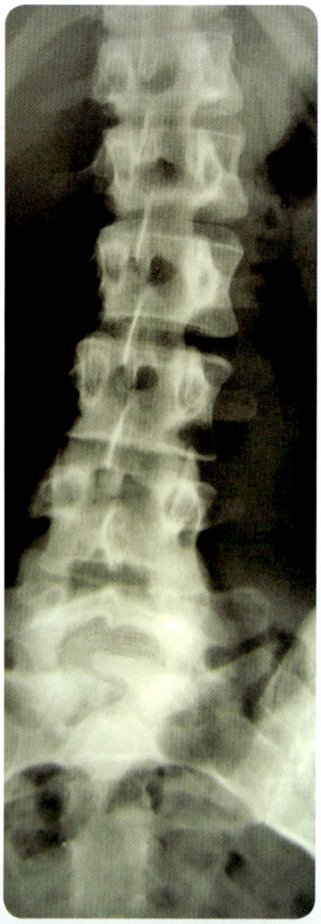

Fig. 2.2.2.
Posterior cleft of the first sacral vertebra with its left-sided articular lumbarization

According to the literature, the most common type (30%–35%) of spina bifida is the incomplete closure of the arch of the 1st sacral vertebra (spina bifida posterior) (Figs 2.2.2 and 2.2.3). The second most common location is the 5th lumbar vertebra (Fig. 2.2.4). Clefts are less common in the cervicothoracic region (Fig. 2.2.5).

One of the rare anomalies of the spine (1%–2%) is the incomplete fusion of the arches of the sacral vertebrae (Fig. 2.2.6). In 3%–5% of cases, the entire sacral canal remains open posteriorly (Figs 2.2.7 and 2.2.8). However, it must be kept in mind that in all children up to the age of 10–12 years, the arch of the 1st sacral vertebra remains unfused in 100% of patients. This is due to late ossification of the arches of the upper sacral and lower lumbar vertebrae, and could be considered normal.

Spina bifida anterior is rare. The anomaly is confined mainly to the level of the lower cervical and upper thoracic vertebrae, but can affect any vertebra in other regions of the spine. Usually, there is splitting of a few adjacent vertebral bodies. In the vast majority of cases, spina bifida anterior is not a single developmental anomaly, but often occurs in conjunction with other severe spinal deformities, such as synostoses (fusion of the vertebrae)

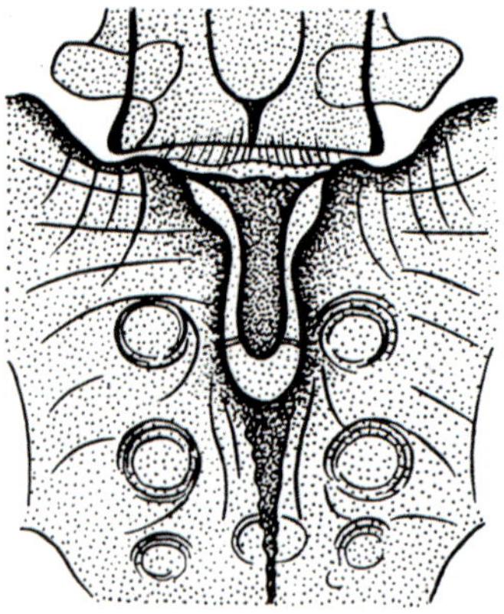

Fig. 2.2.3.
Scheme of congenital sacral arches splitting - *spina bifida sacralis;* elongated spinous process of the 5th vertebra

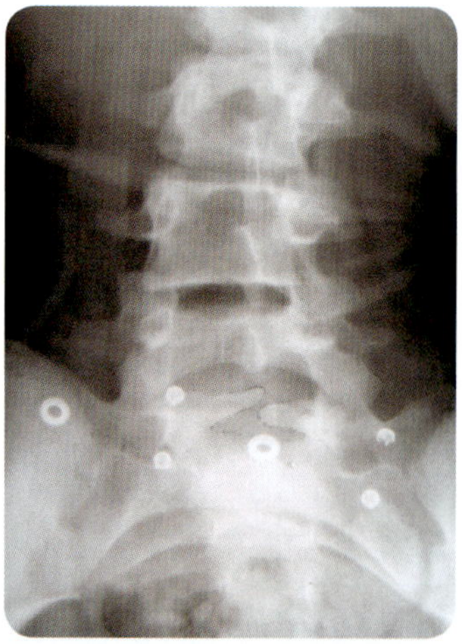

Fig. 2.2.4.
Posterior cleft of 5th lumbar vertebra

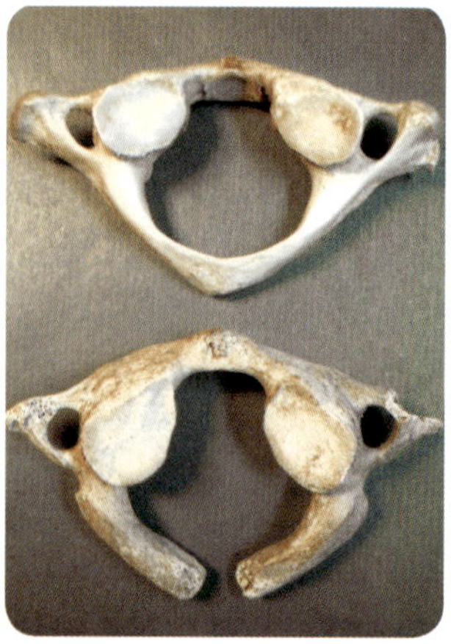

Fig. 2.2.5.
The first cervical vertebra (atlant): A - normal structure; B - posterior cleft (*spina bifida* posterior)

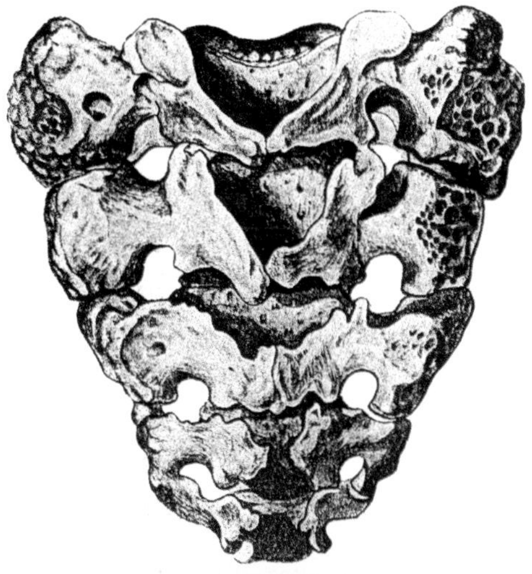

Fig. 2.2.6.
Incomplete fusion of arches of sacral vertebrae

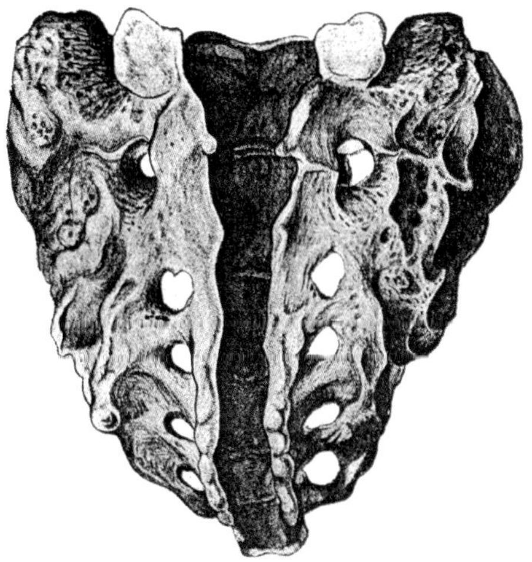

Fig. 2.2.7.
Complete *spina bifida sacralis*

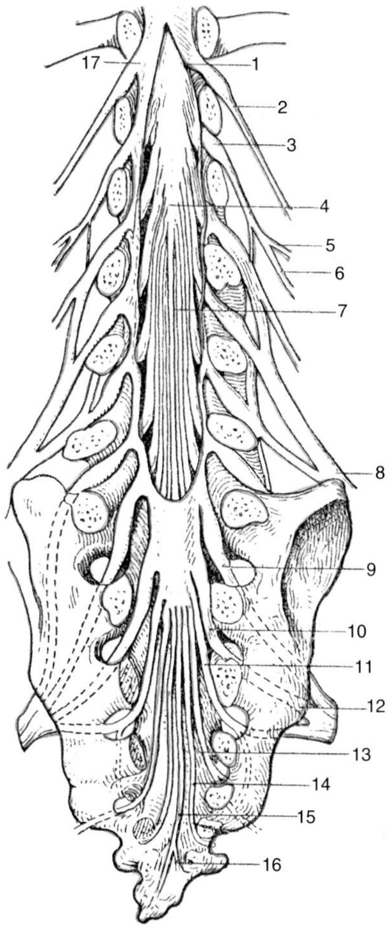

Fig. 2.2.8.
The caudal part of the spinal cord and cauda equina in the spinal canal opened posteriorly and dural sac.
1 - dura mater spinalis; 2 - n. subcostalis;
3 - ganglion spinale lumbale I; 4 - conus medullaris;
5 - n. iliohypogastricus; 6 - n. ilioinguinalis;
7 - filum terminale; 8 - n. femoralis;
9 - n. sacralis I; 10 - n. sacralis II; 11 - n. sacralis III;
12 - n. ischiadicus; 13 - n. sacralis IV; 14 - n. sacralis V;
15 - filum durae matris spinalis; 16 - n. coccygeus;
17 - dura of the spinal cord

and malformation of other organs.

Incomplete fusion of the vertebral bodies leads to the formation of a defect of the posterior wall of the spinal canal, which is clinically manifested as meningeal cysts (meningocele). During clinical examination, one can often observe external signs of incomplete fusion, such as hyperpigmentation of the skin in the area of the defect (Fig. 2.2.9). Limited hypertrichosis (increased pilosity) may also be seen (Figs 2.2.10A and 2.2.10B).

Since the 1920s–1930s, spina bifida has been thought to lead to a wide variety of diseases and several symptoms. These include permanent sacral pain, bedwetting,

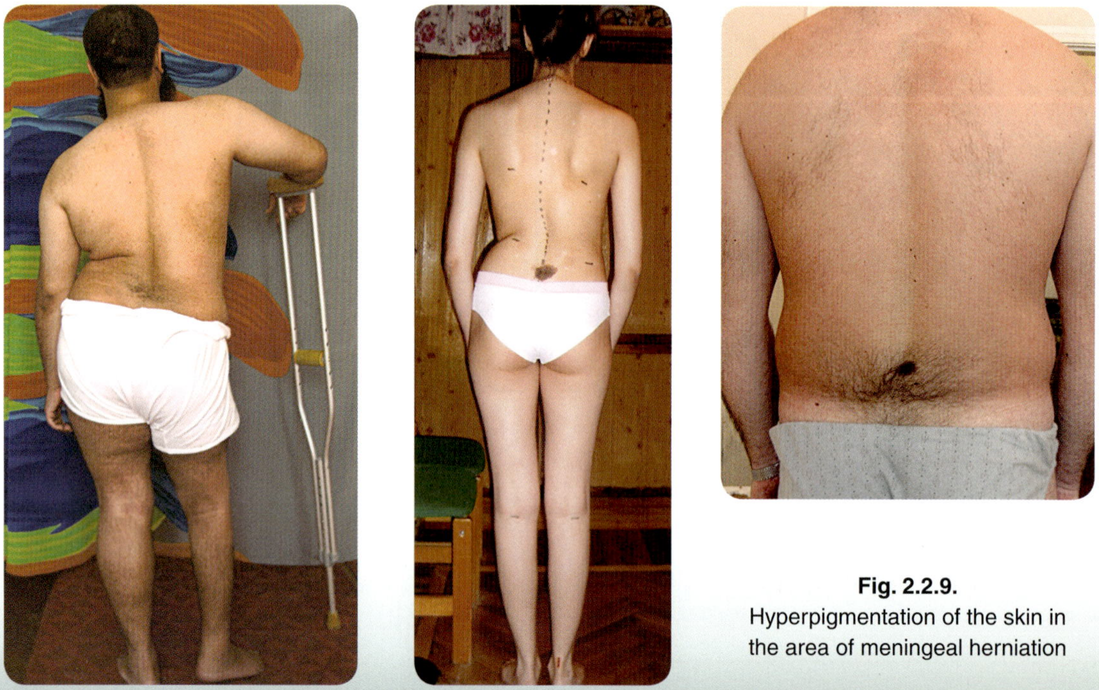

Fig. 2.2.9. Hyperpigmentation of the skin in the area of meningeal herniation

various sexual disorders, menstrual irregularities, chronic constipation, plano-valgus foot, varicose veins of the lower extremities, trophic ulcers and sweating of the feet. However, according to another point of view, all these conditions can occur in the absence of spina bifida.

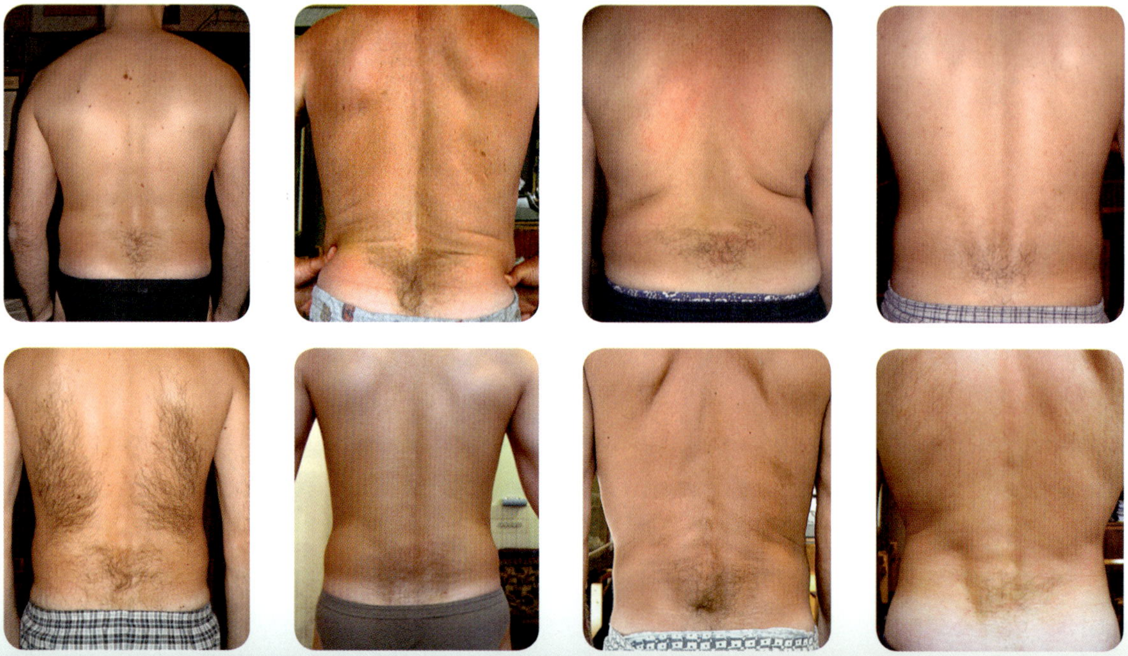

Fig. 2.2.10A. Increased pilosity of the skin (hypertrichosis) in the area of meningeal herniation

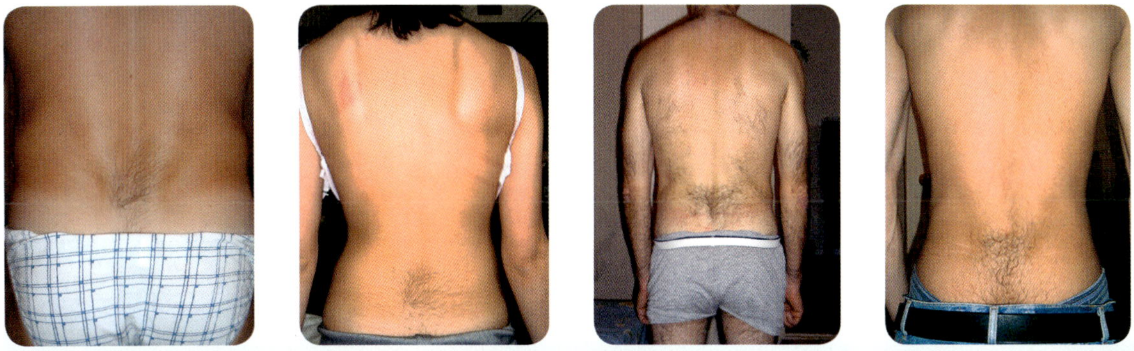

Fig. 2.2.10B. Increased pilosity of the skin (hypertrichosis) in the area of meningeal herniation

On the basis of our considerable clinical experience, we agree with the first point of view on the causal link between the above-mentioned pathological conditions and dysplasia (underdevelopment) of the lumbosacral spine.

2. Wedge-shaped vertebrae

This is a developmental anomaly in which the vertebra is a wedge-shaped bone mass of about half the size that it should be. The vertebra is located between two normal vertebrae (Figs 2.2.11 and 2.2.12). In the thoracic region, an additional unpaired rib often accompanies the wedge-shaped vertebra. Rarely, the wedge-shaped vertebra is located with its base located posteriorly and its apex anteriorly (posterior wedge-shaped vertebra) (Figs 2.2.13 and 2.2.14).

This type of deformity is easily diagnosed by a lateral radiograph. Other than the reduction in the size of the vertebral body, only the posterior part is intact and the

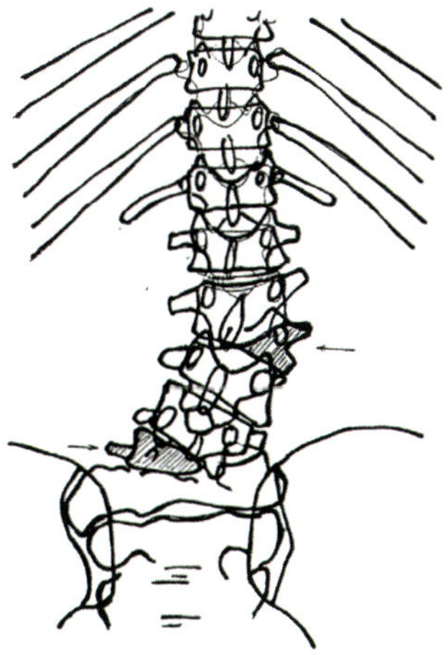

Fig. 2.2.11. Alternating wedge-shaped vertebrae (scheme)

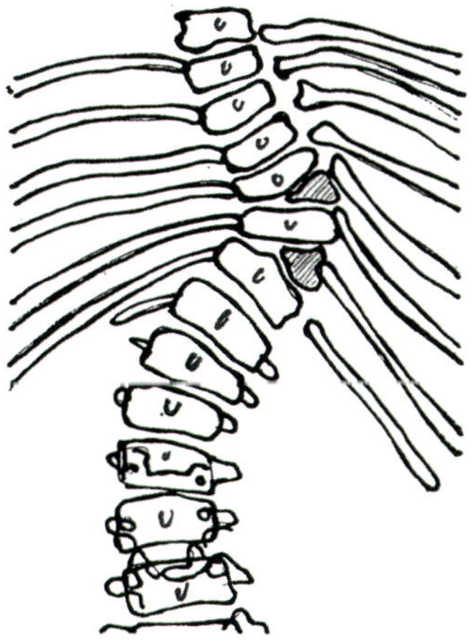

Fig. 2.2.12. Wedge-shaped vertebrae, located unilaterally (scheme)

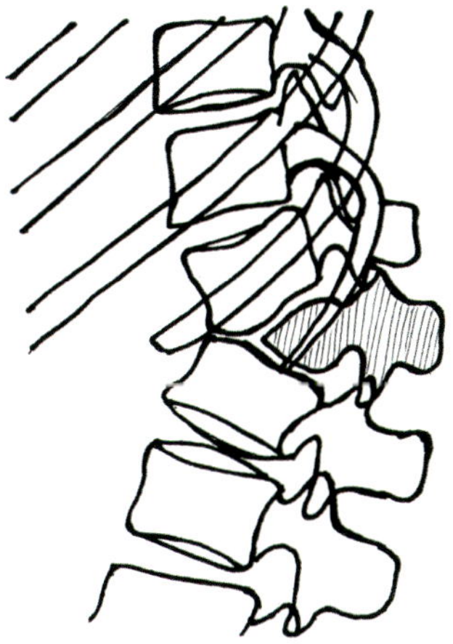

Fig. 2.2.13. Posterior wedge-shaped vertebra (radiographic scheme)

anterior part is underdeveloped. This spinal anomaly is the cause of congenital angular or arcuate kyphosis.

A vertebra may also be formed by two wedges, the apexes of which are directed towards the midline. Such vertebrae are known as 'butterfly' vertebrae. The vertebra is slightly lower and wider than the normal adjacent vertebrae, and its intervertebral cartilage is often slightly narrower (Fig. 2.2.15). This anomaly is usually an incidental finding on radiography.

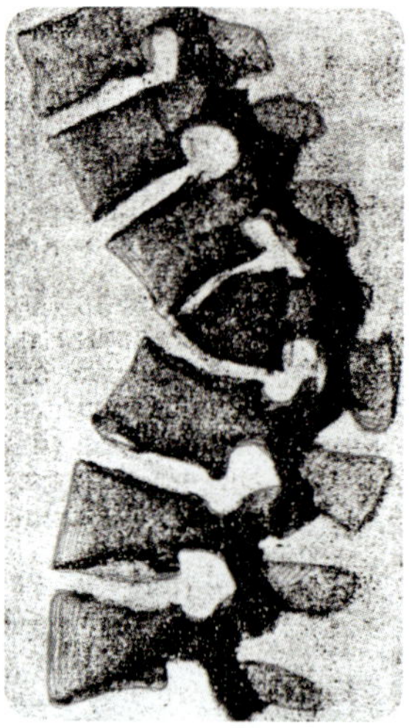

Fig. 2.2.14.
Posterior wedge-shaped vertebra

The presence of one or more wedge-shaped vertebrae, located unilaterally, may cause varying degrees of lateral curvature of the spine. This is known as congenital scoliosis. Scoliosis caused by wedge-shaped vertebrae, as opposed to static scoliosis, is never of great significance. In cases in which the wedge-shaped vertebrae are located on both sides, one scoliosis could compensate for another. On clinical examination of these patients, external deformation of the spine is almost unnoticeable.

Patients with kyphosis and scoliosis typically suffer from spinal pain and dysfunctions of those organs the innervation of which has been impaired. The severity of the complaints depends on the degree of the deformity.

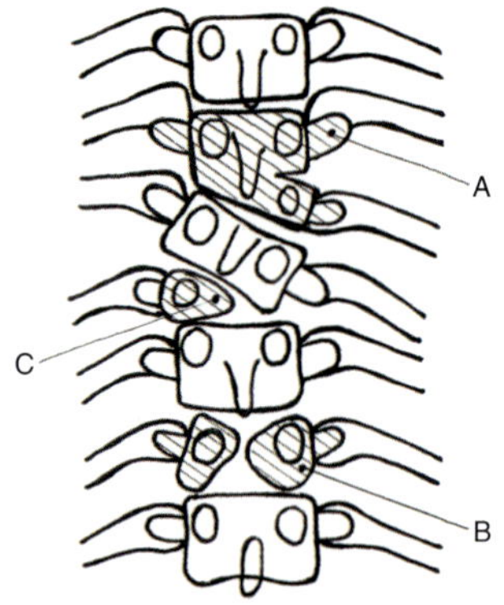

Fig. 2.2.15.
Variations of wedge-shaped vertebrae: **A** - lateral wedge-shaped hemivertebra, assimilated by the overlying vertebra; **B** - butterfly-shaped vertebra (scheme); **C** - lateral wedge-shaped hemivertebra

3. Malformations of the vertebral bodies

This rather large group includes the following:

- Expansion of the diameter of the vertebral body (platispondylia) or flattened vertebrae (Fig. 2.2.16).
- Shortening of the vertebral bodies (brachispondylia) (Fig. 2.2.17). Brachispondylia is clinically important because the shortening of the trunk leads to a reduction in height. When several vertebrae are affected, the decrease in height may be significant (10–12 cm).
- A combination of expansion of the vertebral body and its flattening (platibrachispondilia) (Fig. 2.2.18). The butterfly deformity discussed earlier can be attributed to this type of anomaly.
- 'Fish vertebrae' (codfish vertebrae). In this deformity, the vertebral body has a biconcave appearance due to a varying extent of depression of the central part of the upper and lower borders of the vertebral body. The visible shape of the vertebral

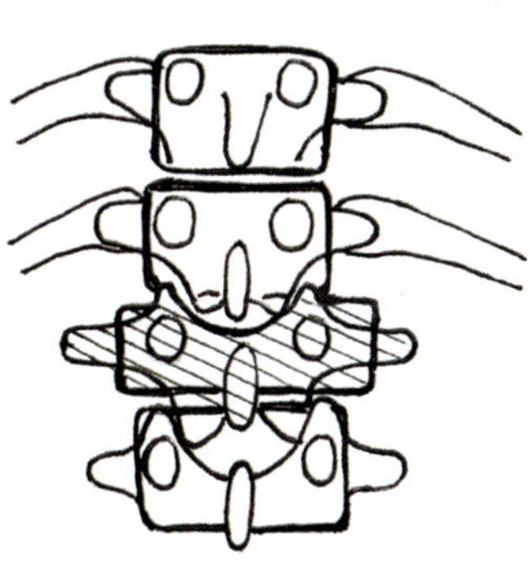

Fig. 2.2.16.
Expansion of vertebral body in diameter (scheme)

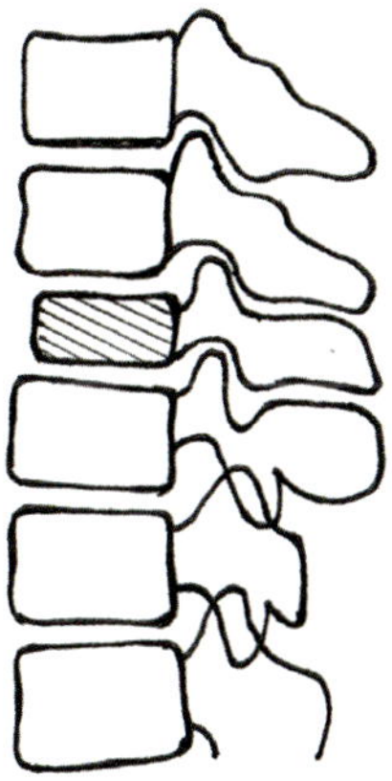

Fig. 2.2.17.
Reduction of vertebral body height with its shortening (scheme)

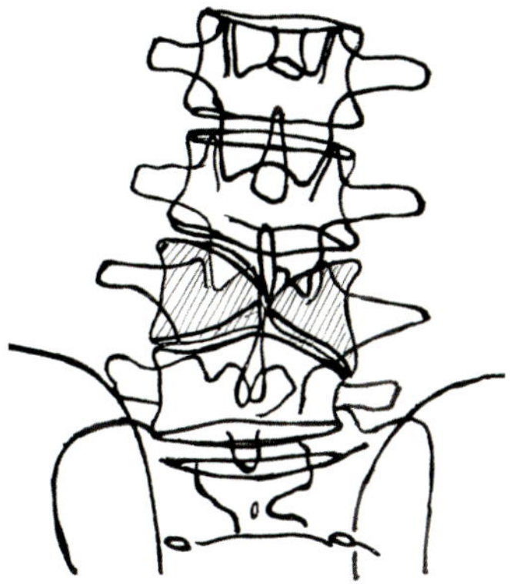

Fig. 2.2.18.
Combination of vertebral expansion with its flattening (scheme)

body does not change, but the upper and lower areas become saucer-shaped or concave. At the same time, the intervertebral discs become thicker, overswollen and biconvex (Fig. 2.2.19).

The clinical manifestations of the anomalies mentioned above include skin diseases (dermatoses) of varying degrees of severity. These are characterized by thickening of the cornified layer of the epidermis. A common manifestation is ichthyosis, or fish skin disease, in which the skin becomes as thick as fish scales.

4. Clefts in the interarticular space of the arch

In persons with spondylolysis, a defect of the vertebral arch, there is a cleft that is 2–3 mm wide in the interarticular area, i.e. between the upper and lower articular processes (Figs 2.2.20 and 2.2.21).

Under certain conditions, spondylolysis can become the cause of complications, such as sliding of the vertebrae or spondylolisthesis. Therefore, spondylolysis is also referred to as 'prespondylolisthesis'. It is caused by the abnormal appearance of two points of ossification, instead of one, in each half of the vertebral arch. These two points do not merge with each other and the vertebral body thus gets separated from the arches, resulting in the formation of a cleft. Spondylolysis, which occurs in 10%–12% of all adults, is observed much more often than spondylolisthesis, and may be unilateral or bilateral. This anomaly is occasionally combined with spina bifida posterior and hypoplasia of the spinous processes (Fig. 2.2.22).

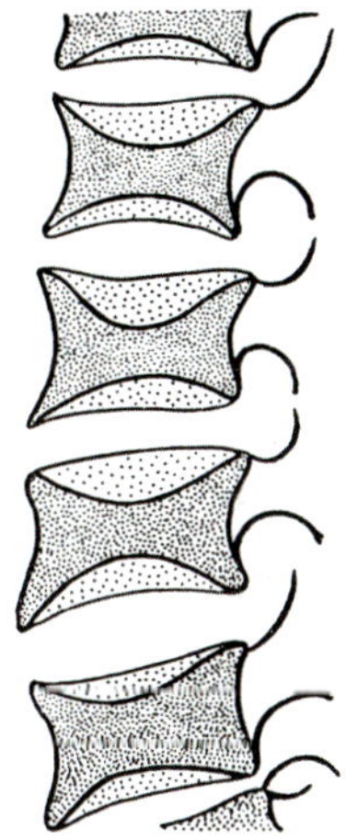

Fig. 2.2.19.
So-called "*fish vertebra*"
This deformation is never congenital, but develops in the setting of severe osteoporosis of any aetiology and in other acquired pathological processes

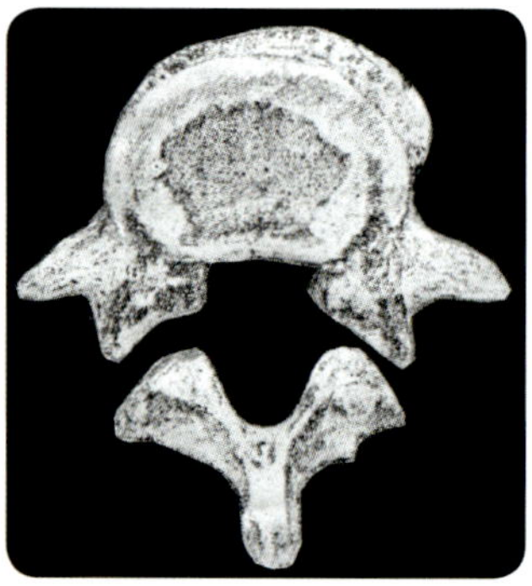

Fig. 2.2.20.
Bilateral spondylolysis of the 5th lumbar vertebra

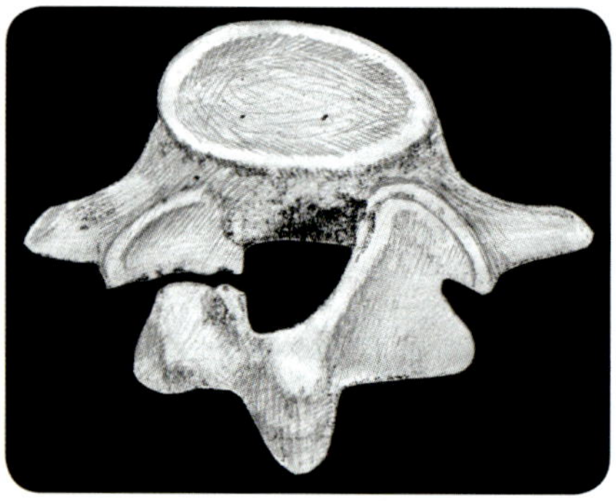

Fig. 2.2.21.
Unilateral spondylolysis

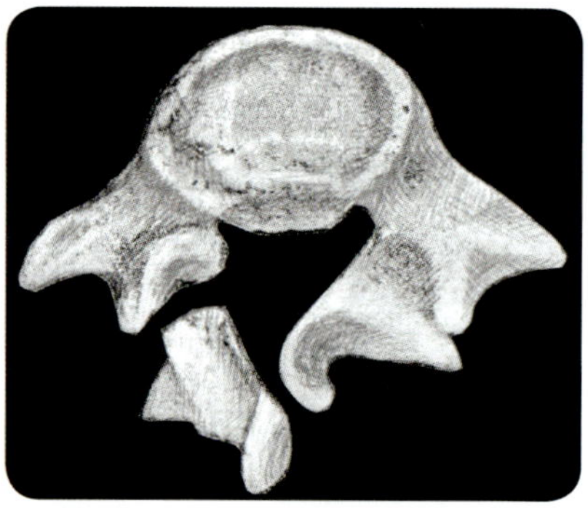

Fig. 2.2.22.
Spondylolysis associated with *spina bifida* of the 5th lumbar vertebra

Among the factors that predispose a person to spondylolisthesis, i.e. sliding of the 5th lumbar vertebra (Fig. 2.2.23), is that the body of this vertebra is normally inclined obliquely forward at about 30 degrees or even more (up to 45 degrees). In addition, the body of the last lumbar vertebra, on which rests the weight of the whole spine, trunk, etc., is wedge-shaped, i.e. its height is greater in the anterior part than in the posterior. Spondylolisthesis affects men twice as frequently as women. The majority of patients are young, between 20 and 35 years of age.

Since the end of the 19th century, various attempts have been made to explain the pathogenesis of spondylolysis and spondylolisthesis. These include theories emphasizing the role of trauma and congenital factors, as well as reconstructive theories. The theory of trauma was shown to be untenable. The congenital theory was also not valid because according to F.L. Neugebauerand and G.I. Turner (cited from S.A. Reinberg, 1964), spondylolysis is not a congenital anomaly of the interarticular isthmus but an acquired disease. If there is a pronounced lordosis and discrepancy between morphological structure and functional overload, articular processes squeeze the pars interarticularis like scissors, which leads to its resorption. Degenerative spondylolisthesis usually occurs among elderly patients and is due to decreased

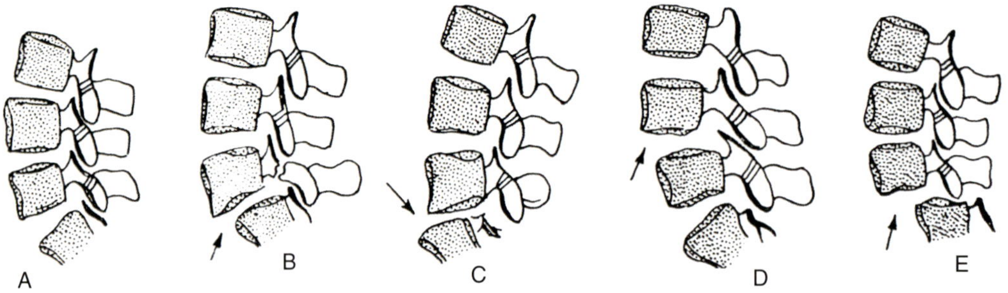

Fig. 2.2.23.
On differential recognition of spondylolisthesis: **A** - normal, **B** - spondylolisthesis; **C** – posterior paradoxical spondylolisthesis; **D** - pseudospondylolisthesis, **E** - true vertebral luxation (dislocation)

connection strength between the articular processes because of the presence of osteoarthritis. Under these conditions, a retrolisthesis may develop.

More than 80% of all patients with spondylolisthesis complain of lumbosacral pain, which may radiate to the lower extremities. Radiography is crucial for a definitive diagnosis (Fig. 2.2.24).

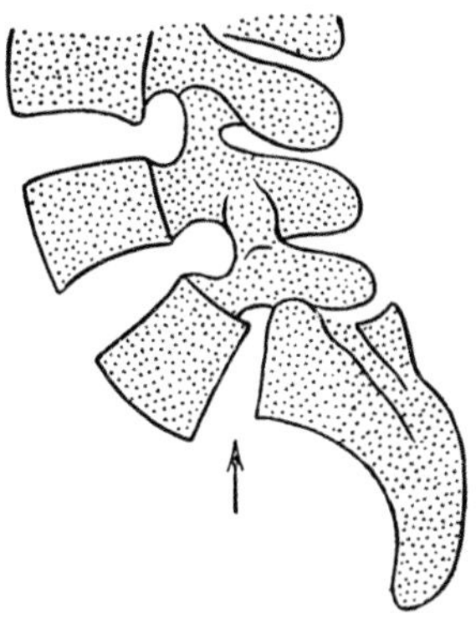

Fig. 2.2.24.
Scheme of lateral radiographs in spondylolisthesis

5. Anomalies of the lumbosacral region

During its development, the foetus has 7 cervical, 13 thoracic and 5 lumbar vertebrae. Then the first caudal (5th lumbar) vertebra fuses with the first sacral vertebra, and the 13th thoracic vertebra becomes the 1st lumbar vertebra after the reduction of the 13th pair of ribs. This process of transformation usually results in the formation of the normal number of vertebrae in the different regions of the spine. However, the process of transformation of the components of the spine may be disrupted at times, resulting in certain permutations of the so-called transitional vertebrae. This is due to acquisition of the characteristics of the adjacent vertebrae.

Variations in the number and size of the lumbosacral vertebrae, various types of fusion between them, etc. can be considered an anomaly. Extensive X-ray studies of this region have shown that a particular anatomical variation may be observed in 60%–75% of cases. It is not for no reason that they say that the features of the lumbosacral region are as unique to a person as is the face.

There is a condition in which the 5th (caudal) lumbar vertebra is modified and acquires the shape of a sacral vertebra. This is usually referred to as 'sacralization' from the Latin 'sacrum'. The development of this last lumbar vertebra may stop at any of the intermediate phases—from the normal lumbar vertebra to the true sacral vertebra (Figs 2.2.25 and 2.2.26). True sacralization refers to the complete bony fusion of the transverse processes of the 5th lumbar vertebra with the sacrum, as well as iliac synchondrosis. Incomplete sacralization refers to only an enlargement of the transverse process. Ossification of the iliolumbar ligament (lig. ileolumbale), which passes from the tip of the transverse processes of the 5th lumbar vertebra to the iliac crest, mimics sacralization and is known as pseudosacralization. In most cases, the various forms of sacralization are bilateral and completely symmetrical. However, unilateral asymmetrical sacralization, mainly left-sided, is not uncommon (Figs 2.2.27 and 2.2.28).

True sacralization is observed in 5%–7% of all cases. The enlargement of the transverse processes should be regarded as a normal anatomical variant, which occurs in about one-third of all patients. Sometimes, there is a combination of sacralization

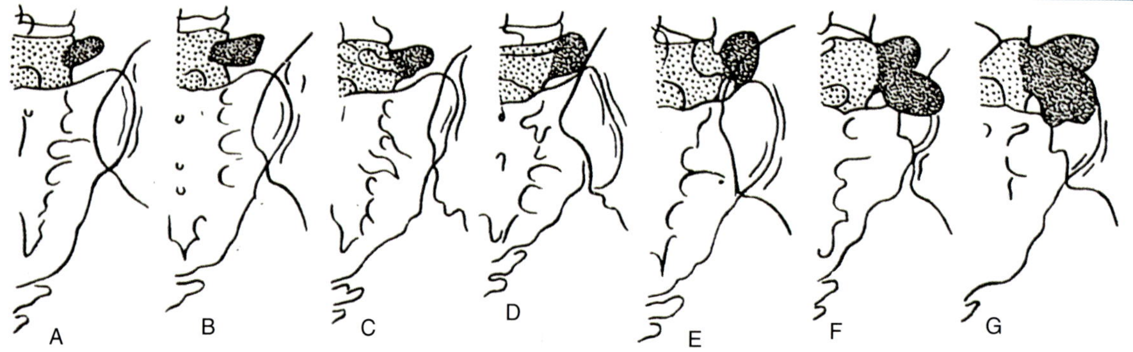

Fig. 2.2.25.
Schematic drawing of different types of sacralization: **A** - normal, **B** and **C** - increased size of transverse processes, **D–G** - synostosis or synchondrosis between massive transverse processes, sacrum and ilium; closure of the intervertebral foramen

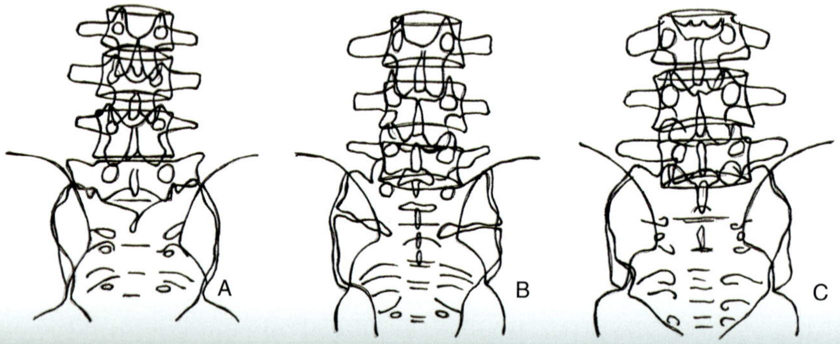

Fig. 2.2.26.
Types of sacralization:
A - incomplete bilateral sacralization;
B - bilateral articular sacralization;
C - bilateral bony sacralization

and spondylolisthesis. The opposite of sacralization is lumbarization of the sacral vertebra, a phenomenon observed less frequently. In order to establish the diagnosis of lumbarization, it must be conclusively proved that the number of sacral vertebrae is 4 rather than 5 and that there are 6 lumbar vertebrae. Since making an accurate diagnosis of sacralization and lumbarization is quite difficult, S.A. Reinberg and others have proposed that the use of these terms be abandoned in favour of the terms 'transitional lumbosacral vertebra' and 'suprasacral vertebra'.

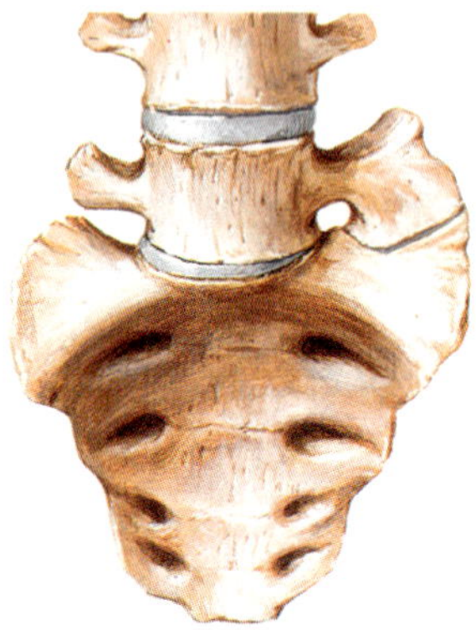

Fig. 2.2.27.
Unilateral (left side) articular sacralization. Increased size of the left transverse process of 5th lumbar vertebra is connected with the left lateral mass of the sacrum via joint

When discussing the causes of lumbarization, clinicians and radiologists should remember that the fusion of sacral vertebrae occurs pretty late. The fusion of the lower vertebrae begins at the age of 13–14 years and the process

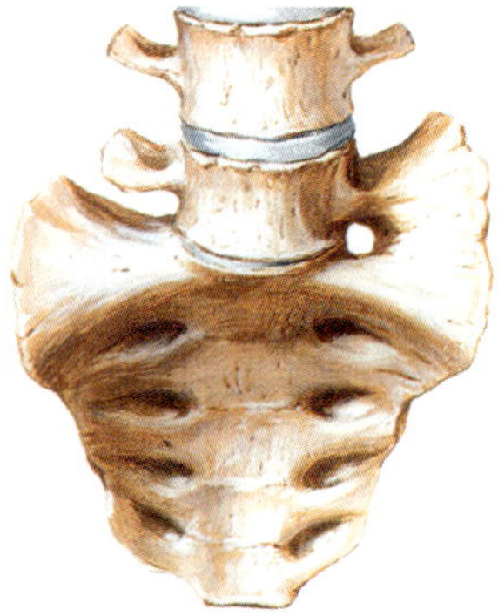

Fig. 2.2.28.
Unilateral complete (left side) bony sacralization

ends by 23–25 years of age, by which time the fusion of the upper vertebrae is complete. Quite often, the 1st, 2nd and even 3rd sacral vertebrae remain unfused lifelong and are functionally the 6th, 7th and even 8th lumbar vertebrae (Fig. 2.2.29). According to V.S. Maykova-Stroganova and M.A. Finkelstein (1952), A.I. Borisevich (1981), cited from V.P. Veselovsky *et al.* (1990), in lumbarization of the sacrum in an adult, even the existence of intervertebral discs between the sacral vertebrae is possible. Two or three upper intervertebral discs are sometimes found to be preserved in the sacrum among individuals aged 25 years and above. This most often occurs among those who have been involved in heavy physical work since adolescence, and can be regarded as an adaptation to increased load.

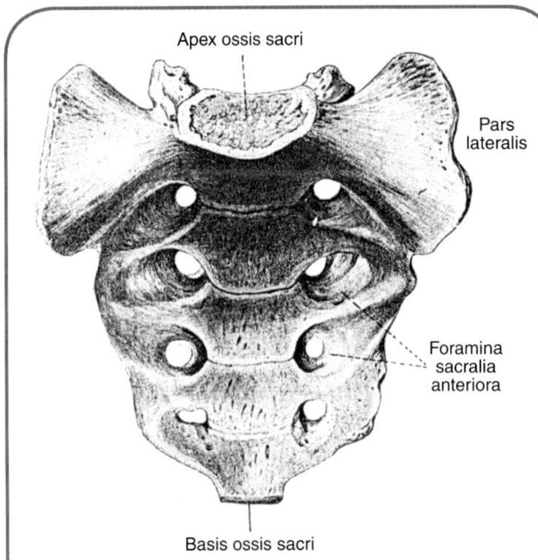

Fig. 2.2.29.
Sacrum, front view; vertebrae are not fused; lineae transversae separate them

Most patients with transitional vertebrae experience lumbar and sacral pain, ischialgia, weakness in the muscles of the lower extremities, fatigue, cramps in the calf muscles, sweating of the feet, etc. Clinicians and radiologists are of the view that transitional vertebrae create some kind of a *lumbosacral spine deficiency, which, however, is not always accompanied by pain.*

Fallenlav and Williams (cited from S.A. Reinberg, 1964) compared a group of 200 individuals who had no lumbosacral complaints for the past 10 years with a group of 200 individuals who were of clinical interest, being patients with low back pain. It is important to note that the authors found various abnormalities of a congenital nature among both groups, and the abnormalities occurred with approximately equal frequency.

The authors came to the logical conclusion that the clinical significance of bony changes, in themselves, is questionable. Lumbosacral pain undoubtedly results not only from intermediate vertebrae, but also certain additional causes. The authors' point is illustrated especially by their observations on athletes, who had various lumbosacral anomalies which, however, were not an obstacle for achieving their goals.

I must add that when analysing my own clinical material, I came to similar conclusions. I shall expand upon these in subsequent chapters of this book.

S.A. Reinberg poses an important question: what exactly compresses and irritates the nerves? His answer is: 'These are primarily bone spurs on the posterior parts of the vertebral bodies, on the posterior surfaces of the edges of their upper and lower areas. Furthermore, there are degenerative and proliferative changes of the intervertebral disc, including so-called posterior hernias located under the yellow ligament near the intervertebral foramen. These are, then, both the thickening of bony articular processes, and in particular joint capsules and ligaments of the intervertebral joints. It is, finally, the displacement of joint elements relative to each other owing to which the nerve "is taken in pincers".'

In our view, the idea that only bony structures are responsible for sacral pain is untenable. We can gain a better understanding of the matter only if we improve our clinical knowledge of the lumbosacral region as a whole, considering the bony, ligamentous, articular, muscular and neural components functioning together. In addition, we need to learn more about the static, mechanical and functional (occupational, household, etc.) aspects. Considering all this, we feel that the surgical removal of an enlarged transverse process of a suprasacral vertebra would be undesirable.

According to S.A. Reinberg (1964), when assessing radiographs, special attention should be paid to the intervertebral joints of the transitional lumbosacral spine. Abnormalities of these joints are more important than many or even all other congenital developmental abnormalities of the lumbosacral spine in terms of the morphological and functional substrates of pain. Anomalies of both intervertebral joints between the 5th lumbar and 1st sacral vertebrae are frequent. Their shape and size vary. As for their location and extent of symmetry, they have a most important functional significance (Fig. 2.2.30). The direction and volume of movements in this part of the skeleton depend on the location of these joints and their relative positions.The joints may be located in an oblique plane, e.g. they may be more displaced inwards or outwards, or they may not be positioned strictly vertically and may thus be inclined towards the horizontal plane in either direction. In more than 30% of cases, there are different combinations of positions of the right and left joints. For example, the right joint may be located vertically and the left, horizontally, or the right joint may be in the sagittal plane and the left

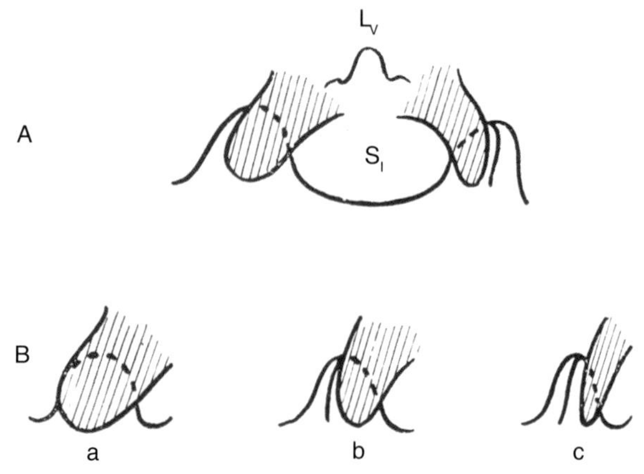

Fig. 2.2.30.
Schematic representation of asymmetrical intervertebral joints between the 5th lumbar and the 1st sacral vertebrae
A - top view—on the right side the joint is located in the horizontal plane (in a standing human); auricular fissure can be observed on plain radiographs; on the left side the joint lies in the sagittal plane; auricular fissure can be seen on anteroposterior radiograph
B - front view—a - the joint is located in the frontal plane, fissure is not visible; c - in the sagittal plane - the fissure is visible; b - an intermediate position between extremes of the transition "a" and "c". In "a" position facet joints are the most unstable, in "c" – most stable

in the frontal plane. It is likely that this is the most frequent cause of unilateral pain.

In view of the above discussion, S.A. Reinberg re-emphasizes an extremely important idea that anomalies are not in themselves the cause of pain. Rather, the pain is a consequence of certain pathological processes which result in complications of the anomalies.

6. Mixed developmental anomalies of the spine

Congenital vertebral synostosis is the fusion of two or more vertebrae. In more than 2% of cases, it may be found in any region of the spine. It occurs most frequently between the 2nd and the 3rd, as well as the 6th and the 7th cervical vertebrae (Fig. 2.2.31). The vertebral bodies, arches and, in some cases, processes may be knitted together. Congenital synostoses are quite diverse (Figs 2.2.32 and 2.2.33). The configuration of the fused vertebrae usually does not change.

In cervical synostosis, secondary spondylosis deformans of a limited area above and below the blocked vertebrae develops even at an early age. This is apparently due to enhanced compensatory movements above and below the fixed segment, and is associated with pain, besides limited mobility of the head and spine. Synostosis may be asymmetrical, a condition which is clinically accompanied by deformation. Radiography is useful in making the correct diagnosis (Fig. 2.2.34).

The existence of various extensive synostoses in the cervical region is called Klippel–Feil syndrome or disease (Fig. 2.2.35). In this condition, some of the cervical vertebrae—most often the lower vertebrae and sometimes the upper thoracic vertebrae as many as 4–6 (Fig. 2.2.36)—are fused together, forming a solid, poorly differentiated bony mass. The number of vertebrae and their height are, therefore, considerably reduced. The neck is shortened or even absent. Simultaneously, one shoulder blade or both

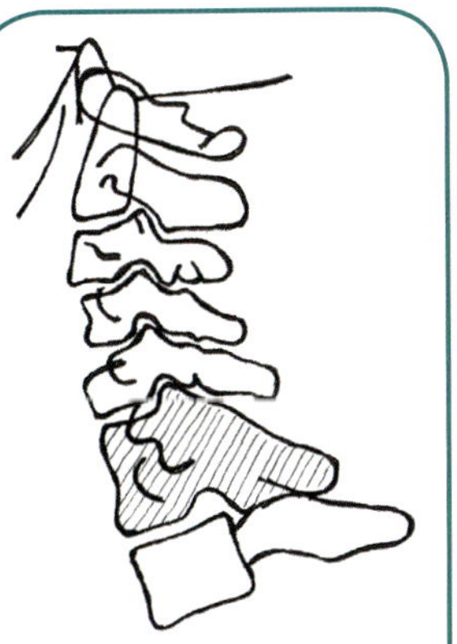

Fig. 2.2.31. Blockage of bodies, arches and processes of two cervical vertebrae (scheme)

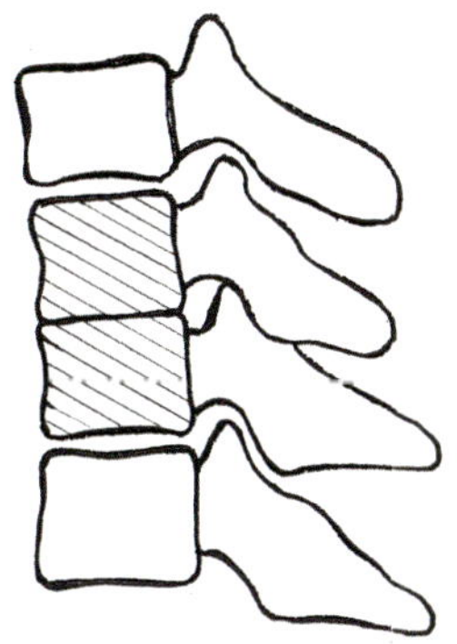

Fig. 2.2.32. Blockage of bodies of two thoracic vertebrae (scheme)

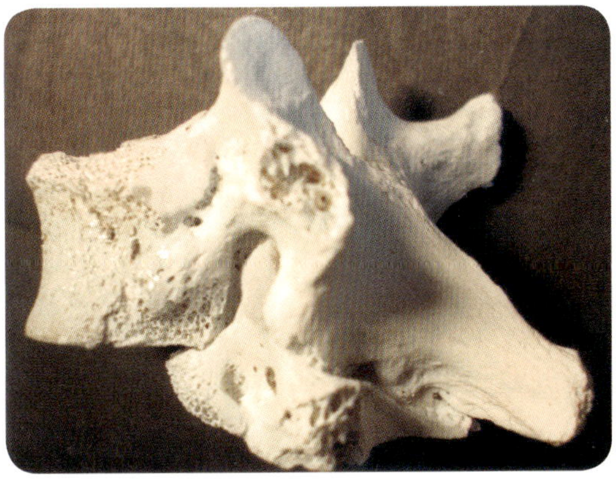

Fig. 2.2.33. Blockage of bodies of two thoracic vertebrae (macropreparation)

may be higher than normal (Sprengel's deformity).

Although most of these anomalies are congenital, they usually come to the clinician's notice only when the patient is 40–60 years of age. The patient complains of local and reflected pain, stiffness and limited mobility of the head and neck, pain in the upper extremities (such as in plexitis), cramps in the fingers and their sweating, which is of great practical importance.

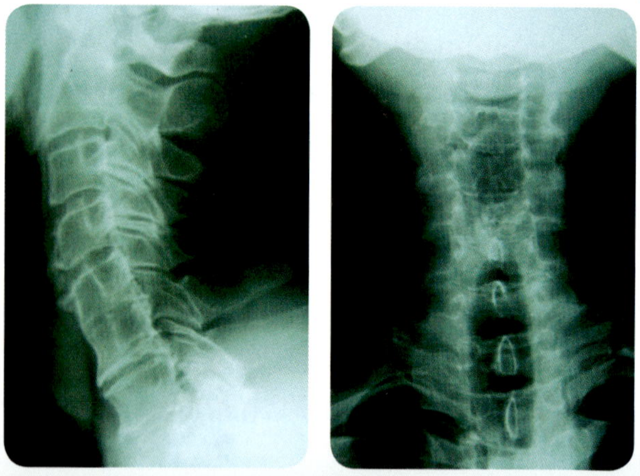

Fig. 2.2.34.
Radiographic picture of V–VI cervical vertebrae fusion

Transitional cranio-cervical border

The abnormalities observed in this region include assimilation and manifestation of the atlas. In assimilation, the lateral parts of the atlas, either on one side or both sides, as well as the arch are partially or completely fused with the occipital bone. The types of fusion are very diverse (Fig. 2.2.37). In cases of assimilation, the atlas may shift anteriorly or laterally, or symmetrically or asymmetrically. This results in deformity and narrowing of the foramen magnum. In manifestation, the elements of the vertebra arise from the occipital bone.

In assimilation and manifestation, the odontoid process of the axis directly compresses the medulla oblongata, which contains the nuclei of the cranial nerves. For this reason, these pathological conditions can lead to serious neurological impairments. The complex of symptoms

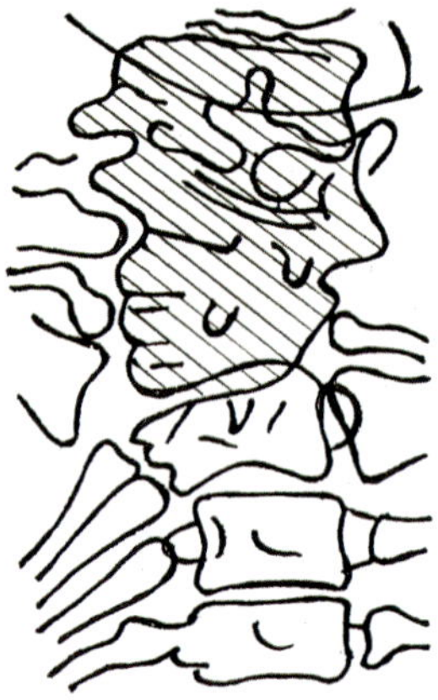

Fig. 2.2.35.
Klippel–Feil syndrome (lateral projection; scheme)

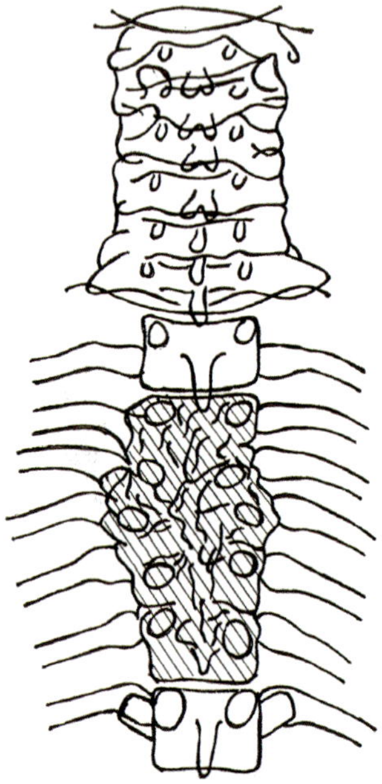

Fig. 2.2.36.
Blockage of bodies, arches and processes of five thoracic vertebrae (scheme)

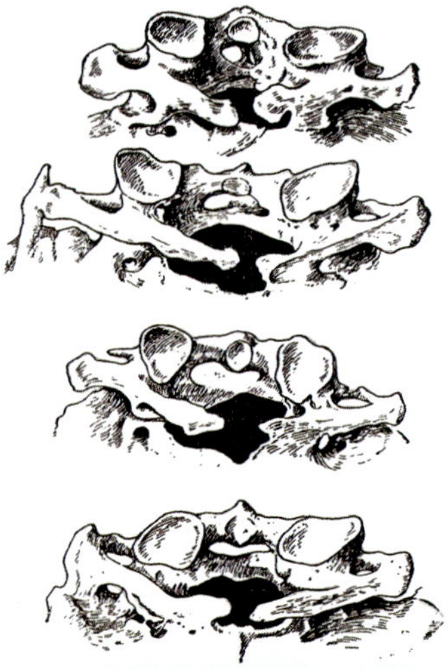

Fig. 2.2.37.
Types of atlas assimilation

may be mistakenly interpreted as arising from amyotrophic sclerosis, syringobulbia, syringomyelia and other diseases of the medulla oblongata and the uppermost part of the SC. Though these anomalies are congenital, they are not apparent in the early stages of life (in newborns, in childhood and adolescence, and even in adulthood). They often manifest in middle age and even old age.

Cervical ribs

Cervical ribs are relatively rare. They can be of considerable size and occasionally articulate with the first rib or manubrium sterni. This anomaly is usually asymmetrical, i.e. a cervical rib can be located on either side (Fig. 2.2.38). In most cases, cervical ribs do not cause pathological symptoms. Sometimes, a deformity is visible and is firm on palpation. Numbness of the fingers and neuropathic pain, such as that in plexitis, may develop. The vascular manifestations include coldness of the hand and weakening of the pulse. Cervical ribs may be associated with other abnormalities (wedge-shaped vertebrae, synostosis, etc.). When there are significant clinical disorders and symptomatic treatment is not effective, surgical removal of the cervical rib together with the periosteum is indicated.

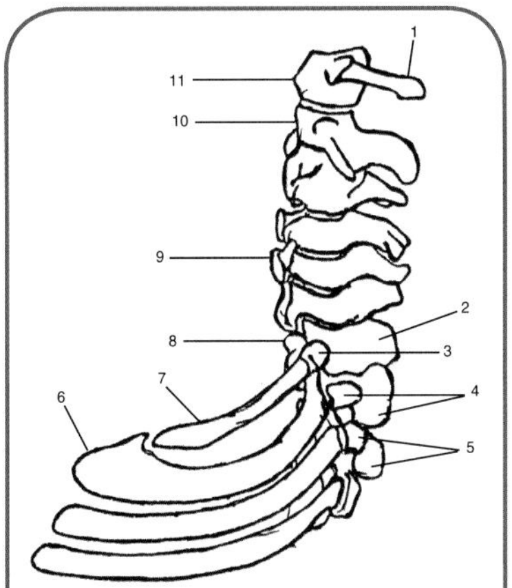

Fig. 2.2.38. Left cervical rib
1 - arch of atlas; 2 - VII cervical vertebra; 3 - transverse process; 4 - Ist thoracic vertebra; 5 - II thoracic vertebra; 6 - I (thoracic) rib; 7 - cervical rib; 8 - head of cervical rib; 9 - tuberculum caroticum; 10 - epistropheus; 11 - body of atlas

Defects of vertebral parts

While performing our own anatomical investigations aimed to find the causes of vertebrobasilar syndrome, weakening of vision, migraine, visual field deficits and short-term loss of consciousness on suddenly turning the head (both among adults and children), we examined the vertebrae of many patients. Though we examined the vertebrae of different regions of the spine, cervical vertebrae were of special interest to us because the description in the literature of the anomalies in this region was clearly inadequate and the information given was also scanty.

The results of ultrasonic dopplerography of the cerebral vessels served as an impetus for us to start our research. Extravasal compression of the vertebral artery and a decrease of 30%–50% and more in the blood flow were observed in all patients with the symptoms mentioned above. This compression was often asymmetrical. While searching for the causes of compression, we first excluded osteochondrosis, spondylosis deformans, specific inflammatory and neoplastic conditions, uncovertebral arthrosis and aseptic inflammation. These conditions could be a reason for extravasal compression. We had examined a few thousand patients and found that these conditions occurred rarely among adults and almost never among children. Thus, we were left with a group of patients whose spinal radiographs did not show any pathological changes, yet these patients suffered from vertebral artery syndrome. So, the question remained: What was the reason of the compression of the vertebral artery?

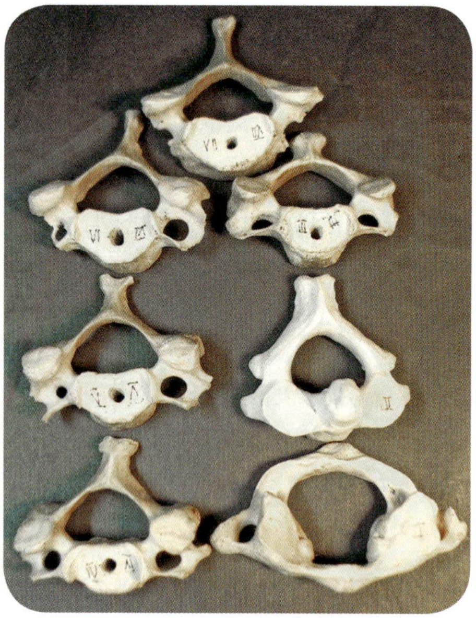

Fig. 2.2.39.
Set of seven vertebrae of cervical spine. Essential difference in the diameter of foramina vertebralia in the transverse processes of the 5th and 6th vertebrae

An examination of the cervical vertebrae revealed that the transverse processes had some defects. In particular, in some cases, foramen transversarium was absent or was doubled, i.e. it was unilaterally or bilaterally divided into two parts by a septum. In other cases, the foramen transversarium was significantly asymmetrical (Figs 2.2.39–2.2.43). Moreover, the shape and size of the articular processes, as well as the size, location and degree of symmetry of the intervertebral joints varied a great deal (Figs 2.2.44 and 2.2.45). Such structural abnormalities, of course, led to violation of permeability of the vertebral artery and accordingly, induced circulatory disorders of the brain.

Concomitant deforming spondylosis, osteochondrosis and post-traumatic adhesion of the bodies and/or processes of the cervical vertebrae (Figs 2.2.46 and 2.2.47) led

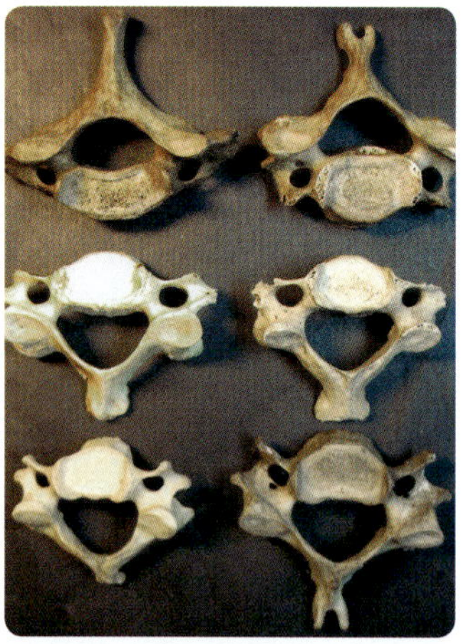

Fig. 2.2.40.

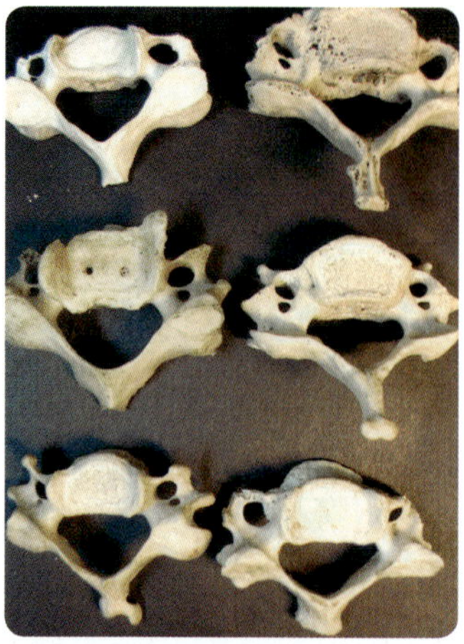

Fig. 2.2.41.

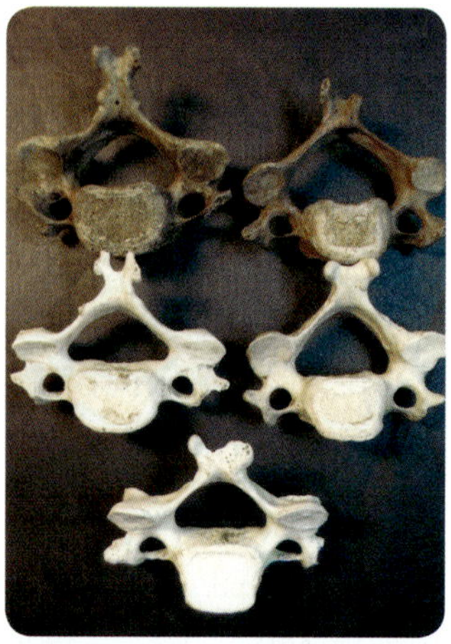

Fig. 2.2.42.

Structural asymmetry of the transverse and articular processes of cervical vertebrae; variations in diameter of the foramina vertebralia

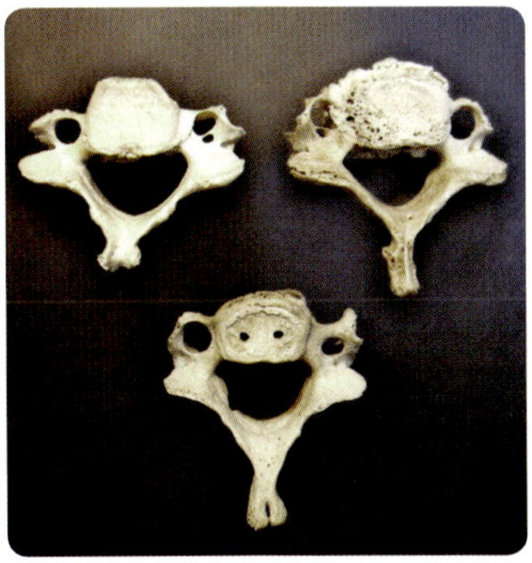

Fig. 2.2.43.

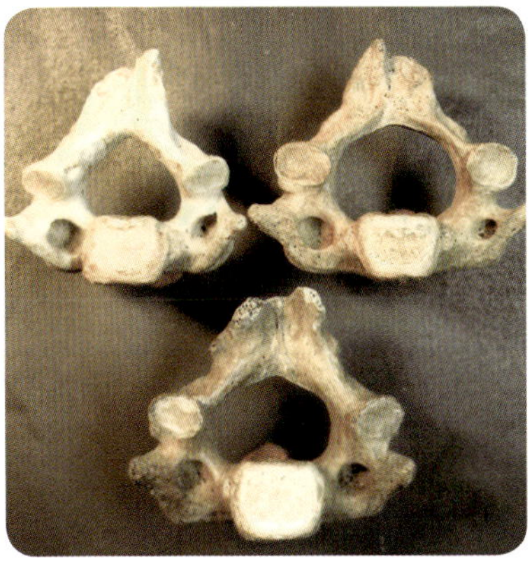

Fig. 2.2.44.

Structural asymmetry of the transverse and articular processes of cervical vertebrae; variations in diameter of the foramina vertebralia

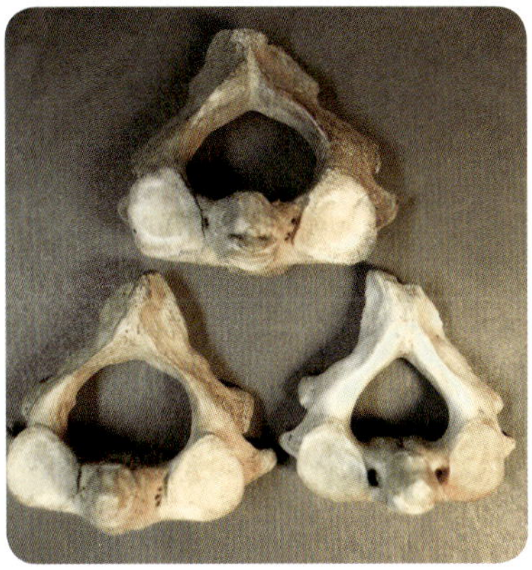

Fig. 2.2.45.
Structural asymmetry of bodies and articular processes of the 2nd cervical vertebra

to further potentiated circulatory disorders of the brain, neurological symptoms, fluctuations in blood pressure, etc. This situation could be associated with increased stenosis of the spinal canal and intervertebral foramina due to deforming changes in the transverse processes and facet joints. However, in our view, the most significant negative factor leading to vertebral artery syndrome was the rotational displacement (torsion) of vertebrae and, in particular, the cervical ones.

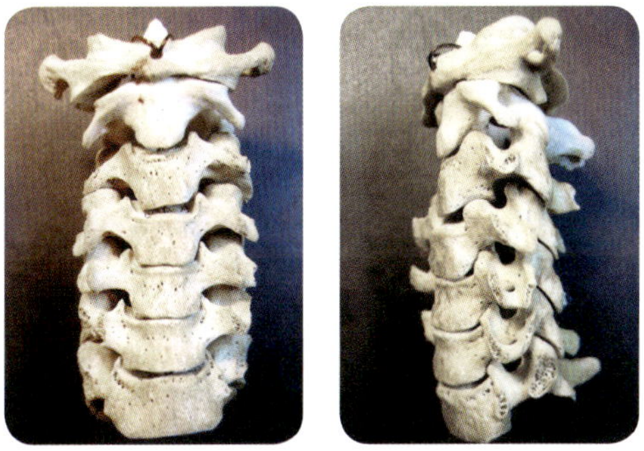

Fig. 2.2.46.
Initial manifestations of deforming spondylosis of the cervical spine; uncoarthrosis

The mechanisms of such displacements will be discussed in subsequent chapters of this book.

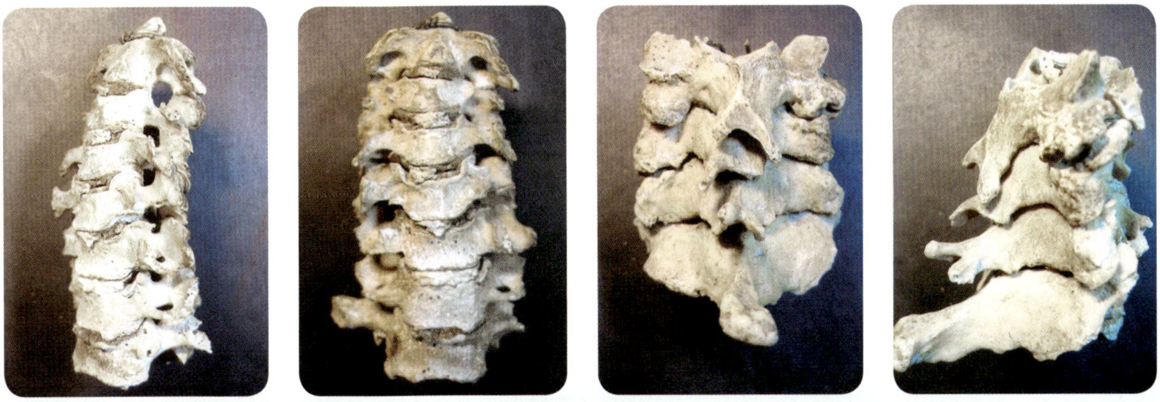

Fig. 2.2.47.
Advanced signs of deforming spondylosis of the cervical spine

2.3 PROPORTIONS, TYPES AND SIGNS OF ASYMMETRICAL ORGANIZATION OF THE HUMAN BODY

Since ancient times, healers, painters and sculptors have given much thought to the regularity of the dimensions of the human body aimed at finding its ideal proportions. The doctrine about the proportions of the body was of great importance to physicians. These ideas made it possible for them to assess the rate of growth of a person's body parts keeping in mind a norm for comparison, and to determine the race or morphological type. This information was taken into account when deciding on preventive or therapeutic measures.

Various 'canons' or theoretical constructs regarding the human form were proposed, in which the ratios of the sizes of the parts of the body were defined. The number of canons is significant. According to Stratz, there were about 80 canons until 1854, and in 1924, Breitman recognized more than 115. Most of them have lost their value, but some are interesting because they give one a glimpse of the criteria regarding the ideal body in different parts of the world and in different periods. For example, the ancient Egyptians were guided by certain rules in the depiction of the human body. The indexing lines carved on the stones in some of their tombs probably served as a measure of the length of various parts of the body. According to Blanc, the length of the middle finger was a unit of measurement in ancient Egypt and the length of the body was supposed to be 19 times this length. In ancient Rome, the sculptor Polyklet Sikionsky (5th century BC), proposed a canon according to which the head must account for 1/8, the face 1/10 and the head and neck together 1/6 of the body length. The width of the palm was adopted as the unit of measure.

Painters and sculptors of the Renaissance as well as later periods (16th–17th centuries) have also used certain canons. These include the canons of Giotto, Alberti, Durer and Rubens. Leonardo da Vinci's canon is of particular interest. Having studied the 'square of the ancients' with the human form included within it, he proposed to similarly inscribe the human figure within a circle in such a way that the outstretched upper and lower limbs should touch the circumference. In this position, the centre of the body corresponded to the umbilicus (Fig. 2.3.1). Leonardo da Vinci's unit of measurement was the height of the head, which, according to his law, corresponded to 1/8 of the length of the body.

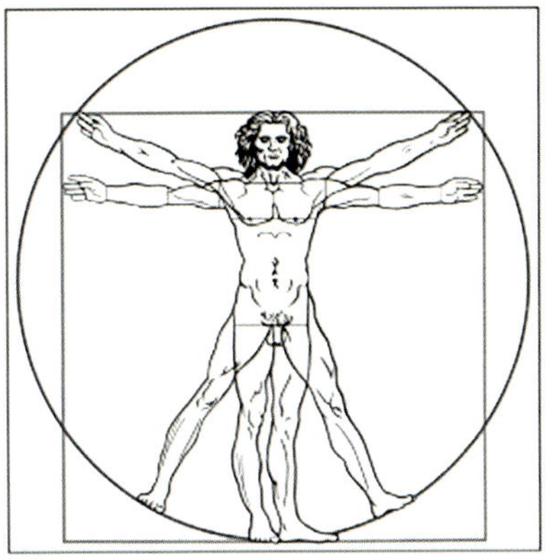

Fig. 2.3.1.
Proportions of the body according to canon of Leonardo da Vinci

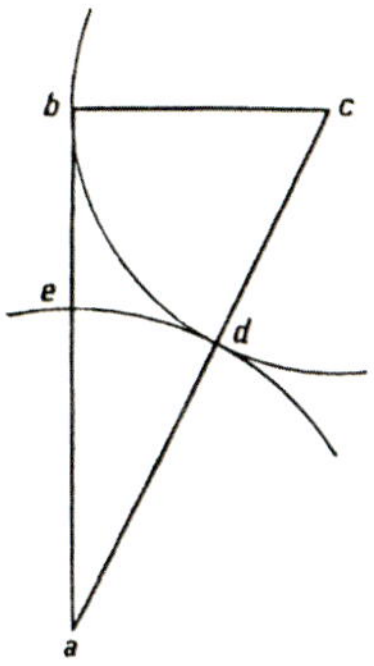

Fig. 2.3.2.
Ratios according to the canon of 'golden section'

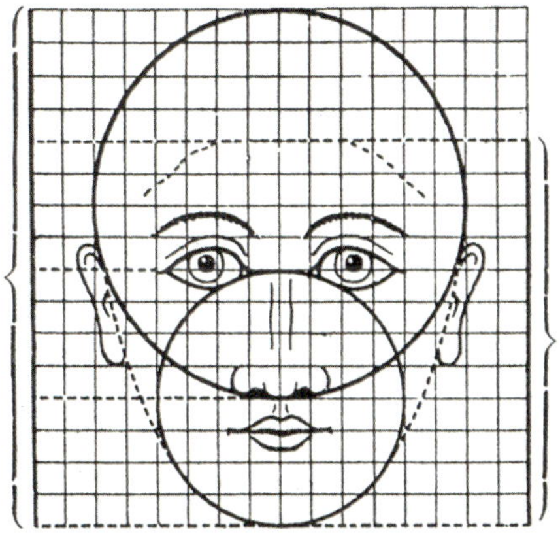

Fig. 2.3.3.
Proportions of the face (according to Stratz)

The canon proposed by Zeising in 1854 became known as the 'golden section'. According to this canon, the body length refers to the distance from the umbilicus to the ground (Fig. 2.3.2). The body length could also be measured by the distance from the top of the head to the end of the hand and that from the latter to the ground. Later, anatomist Carus developed a doctrine on the proportions of the human body. In his work, *Symbolism of the Human Appearance*, he compared the proportions of the body with the length of the spine (excluding the sacrum). It was equal to 18 cm, corresponding to the length of the spine of a newborn and was a basic size for measuring different parts of the body, not only in children but also adults. Schmidt and Fritsch later modified Carus' canon. Subsequently, Stratz clarified Fritsch's data on the proportions of the face (Fig. 2.3.3).

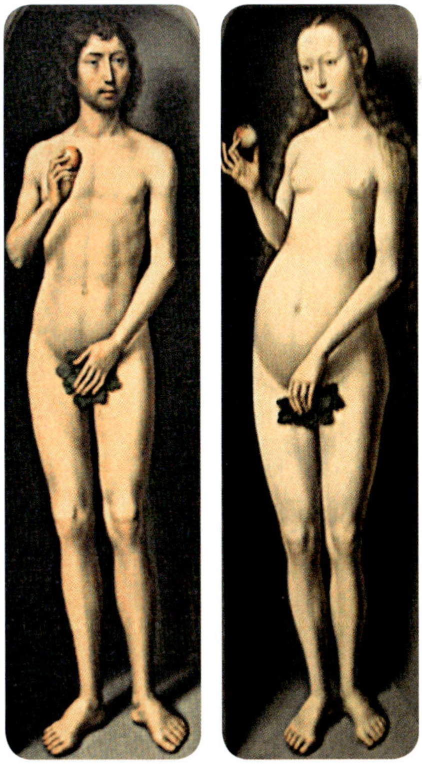

Fig. 2.3.4.
Painting of Adam and Eve by Hanz Memeling (Germany, 1345–1400); from collection of the Museum of Fine Arts in Vienna (Austria)

The purpose of all these canons was to determine the average proportions of the human body, without taking into account any individual differences. This approach cannot be considered correct because when studying the structure of the body, characteristics such as gender, age, race and type of constitution should be taken into account. There are obvious differences in the proportions, as well as the absolute size, of the male and female body. These features have been illustrated by painters since centuries and can be observed quite clearly when examining certain pieces of art (Fig. 2.3.4). Compared to a man, a woman has shorter upper and lower limbs, a longer trunk, narrower shoulders and wider hips. Among women, the facial region is poorly developed compared to the cerebral region. The hands and feet are relatively smaller. The proportions of a woman's body are closer to those characteristic of a child. Age-related changes in the proportions of the body are much more pronounced than sexual differences, according to the Stratz scheme (Fig. 2.3.5). Such changes can be observed clearly when comparing the dimensions of the bodies of individuals of different ages (Fig. 2.3.6).

On the basis of a thorough study of the structure of the body, Sigaud created his own classification of morphological features (Fig. 2.3.7). This is outlined below.

1. The respiratory type is characterized by the predominant development of the respiratory apparatus. This affects a number of features of the frontal part of the head, neck and trunk. The thorax is cylindrical, gradually narrowing towards the waist.
2. The digestive type is characterized by the predominant development of the digestive organs. Of the three facial regions, the lowest, which corresponds to the masticatory apparatus, is the most highly developed. The power of the upper and lower jaws differs. The chewing muscles are highly developed. The abdominal part is noticeably better developed than the thoracic—the stomach bulges out, while the chest is wide and short.
3. The muscular type is characterized by strong development of the musculoskeletal system. This type of constitution is considered perfect. Most antique statues depict subjects with a

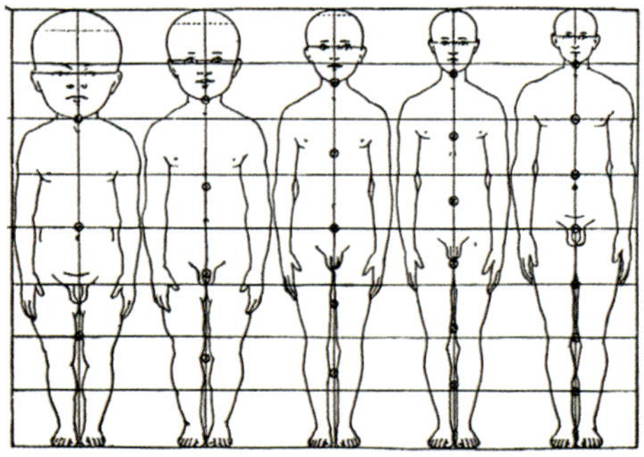

Fig. 2.3.5.
Changes in body proportions from birth to maturity (according to Stratz)

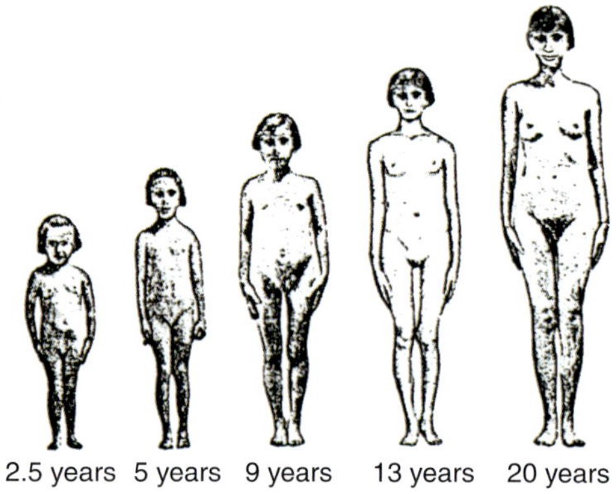

Fig. 2.3.6.
Changing proportions of the female body during the growth process

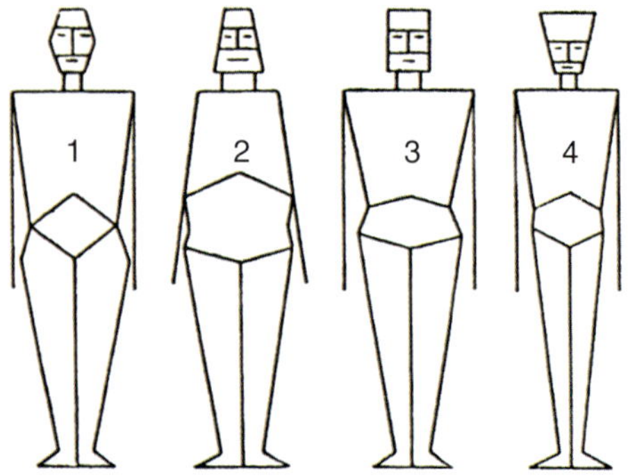

Fig. 2.3.7.
Scheme of body proportions in representatives of four types according to Sigaud classification.
1 - respiratory type; 2 - digestive type; 3 - muscular type; 4 - cerebral type

muscular body structure. The torso of Venus de Milo is a particularly eloquent illustration of this type.

4. The cerebral type is characterized by strong development of the brain, and accordingly, of the cerebral cranium. The forehead, which is high and broad, predominates over the other regions. Due to these features, the person's face acquires a pyramidal shape with the base directed upwards. The cerebral type is observed most frequently among famous people.

Segaud's classification was of great practical significance because it was noted that individuals belonging to a particular category were predisposed to certain diseases. For instance, diseases of the respiratory tract occurred more frequently among individuals belonging to the respiratory type, of the digestive tract among those belonging to the digestive type, of the motor apparatus among those belonging to the muscular type, and of the CNS among those belonging to the cerebral type.

Among the other morphological types proposed, the 'asthenic' constitution described by Schtiller in 1907 is worth mentioning. This type, which is observed frequently, is characterized by poor development of the transverse dimensions of the body relative to its length. The thorax is long and narrow, the trunk is short, and the lower extremities are relatively large. The musculoskeletal system is notably underdeveloped and the subcutaneous fat layer is poorly developed.

In addition to the above-mentioned constitutions inherent to normal subjects, pathological morphological types are distinguished. They are collectively called 'dysplastic' types. Dysfunctions of the endocrine glands are believed to be the cause.

Disproportions of genital origin (eunuchoid type). Gonadal endocrine insufficiency (hypogenitalism) delays the ossification of the epiphyseal cartilage, resulting in excessive tallness or even a gigantic height. This is mainly due to excessive lengthening of the limbs. The trunk, on the other hand, is relatively short and the pelvis is usually wide. Secondary pilosity of the body is weak or absent. In the hypergenital type, increased function of the endocrine glands causes early ossification of the epiphyseal cartilages, resulting in disproportionately short lower limbs, a long trunk and a big head.

Disproportion of pituitary origin. Insufficient pituitary function during the period of active growth leads to a sharp slowdown in growth and premature ageing. Hyperfunction of the cerebral appendage leads to excessive body growth (gigantism). When the disease manifests itself in adulthood, it takes the form of excessive growth of the limbs (acromegaly). In such cases, the growth of the distal ends of the limbs (hands and feet) is particularly active (Fig. 2.3.8). Acromegaly is also characterized by a relatively large oral fissure. Further, the tongue is enlarged (12.5 cm in length, 8.5 cm in width and 4 cm in thickness) and sometimes cannot be placed in the oral cavity, even

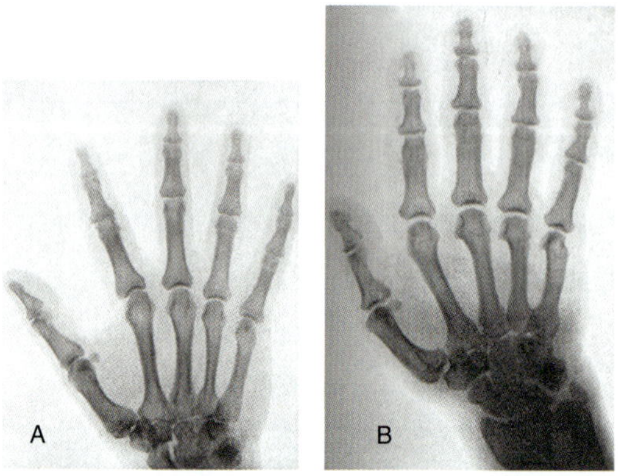

Fig. 2.3.8.
Hand radiographs in acromegaly: **A** - normal hand; **B** - hand of patient suffering acromegaly

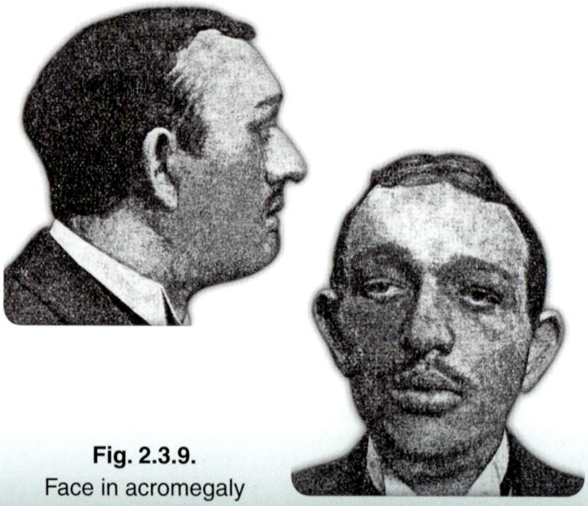

Fig. 2.3.9.
Face in acromegaly

sticking out constantly in some cases. The zygomatic bones and zygomatic processes of the frontal bones are thickened and enlarged, often to the extent that they stand out conspicuously. The edges of the orbits are greatly thickened and bulge out above the eyes. The auricles, particularly near the helices, are also thick and huge (Fig. 2.3.9).

Disproportion of thyroid origin. This refers to congenital hypoplasia of the thyroid gland. It causes marked developmental delay (dwarfism), due to which, in addition to myxoedema, the body retains the proportions of a child. The so-called cretinism among patients suffering from thyroid hormone deficiency due to unfavourable environmental conditions in some mountain areas (endemic cretinism) is characterized by short limbs, a relatively long trunk and a round head, with a markedly depressed root of the nose.

When studying the proportions of the human body, one should also consider the presence of several physiological disproportionalities, particularly the asymmetrical structure of the left and right sides of the body. According to Hasse, 'None of the adult body parts is formed strictly symmetrically. The halves of the head, neck, chest, abdomen and pelvis are not identical; also, the right and left limbs—both upper and lower—are not the same.' This may be observed quite clearly in photographs made in the correct anthropological position. In Fig. 2.3.10A, which shows an adult female as viewed from the back, deformity of the chest, a difference in the length of the arms (the right is lower), hypotrophy of the left gluteal region and pelvic bones, and relative shortening (23 mm) of the left foot are clearly visible. Following the use of a shoe inlaid of the required thickness (in the left shoe), the position of the body returned to normal (Fig. 2.3.10B).

Asymmetry of the head is manifested in various ways. Some typical examples are: the left half of the cerebral part of the cranium is smaller than the right; the right half of the face is longer than the left; the dorsum of the nose is not congruent with the median line; the tip of the nose is displaced to one side; or the distance between the outer corner of the eye and the corner of the mouth is not the same on both sides of the face (Fig. 2.3.11).

Extensive research carried out by the Parisian ophthalmologist, Liebreich, on several thousands of skulls, allowed him to find out that the most common manifestation of asymmetry was in the right zygomatic bone and the lower part of the maxillae being shifted to the right. As a result, the lower edge of the right orbit has a transverse direction and the left orbit slopes backwards. In rare cases, various parts of the facial skull are displaced to the left. Liebreich came to the conclusion that asymmetry of the head may be regarded as a feature that is characteristic of human beings, whatever their race or the period to which they belong.

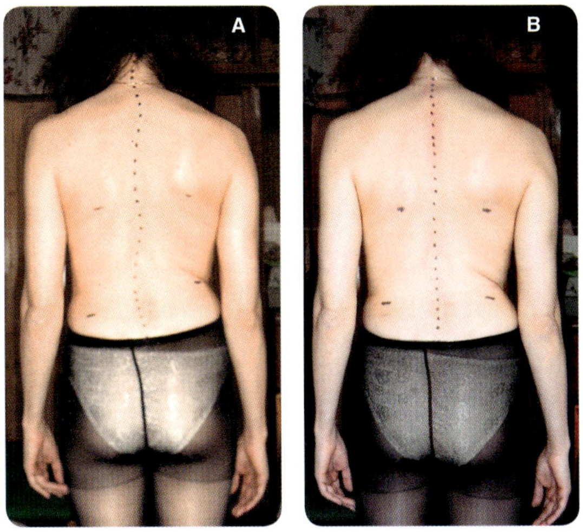

Fig. 2.3.10.
A - marked asymmetry in an adult woman aged 36; relative shortening of the left leg 23 mm; **B** - the same patient with correction of body deformation after insertion of shortening compensator

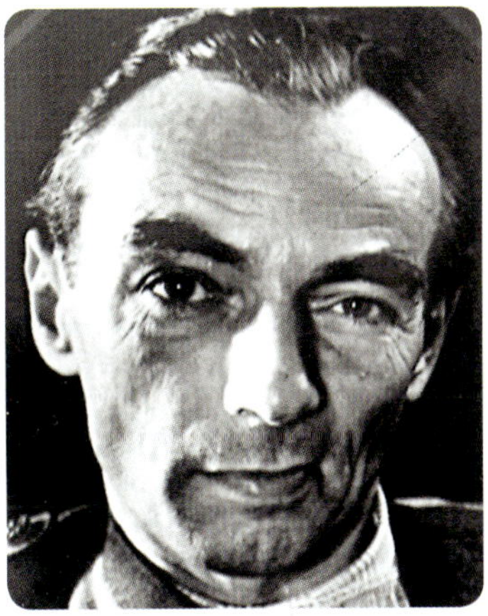

Fig. 2.3.11.
Severe facial asymmetry in an adult patient 50 years of age

Studies by Hasse showed that facial asymmetry could be observed in some of the statues made by Greek sculptors, particularly in the Venus de Milo. If one measures her face using a grid (Fig. 2.3.12), it is evident that only the lower part of the face (lips and chin) is symmetrical. Other parts are asymmetrical on the right and the left sides. The nose is shifted a bit to the right from the median line, the left auricle is higher than the right, the left orbit is located higher than the right. According to Henke, the asymmetrical facial features of the Venus de Milo probably are not the result of a conscious attempt by the artist. He made the portrait in a normal, realistic way depicting usual face structures. The

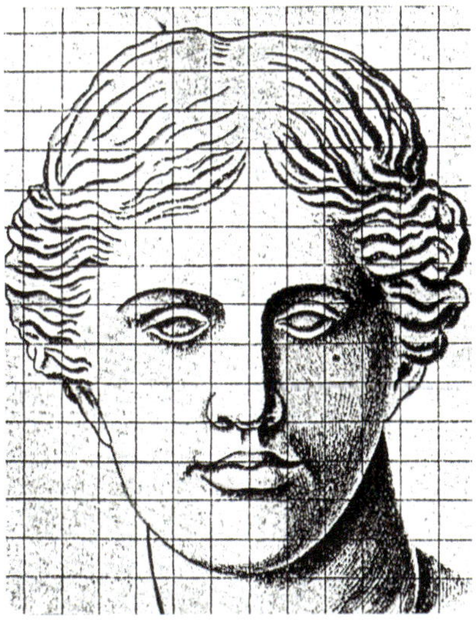

Fig. 2.3.12.
Head of Venus de Milo photographed through a grid

realistic features of the Venus de Milo have made her more natural and human.

Asymmetry is typical not only for the head, but also for the body. In 70% of people, the circumference of the right half of the thorax is greater than that of the left, the difference being 0.5–2.0 cm on an average. Moreover, the ribs on the right side are longer than those on the left, the sternum is asymmetrical (shifted to the left), and the nipples are at different levels.

There is clear evidence of asymmetry even when it comes to the size of the upper extremities. Following their studies on 5141 people, Hasse and Dehner found that in 75% of cases, the right arm is longer than the left. Asymmetry was evident not only in the length of the arms, but also in their circumference, owing to better development of muscles on the right side. As for the lower extremities, their findings were as follows: in 75% of cases, the left limb was shorter than the right; in 18%, both extremities were practically of equal size; and in only 7%, the right limb was shorter than the left. A difference in the length of the left and the right limbs is a characteristic feature even in newborns (Fig. 2.3.13).

In functional terms, asymmetry of the upper limbs is apparent in the marked predominance of right-handedness over left-handedness. On an average, left-handers constitute 5% of adults. Asymmetry of the upper limbs has been observed even in the skeletons of Neanderthals (Neanderthal, La Chapelle-aux-Saints, La Ferrassie). The presence of asymmetry in the length of the limb bones was observed in anthropomorphic apes (Mollison).

There are reasons to believe that there is a certain asymmetry of the limbs even in mammals other than human beings, although the asymmetry in such cases is less pronounced. This is illustrated by the fact that animals, like human beings, move in circles when they lose visual control, as in foggy conditions. This is because of the functional predominance of the motor apparatus of one side of the body over that of the other side. Since the size of the steps taken by the right and left limbs is unequal, the animal or person moves not in a straight line but in a circular path, the diameter of the circle being a few kilometres. This is evident, for example, from Guldberg's observations in Norway of the movements of people in the mist (Fig. 2.3.14). Animals in the same conditions were moving like the people studied. Some hold that circular motion is a general biological feature, which has developed in the course of evolution and can be explained by the fact that the animal cannot go

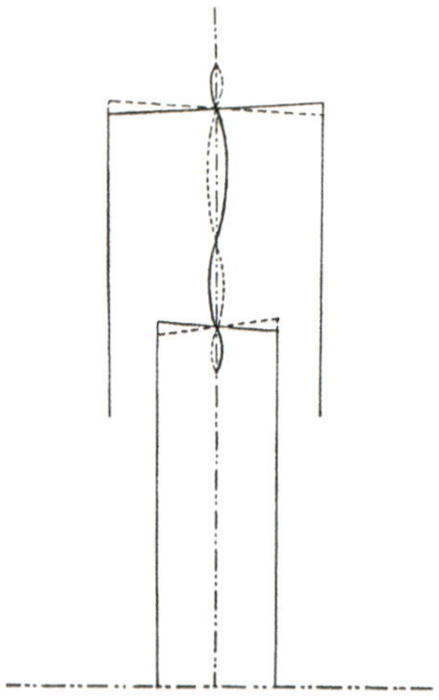

Fig. 2.3.13. Schematic presentation of body asymmetry due to unequal length of lower extremities (according to Hasse)

too far from its habitat. In any case, bilateral asymmetry of the motor apparatus is characteristic not only of humans, but also of all higher vertebrates.

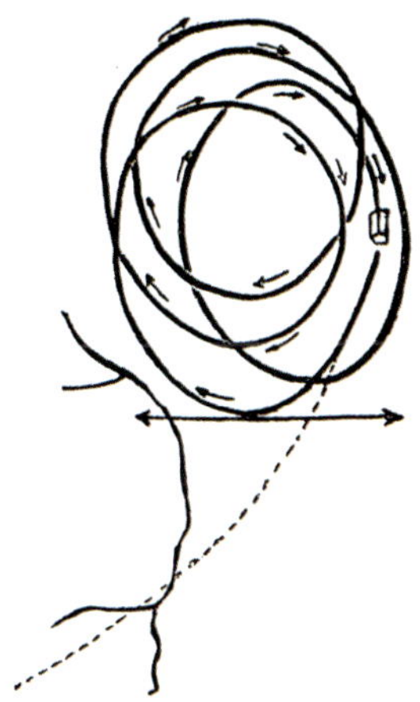

Fig. 2.3.14.
Circular routes that were made by three people travelling in foggy weather, until they reached the hut again, which was the starting point of their journey. The dashed line denotes the intended route (by Guldberg)

1. The contents of these last two chapters, as well as the questions still left unanswered, may be summarized as follows. Asymmetry of the body structure is characteristic of all human beings, without exception, as well as all other vertebrates, i.e. this is the law of nature. Whereas asymmetry of the face, eye slits, eyebrows, ears and arms leads only to cosmetic defects, that of the lower limbs (with difference in length) leads to an imbalance, i.e. sloping of the pelvis towards the shorter side. Most frequently, it is due to differences in the muscle tension of the spinal extensors. In 80% or more, this asymmetry is observed on the left side and in only 20% on the right. It is known as relative shortening. There are also cases of absolute shortening of one leg. This arises from a difference in the length of the femur and/or shinbone of the two sides. These are due to different pathologies of the hip, e.g. congenital hip dislocation and aseptic necrosis of the femoral head. Absolute shortening can occur due to other causes as well, but these are extremely rare. The greater the difference between the length of the legs, the greater is the degree of pelvic tilt.
2. Tilting of the pelvis results in lateral curvature of the spine, as well as rotational displacement of the cervical, thoracic, lumbar and sacral vertebrae.
3. An explanation needs to be found for the facts that have come to light and the questions raised must be answered. What causes asymmetry of the trunk muscles, not only in adults, but in the newborn as well? Why are the muscles on the right side of the trunk stronger than those on the left in the vast majority of cases? What causes torsion (turning) of the vertebrae and why does it occur strictly in particular places? Is this an accident or a rule? Which changes occur when the medulla oblongata and spinal cord are compressed, and when the vertebral arteries and veins, nerves and plexuses are clamped? How do various diseases of the internal organs, skin, etc. emerge? Finally, how does one explain the emergence of spinal pain?

The next chapter attempts to answer these questions, as well as throw light on the mechanism of asymmetrical positioning of the trunk and the formation of scoliosis deformity.

3 Body asymmetry, its causes and consequences

(principles of formation of lateral spine curvature)

THE MAIN QUESTIONS DEALT WITH IN THIS CHAPTER ARE:

- What causes body asymmetry?
- How does lateral curvature of the spine develop?
- What comes first—lateral curvature or muscle asymmetry? What is the relationship between the two?
- Are there any regularities in the formation of spinal curvatures? What are the stages of this process?

While trying to answer these questions, we found ourselves in a difficult situation because the required information was not available in the literature, and that which was available had not been put together in a systematic manner. Therefore, along with clinical work, aimed mainly at helping patients with spinal pain of various kinds and treating children with scoliosis, we decided to study special publications. The information in this chapter was collected literally brick by brick, or in fragments, from a wide range of sources of information. When the diverse pieces of information were put together, we were able to form a complete picture of scoliosis and other spinal deformities. The relation between spinal deformities and spinal pain as well as a variety of other diseases that affect all age groups will be discussed in subsequent chapters.

It is spinal pain that causes patients to seek help in clinics and hospitals. Most often, the pain is accompanied by spinal deformities, such as scoliosis, kyphosis, kyphoscoliosis, spondylosis and spondylitis, spondylolisthesis and degenerative disc disease. However, the causes of radicular pain in different regions of the spine are extremely diverse, and may include trauma, the presence of benign or malignant processes, osteoarthritis, osteoporosis, and the presence of specific or non-specific inflammatory processes. Spinal pain may be a reflection of a large variety of internal diseases.

It must be noted, however, that the number of patients with the pathologies mentioned above is significantly smaller than that of those who do not have these pathologies but nevertheless suffer from spinal pain without any apparent cause.

They may suffer pain, for example, while stooping over the sink or rotating the body when lifting loads. This occurs more frequently among adults. However, children, adolescents and physically strong young people may also suffer such pain. We worked on determining the causes of spinal pain in these individuals and, at the same time, discovering the reasons why these 'beginners' develop serious diseases later in life. While trying to unravel this mystery, we also gained an understanding of the significant role of degenerative disc disease (spinal osteochondrosis) in the development of pain. Due to its high prevalence, spinal osteochondrosis is called 'the disease of the century'. In an adult with spinal pain, osteochondrosis, along with various other spinal deformities, may certainly play an important pathogenic role.

And what about the occurrence of spinal pain in a child of 1.5–2 years of age? What causes it? In recent years, the term 'paediatric osteochondrosis' has come into use. As discussed in the next chapter, osteochondrosis exists among children and adolescents, but its prevalence is low and the condition is associated with hereditary abnormalities of the spine. Here, we will discuss an everyday situation in which a physician observes some sign of spinal pain while examining a child.

I often see patients who have cervical pain and pain in the interscapular region, and who have been diagnosed with 'osteochondrosis' by their physicians without even getting a radiography done. The idea that the pain is associated with spinal osteochondrosis is firmly lodged in the mind of doctors and patients. This diagnosis allows the physician to explain the lack of effectiveness of the treatment prescribed by him. Further, having made this diagnosis, he is not compelled to search for the true cause of the disease. We perform detorsional correction in such patients and the pain immediately resolves. Detorsional correction is preceded by an obligatory analysis of radiographs and, if necessary, CT scans. In some cases, these do show signs of degenerative disc disease, but this is not so in the majority of patients. Does the success of detorsional correction mean that osteochondrosis can be healed with simple and non-traumatic movement of the body or 10 minutes of cervical traction using a pneumatic rubber collar? Of course not! Rather, it means that the pain has some other cause, which may be found in young children, adolescents, adults, and even very old people.

When the door to my office opens and the next patient comes in, I know in advance that the reason for the consultation is one of the two following problems.

1. If the patient is a child, he has usually been brought for consultation because of a scoliotic spinal deformity. The standard complaints that accompany this deformity include headaches and/or dizziness, impaired vision and/or hearing and/or memory, fatigue in the legs, cramps in the calf muscles at night, emotional

lability, sweaty hands and feet, tendency to constipation and allergies. Bedwetting may also be observed. The number of complaints and their severity depend on the degree of deformation, age, skeletal anomalies, etc.

2. Among adult patients, the usual complaints include spinal pain in its various manifestations, in the backdrop of scoliotic posture, as well as degenerative disc disease and spondylosis of varying degrees of severity. There may be muscle pain and tightness in the cervicothoracic region. Fluctuations in the blood pressure are characteristic; the patient may suffer from numbness and spasms of the fingers. If the thoracic region is affected, there may be retrosternal pain, shortness of breath, arrhythmia, extrasystoles, etc. (The characteristics of the pain and associated symptoms, which depend on the localization of the pathological process, will be discussed in detail in subsequent chapters.)

Our data on spinal deformities and spinal pain can be of great practical value, both for the enquiring patient and the ordinary physician. It can also be of use to those living and working in rural areas. Understanding the problem may improve the quality of care for people suffering from these conditions. As mentioned earlier, we have observed that the clinical picture is the same in all individuals, regardless of age and sex. In this context, I would like to bring to the reader's notice that the youngest patient we have treated was two-and-a-half months old and the oldest, 89 years old.

Among our patients was a child who had just learnt to walk. He already had a slight deformation of the chest (scapula protruding posteriorly), which could be felt even through his thin clothing. In the majority of cases the right scapula is protruding. When the child was placed in a prone position and his clothes were taken off, rotational displacement of the spinous processes of the 5th–7th thoracic vertebrae was clearly visible. The processes were located above and below the deformity. Similar curves were observed in the upper thoracic and lumbosacral regions.

When examining infants, palpation of the spine shows that the overall width of the m. erector trunci varies substantially at the site of its attachment to the sacrum. In most cases, the right part is wider than the left. According to Professor I.A. Movshovich (1964), this is not due to muscle hypertrophy but due to posterior protrusion of the muscle, caused by deviation of the transverse processes of the lumbar vertebrae as a result of torsion. This explanation is acceptable in the case of a person who is walking, but not in the case of one who is lying down. Also, it does not apply to babies, who cannot walk. How do muscle asymmetry and lateral curvature of the spine appear? What comes first—lateral curvature of spine or asymmetry of the muscles? How do they depend on each other? What is the interrelation, if any, between them?

In this context, an interesting fact is that muscular asymmetry and spinal deformities are observed not only among infants but also among newborns. Does this mean that everything begins during intrauterine development? We have observed asymmetry of the m. erector trunci in all the adult patients we have examined (*see* Chapters 1 and 2).

The fact that this muscular asymmetry was always associated with lateral curvature of the spine is of great importance. Left-sided thoracic curvature was observed in cases in which the width of the left extensor of the spine was increased. When the width of the right extensors was greater, the trunk curved in the opposite direction (*see* Chapter 1). Among children, the curvature of the trunk was manifested minimally, but it progressed with age.

Asymmetry of the trunk muscles and lateral curvature of the spine were observed among absolutely all patients and even among healthy people who did not have any complaints. In view of this, we believe that it is not unreasonable to suggest that the coexistence of asymmetry of the trunk muscles and lateral curvature of the spine is the law of nature. Also, these two features are often associated with a third one—spinal pain.

It is not only one particular part of the trunk that is characterized by asymmetry. As mentioned earlier, it is typical of the whole body and can be clearly observed in the face as well as the pelvic area. From the frontal view, all individuals, regardless of nationality and without exception, have an asymmetrical face (one eyebrow is higher than the other). Watching the faces of students hurrying to class in the morning would be enough to illustrate my words. If the reader wishes to notice the signs of asymmetry in the pelvic region, it is best to observe people during summer, when they are wearing thin clothes. Viewed from the posterior all people have a body asymmetry—one scapula protrudes more posteriorly than the other, similarly there is a difference in the sizes of the buttocks.

3.1 Origin of body asymmetry

By now, we have seen that asymmetry of the body muscles and lateral curvature of the spine are present among all individuals, and that these are often associated with pain. In the previous chapter on the anatomy of the spine, we mentioned that the spine of each individual has a curvature and some scientists consider this to be the norm. But if this is the norm, where does the pathology begin? We already know that spinal pain always appears with scoliotic deformity in the background. Therefore, it was logical to start searching for answers about their origin not in pain as a consequence, but in the initial cause(s) of the lateral curvature of the spine. In our view, the development of spinal pain is preceded by the development of asymmetry of the trunk muscles. For this reason, we have arranged the issues raised in the beginning of this chapter in the following sequence:

- What causes asymmetry of the body?
- How does lateral curvature of the spine develop?
- What comes first—lateral curvature or muscle asymmetry?
- What is the interrelation between them?

While searching for the answers, we studied the issue in depth and familiarized ourselves with the classic works of national and foreign orthopaedic experts, as well as experts in anatomy and physiology (V.D. Chaklin, 1958; I.A. Movshovich, 1964; V.Y. Fischenko, 2005; D. Stillwell, 1962; D. Hubel, 1979; R.F. Schmidt and G. Thews, 1983; F. Bloom, A. Lazerson and L. Hofstadter, 1988, etc.). Our study of the subject yielded the following information.

3.1.1 Anatomy and physiology of interhemispheric differences

In 1968, on the basis of a detailed post-mortem examination of the brain of 100 individuals, Norman Geschwind and Walter Levitsky (cited from *Brain*, *Mind* and

Behavior by F.E. Bloom, A. Lazerson and L. Hofstadter, 1988) reported significant anatomical differences between the hemispheres. In 65% of cases, the area of the temporal cortex, which overlaps the Wernicke's area (also known as the planum temporale and is responsible for semantic speech), was greater in the left hemisphere (Group 1), and only in 11% of cases was it greater in the right hemisphere (Group 2). In 24% of cases, such interhemispheric differences were not observed (Group 3).

In later years, the same researchers studied and measured hundreds of other post-mortem brains. Their findings were similar to the earlier ones. In approximately 70% of cases, the planum temporale of the left hemisphere was significantly larger than that of the right (Figs 3.1.1 and 3.1.2). This asymmetry was characteristic of the brain of the foetus as well. It was also found that the Sylvian fissure, a deep sulcus in the cerebral cortex that separates the temporal lobe from the rest of the cortex in the left hemisphere, is longer and straighter. In the right hemisphere, the same Sylvian fissure is curved upward to a greater degree. This asymmetry had been identified in studies of human fossil skulls (Neanderthals), on the basis of which the authors suggested that asymmetry of the hemispheres is likely to be a part of the human genetic heritage.

Stephen Wilson and Jenny Regan, scientists from the University College of London, have also reported on asymmetry of the cerebral hemispheres, as well as unequal distribution of functions between them, with the left hemisphere predominating.

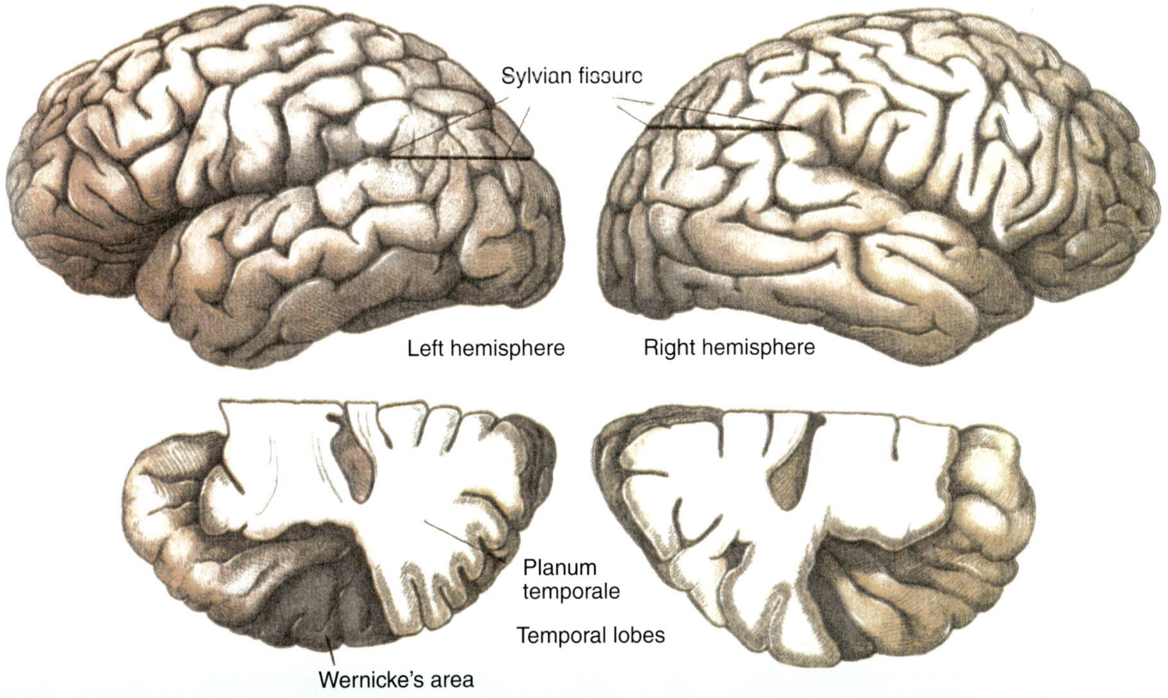

Fig. 3.1.1. Anatomical asymmetry of cerebral hemispheres. **Above:** Sylvian fissure in the right hemisphere is deflected upward at an acute angle. **Below:** posterior part of the planum temporale is usually much larger in the left hemisphere, which is associated with speech.

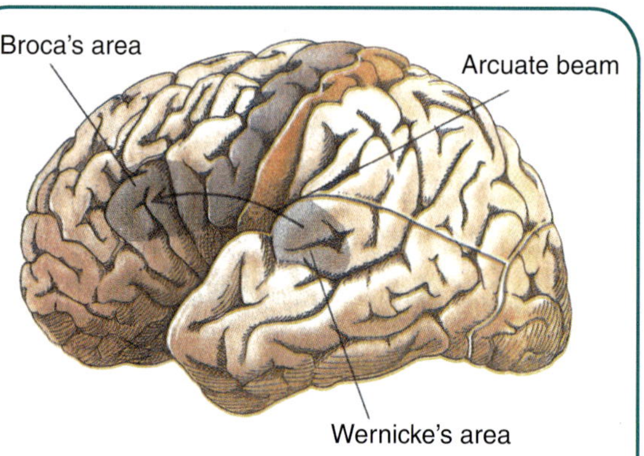

Fig. 3.1.2.
Areas of the left hemisphere involved in speech and its perception; Wernicke's and Broca's areas are interconnected via a fibrous tract — so-called fasciculus arcuatum (arrow), because this structure is not visible from the outside

The specimens were obtained from experiments with the zebrafish species ('Cerebral hemispheres are having a real war for neurons', *News of Medicine and Pharmacy,* Ukraine, No. 3–4 [269–270], February 2009, p. 11).

It may be noted that the right hemisphere controls the sensory and motor functions of the left side of the body, while the left controls those of the right side. In 95% of right-handed persons, the left hemisphere is responsible for language and speech, and is thus known as dominant. The right hemisphere controls skills associated with visual and spatial experience. It is called non-dominant.

The psychological research carried out by the authors mentioned above revealed other important details of the physiology of the brain. For example, it was shown that in most cases, women are superior to men in verbal skills but are inferior to them with respect to mathematical and 'spatial' abilities. These differences are already noticeable in childhood. Girls begin to talk and read earlier than boys. Among children who are unable to read, the number of boys exceeds that of girls by four times.

We shall now discuss the structure and functioning of the hemispheres of the brain in the prenatal period (intrauterine development). As Norman Geschwind (1982) (cited from *Brain, Mind* and *Behavior* by F.E. Bloom, A. Lazerson and L. Hofstadter, 1988) showed, the gonads or sex glands are formed in the sixth week after fertilization; initially, they are the same in both sexes. If the foetus is male, then in the third month of intrauterine development, under the influence of one or more genes of the Y-chromosome, the gonads start to differentiate into testes and secrete the male hormone, testosterone. Although testosterone is present in a low concentration in the female foetus (since a certain amount of it is produced by the mother), the level of this hormone increases greatly in the male foetus after the formation of the testes. The high level of testosterone during intrauterine development inhibits the growth of the left hemisphere in the male foetus as compared to the female, and facilitates the relatively greater development of the right hemisphere in males.

If it is true that testosterone has an inhibitory effect on the development of the left hemisphere, then it can possibly explain the differences between the cerebral hemispheres of the two sexes.

The information obtained by us can be summarized as follows:

1. The left and right cerebral hemispheres are asymmetrical, a characteristic which is predetermined genetically.
2. In 95% of people who are right-handed, speech and language are controlled by the left hemisphere, while in the remaining 5% who are left-handed, they are controlled by the right hemisphere.
3. Broca's area is a specific part of the left frontal lobe that controls all the muscles of the face, tongue, jaws and throat. This is achieved through connections of this area with the anterior central gyrus, the cortical area responsible for motor functions of the right side of the body. Broca's area can be called the motor centre for speech.
4. Wernicke's area, the posterior part of the first temporal gyrus, is responsible for semantic speech. In 65%–70% of cases, this area is larger in the left hemisphere (1st group).
5. Wernicke's and Broca's areas are interconnected by a fibrous tract that allows them to function in a synchronized manner, i.e. motor and semantic speech constitute a single process.
6. Taking into consideration the functional connection of Broca's area and Wernicke's area, one can assume that both of them function more actively in the left hemisphere (1st group) than the right. This leads to an increase in muscle tone on the right side of the body. This applies not only to the muscles of the head and neck but also to the spinal extensors (Fig. 3.1.3). The asymmetrical contractile ability of the spinal extensors results in relative shortening of the left lower limb on the weaker side, as well as left-sided scoliosis of the trunk in the lumbar area. It is interesting to note that mimetic spasm is the cause of facial asymmetry (*see* Chapter 1).
7. Among those people (11%) in whom the planum temporale is more developed in the right hemisphere (2nd group), hypertonus of the spinal extensors is greater on the left side, leading to a curvature of the body to the right. This results in relative shortening of the right leg (Fig. 3.1.4).
8. In 24% of cases, the volume of the planum temporale is the same (3rd group) and, therefore, the face and other parts of the body should be symmetrical. However, our clinical observations have shown that this is doubtful, as there is no symmetry in nature. Thus, there is a need for physiologists to confirm the veracity of this information.
9. During the development of the male foetus, the growth of the left hemisphere is inhibited by the secretion of a high level of testosterone. In boys, such underdevelopment of the left hemisphere, particularly of Wernicke's area, explains why there are four times as many boys as girls among the population of children who are unable to read, and why girls have better verbal skills than boys.
10. If we agree with the fact that Broca's and Wernicke's area are four times more

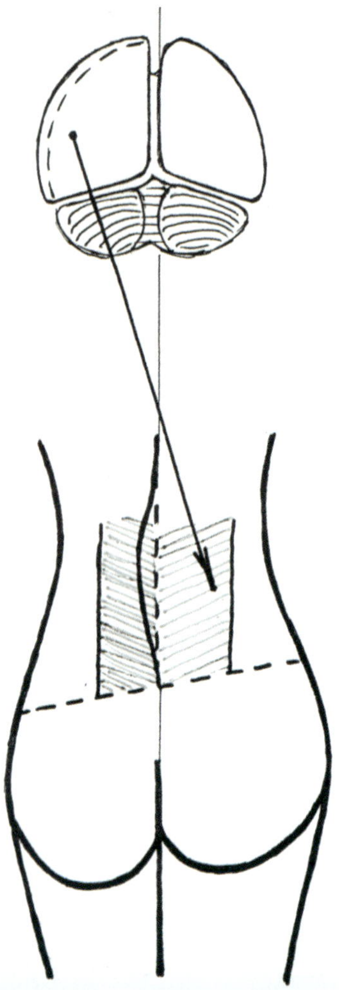

Fig. 3.1.3.
Hypertonus of extensors of spine on the right is caused by increased functional activity of gyrus centralis anterior of the left hemisphere

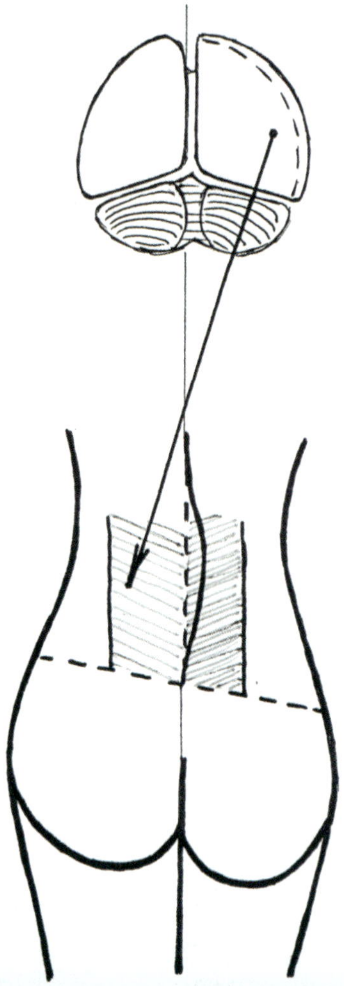

Fig. 3.1.4.
Hypertonus of extensor muscles of spine on the left is caused by increased functional activity of gyrus centralis anterior of the right hemisphere

active among girls than boys, it means that tonus of the spinal extensors, especially on the right side, is four times more pronounced among girls. Further, if the left hemisphere is smaller in boys than in girls, the difference in tone of the trunk muscles would increase even more. This probably explains the universally known fact, which has been mentioned in the literature, that lateral (scoliotic) curvature occurs 5–6 times more frequently among girls than boys.

11. As the newborn grows, asymmetry of the trunk muscles gets imprinted in the cerebellum, which controls all movements. Indeed, the cerebellum is called the 'keeper of conditioned reflexes'. In our view, the conditioned reflex that keeps the vertical body position develops from the time when a child takes her or his first steps, and then during the following months when the child becomes capable of standing in a stable upright posture and walking steadily.

12. In girls, this process occurs faster than in boys, which is why they begin to walk earlier. However, unfortunately, this conditioned reflex—let us call it 'vicious'—preserves the wrong body posture, either leaning to the right or to the left. This is how a child enters life and this is how he remains in all subsequent periods of his life, unless he meets a competent orthopaedic surgeon.

This is why anatomists consider body curvature to be normal. In fact, it is characteristic of all individuals.

Thus, it may be said that asymmetry of the body occurs due to certain features of the development of the brain, and begins to develop as early as the foetal stage. Newborns have asymmetry of the trunk muscles. Later, when they begin to walk, different degrees of tension of the spinal extensors on the two sides lead to the formation of a lateral curvature of the spine, which should be called a physiological scoliotic posture.

The degree of inclination of the body and the transition from the physiological to the pathological state (scoliotic disease) depends both on the tone of the trunk extensors and the structural features of the spine, which in most cases are genetically determined. In the situation which we describe, we do not consider a variety of specific and non-specific pathological processes that may affect the structure of the musculoskeletal system.

The preceding information suggests that during the intrauterine period up to birth, *it is only the cerebral mechanism that is responsible for lateral curvature of the spine.* However, after birth, other than cerebral factors are involved as well. Various theories on the aetiology of scoliosis proposed by numerous authors and our analysis of them are presented next.

3.2 Scoliotic disease

We shall now look into the causes and mechanisms of the development of scoliotic disease. Without this knowledge, we cannot understand the aetiopathogenesis of spinal pain. To tell the truth, when I began writing this book on spinal pain, I had not expected that we would need to make a thorough study of scoliosis. However, it is now clear that spinal pain is inextricably linked with scoliosis and vice versa, and scoliosis is the leading cause of spinal pain. This extremely complicated issue will be tackled step by step in the following pages.

Scoliosis as a disease is considered one of the most difficult areas of orthopaedics. As the eminent German orthopaedist A. Schantz said, spinal diseases are among the most obscure areas of pathology. The problem of scoliosis has been, and remains, a subject of keen interest in all orthopaedic clinics in the world. We had to muster up considerable courage and work tenaciously, on the basis of our own extensive clinical material, to try and uncover from a new angle the essence of the disease and the mechanisms of its occurrence. The fact that such attempts have been made by many highly qualified professionals was also daunting.

The first precise description of scoliosis was given by Ambroise Paré (1510–1590), the famous French surgeon who was also the first to propose treating the condition with a cast made of perforated plates that immobilize the chest. Hippocrates knew of scoliosis and placed it the category of serious disorders that significantly shorten the life of a patient. This problem was studied thoroughly in the early medieval period. Hippocrates treated scoliosis with respiratory gymnastics, singing and bandaging the chest. He is the one who coined the terms scoliosis, kyphosis and lordosis. Glisson, Fabricius and Hildanus used medical gymnastics and various devices for treatment.

It is with deep respect and appreciation that I make a mention of many prominent national and foreign orthopaedic surgeons who made great contributions to investigations of the aetiology, pathogenesis, morphology and pathology of scoliosis. These include E.A. Abalmasova, F.R. Bogdanov, M.V. Volkov, R. Voronovich, R.R. Vreden, I. Herzen, G.H. Gruntovsky, D.A. Ivashchenko, A. Kazmin, I. Cohn, A. Korzh, M.I. Kuslik, Z.A. Lyandres, V.O. Marks, I.M. Mitbreyt, I.A. Movshovich, N.P. Novachenko, E.K. Nikiforova, E.Y. Osten-Sacken, N. Prior, A.K. Prikhodko,

T.A. Revenko, G.I. Turner, V.Y. Fischenko, N.I. Hvisyuk, Y.L. Tsivyan, W. Chaklin, S.D. Shevchenko, L.I. Shulutko, A. Farkas, Frejk, Jaroz, Hnevkovsky, A. Gruca, C. Nicoladoni, K. Lindemann, L. Lorenz, K. Matzen, G. Muller, I. Ponseti, Radulesku, R. Roaf, A. Schanz, W. Schulthess, *et al.*

Though we examined the literature extensively, I would like to particularly mention some of the studies that gave us a deep understanding of the aetiology and pathogenesis of scoliosis, which subsequently allowed us to draw our own conclusions. These works are: G. Muller, *Orthopaedics for Practicing Physicians*, SPb, 1913; A. Schantz, *Practical Orthopedics*, Moscow, 1933; I. Movshovich, *Scoliosis. Surgical Anatomy and Pathogenesis*, Moscow, 1964; V.Y. Fischenko *et al. Non-surgical Treatment of Scoliosis*, K, 1994; V.Y. Fischenko, *Scoliosis*, Makeevka, 2005, etc. In the ultimate analysis, our conclusions were based on our own extensive clinical experience with more than 8000 patients who were of different ages and suffering from spinal pain.

It is not possible, and perhaps not necessary, to present a deep analysis of each of the works we studied. Therefore, these works will be discussed briefly, only to the extent necessary for understanding the major aspects of the problem. Moreover, the discussion will be simple enough because this book is intended not only for professionals (orthopaedic surgeons and medical students), but also for the ordinary reader who has basic medical knowledge. Before proceeding to analyse the causes and mechanisms of the development of scoliosis, it would be useful to describe the anatomical and physiological features of the spine in this condition.

Anatomical and physiological features of the spine in scoliosis

The human spine consists of 24 vertebrae (excluding the sacral and coccygeal vertebrae), which are more or less firmly interconnected with each other. Seven of them are cervical, 12 thoracic and 5 lumbar. Twelve pairs of ribs (7 pairs of true and 5 pairs of spurious ribs) are connected with 12 vertebrae. The pairs of true ribs are connected with the sternum frontally, the 8th–10th pairs meet anteriorly to form the costal arch, and the 11th–12th pairs end freely without connection to the sternum. The 24 vertebrae and the discs are surrounded by a framework of dense ligaments and together, these form a strong pillar that supports the body. Despite the fact that the vertebrae are held together very tightly, the junctions between successive vertebrae allow for a slight degree of mobility. As a result, the whole spine is characterized by a certain degree of flexibility. This can be increased significantly through exercise, such as in the case of acrobats, gymnasts and circus performers. Bending forward, backwards and sideways, as well as lateral rotation, are known to increase the flexibility of the spine.

The spine is not straight and has bends, which are considered merely physiological as long as they are within certain limits and are located in the frontal plane. The following curvatures of the spine are recognized: anterior curvature of the cervical spine (lordosis), posterior curvature of the thoracic spine (kyphosis), lumbar lordosis and finally, kyphosis of the sacrococcygeal region.

Let us now discuss the reasons for the formation of these physiological curvatures, which are not present in a newborn. As long as a baby is in the prone position, the entire spine forms a straight line. The spine bends backwards during the initial attempts to sit up. Once the child begins to stand or walk systematically, the posterior convex curvature is replaced by the curvatures described above. This process is as follows.

In the caudal region of the spine, the sacral bone, which rests between the two iliac bones, is not free to move, while the rudimentary tailbone ends freely. While sitting, the body rests on three points on the tubera ischii and coccyx (rear sitting) or on the tubera ischii and lower surfaces of the thighs (front sitting). In either of these positions, the surface area on which the spine rests is adequate for it to support itself and, therefore, it does not require balancing. Both in children and adults, when sitting, the spine is in a vertical position in the case of those who are not tired, and forms a single convex arch in the case of those who are in a state of fatigue.

When standing or walking, the conditions are different. The spine no longer has the three points of support and must depend on only one point, located in the middle of an imaginary line connecting the two hip joints. The situation is further complicated by the fact that this point is located in front of the spine; thus if a person tries to get up and follow his centre of gravity, he would fall forward. The entire upper body would be bent and would fall forward due to the vertical position of the pelvis and the fact that the joints between the sacral and iliac bones are not mobile if there is no flexion of the lumbar spine. It is only due to the formation of lumbar spine curvature (lordosis) that lumbar spine flexion is possible. The process of development of this curvature occurs at two more points. The upper part of the body would become too heavy and fall backwards were it not for a kyphotic curvature, i.e. if we did not bend the head and neck forward. The head would fall forward if it was not supported by cervical lordosis. Therefore, these three physiological curvatures serve a purpose. They are necessary to move the pivot point on the sheer line. These physiological curves are formed during the first two years of life.

As for the kyphotic configuration of the sacrum, it probably makes for optimal location of the large and small pelvis, besides facilitating childbearing function in women.

Apart from the fact that these physiological curvatures are a necessity, they also have an aesthetic value. It is because of these curvatures that the spine and, therefore the back, form a winding line that lends beauty to the structure of a normally built individual. Of course, such beauty is possible only if the degree of the curves is moderate. Curvatures that are too pronounced or too weakly accentuated should not be considered physiological but pathological. Also, curvatures should not be considered normal if they are not located in the frontal plane and if the spine forms at least one slight lateral curvature. Then it becomes scoliotic or kyphoscoliotic curvature of the spine. A more pronounced posterior curvature in the thoracic region is known as accentuated kyphosis (slouching), and when this is combined with accentuated lordosis (forward curvature), it is termed 'roundback'.

The preceding sentences might seem to imply that the distinction between physiological and pathological spinal curvature is based on the concept of beauty and, therefore, the whole question of scoliosis is a matter of aesthetics. However, it is known that the development of forms in nature is determined by expediency and, thus, beauty of form and expediency are closely linked. In the case of spinal deformities, pathological formations not only lack beauty, but are also not expedient and, in some cases, are even dangerous to the life and health of an individual. Dealing with scoliosis is, therefore, not only a problem of aesthetics, but is also extremely important from a medical point of view. Other than attempting to keep the beauty of the human body intact, a physician's aim is to protect people from serious illness and premature death.

Asymmetry of the trunk

During clinical examination of a patient with scoliosis, it is the asymmetry of the body that first draws one's attention. Usually, the primary reason for which parents visit an orthopaedic surgeon is that they have noticed asymmetry of the trunk in their child.

The features of the deformities of the trunk depend on the location of the curvatures of the spine and their number. Thus, in scoliosis of the upper thoracic spine, there is a marked inclination of the head towards the concave side; the shoulder girdles are at different levels and the contours of the neck are asymmetrical. In the case of a single curvature in the thoracic spine, the distance between the shoulder blades and the spinous processes remains almost the same on both sides, and their lower angles are located at the level of one pair of ribs (Fig. 3.2.1). Thus, in a solitary thoracic spinal curvature, the position of the arc of the shoulder blades is symmetrical.

Two adjacent curvatures in the thoracic region give rise to asymmetry, with the shoulder blades being located at different levels relative to the vertical line that may be drawn through the spinous process of the 7th cervical vertebra (Fig. 3.2.2). Analysing the mechanism of the asymmetrical positioning of the shoulder blades, I.A. Movshovich concluded that the rhomboid and trapezius muscles play the main role in such cases (Fig. 3.2.3). It was this author who proposed and described the 'symptom of shoulder blades positioning'. Looking out for this symptom is of great importance in the clinical examination of patients with scoliosis.

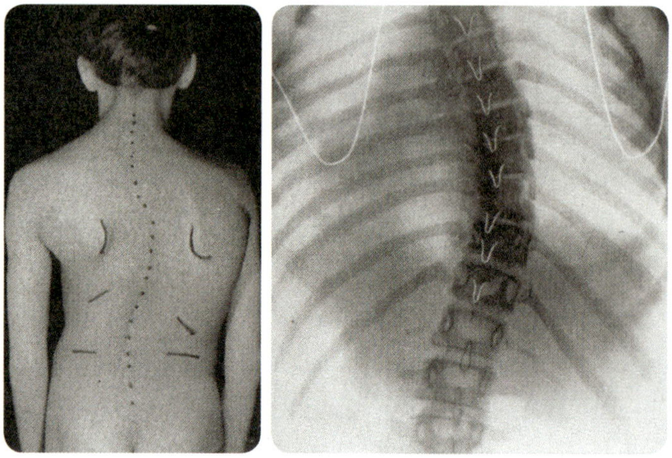

A B

Fig. 3.2.1.
Right-sided thoracic scoliosis; inferior angles of scapulae are located at the level of 7th pair of ribs and at the same distance from the spinous processes (negative 'symptom of scapulae positioning'): **A** - patient photo, **B** - plain radiograph

In second- and sometimes first-degree lumbar scoliosis, a muscular cushion is formed on the convex side of the curvature. This is the so-called 'Chaklin symptom' which indicates the presence of torsion of the spine due to a change in the volume of the m. erector spinae. Curvature of the lumbar spine also leads to flattening of the waistline on the convex side of the curvature and the waistline becomes more pronounced on the concave side. Sometimes a transverse line is formed (Fig. 3.2.4).

As in the lumbar region, a muscle ridge is also formed on the convex side of the thoracic curvature resulting in torsion of the spine, but the formation of the rib hump masks this cushion. How do we explain the emergence of a 'massive' m. erector spinae on the convex side of the curvature? Should it be seen in terms of muscular hypertrophy or should it be considered a mechanical protrusion caused by the underlying bony structures? Morphological studies of the trunk muscles by I.A. Movshovich showed that there is no muscular hypertrophy on the convex side of the spinal curvature; on the contrary, there is a degenerative process. Thus, the bulging of the muscle is a result of torsion of the lumbar vertebrae and posterior deviation of the transverse processes (Fig. 3.2.5). The obligatory condition (*sine qua non*) for the identification of this symptom is symmetrical positioning of the legs (the feet are together). Bending and rotation of the body are also related to the functioning of the m. erector

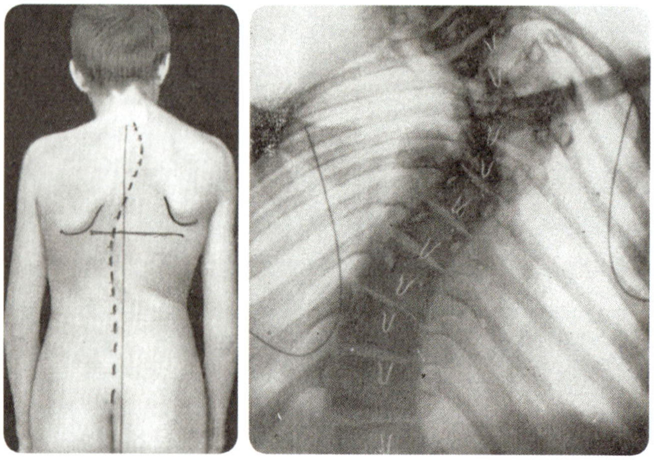

A B

Fig. 3.2.2.
Right-sided upper thoracic and left-sided lower thoracic scoliosis; right scapula is located farther from the spinous processes of lower thoracic curvature and higher than the left scapula (positive 'symptom of scapulae positioning'): **A** - patient photo, **B** - plain radiograph

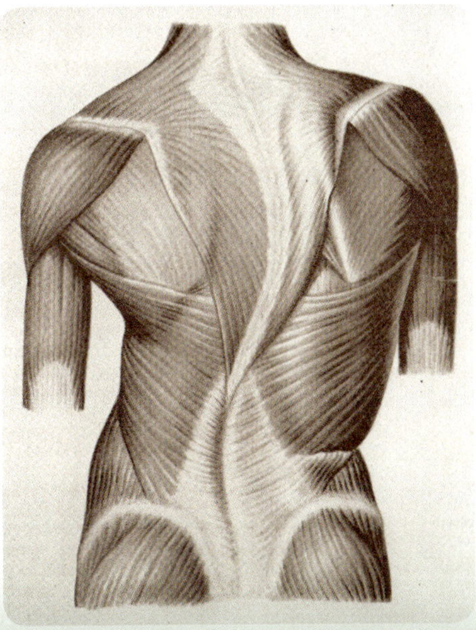

Fig. 3.2.3. Superficial muscles of the spine in S-shaped scoliosis; on the convex side of thoracic and lumbar curvatures of the spine, bulging of muscles is observed which is caused by typical deformation of the spine and ribs

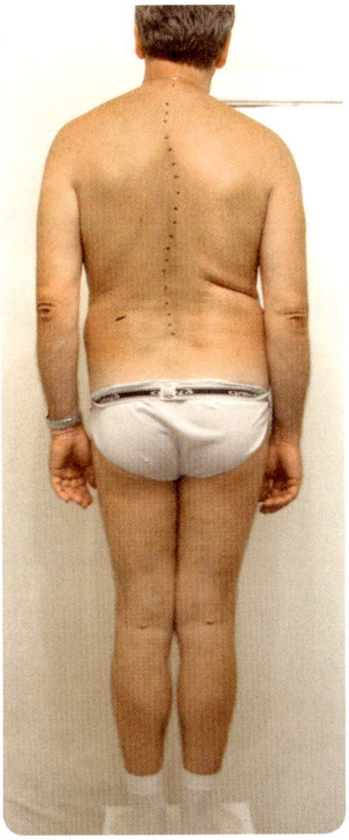

Fig. 3.2.4. Relative shortening of the left leg to 25 mm; right-sided scoliosis; smoothing of the waist with formation of transverse skin fold

spinae, as well as of the m. psoas major (Fig. 3.2.6) and m. quadratus lumborum (Fig. 3.2.7).

According to I.A. Movshovich, asymmetry of the trunk muscles is a result of torsion of the vertebrae. This explanation is acceptable in the case of adult patients, but not in the case of children, especially infants. It would be useful to refer to Section 3.1.1. 'Anatomy and physiology of interhemispheric differences', which describes how asymmetry of the spinal extensors is associated with certain aspects of the functioning of the brain. It is possible that the cerebral mechanism responsible for asymmetry of the spinal extensors is prevalent in early childhood. As an individual gets older, torsion of the vertebrae (spinal mechanism) occurs, resulting in the formation of a muscular cushion.

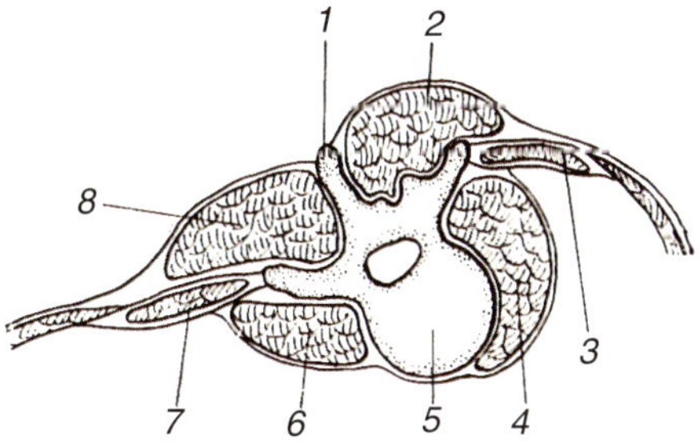

Fig. 3.2.5. Positioning of paravertebral muscles on convex and concave sides of lumbar curvature; on the convex side, muscle stands out against the underlying bone due to torsion of vertebrae — the muscular cushion is formed (2)
1 - spinous process, 2 and 8 - m. erector spinae; 3 and 7 - m. quadratus lumborum; 4 and 6 - m. psoas major; 5 - vertebral body

Surgical anatomy of the vertebral canal and the spinal cord

The spinal cord is surrounded by meninges and is located centrally in the spinal canal. It reaches only the upper margin of the second lumbar vertebra. The space between the

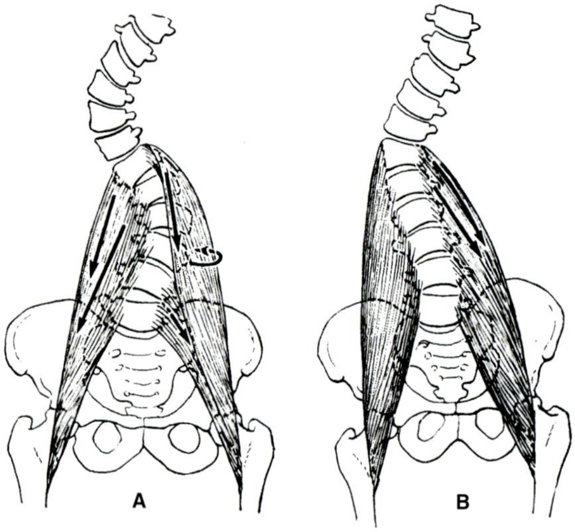

Fig. 3.2.6.
Position and functional axis of m. psoas major in lumbar and thoracolumbar scoliosis
A - in lumbar scoliosis unilateral muscle contraction on the convex side increases torsion of the spine and increases the degree of lumbosacral curvature; **B** - in thoracolumbar scoliosis unilateral muscle contraction on the concave side reduces curvature of the spine

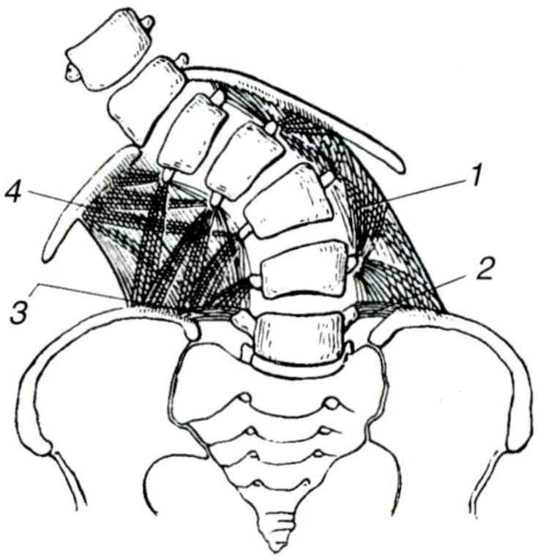

Fig. 3.2.7.
Position of m. quadratus lumborum (1, 4) and lig. iliolumbale (2, 3) in left-sided lumbar scoliosis (scheme)

periosteum, which lines the walls of the canal and the dura, is filled with adipose tissue and epidural venous plexuses. On the basis of his morphological studies, I.A. Movshovich showed that there are certain typical and significant changes in the shape and position of the spinal canal in scoliosis. These changes are especially pronounced among people with severe scoliotic deformities at the top of the thoracic or lumbar curvature (Fig. 3.2.8), and may cause paresis of the lower limb. This problem has been discussed extensively in the literature. R.R. Vreden, T. Vitvitsky and others suggest that paresis is caused by 'stretching, bending and twisting of the spinal cord'. On the other hand, Mac Kenzie, Dewar, Langenskild, Kleinberg and Caplan (cited from I.A. Movshovich '*Scoliosis. Surgical Anatomy and Pathogenesis*', Moscow, 1964) consider that paresis is caused by longitudinal tension of the dura due to the fact that the growth of the dura is unequal when the spine is curved.

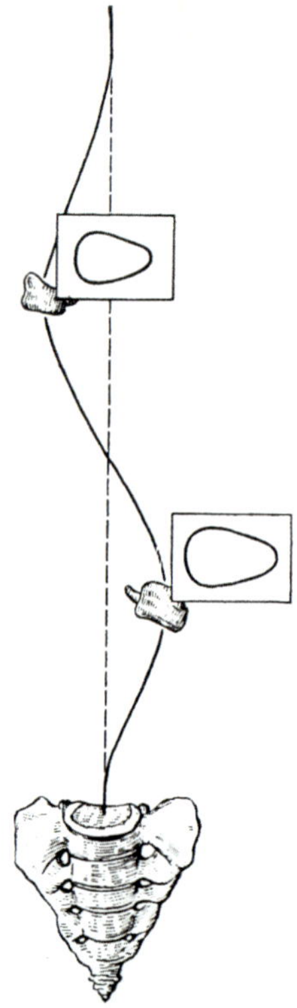

Fig. 3.2.8.
Form of the spinal canal in thoracic and lumbar curvature arcs

However, the studies carried out by I.A. Movshovich (Fig. 3.2.9) showed that a slight rotation of the spinal cord about the frontal plane of the body cannot cause paresis of the lower extremities, especially considering that this rotation occurs gradually over a long period of time. According to the author, the mechanism of this complication is that during the formation of curvature, the dura compresses the vessels supplying the spinal cord and, to a lesser degree, the tissue of the spinal cord (Fig. 3.2.10).

An understanding of the causes of paralysis allowed I.A. Movshovich to create an original and highly effective method of surgical treatment of paresis of the lower extremities. It involves excision of the thickened and inelastic dura on the concave side of the curvature, as well as translocation of the spinal cord into a new bed (Fig. 3.2.11).

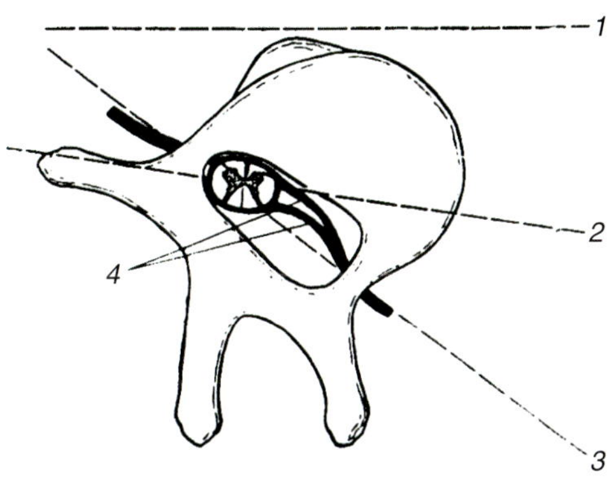

Fig. 3.2.9.
Location of spinal cord and its meninges with respect to frontal plane of the spinal canal and frontal plane of patient's body (scheme)
1 - Frontal plane of the patient; 2 - frontal plane of the spinal cord; 3 - frontal plane of the spinal canal; 4 - roots, surrounded by outgrowths of the dura

Surgical anatomy of the spinal and intercostal nerves, and lumbar and sacral plexuses

On the concave side of the deformity, even in the 4th grade of scoliosis, the location of the spinal and intercostal nerves is hardly pathological. On the convex side, these nerves and blood vessels lie close to the lower edge of the rib. On the concave side of the lumbar spine the situation is

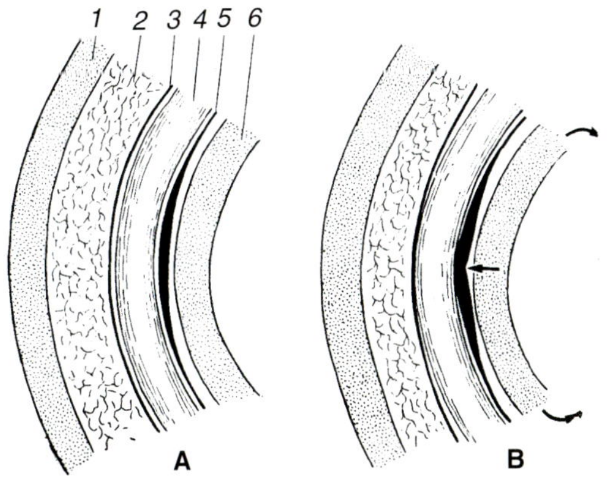

Fig. 3.2.10.
Changes of anatomical interrelations of the dura and the spinal cord in increasing curvature of the spine in severe scoliosis (scheme)
A - spinal cord is shifted towards the concave side—the dura on this side is thickened and has lost its elasticity; **B** - in increasing curvature arc a thickened part of the dura bends over and compresses the spinal cord with its vessels at this level
1, 6 - wall of the spinal canal; 2 - epidural adipose tissue; 3, 5 - dura mater; 4 - spinal cord

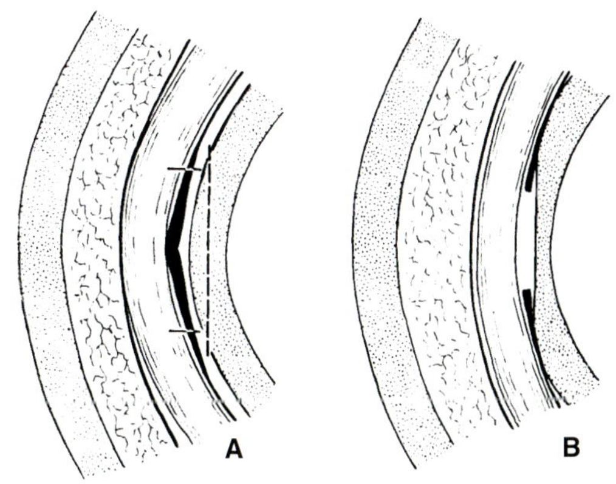

Fig. 3.2.11.
The scheme of surgery in lower limb paresis that develops in severe scoliosis
A - area of tangential resection of the spinal canal wall and borders of dura excision; **B** - the spinal cord has been transposed to a new bed and the thickened portion of the dura is removed

different because the size of the intervertebral foramina is decreased, occasionally by 1.5–2 times. As scoliosis progresses, a fibrous ring of intervertebral disc bulges laterally towards the arc of the curvature and invades the lower part of the intervertebral foramen on the concave side. Posteriorly, the articular processes with the yellow ligament invade the foramen (Fig. 3.2.12).

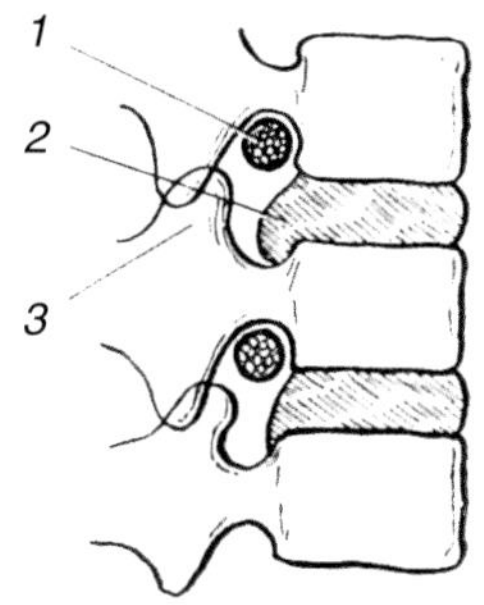

Fig. 3.2.12.
Left-sided lumbar scoliosis (view from the concave side); deformation of intervertebral foramina in the top curvature arc; the lower part of intervertebral foramen is narrowed due to displacement of the disc and superior articular process of an underlying vertebra, covered with yellow ligament
1 - spinal nerve; 2 - disc; 3 - articular process

However, compression of the spinal nerve is not observed in these circumstances. This is primarily because *under normal conditions, the diameter of the intervertebral foramen is 2–3 times greater than that of the neurovascular bundle that lies within.* Second, *narrowing of the intervertebral foramen occurs gradually and causes the neurovascular bundle to shift upwards accordingly.* Under certain functional conditions of the spine, such as sudden extension, the articular processes of an underlying vertebra and yellow ligament can penetrate into the intervertebral foramen (at once), causing compression of the neurovascular bundle.

Let us now discuss spinal pain in adults with scoliosis. Most patients suffer from pain in the lower back. In I.A. Movshovich's experience, osseous elements of the vertebrae were never seen to cause neural compression in the intervertebral foramina. The diameter of the nerves was always at least two times less than that of the foramina. According to the author, lumbar pain in scoliosis is related to congestion in the intervertebral veins due to their narrowing, and is not the result of compression of the spinal nerves in the intervertebral foramina.

In scoliosis, the lumbar plexus is shifted anteriorly on the convex side of the deformity and lies adjacent to the torsioned vertebral bodies. To prevent damage to the plexus, this fact should be kept in mind when performing anterior spondylodesis. As for the sacral plexus, its topographical anatomy remains practically unchanged in scoliosis.

Morphological changes of the spine

I.A. Movshovich's study of the spines of 50 people with scoliosis of dysplastic, idiopathic, congenital and paralytic origin yielded the following data.

In functional or physiological scoliosis (FS), no changes were observed in the normal anatomy of the spine. In structural scoliosis (SS), on the other hand, changes were evident in the bodies of the vertebrae and intervertebral discs with decrease in their stabilizing role. Single-sided decrease in height of the intervertebral discs was one of the main causes of disturbance of the static of the spine in scoliosis. Both in the case of thoracic and lumbar curvature arcs, the nucleus pulposus was displaced towards the convex side; there was a unilateral narrowing of the fibrous ring, making it significantly enlarged on the concave side (Fig. 3.2.13). Torsion is the most marked at the top of the curvature arc. Spinal deformity is accompanied by typical deformities of the ribs.

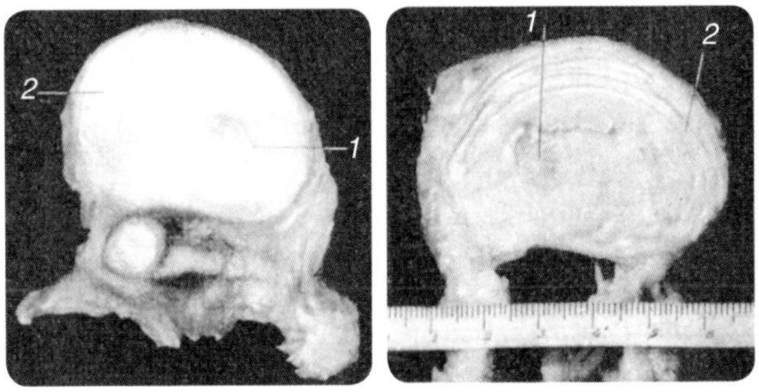

A B

Fig. 3.2.13.
Changes of the intervertebral disc in scoliosis of 3rd degree
A - thoracic vertebra in right-sided bending (15-year-old female); **B** - lumbar vertebra in left-sided bending (73-year-old female); gelatinous core (1) is shifted towards the convex side, annulus fibrosus is widened on the concave side (2)

The type of scoliosis depends on the number of curvatures (Fig. 3.2.14–3.2.16). The most common types are:

1. C-shaped left-sided scoliosis
2. C-shaped right-sided scoliosis
3. S-shaped scoliosis with two curvatures (left-sided thoracic and right-sided lumbar)
4. S-shaped reverse scoliosis with two curvatures (right-sided thoracic and left-sided lumbar)
5. S-shaped scoliosis with three curvatures (thoracic, lumbar and lumbosacral)—right-sided deformity in the thoracic region
6. S-shaped scoliosis with three curvatures—left-sided deformity in the thoracic region

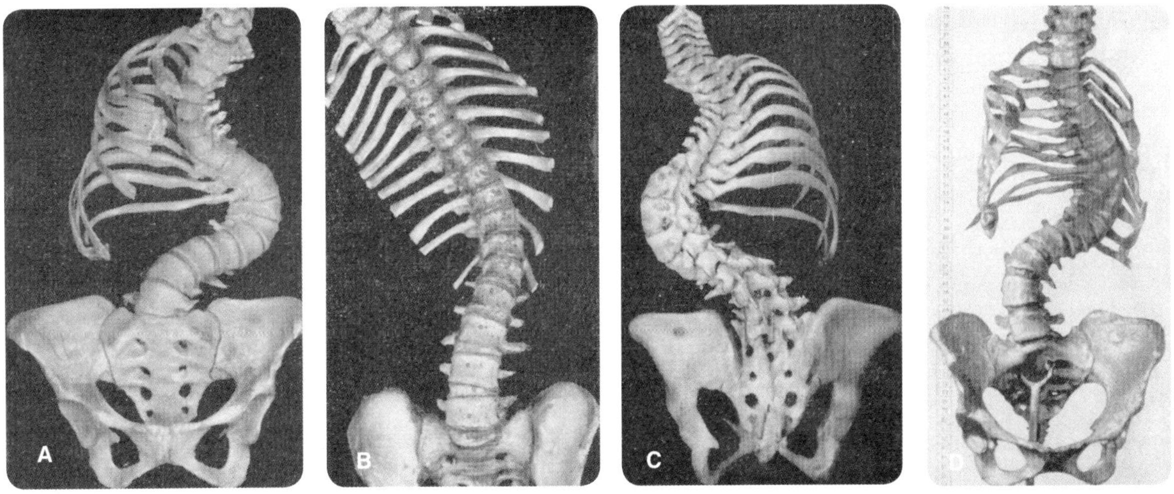

Fig. 3.2.14.
Forms of scoliosis depending on the number of curvatures
A - C-shaped scoliosis; **B** and **C** - S-shaped with two arcs (front and rear view); **D** - S-shaped with three arcs (thoracic, lumbar and lumbosacral)

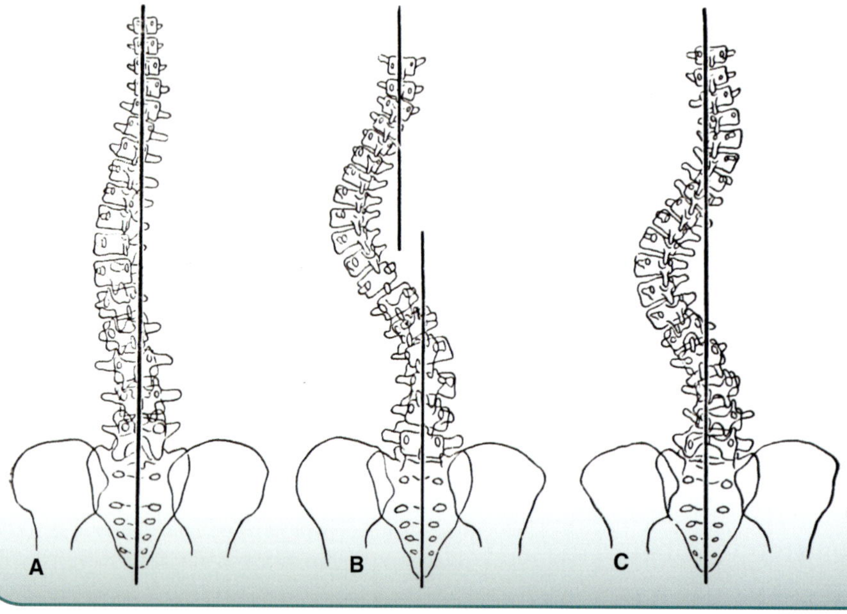

Fig. 3.2.15.
A - scoliosis with a single curvature arc;
B - scoliosis with two arches;
C - scoliosis with three arches
True scoliotic arches, unlike anticurvatures, are more towards the opposite side of the vertical line drawn through the non-deformed spine

I. Ponseti and B. Friedman (1950) classified dysplastic, congenital and neurogenic scoliosis into the following types on the basis of their location:

1. Cervicothoracic
2. Upper thoracic
3. Thoracic
4. Thoracolumbar
5. Lumbar
6. Lumbosacral
7. Total (C-shaped)
8. Combined (S-shaped)

Morphological changes of the thorax

While studying the shapes of discs and vertebrae in the arc of the thoracic curvature, one may observe slight wedging of the discs and significant wedging of the vertebrae. This is one of the early signs of structural scoliosis (Fig. 3.2.17). At the same time, a wedge-shaped deformity of

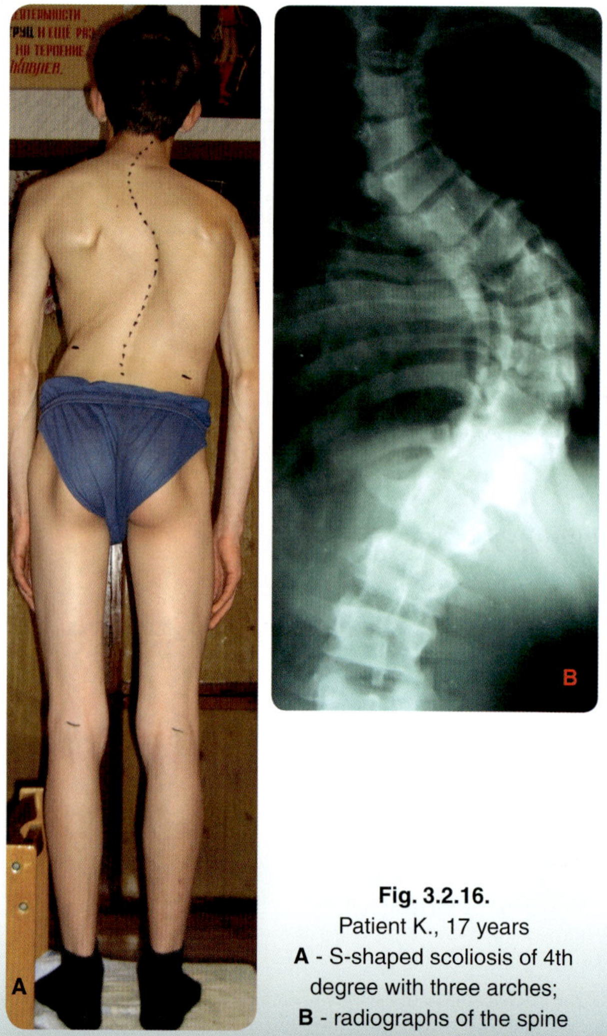

Fig. 3.2.16.
Patient K., 17 years
A - S-shaped scoliosis of 4th degree with three arches;
B - radiographs of the spine

the vertebral bodies, located on top of the arc of the curvature, is already present in second-degree scoliosis. The causes of these changes are not yet known. Some theories suggest that these changes are due to increased pressure on the concave side, adaptation to new conditions and abnormally soft bones.

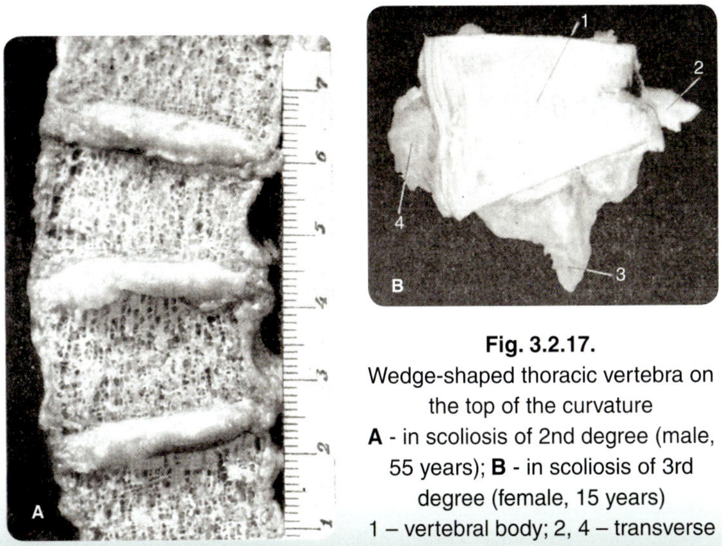

Fig. 3.2.17.
Wedge-shaped thoracic vertebra on the top of the curvature
A - in scoliosis of 2nd degree (male, 55 years); **B** - in scoliosis of 3rd degree (female, 15 years)
1 – vertebral body; 2, 4 – transverse processes; 3 – spinous process

On radiographs of the scoliotic spine in the initial stages of deformity (even in children), one can observe the formation of coracoid outgrowths originating from the lower and part of the upper margins of the vertebral body on the concave side of the curvature. According to I.A. Movshovich, these outgrowths are formed due to the displacement of vertebral apophyses and intervertebral discs towards the concave side, and their subsequent ossification and synostosis.

With age, the coracoid outgrowths lengthen and part of the fibrous ring of the intervertebral disc lying between them becomes thinner. As a result, a semi-mobile junction between the bodies of adjacent vertebrae is formed. In old age, coracoid outgrowths usually merge into a conglomerate that includes parts of vertebral bodies, transverse processes and ribs, resulting in synostosis (Fig. 3.2.18).

Thus, the formation of coracoid outgrowths is a result of adaptation of the spine to changed static conditions.

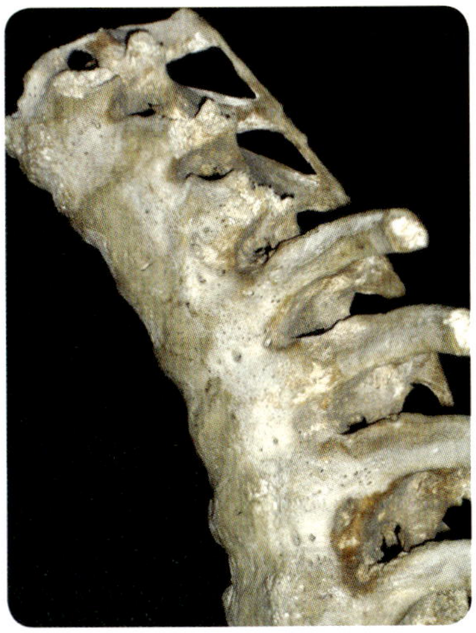

Fig. 3.2.18.
Vertebral osteophytes are fusing into one bony conglomerate, which consists of parts of vertebral bodies, transverse and spinous processes and ribs

A. Schantz (1933) also studied the nature of coracoid outgrowths (exostoses). His conclusion was identical to that of I.A. Movshovich. However, his explanation was different. It was by studying one of the complications of scoliosis that he gained an understanding of the nature of exostoses. This was the *static insufficiency of the spine*. According to Schantz, this complication is a result of chronic overwork and is characterized by a sense of fatigue, as well as back pain radiating to the chest and abdomen. Headaches, reduced mental alertness, insomnia, depressed mood,

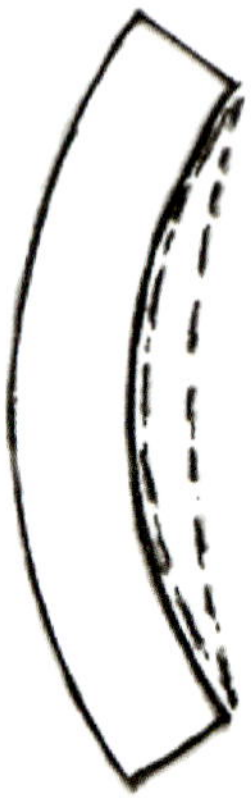

Fig. 3.2.19.
The bar bent under congestion can protect against further deformation by a supporting arch, inserted into the concave part

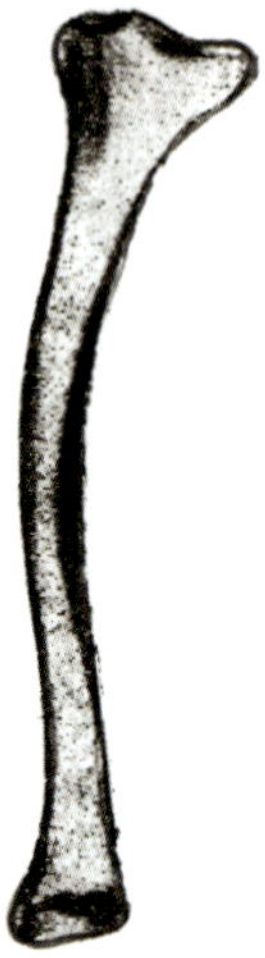

Fig. 3.2.20.
Rachitic deformation of the tibia. Supporting arch on the concave side

neurasthenia and severe hysteria are common. Radiating pain in the form of neuralgia, neuritis of the femoral and sciatic nerves, and intercostal neuralgia, as well as cardiac and digestive disorders, and diseases of the reproductive organs in women occur frequently.

Analysing the causes of insufficiency of the spine, A. Schantz concluded that it is the result of impaired physiological relation between the load on the spine and the endurance of the spine. The law governing the development of deformity caused by static overload comes into force. The following two examples illustrate this.

The overloaded vertebral column (Fig. 3.2.19) can be supported by inserting a supporting arch into the concave part of the deformity. How the body uses such technical support in rachitic limb deformities is shown in Fig. 3.2.20.

The law of deformation also extends to the spine. For example, one of the manifestations of spinal functional insufficiency is spondylosis deformans (Fig. 3.2.21). At first glance, in severe forms of this disease, deformity of the vertebrae seems to be chaotic and haphazard (Fig. 3.2.22). However, if one assumes that spondylosis deformans develops to protect the spine from injury due to overload, the change in the interrelationship between the vertebrae would seem to have a valid purpose.

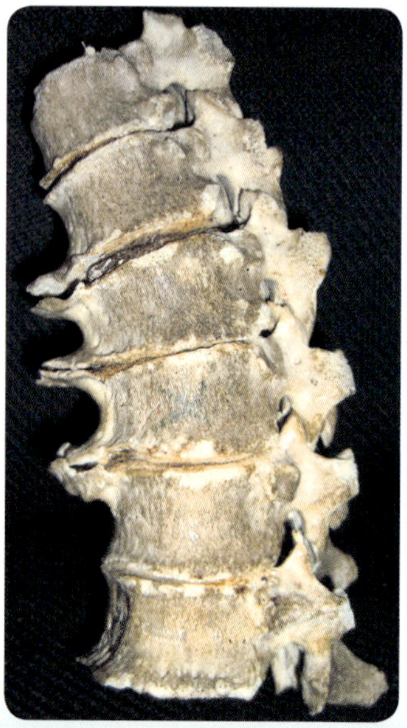

Fig. 3.2.21.
Advanced signs of deforming spondylosis

The spine is a loaded column, consisting of separate parts interconnected by mobile ligaments and intervertebral discs. To prevent the possibility of distortion of the column due to overloading, as shown in Fig. 3.3.23, nature, like a technician, provides local supports between different parts of the column. This is how osseous outgrowths, also called coracoid outgrowths, exostoses and osteophytes, are formed (Figs 3.2.24 and 3.2.25). *Consequently, exostoses are not a sign of pathological vertebral restructuring, as many physicians and patients believe, but are formations that serve to protect the spine from curving due to static overload.*

Proceeding from the above, we can conclude that the mechanism of the formation of exostoses is more

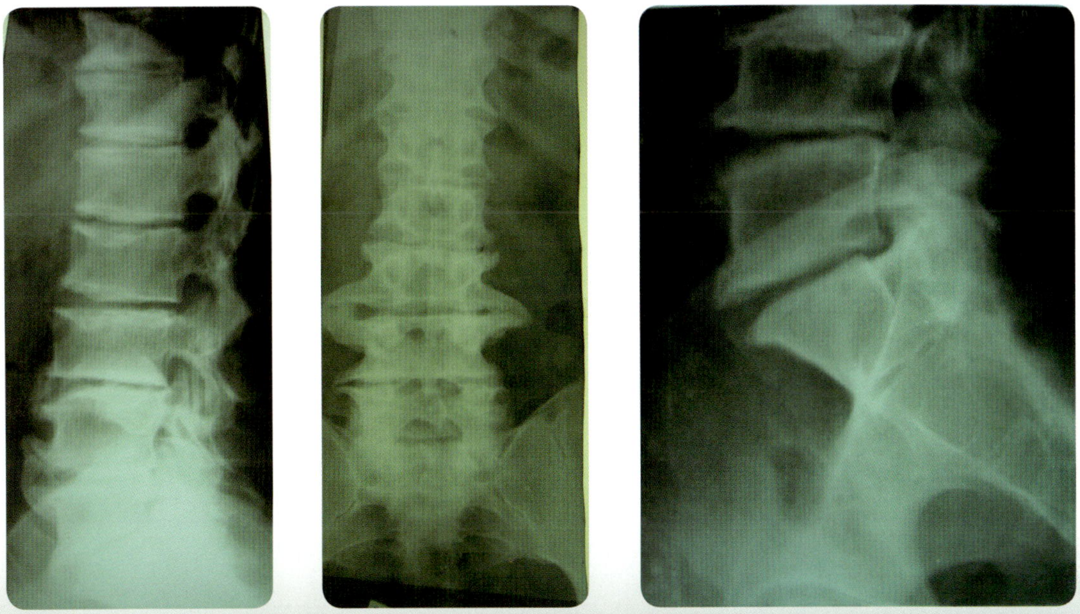

Fig. 3.2.22. Radiographic images of disfiguring spondylosis

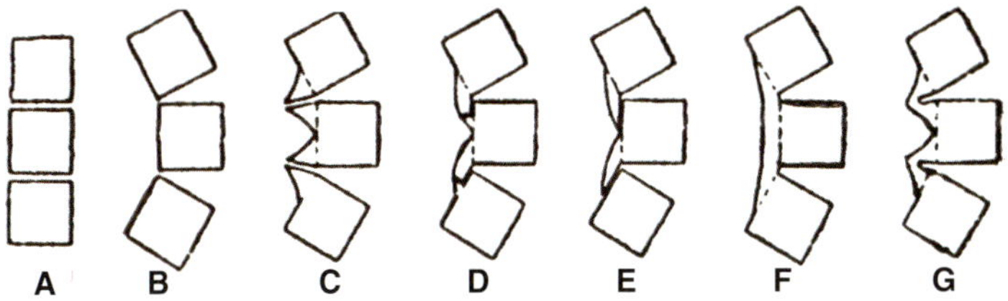

Fig. 3.2.23.
Schematic presentation of column **A** consisting of interconnected moving parts; **B** shows how a column is bent under overload; **C–G** depict how to support a curved column using technical devices

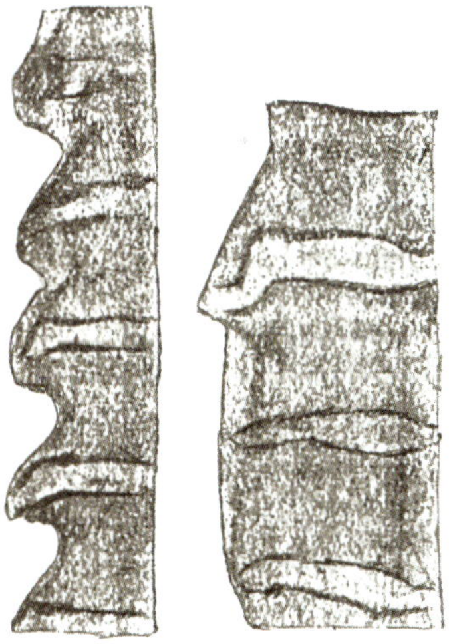

Fig. 3.2.24. **Fig. 3.2.25.**
Vertebral bodies affected by disfiguring spondylitis; figures show the development of constructive forms of support by a living organism, shown in Fig. 3.2.23 C–G (according to Beneke)

complicated than what I.A. Movshovich thought. It is based both on the law of deformity and on the displacement of the vertebral epiphyseal plates. I.L. Krupko (1975), who studied these mechanisms, came to similar conclusions.

Static insufficiency causes extremely complex changes not only in the spine but also in other parts of the human skeletal system (hips, knees, ankles, etc.). This will be discussed later.

There is significant deformation of the ribs in scoliosis. A costal hump is formed posteriorly, on the convex side of the spinal curvature, and there is retraction of the chest on the concave side. The situation is the opposite on the anterior side: there is retraction of the chest on the convex side and protrusion of the ribs on the concave side (anterior costal hump). This also includes the sternum. Depending on the extent

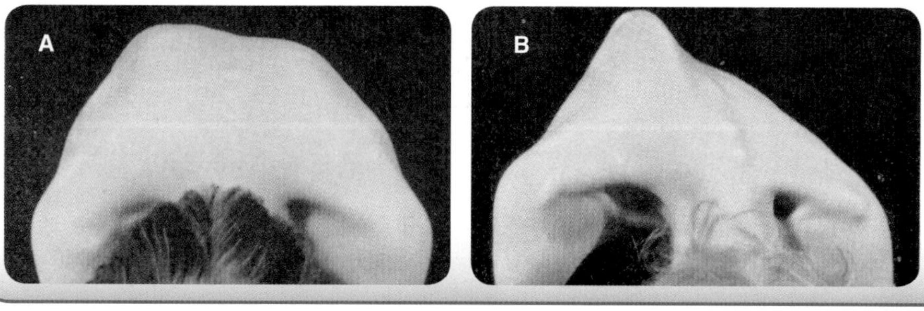

Fig. 3.2.26.
Costal hump
A - flat;
B - pointed

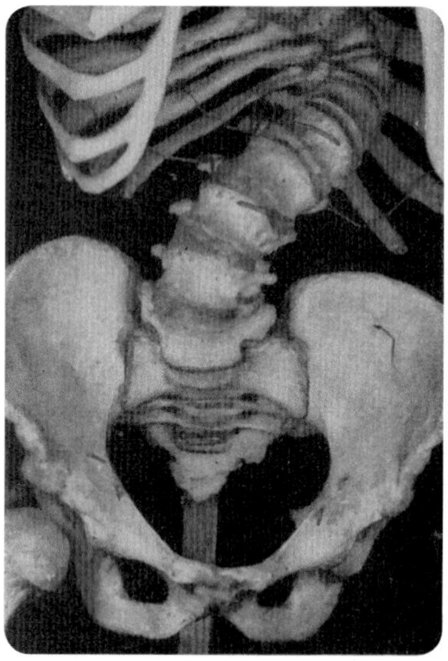

Fig. 3.2.27.
Left-sided thoracolumbar scoliosis of 3rd degree; lower ribs on the concave side lie parallel to the upper lumbar spine

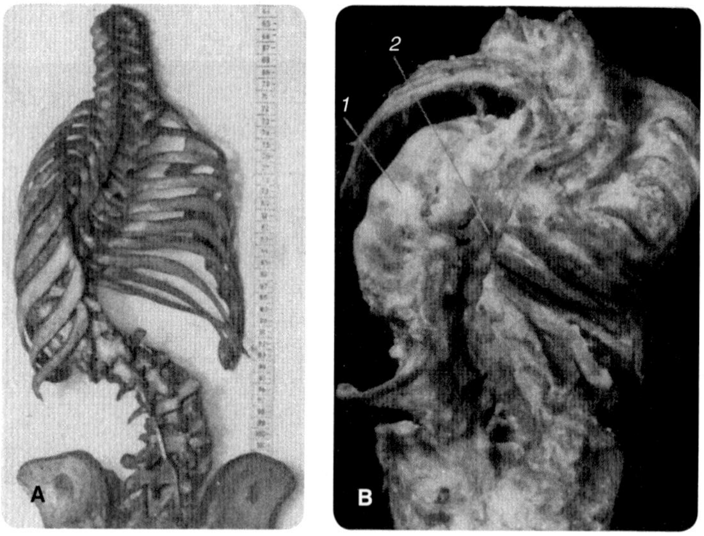

Fig. 3.2.28.
Deformation of the thorax in severe scoliosis
A - left-sided thoracic and right-sided lumbar scoliosis of 4th degree: significant deformation of the spine;
B - two curvature arcs of the thoracic spine which are located near each other; scoliosis of 4th degree in 58-year-old woman: on the left side some ribs are removed, the torsioned vertebral bodies are visible (1); 2 - spinous processes

and nature of vertebral torsion, the costal hump may be flat or peaked (Figs 3.2.26–3.2.28). It begins to form at the same time as the onset of spinal torsion, and possibly only during the period of skeletal growth (Fig. 3.2.29).

On the basis of his morphological, clinical and radiographic observations, I.A. Movshovich came to one more conclusion that changes of the thorax in scoliosis do not depend on the aetiology of the condition. Deformities of the vertebrae are similar in dysplastic, idiopathic and paralytic scoliosis. Even in the presence of developmental abnormalities, deformity develops according to the same rules as in scoliosis of other aetiologies. Usually, the progression of scoliosis is the greatest during the period of rapid skeletal growth.

If we compare the direction of rotation of the thorax with that of pelvic rotation in an S-shaped scoliosis, we find that the directions are mutually antithetical (Fig.

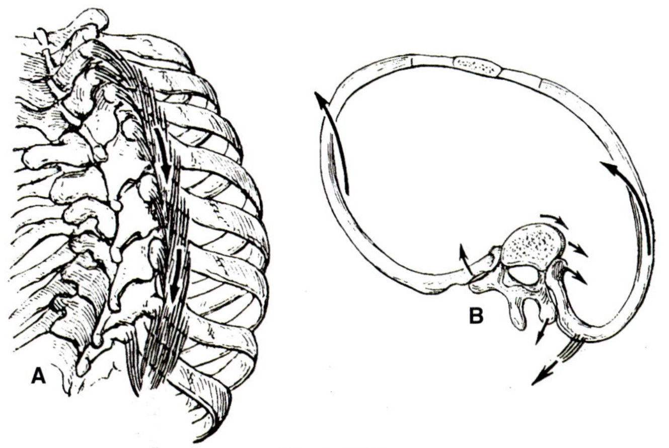

Fig. 3.2.29.
Scheme illustrating costal hump formation in scoliosis
A - effect of m. erector spinae on vertebral parts of ribs on the convex side of spinal curvature; **B** - shape of the thorax and direction of forces in formation of costal hump

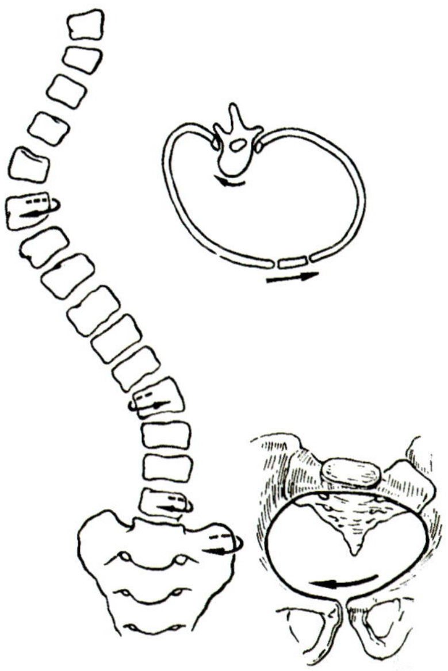

Fig. 3.2.30.
The scheme shows mutual antithetical rotation of the thorax and pelvis in right-sided lumbar and right-sided lumbosacral scoliosis; arrows indicate the direction of rotation and torsion of vertebrae, thorax and pelvis

2.3.30). This is due to the fact that the rotation of the thorax occurs in a direction opposite to the torsion of the thoracic vertebrae, while pelvic rotation corresponds to torsion of the proximal part of the sacrum. In addition, torsion of the thoracic vertebrae and that of the lumbosacral vertebrae occur in the same direction, as long as there are lumbar vertebrae lying between them with the opposite direction of torsion.

Morphological changes of the lumbar spine

The conditions in which lumbar scoliosis develops are different from those in which thoracic scoliosis develops. These primarily include the presence of lordosis, absence of ribs (in the lumbar region), greater height of the intervertebral discs and originality of structure in the ligamentous and muscular systems. Owing to the presence of lordosis in the lumbar spine, the basic static load falls on the posterior part of the spine, i.e. the arches, articular processes and, partially, the spinous processes.

The bodies of the lumbar vertebrae are less loaded than those of the thoracic vertebrae and, therefore, are less deformed in scoliosis. In particular, the wedge shape is barely marked. At the same time, there are considerable deformities in the posterior parts of the lumbar vertebrae. Thus, curvature of the lumbar spine is largely due to changes in the shape of the intervertebral discs.

3.2.1 Aetiology of scoliosis

The first and basic question that attracts attention in studying scoliosis is to determine the causes of this deformity. Scoliosis is a lateral curvature of the spine, i.e. the spine is curved in the frontal plane. However, this definition may be applicable only in the initial stage of the disease (physiological scoliotic posture), or in the so-called functional scoliosis (such as idiopathic scoliosis, dysplastic scoliosis, habitual scoliosis, static scoliosis, rachitic scoliosis, paralytic scoliosis, osteopathic scoliosis, discogenic scoliosis, congenital scoliosis, musculo-ligamentous insufficiency scoliosis, constitutional scoliosis, neuromyogenic scoliosis, endocrine and metabolic disorders, etc.) that is not accompanied by structural changes of the vertebrae. On the other hand, true scoliosis (SS) is characterized by a complex deformity of the vertebrae with torsion (rotation of the vertebra around its axis) and the development of spinal curves in three planes: frontal, sagittal and horizontal. This is not just a spinal deformity; it is a disease with a different aetiology but characteristic clinical signs.

According to various authors, scoliosis occurs very often. However, their figures differ significantly, ranging from 1.3% (Z.A. Lyandres, 1966) to 53.2% (I.I. Vanovsky, 1906 cited by V.Y. Fischenko *et al. Conservative Treatment of Scoliosis*. Kiev, 1994) and even higher. This wide range can be explained by two factors. First, the patients studied were of different ages and second, the approaches adopted for the assessment of spinal curvature were also different. For example, some authors considered only advanced forms of scoliosis, starting from Grade 2 (according to V.D. Chaklin's classification), while others included all cases of scoliosis, starting from Grade 1. The latter covered a large group of children with functional scoliosis, and it must be remembered that in most of these cases, the curvature disappears later.

The study of the aetiology of scoliosis is a very complicated task. The most frequent form of the disease is scoliosis of unknown aetiology (idiopathic) which, according to J.R. Cobb (1960), comprises up to 90% of all cases of lateral curvatures. Often, dysplastic, habitual and static scoliosis are observed. There are also more rare forms—rachitic, cicatricial, paralytic, reflex, hysterical, emphysematous, hereditary and post-traumatic scoliosis. Spinal curvatures in systemic diseases of the skeleton, such as neurofibromatosis (hyperparathyroid osteodystrophy) and Marfan's syndrome (congenital disorder of mesenchymal tissue), should also be considered rare forms of the disease.

Interesting data were obtained by V.P. Skrygin (1949) cited by I.A. Movshovich (*Scoliosis*, 1964), who examined 54 patients with idiopathic scoliosis. Extensive X-ray and neurological examination revealed the presence of gliomatosis and gliomatous syringomyelia in 29 patients, myelodysplasia in 11 and myopathy of the back muscles in 6. In 8 patients, the aetiology remained unknown. Thus, the author showed that in most cases, idiopathic scoliosis has a neurological basis, which a physician must be able to identify. V.P. Skrygin's findings were fully confirmed by the work of other orthopaedic surgeons and neurologists (E.A. Abalmasovoy, S.N. Davydenkova, A.V. Kogan, J.A. Ratner, M.O. Friedland, V.D. Chaklin, etc.). It should be mentioned that the fact that there is an association between scoliosis and changes in the central nervous system is not new, but it certainly requires further study.

According to Professor V.Y. Fischenko (2005), the clinical, radiological and morphological manifestations of idiopathic and dysplastic scolioses have much in common. On the basis of detailed analysis of the literature, as well as his own clinical material, V.Y. Fischenko (1994) suggested that idiopathic and dysplastic scolioses should be put under one group. His data have led him to conclude that the frequency of these types of scoliosis is 65.4%, followed by a group of congenital scolioses (21.2%).

A. Kozlovsky was the first to classify dysplastic (congenital) scolioses as an independent group in 1927. He believed that dysplasia of the lumbosacral spine is the cause of these types of scolioses. These scolioses manifest themselves as partial or complete lumbarization and/or sacralization, incomplete fusion of the posterior parts of the lumbar and/or sacral vertebrae, and longitudinal slit of the 4th and 5th lumbar vertebrae (rachischisis), which weakens the base of the spine.

Congenital anomalies include anomalies of the articular processes, unilateral costal synostosis, butterfly (Fig. 3.2.31) or wedge-shaped vertebrae and hemivertebrae (Fig. 2.3.32). This group also includes blocked vertebrae (fusion; *see* Fig. 3.2.33) in different regions of the spine and scoliosis caused by an additional vertebra (Fig. 3.2.34).

These changes lead to the development of the primary

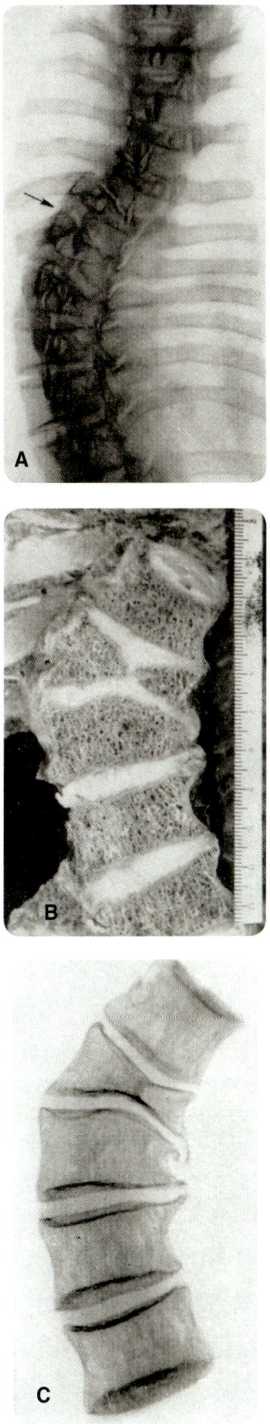

Fig. 3.2.31.
Congenital right-sided thoracolumbar scoliosis of 3rd degree in a 57-year-old woman
A - radiograph of the spine;
B - cutting across the curvature arc;
C - radiograph of fragment of macropreparation

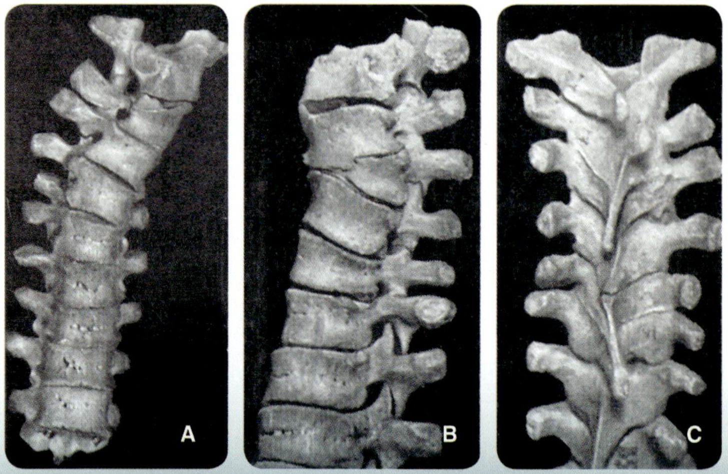

Fig. 3.2.32.
Congenital right-sided 'local' scoliosis with the presence of wedge-shaped vertebrae
A - front view; **B** - lateral view; **C** - rear view

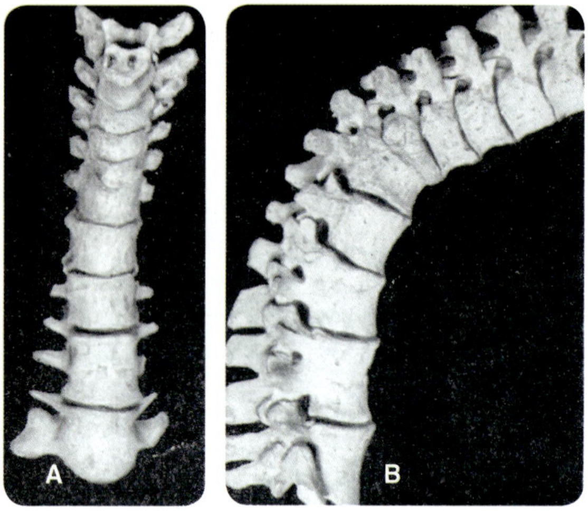

Fig. 3.2.33.
Blockade (concrescence) of vertebrae (lumbar and thoracic regions); in the thoracic region, anterior parts of vertebral bodies are blocked and as a result there is kyphosis
A - macropreparation, front view; **B** - view from the right

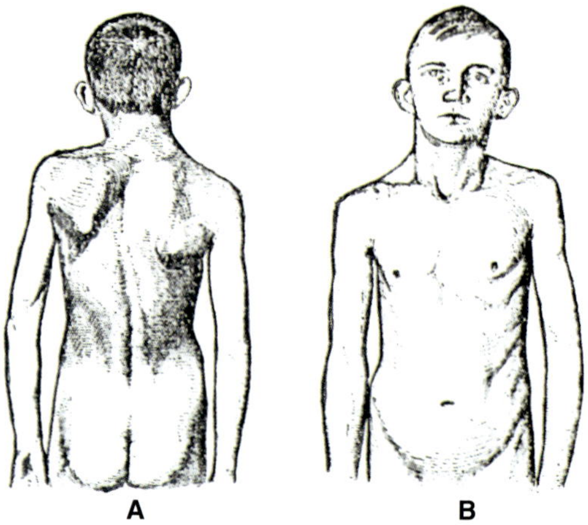

Fig. 3.2.34.
Scoliosis caused by an additional vertebra
A - rear view; **B** - front view

curvature in the anomalous zone, and then to the development of a secondary compensatory curvature in the thoracic and/or lumbar regions. Clinically, dysplastic scolioses often manifest as myelodysplasia with paresis of the lower extremities. The characteristic external pathological signs include hypertrichosis (increased pilosity [Fig. 2.2.10A and Fig. 2.2.10B] in the area of the first sacral vertebra) and hyperpigmentation of the skin in this region (Fig. 2.2.9).

Selective supporters of this hypothesis were G.I. Turner (1929), R.R. Vreden (1931) and E.A. Lyandres (1959). In subsequent studies, E.A. Abalmasova (1965) reviewed the theory that bone dysplasia is a leading causative factor of scoliosis and concluded that it is an associated factor. To an extent, habitual scoliosis should be considered an occupational disease that is associated with sitting for long periods of time. There was a time when scoliosis was regarded as a direct result of attending school and was simply known as 'school disease'. However, this cannot be considered correct in view of the fact that scoliosis may develop even in pre-school years, when children have not yet begun sitting at desks. Moreover, a person can develop scoliosis a long time after graduation and the completion of growth. A question that requires an answer is why scoliosis does not develop among all children living in similar harmful conditions, and why girls are affected 5–6 times more often than boys. In G. Muller's opinion (1913), boys are less susceptible because they are often physically stronger than girls (*see* Section 3.1.1. 'Anatomy and physiology of interhemispheric differences').

A.M. Schantz (1933) made some interesting observations on examining a large number of children of schoolgoing age. He found that many of the children's skeletons did not have any anatomical abnormalities, although bending of the trunk was observed. Studying the dynamics of treatment in children, the author found that new deformities did not always form as a consequence of poor posture. He concluded that poor posture is not an obligatory preliminary stage of deformation; scoliosis may occur even in a child with perfect posture.

The Polish physician, A. Shlumsky (1933) (cited from A.M. Schantz, *Practical Orthopedics* [translated from German], Moscow: State Medical Publishing House, 1933), compared children attending school with those not attending school in Krakow, and found that the frequency of scoliosis was almost the same in both the groups. Moreover, deformities were more severe among those not attending school.

A.M. Shantz (1933) made a distinction between benign and malignant deformities. The forms of scoliosis that develop over the school period are mostly benign. The later the appearance of scoliosis during childhood, the greater are the chances of its being of a benign nature, as supported by data. Malignant deformities usually develop after the schoolgoing years. Malignant scoliosis occurs among children who are born with a weakened spine. This form of scoliosis, first described by W. Schulthess, is called *constitutional*. Its true cause is not known yet.

There is a difference between malignant and benign deformities. In most cases, benign deformities disappear or remain as minor growth defects (high thigh or shoulder) when the person reaches maturity. Malignant deformities have a tendency to worsen after the school years and at the end of the period of growth, as well as throughout life. When patients suffer from new diseases later in life, malignant scolioses respond rapidly and benign ones may become malignant. This needs to be emphasized because patients, and often physicians, believe that scolioses will not deteriorate after the school years, or at least after the end of the period of growth.

Instead of the term 'school scoliosis', A.M. Schantz proposed the term 'spinal deformity due to overload during childhood' (from early childhood to the end of the school period). It is mainly during this period that longitudinal growth of the spine occurs. During these years, most children suffer from several childhood diseases and also bear the physical workload associated with going to school. In the later school years, they graduate from childhood to puberty. All these factors can lead to an imbalance in the load on the spine.

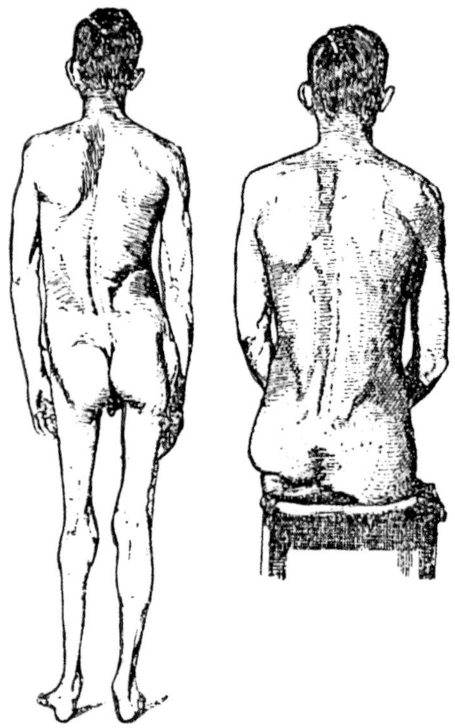

Fig. 3.2.35.
'Static scoliosis'—The difference in leg length is the cause of spinal and pelvic distortion; when the patient sits on a horizontal plane, pelvis and spine straighten

Static scoliosis is characterized by a lateral curvature of the spine due to impaired statics (vertical positioning of the body) (Fig. 3.2.35). However, it should be clarified that the division of scolioses into habitual and static must be acknowledged as conditional. The two types reflect the same process—uneven loading of the spine while standing or sitting. The concept of vicious posture has its origins in the works of Hueter and Volkmann. In 1862, after studying the articular ends of bones in children, Hueter concluded that among growing individuals, epiphyseal growth is intensified in areas where there is no match of cartilaginous surfaces. Volkmann applied this concept to scoliosis. Since then, the so-called Hueter–Volkmann law has gained recognition in the literature. According to this law, areas of the bone where the epiphyseal cartilage is exposed to strong and long-term compression grow slower; growth is accelerated in areas where the epiphyseal cartilage is less loaded. As a result of the asymmetrical growth of the bone, a deformity develops.

Thus, *if we proceed from this concept, the presence of an asymmetrical load on the spine is sufficient for the appearance of a curvature*. This supposition led many to believe that *vicious posture is a major aetiological factor in the development of most forms of scoliosis*. Many studies have concluded that incorrect position of the child's spine during school hours is the main cause of scoliosis.

Many experiments were conducted on growing animals in the 19th–20th centuries to determine the impact of asymmetrical load on the development of spinal deformity. A. Lesser and D. Wullstein tried to prove that prolonged forced position of the spine leads to deformity. Moreover, although it was later recognized that school load could not be the sole aetiological factor in the development of scoliosis, it became clear that asymmetrical static load on the growing spine could result in true scoliosis, with structural changes of the vertebrae (V.D. Chaklin, G.I. Turner, J. Yuk and W. Brizard). The development of static scoliosis in childhood has been proven.

Development of static scoliosis may be also initiated due to a number of diseases, which lead to unilateral inclination of the pelvis and consequently to deviation of the spine. Some such diseases are: true shortening of the leg after bony resection, underdevelopment of one of the lower extremities in cerebral palsy or due to the consequences of poliomyelitis, etc.

Now we propose to discuss the mechanism of formation of lateral curvature of the spine in different lengths of the lower extremities. According to G. Muller (1913): '... Let us assume that the left half of the pelvis is for some reason located lower than the right. In this case, the spine, being perpendicular to the line passing through the intertrochanteric area of the thighs (linea intertrochanterica), must bend to the left. As a result, the trunk would have to fall to the left if the body would not balance so that the upper body would bend to the right and the head to the left. As a result, the balance is restored. However, the process of balancing in the sagittal plane leads to the normal position of the body, in the frontal plane it leads to the formation of scoliosis. Thus, actually the picture is the same as in the formation of physiological curvatures... .'

It is important to note that we reached a similar conclusion in the initial stage of our research, devoted to spinal deformities without even knowing at that time about G. Muller's publication (see Chapter 1).

Not by coincidence a Nobel laureate, professor of physiology, Ivan Pavlov (Russia), said: 'Pathology is such a state of health when primarily normal physiological processes are developing in new abnormal conditions.' Some national manuals on orthopaedics recognize the rachitic form of scoliosis, which develops in the first 2–3 years of life or even later. The course of the disease is very rapid and it is also called malignant scoliosis (V.D. Chaklin, N.P. Novachenko, T.S. Zatsepin, M.O. Friedland and others). I.A. Movshovich thought that it is more appropriate to classify rachitic scoliosis as idiopathic, since the origin of this form of the disease is highly unclear.

When discussing aetiology of scoliosis, it is necessary to recognize the existence of predisposing factors. First, genetics plays a big role and the condition is often a 'game of nature'. The children of those suffering from scoliosis do not always have the disease, and often it is the grandchildren who are affected. Sometimes, when one of two sisters has scoliosis, she has healthy children while her sister's children suffer from scoliosis. Various authors have come across such situations, but have been unable to find any explanation.

The frequency of congenital (hereditary) scolioses ranges from 15% to 30% (V.P. Skrygin [1949], E.A. Abalmasova *et al.* [1978], G. Frontino, R. Scarponi [1980]) (cited from V.Y. Fischenko *et al. Non-surgical Treatment of Scoliosis*, Kiev, 1994). According to these authors, scoliosis itself is not inherited, but metabolic disorders of connective tissue are inherited, which provoke the development of scoliosis.

According to R. Hodjaev (1970), transmission of scoliosis from mothers to daughters was observed in 91% of cases. Fathers were 2.5 times more likely to transmit deformities to their daughters than sons. The period of greatest progression of scoliosis was between 11 and 14 years in girls and 13–15 years in boys.

A discussion of the problem of vicious posture involves a number of issues related to the assessment of the musculo-ligamentous apparatus of the spine and the state of the vertebrae and intervertebral discs. Many authors of the past two centuries, as well as the current century (N.F. Gagman, Malgaigne, Lovett, Abbot, Shede, etc.), put forward the theory of musculo-ligamentous insufficiency to explain the cause of scoliosis. After its emergence in the 1900s, this theory was developed further in the 1930s by R.R. Vreden, A. Kozlowski, Niederhoffer, Rogers, Carey and others. During at the same period, Hauser even expressed the view that adolescent scoliosis is due solely to muscular insufficiency, which may be caused by hereditary factors, rapid growth of the skeleton during certain periods, overload, various diseases, etc. In such conditions, according to the above-mentioned authors, *first a vicious posture forms, followed by the development of scoliosis.*

Paralytic (neurogenic) scoliosis may be a consequence of polio and is rare, occurring in 8%–20% of patients. Impaired muscular balance plays a certain role in the pathogenesis of paralytic scoliosis. From the perspective of pathological anatomy of the spine, structural changes of the spine even in patients with severe paralytic scoliosis are identical to the morphological changes seen in the dysplastic and idiopathic forms of the disease. Paralytic scoliosis may also occur among those with cerebral palsy, but its severity as well as frequency are considerably lower than in cases of poliomyelitis.

Parallel to the theory of musculo-ligamentous insufficiency emerged the osteopathic theory, aimed at explaining the causes of the changes in the shape of the vertebrae in scoliosis. Dolega and Shultes suggested that increased static load makes the vertebrae softer and pliable due to decreased strength of the vertebral bone structure. Shultes proposed the term 'constitutional scoliosis', as was already mentioned earlier, and attributed this situation to 'a congenital bone softening'. Kirmisson, Albert, Lorenz, etc. emphasized on weak resistance to deformity of the vertebrae and their increased plasticity in systemic diseases. The authors attributed this not only to certain constitutional features of the skeleton, but also to the complications of various diseases. The osteopathic theory, although not comprehensive and universal, still has its own merits. Volkman and Nikoladoni also associated the imbalance of the entire spinal column in scoliosis with asymmetrical growth of the vertebral bodies.

Disharmony of endocrine processes, especially during puberty (theory of endocrine and metabolic disorders) is of great importance in scoliosis. Decref, Yuk and Brizard linked the development of scoliosis with impaired functioning of the thyroid and pituitary glands, as well as ovaries. Endocrine insufficiency results in the impairment of mineral and protein metabolism, which leads to softening of the skeleton. To prove this hypothesis, Baird conducted a number of experiments on young rats and showed that impairments in hormonal function and metabolism of mucopolysaccharides in animals lead to typical alterations of the skeleton, which cause secondary deformities.

Another theory focuses on discogenic scolioses. According to this, impaired metabolism of the connective tissue of the intervertebral discs decreases the strength of the discs during torsion of the vertebrae and favours an early migration of nuclei pulposus. This leads to a wedge-shaped deformity of the vertebral bodies and discs which, in turn, results in the development of structural scoliosis.

A significant contribution was made to the development of this theory by Professor V.Y. Fischenko and his colleagues, V.A. Uleschenko, N. Vovk, G.A. Pokidalov and G.V. Blokhintsev (Scientific Research Institute of Orthopaedics and Traumatology, Kiev). The authors' views on the aetiology and pathogenesis of scoliosis were based on their studies of the clinical and radiographic signs of dysplastic and congenital scoliosis, the morphological and ultrastructural changes in the intervertebral discs, as well as the results of electron microscopy and histochemical and biochemical studies of the contractile proteins of the paravertebral muscles. The results of these studies were stated in the authors' seminal research work, *Non-surgical Treatment of Scoliosis* (Kiev, 1994). In their view, the primary cause of scoliosis is dysplasia of the intervertebral disc (Table 3.2.1).

The identification of the discogenic component in the pathogenesis of scoliosis enabled the authors to develop pathogenetically based methods of surgery on the intervertebral disc (discotomy, enucleation of nuclei pulposus, papainization of intervertebral discs). In severe forms of scoliosis, when there were changes in the soft tissues of the spine, accompanied by gross structural changes in the bony elements of the vertebrae, surgeries were performed on the vertebral bodies. These included wedge-shaped resection of the spine, as well as vertebrotomy followed by

Table 3.2.1. Scheme of scoliosis aetiology and pathogenesis (according to V.Y. Fischenko *et al.*)

Period of anlage of the spine Adverse effects of exogenous or endogenous agents
Period of postnatal development Dysplasia of the disc, which is manifested by the presence of immature nucleus pulposus cells – chondrocytes
Impaired lysosomal apparatus of immature chondrocytes
Release of large amounts of lysosomal enzymes
Metabolic changes in connective tissue
Impairment of intervertebral disc structure
Early degeneration of tissues
Loosening of the fibrous ring
Lateral migration of nucleus pulposus
Development of structural changes of vertebrae (wedge-shape and torsion)
Activation of compensatory mechanisms and formation of structural changes in lateral and posterior elements of vertebrae
Development of spinal anticurvatures

stabilization of the deformed regions, using various metal structures in conjunction with bone grafting.

Scoliotic deformity can be identified at different ages (I.V. Ponseti, B. Friedman, 1950; J.I. James, 1967; R. Heine, H. Reher, 1975). Depending on the age of onset of scoliosis, patients can be divided into the following clinical groups: infantile (from birth to 3 years of age), juvenile (4–10 years of age) and adolescent (over 10 years of age). The age of onset and the age which the disease is identified, which often occurs later, should not be confused. At the time of diagnosis, the curvature may be in an advanced stage such as the 3rd or even the 4th degree. In view of this, it is important for children to be taken for regular check-ups, and attempts should be made to increase health literacy among parents. This would reduce the difference between the age of onset and the age of diagnosis.

Special attention should be paid to infant (infantile) scolioses. This group was first distinguished and described by R.J. Harrenstein in 1933. Infant scolioses usually develop in the first year of life and have a tendency to progress. These scolioses are not covered adequately in the literature. V.Y. Fischenko *et al.* (1994) have come across only one publication on this subject, by G.A. Yukina and L.K. Mikhailova (1984). The authors observed 117 children, the majority being girls (ratio 2.4:1). In most patients (57.3%), the curvature was C-shaped and left-sided. In 69.3% of cases, at the end of the first year of life, there were already no clinical signs of scoliosis and the X-ray revealed a decrease in the degree of curvature. Other studies designed to address the causes of infantile scoliosis were conducted. No doubts were raised in cases of paresis of trunk muscles after poliomyelitis. However, there were cases of infantile scoliosis in which the deformity developed without paresis and asymmetrical load on the spine. It was even believed that scoliosis develops in newborns as a result of spiral bending of the embryo. However, this remains merely an unsubstantiated hypothesis.

According to Enchura, during the first year of life, scoliosis develops due to early torsion of the vertebrae and by the age of 2 years, due to the marked change in the shape of the vertebrae. The resulting scoliotic deformity changes the spinal load and shifts the common centre of gravity. Initially, this imbalance is sought to be rectified through increased activity of the muscles on the convex side of the body, but since this is not successful, a secondary (compensatory) curvature begins to form. The very fact that compensatory curvatures should be formed in children with infantile scoliosis is considered by J. James (1967) as a sign of irreversible deformity. As a rule the compensatory curvatures are of two kinds—above or below the major one. Only in lumbar scolioses (usually right-sided) there is an upper compensatory curvature. As for a tilt of the pelvis, it is often regarded as a curvature of the lower part.

Here, it is worth mentioning the important publication, *Scoliosis* (2008), of M.T.

Sampiev, A. Luck and N.V. Zagorodniy of the Scoliosis Correction Centre in Moscow. On the basis of the results of the latest research, the authors believe that the most objective theories regarding the aetiology of idiopathic scoliosis (IS) are those that point to genetic, endocrine and neuromuscular factors. According to the authors, the main cause of scoliosis is an imbalance of the muscles supporting the spine. The causes of this impairment are insufficiency and weakness of the muscles and ligaments (A. Grutsa, 1959), asymmetrical and weakened growth of separate muscular groups (R.R. Vreden, 1936), and congenital (meningocele) or acquired diseases of the spinal cord (A.J. Ratner, 1985) and paraspinal muscles (R. Yaromet *et al.*, 1978).

In recent years, the term 'myogenic scoliosis' has been replaced with 'neuromyogenic scoliosis' (P. Touzet and P. Rigault, 1983), which emphasizes the role of the nervous system in the genesis of IS. An experimental study by W.F. Enneking and P. Harrington (1969) is of particular interest. The authors believed that the cause of IS lies outside the spine and that all bony changes typical of scoliosis are secondary. K. Yamada, H. Yamamoto and Y. Nakagava *et al.* (1984) studied the association of IS and vestibular dysfunction in experimental animals and patients. Their main conclusion was that scoliosis may be the result both of functional and organic lesions of the brainstem.

Thus, there is compelling evidence in favour of the idea that dysplasia of the nervous system is an important aetiological factor in the development and subsequent progression of scoliotic spinal deformity. Only the level of dysfunction remains controversial.

Now that we have discussed the various theories on the causes of scoliosis, we shall go on to analyse them and list the premises that are accepted by all researchers.

1. The development of lateral curvature of the spine in a child from the first few days after birth and until the end of the first year of life is due to early torsion of the vertebrae.
2. In the case of children with insufficiency of the endocrine glands, the metabolism of mucopolysaccharides, minerals and proteins is impaired, resulting in changes in the strength of the skeleton.
3. Underdevelopment of nucleus pulposus cells as a consequence of metabolic disorders results in structural changes in the intervertebral disc. As a result, in addition to the physiological scoliotic deformity, wedge-shaped discs and vertebral bodies appear. Evolving torsion leads to the development of structural scoliosis.
4. Vicious posture is the main aetiological factor in the case of most scolioses. According to the Hueter–Volkmann law, asymmetrical load on the spine is sufficient to cause its bending and subsequent torsion of the vertebrae.
5. Absolute or relative shortening of one leg at a young age leads to the formation of

a lateral curvature. Again, the formation of this deformity is caused by rotation of the vertebrae in addition to the scoliotic deformity.

So what have we found after analysing theories on the causes of scoliosis? Though various authors have approached the issue from different perspectives, the overall belief is that *scoliosis develops only during the period of skeletal growth and that it is based on the asymmetrical growth of the vertebrae. It leads to lateral bending of the spine and the subsequent inevitable rotation (torsion) of separate vertebrae or entire segments about its axis.* The progression of scoliosis stops after the completion of skeletal growth.

This was why Professor I.A. Movshovich (1964) said that understanding the causes of vertebral torsion means revealing the mechanism of the disease.

What is the mechanism of torsion? Why does rotation or torsion of the vertebrae occur? Is the process haphazard or logical? What is the role of muscular asymmetry in the mechanism of torsion? At what levels of the spine does it occur and why exactly at these levels? We will attempt to answer these and other questions by presenting some interesting information yielded by the research of many investigators who have focused on the mechanisms of scoliosis.

3.2.2 Pathogenesis of scoliosis

We will begin this section by restating the idea that is recognized by all orthopaedic surgeons: torsion of the vertebrae plays an essential role in the pathogenesis of scoliosis. In 1913, Lange and Schede (cited from I.A. Movshovich, *Scoliosis*, 1964) used the word 'scoliosis' to denote a deformity of separate vertebrae, and the word 'rotation' to denote rotation of the spine about its longitudinal axis. Lindemann (1958) understood 'torsion' as pathological twisting of the vertebrae against each other, accompanied by structural changes of the vertebrae. I.A. Movshovich (1964) used the term rotation to mean physiological rotation of the normal (non-deformed) spine about the vertical axis. He applied the concept of torsion only to structural scoliosis.

Despite the differences in the authors' understanding of 'torsion' and 'rotation', all of them wanted to find the causes of this process. One of the earliest studies aimed at explaining the mechanism of torsion was that conducted by Bigelow in 1844 (cited from I.A. Movshovich, *Scoliosis*, 1964). He found that bending a flat flexible plate width-wise would entail rotating the middle of it around its longitudinal axis. However, Lovett (1905) thought that it was more appropriate to compare the spine with a flexible elastic rod, curved in the anteroposterior direction, than with a flat body. That is why due to motion in two planes its lateral bending inevitably led to a rotation in addition to the deformity.

Other authors have developed Lovett's ideas on the nature of torsion further. For example, in 1926, Heuer proposed a theory on the development of scoliosis on the basis of an assessment of the difference in height between the column of vertebral bodies and that of arches. According to the author, scoliosis develops because the column of vertebral bodies grows faster than that of the arches, and since they are interconnected, the longer column makes the shorter one take a position on the concave side. The correlation between the row of the vertebral bodies and the arches is shown schematically in Fig. 3.2.36. The round bar represents the column of vertebral bodies and the adjacent longitudinal stripe, the column of arches. In cases of overload, the column bends parallel to the line joining the supporting bands, if any other force hinders the process of bending or pushes it to the other side. This is the author's explanation of how static deformities due to load very often manifest as lateral curvatures.

When a load on the spine exceeds the strength of the spine, a curvature forms simultaneously on all units on cross-section of the spinal column. The curvature may be formed in more distant parts of the strip than those which are less distant. The curvature leads to rotation of the column, i.e. a certain part of the column on the top of the deformity rotates towards the convex side of the curvature. This experiment (Fig. 2.3.37) was designed to explain the mechanism of torsion of the vertebrae in scoliosis (Fig. 3.2.38).

In subsequent years, research on the pathogenesis of scoliosis continued, but the conclusions of the scientists often did not coincide. For example, Rogers (1933) and Arkin (1950) objected to Heuer's theory, describing it as a mechanistic approach to the problem of scoliosis. They said that the behaviour of the 'living' spine is too complex to be accounted for by any model of deformity. The supporters of Heuer's theory were Somerville (1952) and

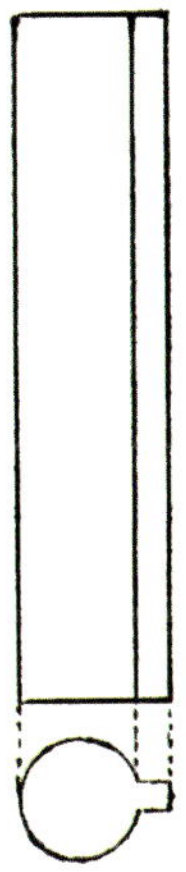

Fig. 3.2.36.
Schematic presentation of the column, strengthened with a strip attached to its periphery

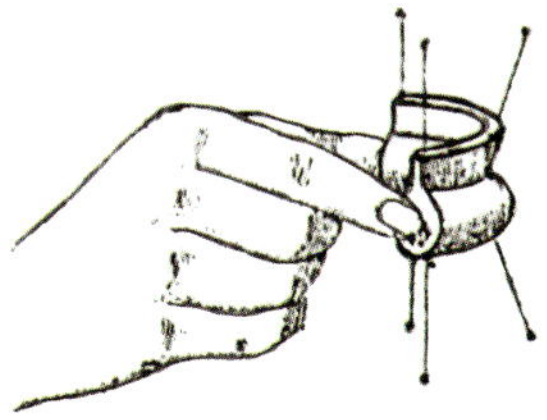

Fig. 3.2.37.
Column in which rotation occurs under overload; through the insertion of pins in a column this movement becomes apparent

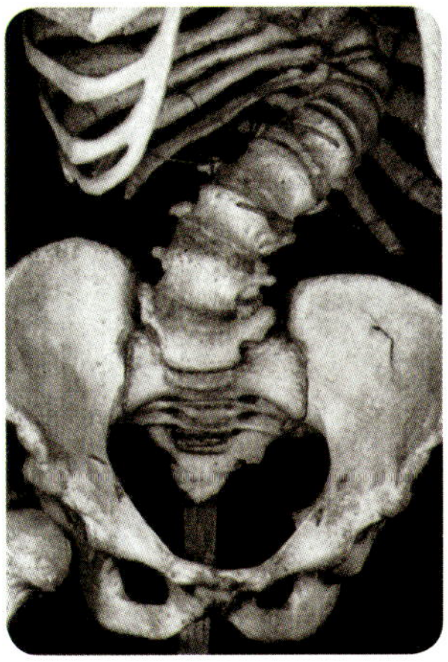

Fig. 3.2.38.
Left-sided thoracolumbar scoliosis of 3rd degree Torsion of lumbar and thoracic vertebrae

Farkas (1954). Later, Heuer developed his theory of pathogenesis, according to which the body turns during walking and simultaneous rotation of the pelvis relative to the lumbar spine are the leading causes of scoliosis.

Roaf (1958) studied the movement of different parts of the spine under normal conditions and their relationship to the lateral tilt, rotation and deformity of the spine in scoliosis. The study analysed the spines of stillborn children released from muscles, and radiographs of the spines of normal children. The author's main conclusion was that rotation is the predominant pathogenetic factor in scoliotic deformity.

A.M. Schantz, a faculty with the Dresden Medical Academy, made a significant contribution to the understanding of the pathogenesis of scoliosis in his book, *Practical Orthopaedics* (1933). Earlier, in Section 3.2.5.1 (Morphological changes of the thorax), we have discussed the research done by A.M. Schantz on the mechanism of the formation of vertebral exostoses. The author believed they were the result of static overloading. He also devoted much of his time to the study of the essence of the law of curvatures and anticurvatures of the spine. From the perspective of static load, the spine is loaded from the top, and is a vertical column (Fig. 3.2.39) that does not stand firmly and continuously changes position, with the range of positions being wide.

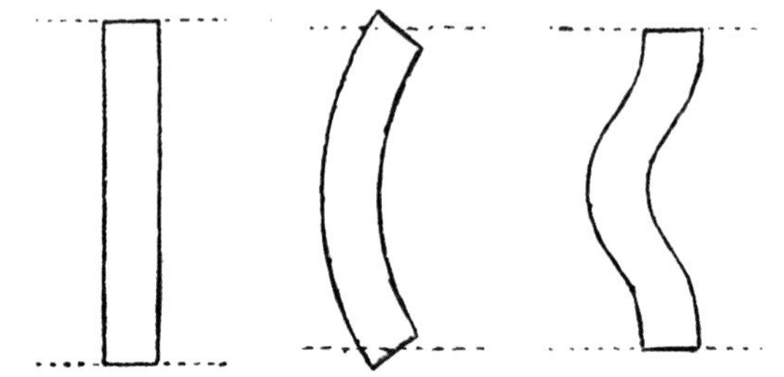

Fig. 3.2.39. Vertically standing column

Fig. 3.2.40. Vertical column with free ends in cross-section is bent under load as a simple bending

Fig. 3.2.41. Column in which cross-section ends are lying in a horizontal plane bends under overload, thus forming one main curvature and two anticurvatures

In the *mid-functional position*, terminal cross-sections of the spine touch two horizontal planes: the ground plane at the bottom and the plane of the line passing through both eyes. *Under load*, a vertical column with free ends undergoes simple bending (Fig. 3.2.40). *Under overload*, a column whose cross-sectional ends lie on a horizontal plane bends to form one main curvature and two anticurvatures (Fig. 3.2.41). The main curvature forms in the middle of the column, while the other two form towards its ends.

The essence of the law of curvatures and anticurvatures is that along with the main curvature of the spine, two anticurvatures will always form and these together will be equal to the main curvature (Fig. 2.3.42).

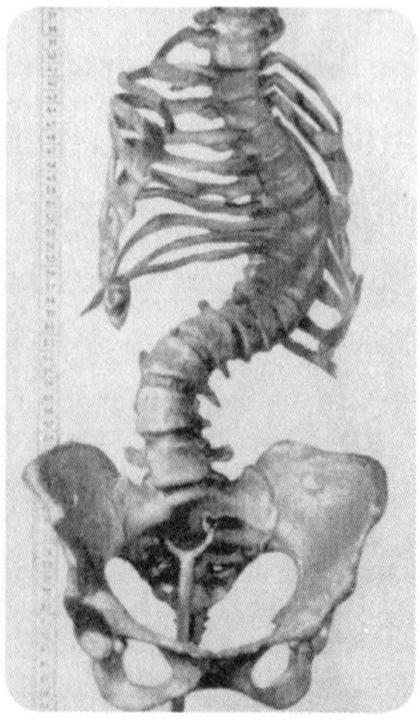

Fig. 3.2.42. Scoliotic spine that has one main curvature and two anticurvatures

The presence of a main curvature with anticurvatures has also been observed in other deformities of the spine that are caused by static load, such as senile kyphosis (Fig. 3.2.43). In this case, the deformity is significant and affects the entire spine, up to the top of the neck. Cervical lordosis is the upper anticurvature, while the different positioning of the feet serves as the lower anticurvature.

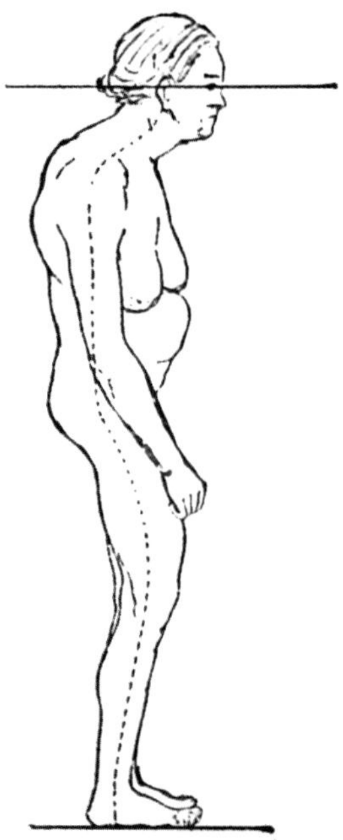

Fig. 3.2.43.
Senile kyphosis is also a combination of main curvature and two anticurvatures

The legs are the link between the lower part of the spine and the ground. Various positions of this link correspond to spinal curvature. Senile kyphosis is an example of such a lower anticurvature. If the upper anticurvature does not form, then different positioning of the eyes is an equivalent. (According to the author, maybe this is the cause of fixative strabismus, which is characteristic of all human beings and is interpreted by ophthalmologists as a physiological norm.) Oblique position of the pelvis, which so often occurs in scoliosis, is equivalent in relation to lateral curvatures.

Our understanding of the mechanism of static deformities of the spine due to excessive load has been facilitated by the law of curvatures and anticurvatures, as well as the law of deformity depending on static load, as described by A.M. Schantz.

In the following sections of this book, we will focus on the clinical manifestations of this condition. As for the pathogenesis of scoliosis, the author concluded that insufficiency of the spine is the result of an altered ratio between the load on the spine and the endurance of the spine, and that it develops in actual disequilibrium. In other words, insufficiency of the spine is a result of impaired normal physiological relationships. This may explain why, in childhood and adolescence, scoliosis may occur even among those with well-developed muscles of the trunk and initially perfect posture. According to the author (A.M. Schantz), this is caused by an increasing unilateral spasm of the long extensors of the spine which, in turn, is due to growing asymmetry between the lengths of the lower extremities.

On the basis of the laws of mechanics, A.M. Schantz explained not only the mechanism of torsion and rotation of the vertebrae, but also the formation of the costal hump, as well as reduction in the height of the anterior part of a vertebral body in kyphotic curvature.

Static deformities of the spine due to excessive load can develop at any time in life, in the presence of certain necessary conditions. A knowledge of the law of spinal deformities due to loading is of practical significance, in that it can help us in preventing progression of the disease. In this context, the following two points should be noted:

1. The progression of the disease may be stopped by restoring the balance of the load.
2. The more severe the deformity and the older the patient, the more difficult it is to achieve favourable results.

The pathogenesis of structural scoliosis can be traced to asymmetrical growth of the vertebrae. This point of view has been endorsed by Nicoladoni (1909), Folkman, etc. However, there is a debate over the causes of this asymmetry and the order in which symptoms occur, i.e. whether lesions of the musculo-ligamentous apparatus of the spine (myopathic theory) appear first or changes in the bone structure (osteopathic theory).

Ponseti (1962) (cited from I.A. Movshovich, *Scoliosis,* 1964), who subscribed to the myopathic theory, suggested that slippage and torsion of vertebrae are caused by metabolic disorders, including those affecting the metabolism of hormones and mucopolysaccharides, which impair the development of the muscles and ligaments of the spine. The development of scoliosis is the result.

According to I.A. Movshovich (1964), myopathic and osteopathic factors are equally involved in the pathogenesis of scoliosis. The theory of musculo-ligamentous insufficiency, however, did not provide a comprehensive explanation and it was necessary to look for some other primary pathological factor that underlies asymmetrical growth of the spine. Exploratory research is being continued.

In his publications of 1960 and 1961, I.A. Movshovich stated that vertebral torsion is closely linked with the vertebral bodies being wedge-shaped. He considered this process an interdependent one. A similar view had been expressed in 1950 by Arkin, who created a model of wedge-shaped vertebra (Fig. 3.2.44). His conclusion was that elements of torsion are already present in a wedge-shaped vertebral body, and these signs of torsion become fully manifested during pathological (asymmetrical) growth of the spine. As the degree of curvature increases, so does vertebral shifting. The process of asymmetrical progression of scoliosis depends not only on the action of the muscles, but also on an increasing asymmetrical workload. Despite the fact that the studies mentioned above are of undoubted value, they do not give a definitive

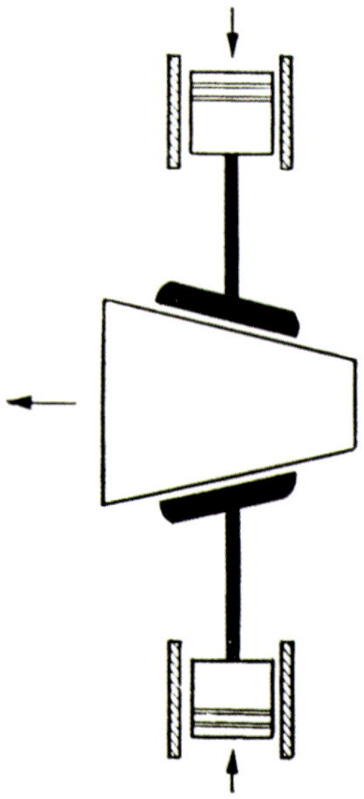

Fig. 3.2.44.
Arkin model illustrating the significance of wedge-shape of vertebral body during torsion

answer to the questions of what causes torsion and what is the mechanism of its occurrence.

Therefore, the work of D. Stilwell (1962) was of considerable theoretical and practical interest. The author experimented on young monkeys, of the ages of 1–1.5 years. Surgery consisted of unilateral extirpation of the common extensor of the trunk (m. erector trunci), from the sacrum to the lower part of the chest. No more than a month later, a lateral curvature of the spine developed. In 3–4 weeks following surgery, wedge-shaped vertebrae appeared as a result of asymmetrical growth. The author reported that the X-rays of the spines of these monkeys resembled those of people with scoliosis.

We shall take up these findings in greater detail and link the author's conclusions with our own. D. Stilwell found that the only but very important cause or first link in the pathogenesis of scoliotic deformity in the experimental animals was unilateral spasm of the preserved common spinal erector (m. erector trunci). The spasm caused the pelvis to tilt towards the weak muscles.

It must be noted that we came to a similar conclusion independently when examining the backs of babies. During the discussion of the origins of body asymmetry we have already mentioned that we observed one-sided asymmetry of the common back extensor among infants who were just a few months old, long before they began to walk. By the time they were six months old, we also clearly identified vertebral torsion in the thoracic region of the spine. This, however, was easily eliminated with the help of detorsional movements. Several motions were enough to do away with an emerging lateral curvature and muscle asymmetry. Subsequent detorsional gymnastics led to the disappearance of muscular asymmetry and lateral bending. *Therefore, muscular asymmetry is the principal factor in the development of torsion.*

D. Stilwell created such asymmetry artificially by unilaterally cutting off the entire common back extensor, beginning from the sacrum. However, in a child as we have established, this process occurs due to a cerebral mechanim resulting in asymmetry of the body muscles (*see* Section 3.1.1). When the child grows up and starts to walk, the spinal mechanism of trunk asymmetry also comes into play.

Lindemann (1958) emphasized the importance of contractures of the spinal muscles as one of the first signs of the progression of scoliosis in infancy.

According to V.Y. Fischenko (1994; 2005), degenerative changes of the intervertebral discs play a key role in the pathogenesis of scoliosis. These begin to manifest themselves during post-natal development. However, the beginning of the process goes back to the pre-natal period, when impaired anlage of the spine is associated with the negative influence of endogenous and exogenous factors. Metabolic disorders lead to structural changes in the intervertebral discs and underdevelopment of the nucleus pulposus cells. Disc dysplasia occurs in addition to the main curvature of the spine. *Hence development of this curvature precedes changes in the disc and it is the progressive spinal curvature caused by muscular asymmetry which is the negative exogenous factor mentioned above.*

Many authors have conducted clinical, radiological and morphological studies to discover the pathogenesis of scoliosis. An example is the important monograph, *Scoliosis: Surgical Anatomy and Pathogenesis*, written by I.A. Movshovich in 1964. The author's long-term observation of patients with scoliosis led him to conclude that *certain conditions are required for the development of progressive idiopathic and dysplastic scoliosis*. These are as follows:

1. There needs to be a primary pathological factor that impairs the normal growth of the spine, e.g. dysplastic changes in the spinal cord and/or vertebrae and/or discs, etc.
2. There must be a metabolic or hormonal disorder which creates a common pathological background for the manifestation of the first factor.
3. Another condition is the presence of static and dynamic disorders that are of particular relevance during the active growth of the spine (e.g. pelvic tilt in hip ankylosis with a vicious hip position, scars that tighten the skin and cause distortion of the body, asymmetry of muscle strength, etc.).

Under the influence of these factors, the epiphyseal growth of the vertebrae may be disrupted and a lateral curvature of the spine may develop. A comparison of the consequences of the presence of each of these factors showed that it was not one factor alone that was not responsible for the child to develop scoliosis. *Only a combination of all three factors could cause progressive coliosis* (Fig. 3.2.45).

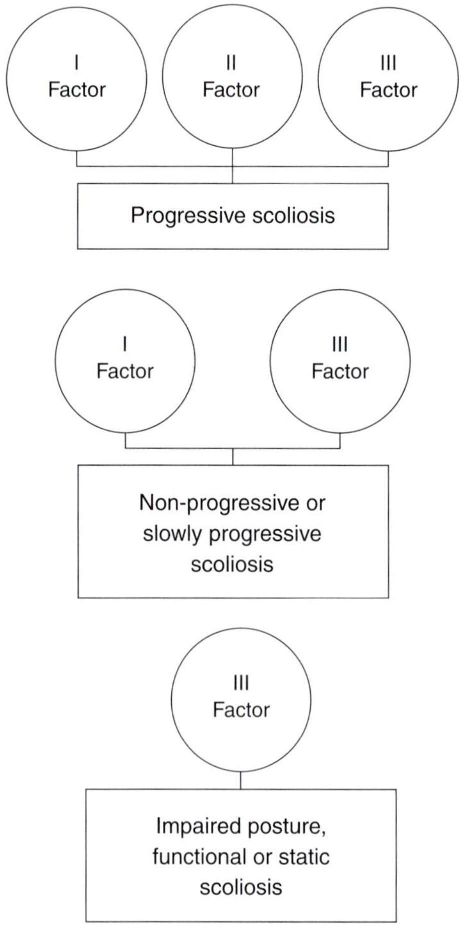

Fig. 3.2.45.
Interrelations of factors contributing to the development of scoliosis (scheme)
Presence of all three factors causes progressive scoliosis; presence of only two factors (I and III) causes non-progressive or slowly progressive scoliosis; the isolated action of the 3rd factor leads to impaired posture, as well as to development of functional or, during the period of skeletal growth, static scoliosis

According to I.A. Movshovich, the initial period of the development of structural scoliosis consists of several features, which are in the following sequence:

1. Lateral tilt of the spine leads to reflex contraction of the paravertebral muscles (muscular contracture), which gradually becomes persistent. *Progressive contracture, which is observed in scoliosis even in infants, provokes structural changes of the spine.*
2. The development of structural scoliosis is the result of asymmetrical growth of the vertebrae.
3. Even if there is a slight curvature, it immediately has an adverse effect on the conditions required for dynamic equilibrium of the spine. The pressure on the concave side of the curvature becomes greater than that on the convex side.

It is necessary, however, to point out that the situation outlined by I.A. Movshovich begins to manifest itself only when the child starts walking, and it persists in the later years of the child's life. *In our opinion, before a child starts walking, contracture of the trunk muscles, a phenomenon which has a cerebral origin, precedes the lateral tilt of the spine and is thus the primary cause of deformity.*

When lateral scoliotic curvature is initially formed, the first victim is, of course, the intervertebral disc, which normally provides elasticity and helps to reverse dynamic disorders. Later, a prolonged and even increasingly asymmetrical load causes a series of structural changes in the disc.

In lateral curvature of the spine, the forces of compression are more pronounced on the concave side of the arc of curvature. Therefore, the fibrous ring on this side experiences not only horizontal (due to the nucleus pulposus) but also vertical pressure. Since the nucleus pulposus is incompressible, as the curvature progresses, it gradually shifts towards the lowest vertical load, i.e. towards the convex side of the arc of curvature (Fig. 3.2.46).

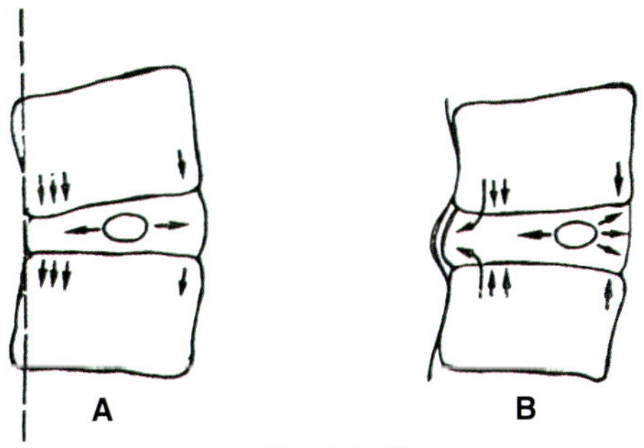

Fig. 3.2.46.
Forces acting on intervertebral disc in process of development of scoliosis
A - at the initial stages of spinal curvature formation; **B** - in process of development of scoliosis, the gelatinous nucleus shifts towards the convex side and the annulus bulges towards the concave side

We have already mentioned that according to the Hueter–Folkmann law, there is a slowing down of growth in areas of the bone where the epiphyseal cartilage undergoes severe and prolonged compression, and the growth of bones is accelerated in less loaded areas of the epiphyseal cartilage. Thus, wedge-shaped vertebrae are formed. The fact that the progression of scoliosis is maximally evident during the period of skeletal growth may be regarded as an evidence of the Heuter–

Folkmann law. As the arc of curvature of the thoracic spine develops, the forces of vertical load increase further and suppress epiphyseal growth of the vertebrae on the concave side.

Thus, *continuous and increasing asymmetrical load on the spine during the period of active skeletal growth, especially in cases of progressive scoliosis, creates the so-called 'vicious cycle'*. The essence of the matter is that growing pressure on the spine makes the wedge-shaped deformity of the vertebrae more pronounced, which increases the curvature of the spinal segment, resulting in a further increase of asymmetrical load.

It is necessary to mention other theories on the pathogenesis of scoliosis. According to R. Burwell and P. Dangerfield (1998), progressive asymmetrical development of the human skeleton may play a major role in twisting of the pelvis and lumbar spine, and consequently, rotation of the thoracic region in the opposite direction.

The Swedish physician, J. Sevastik (1993), proposed a theory on the pathogenesis of idiopathic scoliosis. According to this, asymmetry of blood supply to the right and left halves of the chest, which occurs for some unknown reasons, results in accelerated growth of the ribs on one or the other side of the body. However, this hypothesis could not be validated by studies carried out by P. Korovessis *et al.* (2003). Our understanding of the pathogenesis of progressive scoliosis is shown in Scheme 3.2.1.

We arrived at our conclusions after going through a significant volume of material on different aspects of asymmetry of the human body as well as the aetiology and pathogenesis of scoliosis. We have presented data to support our view, and have also provided data supporting the views of other researchers. To help the reader better understand the points made in this chapter, we present a comprehensive summary.

1. The initial manifestations of asymmetry of all body structures, including the muscles of the trunk, appear during foetal development due to asymmetrical functioning of the cerebral cortex (*cerebral mechanism of asymmetry*).
2. In the first months of life, the asymmetry of the body that has formed becomes

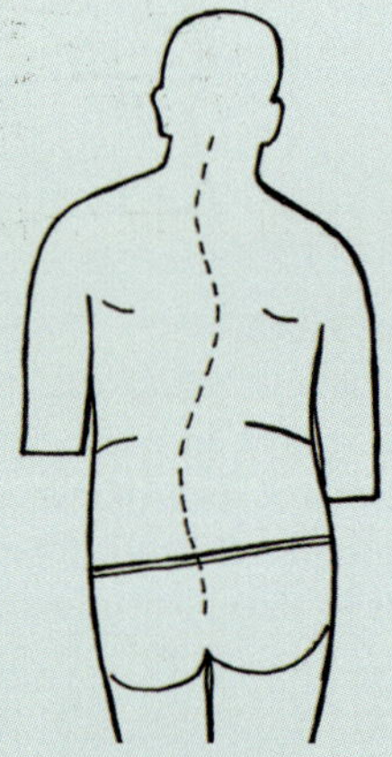

Scheme 3.2.1.

Pathogenesis of progressive scoliosis

Stages of development

- Brain asymmetry
- Asymmetry of trunk muscles; unilateral spasm of spinal extensors
- Lateral curvature of the spine with elements of rotation
- Impairment of dynamic equilibrium of the spine with development of insufficiency
- Asymmetrical growth of vertebral bodies and discs; their wedge-shaped deformition
- Torsion of vertebrae
- Progressive scoliosis

persistent. The back muscles are fixed in a state of unilateral spasm, which gradually leads to the development of lateral spinal curvature with rotation of elements of the spine. *Thus, in addition to the cerebral and spinal mechanisms of asymmetry,* there is also the resulting development of *functional scoliosis*, which is not yet characterized by structural changes of the vertebrae.

3. Humans do not start walking upright immediately after birth, unlike animals (colts, calves, kids, etc.). Within 6–9 months, a child gradually gets used to the upright position, learning to rise to his feet, stand and then walk. The vertical body position is controlled by the cerebellum, which is the centre that controls the skeletal muscles involved in the execution of movements. The cerebellum also receives signals from the vestibular system, which is located in the pyramid of the temporal bones and helps to maintain static sense. Since the cerebellum is responsible for various conditioned reflexes, we can assume that asymmetry of the body muscles and the trunk being skewed to one side are *features that are imprinted in the cerebellum when a child begins walking, and can be considered a conditioned reflex of vertical posture.*
4. Even a slight lateral curvature of the spine causes impairment of its dynamic equilibrium and the development of insufficiency.
5. Prolonged and growing asymmetrical load on the spine during the period of growth leads to progressive bending of the spine which, in turn, increases the asymmetrical load further. This is how the *'vicious cycle'* develops. As a result, due to impaired growth of the vertebrae and discs, as well as their unilateral deformation, wedge-shaped vertebrae are formed.
6. One-sided spasm of the spinal erectors causes the vertebrae at the top of the deformity to turn. This condition leads to development of structural scoliosis, which is characterized by lateral curvature, wedge-shaped vertebrae and vertebral torsion.
7. Tilting of the body to one side may be caused not only by unilateral spasm of the trunk muscles, which is always present, but also by an additional factor, i.e. unequal length of the lower extremities due to their shortening as a consequence of fractures, polio, joint ankylosis in the wrong position, etc. Such shortening is known as absolute. In the vast majority of cases, however, the shortening is relative and is caused by spasm of the trunk muscles and not by bone deformities. In all the patients examined by us, we found that this type of shortening tends to increase from a few millimetres in early childhood to centimetres in adulthood. The greater the shortening, the more pronounced the lateral curvature.
8. The law on curvatures and anticurvatures (A.M. Schantz, 1933) allowed us to explain the mechanism of the formation of curvatures and anticurvatures not only

in the cervical, thoracic and lumbar regions of the spine, but also in the transitional levels between the cervical and thoracic, thoracic and lumbar, as well as lumbar and sacral regions. Torsion also occurs at the junction of the skull with the cervical spine (C_1–C_2), at the transition between the fifth lumbar and first sacral vertebrae (L_5–S_1) and even between the sacral vertebrae (in cases in which they are not fused).

But what causes these rotations? For good reason, I.A. Movshovich like other researchers, emphasized that vicious posture or one-sided pathological changes of the vertebrae and disc growth are not enough for the development of extensive progressive scoliosis. *Some other factor is required to cause reversal of a whole segment of the spine or even of the entire spinal column*. The search for this factor has forced us to go back to the study of the biomechanics of the human body. Before discussing this, it is appropriate to describe the features of the structure of the spine and their association with the formation of lateral curvature.

We have had numerous visits from the parents of children between the ages of 12 and 14 years (mostly girls) who had progressive scoliosis despite the fact that they were actively engaged in sports. The reason for their visits to me was increasingly visible deformation of the chest with formation of hump back. Often, there were no complaints from the children. It was natural to ask why and when progressive scoliosis appeared.

It was logical to assume that along with the laws discussed above, there is some other mechanism which provokes the growth of lateral spinal curvature and acts the same way in adolescent children as in adults. While searching for an answer, we noticed that in all clinical cases of scoliosis, the first and second sacral vertebrae were not fused, which is known as lumbarization of S_1–S_2.

In his textbook of anatomy, G.F. Ivanov (1949) informed us that unfused sacral vertebrae are observed among all people between the ages of 24 and 25 years. At older ages, according to S.A. Reinberg (1964), unfused vertebrae are observed in 20%–25% of cases. We established that during adolescence, such people were actively engaged in sports and experienced spinal injuries, etc. So, probably traumatic injuries of the sacral vertebrae in the period of active growth of the skeleton were the cause of lumbarization in the coming years.

In our opinion, unfused sacral vertebrae are the weakest region of the entire spine. In fact, this region experiences the maximum vertical load, equal to the body weight, and there are no powerful muscles and ligaments in this region that can prevent displacement of the sacral vertebrae. *Therefore, the presence of a mild pelvic tilt is sufficient to cause turning of the sacral vertebrae, which triggers torsion and leads to development of the structural scoliotic deformity.*

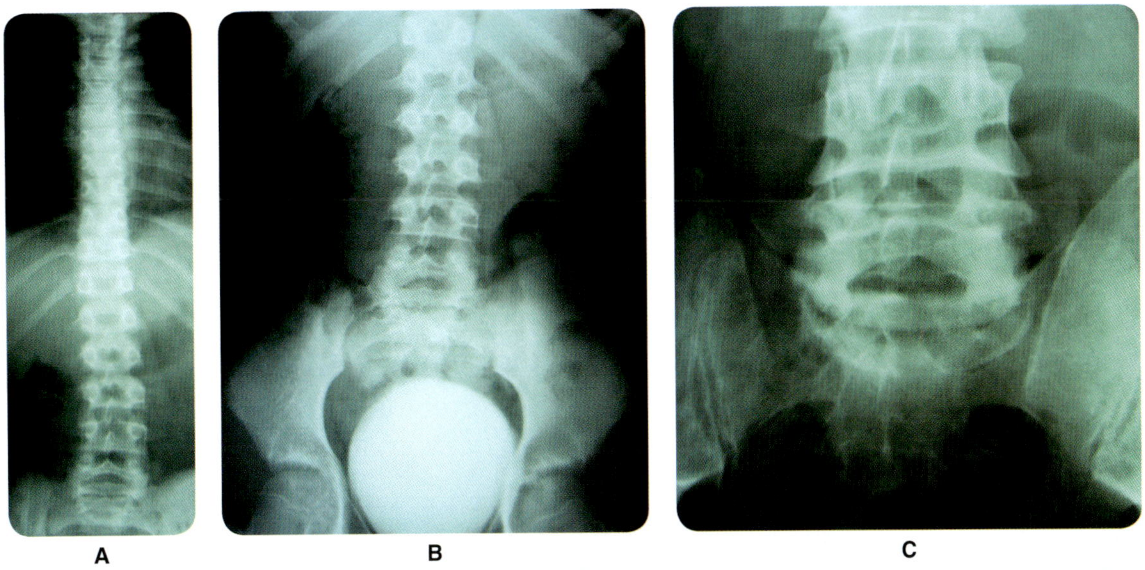

Fig. 3.2.47.
Spondylosis deformans at the level of first and second sacral vertebrae
A - 7.5-year-old child; **B** - 11-year-old child; **C** - adult patient, 49 years of age

When we talk about deforming spondylosis, we are usually referring to an average middle-aged or, more often, older person. However, radiographs of the lumbosacral region of children and adolescents with progressive scoliosis show the presence of deforming changes at the level of the first and second sacral vertebrae, as well as complete absence of deforming changes at other levels of the spine (Figs 3.2.47A and B). Figure 3.2.47C shows a similar example of deforming spondylosis at the level of L_5–S_1–S_2 in an adult patient with lumbarization of S_1.

The presence of deforming changes at the above-mentioned levels indicates that repeated and even continuous rotational displacement of these vertebrae causes traumatization of the closing plates of their bodies and discs. It is quite possible that this is the cause of local deforming spondylosis at the level of L_5–S_1–S_2 among both children and adults. Exactly at this level, a zone of primary spinal instability arises, which subsequently leads to torsion of the vertebrae at all levels and ultimately, the formation of structural scoliotic deformity.

The more strenuous the teenager's movements and the more intense the training and exercises done by him, the greater the progression of the existing spinal deformity due to increasing unilateral spasm of the spinal extensors.

Deformity of the spine begins in the presence of the above factors and shortening of one leg plays a major role. It should be remembered that during rapid growth among teenagers, there is an increase in the difference between the lengths of the legs. The insufficiency that develops causes the progression of deformity.

The sacrum appears to play the most important role in the development of scoliosis.

It is probably for this reason that the anatomists of ancient days named this bone the 'sacrum', which means 'sacred' or 'object of worship'. An understanding of the role of the sacrum in scoliosis allowed us to develop a highly effective method of treating the disease. An understanding of the role of the instability of sacral vertebrae enabled us to uncover the mechanism of persistent pelvic pain syndrome and to provide effective treatment to hundreds and even thousands of patients with sacral pain.

So, we have by now managed to answer all the questions that were posed earlier. Only one question remains: What makes the vertebrae rotate relative to each other in all regions of the spine, including the sacrum, and why does lateral flexion of the spine inevitably lead to rotation–torsion of the vertebrae? This question is answered in the following section, which is based on our study of the biomechanical aspects of the process. (This section was written in collaboration with Y.N. Svinarev, Associate Professor of Theoretical Mechanics and Mechanical Engineering of Odessa National Polytechnic University.)

3.3 JUSTIFICATION ON BIOMECHANICAL GROUNDS OF ROTATORY DISPLACEMENT OF VERTEBRAE RELATIVE TO EACH OTHER IN BENDING OF THE SPINE

'No human investigation can claim to be scientific if it does not pass the test of mathematical proof.'

—Leonardo da Vinci

When examining a patient (child or adult) with progressive scoliosis and spinal pain syndrome and wondering how to help him, the most important conclusions of my work immediately come to mind, as these have made it possible to successfully treat patients. These conclusions are as follows:

1. The development of scoliotic posture in a child below the age of one year is caused by early torsion of the vertebrae, owing to unilateral spasm of the back muscles. The latter is of cerebral origin.
2. In most cases, the progression of scoliosis in infancy is associated with an increasing difference between the length of the legs.
3. In patients of all ages (children, adolescents, adults and even the elderly), dysplastic changes of the lumbosacral spine (lumbarization of S_1–S_2, sacralization of L_5, spina bifida, asymmetry of articular processes, etc.) weaken the basis of the spine. As a result, a primary zone of instability is created.
4. The combined effect of the factors mentioned above impairs the equilibrium of the spine. Given the presence of wedge-shaped deformity of the vertebral bodies and discs, first functional scoliosis develops and then structural scoliosis.

According to the laws of mechanics, an object will remain stable only if the projection of its centre of gravity lies within the area delineated by the bearings of the object (Fig. 3.3.1). The object shown in Fig. 3.3.1A will be stable, while that shown in Fig. 3.3.1B will tip over. This law holds good even in the case of the biomechanics of the

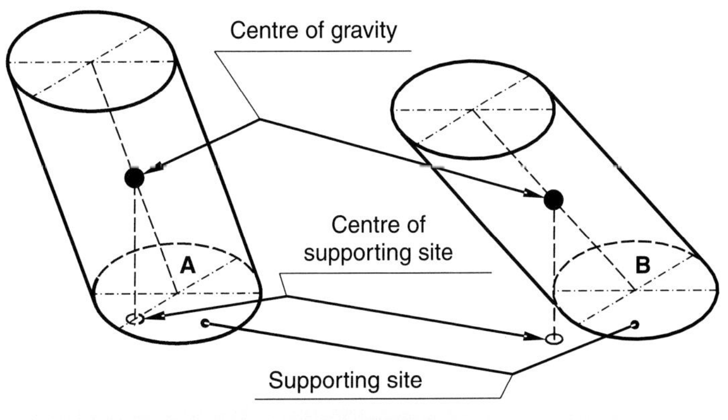

Fig. 3.3.1.
Stability of an object: **A** - stable object; **B** - unstable object

human body. The cerebellum and vestibular apparatus of the inner ear, which maintain the vertical position of the body and control its movement in space, project the body's centre of gravity within the supporting area, bounded by the feet, to provide maximum stability (Fig. 3.3.2).

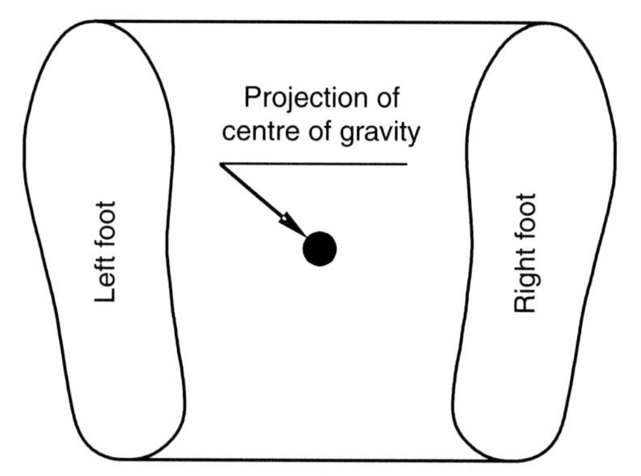

Fig. 3.3.2.
Supporting site

In bending of the trunk and pelvic tilt caused by an absolute and/or relative shortening of one leg, the axis of the spine (Fig. 3.3.3A) deviates from the vertical axis, shifting the centre of gravity towards the tilt (Fig. 3.3.3B). At the same time, to preserve the balance, the back muscles bend the spine in the direction opposite to the deviation of the centre of gravity (Fig. 3.3.3C).

If the tilt could be eliminated by rotation of only one vertebra relative to another in a vertical plane, then the spine would come back to the vertical position and bend at point *O*, as shown in Fig. 3.3.3C. The centre of gravity would return to the axis of symmetry A–A, the stability of the body would be restored and the spine above point *O* would become straight.

In fact, possible relative motions of the vertebrae allow the spine to bend to a desired angle only through the simultaneous rotation of a few adjacent vertebrae. As a result, the spine, bending in the region c over some radius r_c and assuming a vertical position, will not return to the centre of gravity on the axis of symmetry A–A (Fig. 3.3.3D). So

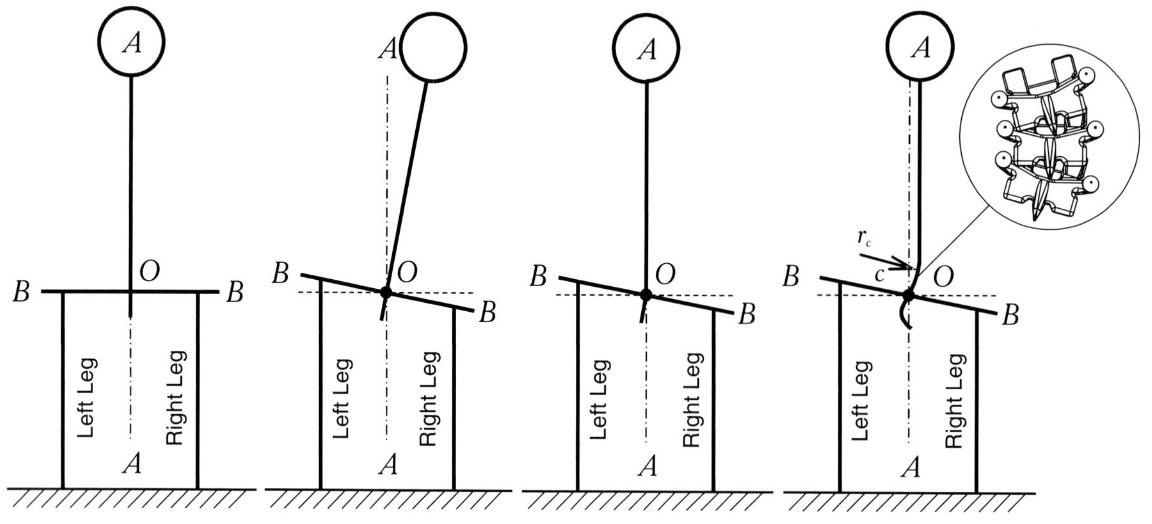

Fig. 3.3.3.
Curvature of the spine in shortening of the right leg

in reality, in region c the spine rotates at a greater angle so that the axis of the spine intersects the vertical line A–A (Fig. 3.3.4A).

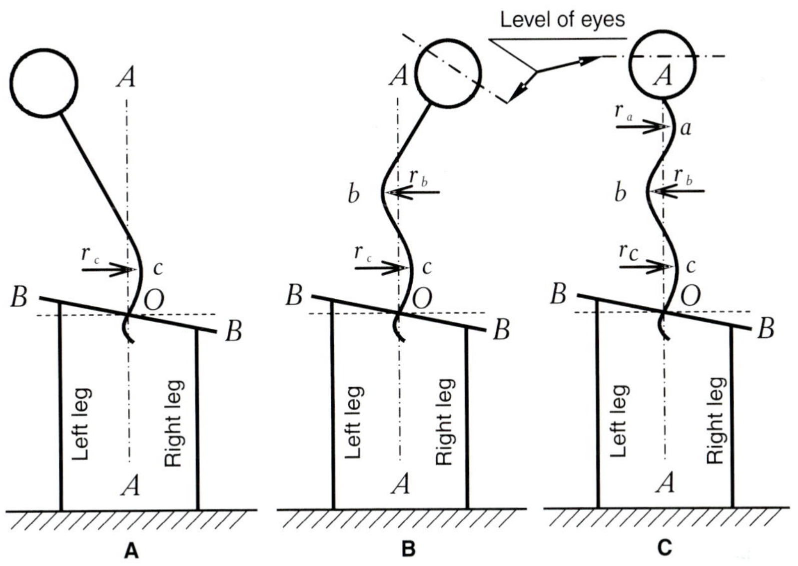

Fig. 3.3.4.
Formation of typical curvatures of the spine in cervical, thoracic and lumbar regions of the spine in shortening of the right leg

At the same time, under the direction of the cerebellum and the vestibular system, the spine tends to assume a vertical position, due to which it bends in region *b* over a radius r_b (Fig. 3.3.4B). In this position, the centre of gravity will be projected close to the centre of the supporting area, maintaining the equilibrium of the body. However, the resulting tilt is not physiological, so it is reflexively corrected through bending of the spine in region *a* over some radius r_a (Fig. 3.3.4C). The head also tends to turn reflexively so that the line of the eyes assumes a maximally horizontal position.

Thus, spinal deformity is not limited only by lateral curvature. Simultaneously there is turning of separate vertebrae about their axis—that is what we call rotation, resulting in subsequent reversal of individual segments of the spine—its torsion. As a result of all the above factors, the characteristic regions of the spine are formed (*a*, *b* and *c*), with the vertebrae rotating relative to each other in a vertical plane (Fig. 3.3.5). However, in all people of up to 24–25 years of age and in 20%–25% of older people, the fifth lumbar and upper sacral vertebrae also rotate relative to each other in region *d* (Fig. 3.3.6). This is due to the presence of unfused sacral vertebrae. Figures 3.3.5 and 3.3.6 show the areas of bending of the spine in cases of shortening of the right leg. If it is the left leg which is shortened, rotation occurs in the opposite direction.

To throw light on the causes of the rotation of two adjacent vertebrae relative to each other, we will examine the details of the process of their interaction. When the spine is not bent (Fig. 3.3.7), compression or stretching of the ring-shaped cartilage (meniscoids) covering the articular processes of the vertebrae in areas *L* and *P* (left and right, respectively) is equal (to illustrate deformities, the figures show meniscoids of exaggerated thickness in zones *L* and *P*). In bending of the spine, due to contraction of the spinal muscles, the bending moment M_u is applied to the vertebrae (Fig. 3.3.8). This

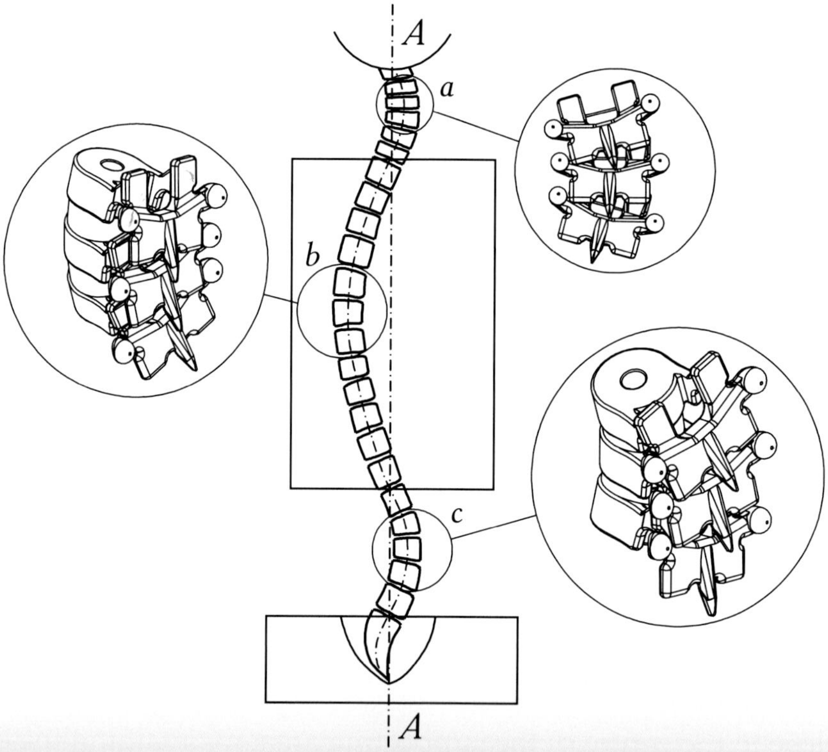

Fig. 3.3.5.
Regions of typical curvatures of the spine in an adult human with normal sacrum; shortening of the right leg

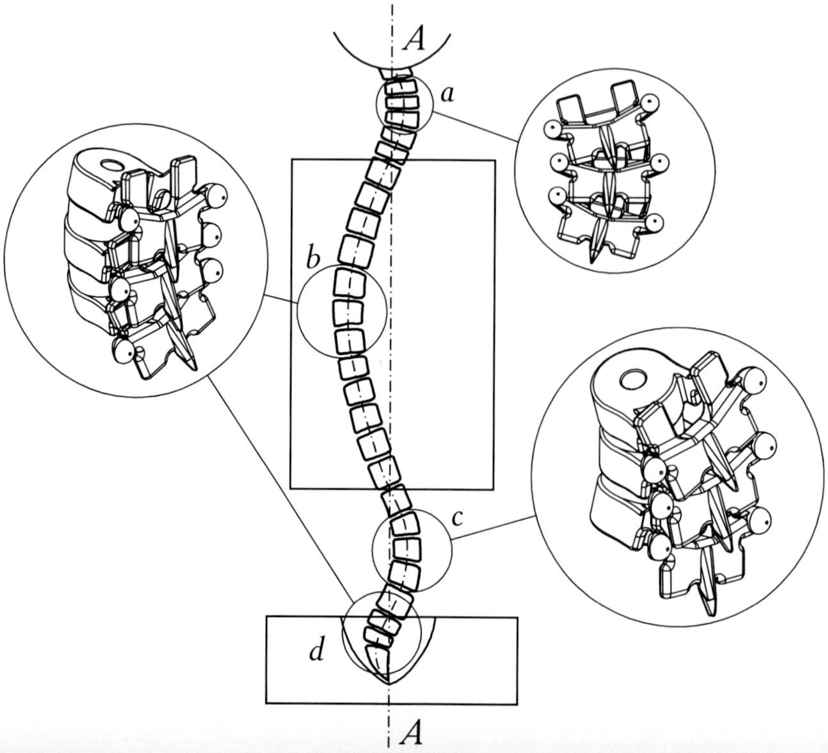

Fig. 3.3.6.
Regions of typical curvatures of the spine in unfused sacral vertebrae; shortening of the right leg

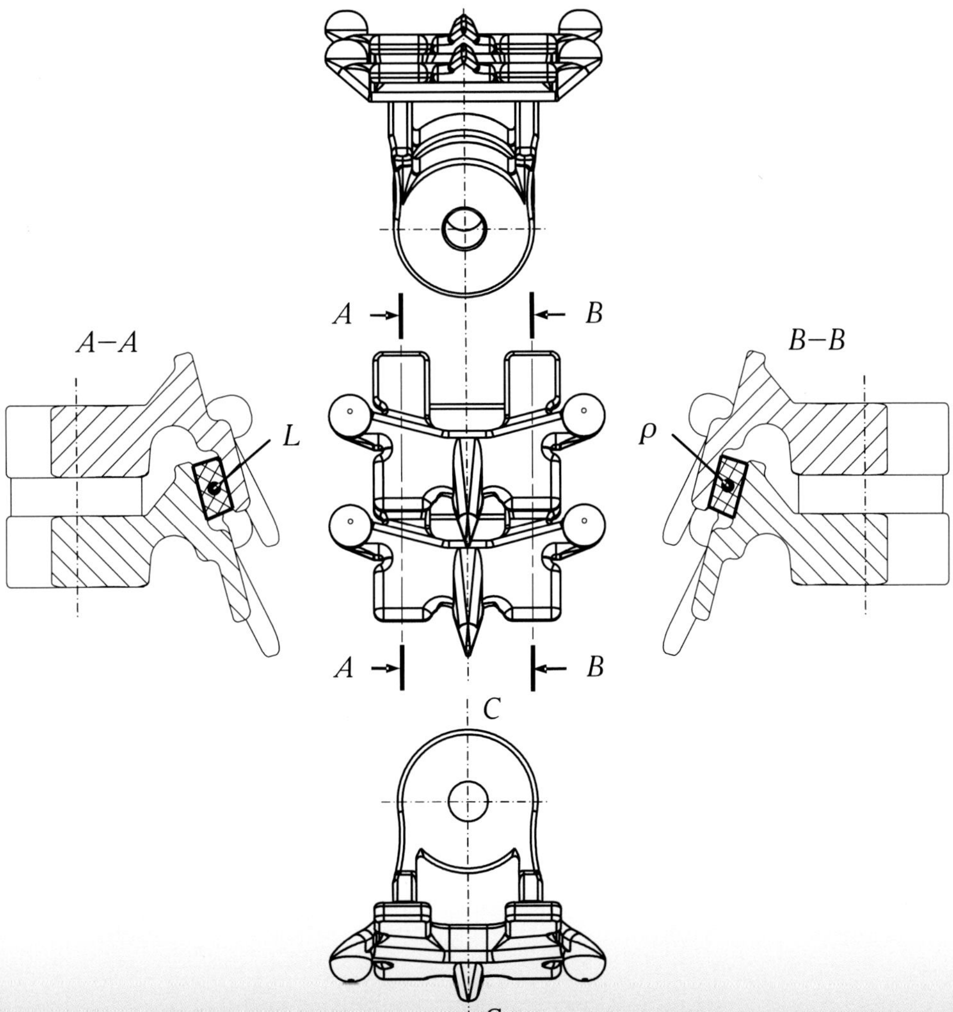

Fig. 3.3.7. Vertebrae in non-bent area of the spine

causes rotation of adjacent vertebrae relative to each other in a vertical plane at an angle α. While rotating, the distance between the adjacent processes of the vertebrae in area *L* decreases and that in area *P* increases. Accordingly, the meniscoid is compressed in zone *L* and stretched in zone *P*.

The cartilaginous tissue and synovium in zone *L* of the articular processes of the vertebrae will resist compression and apply a force $\overline{F}_{com}$ which should push the articular processes to their original position. In zone *P*, these tissues resist stretching and exert force $\overline{F}_p$ on the articular processes, seeking to bring them closer to each other (Fig. 3.3.8).

According to Newton's third law, the forces $\overline{F}_{com}$ and $\overline{F}'_{com}$ acting on the adjacent vertebrae in zone *L* (Fig. 3.3.8) are equal and forces $\overline{F}_p$ and $\overline{F}'_p$ acting on the adjacent vertebrae in zone *P* are also equal. Their values depend on the extent of the deformation of the meniscoids and their elastic properties.

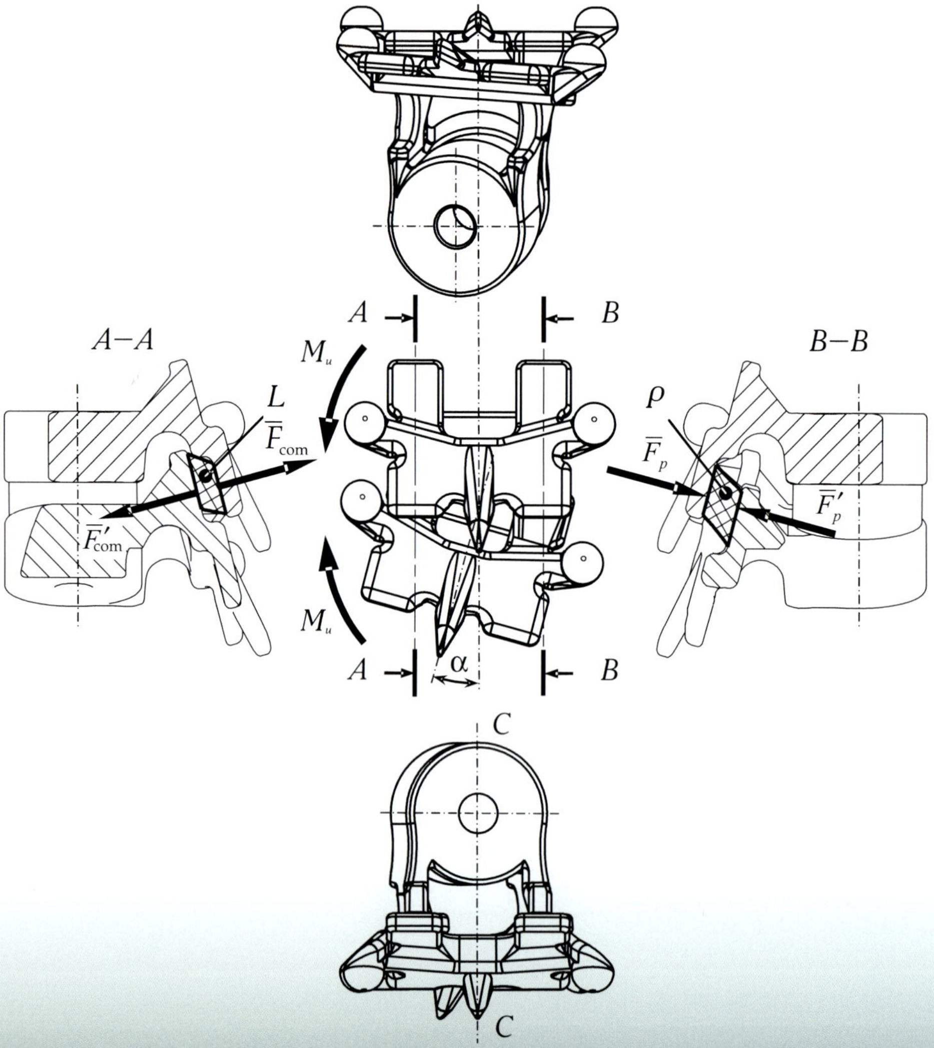

Fig. 3.3.8. Vertebrae in bent area of the spine

To gain a better understanding of the mechanism of the interaction of forces between vertebrae which causes rotation, one could consider the equilibrium of one vertebra (Fig. 3.3.9). Since the articular processes of vertebrae are tilted in the vertical direction at an angle β, the forces $\overline{F}_{com}$ and $\overline{F}_p$ in projections on the X- and Y-axis resolve into two components each (Fig. 3.3.9):

The force component F_{com} would give the following projections:

$$F_{comZ} = F_{com} \cdot \cos\beta \quad \text{and} \quad F_{comY} = F_{com} \cdot \sin\beta$$

The force component F_p would give the following projections:

$$F_{p_Z} = F_p \cdot \cos\beta \quad \text{and} \quad F_{p_Y} = F_p \cdot \sin\beta$$

Forces $\overline{F}_{comY}$ and $\overline{F}_{p_Y}$ will create a moment of resistance (or restoring moment) in the vertical plane (X–Y), and this will counteract the moment M_u which bends the

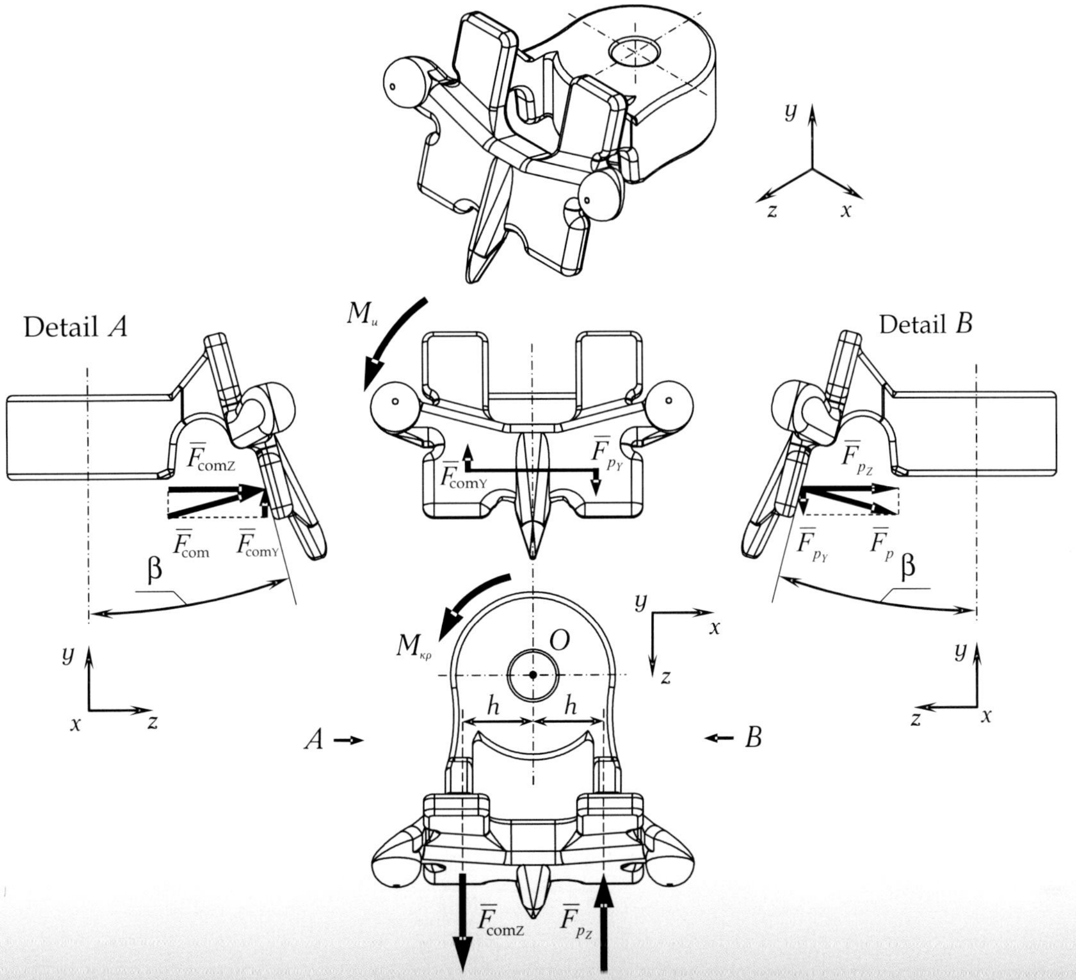

Fig. 3.3.9. Force impacts on the vertebra in bending of the spine

spine. These two factors will counterbalance each other and not affect the rotation of the vertebra, so they shall not be considered further.

Forces $\overline{F}_{comZ}$ and $\overline{F}_{p_Z}$ will create a torque that is not balanced, M_{kp}, in the horizontal plane (Fig. 3.3.9):

$$M_{kp} = F_{comZ} \cdot h + F_{pZ} \cdot h = (F_{comZ} + F_{pZ}) \cdot h$$

The moment M_{kp}, being unbalanced, will cause rotation of the vertebra relative to the adjacent vertebrae at an angle γ (Fig. 3.3.10) and around an axis Y, passing through the relative centre of rotation *O*. During the rotation of the vertebra, the distance between the articular processes of the adjacent vertebrae will equalize (Fig. 3.3.10, zones *L* and *P*), the forces of compression and stretching of the cartilage and synovial membrane will disappear or become equal, the torque M_{kp} will disappear and the vertebrae will remain rotated relative to each other at an angle γ (Figs 3.3.10– 3.3.11).

Thus, we can draw the following conclusion: if any vertebra is linked with a Cartesian coordinate system oriented as shown in Fig. 3.3.12, and any adjacent

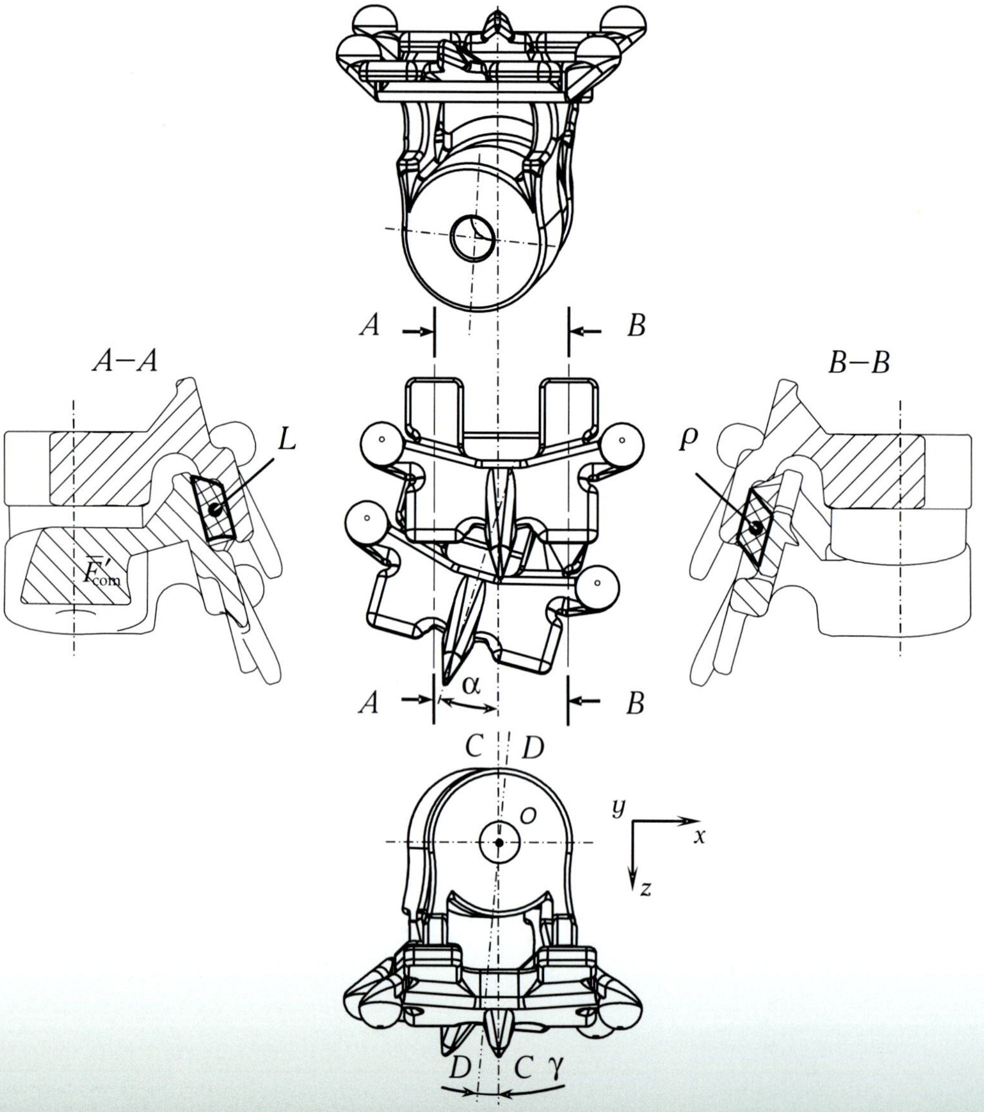

Fig. 3.3.10.
Rotation of vertebrae in horizontal plane

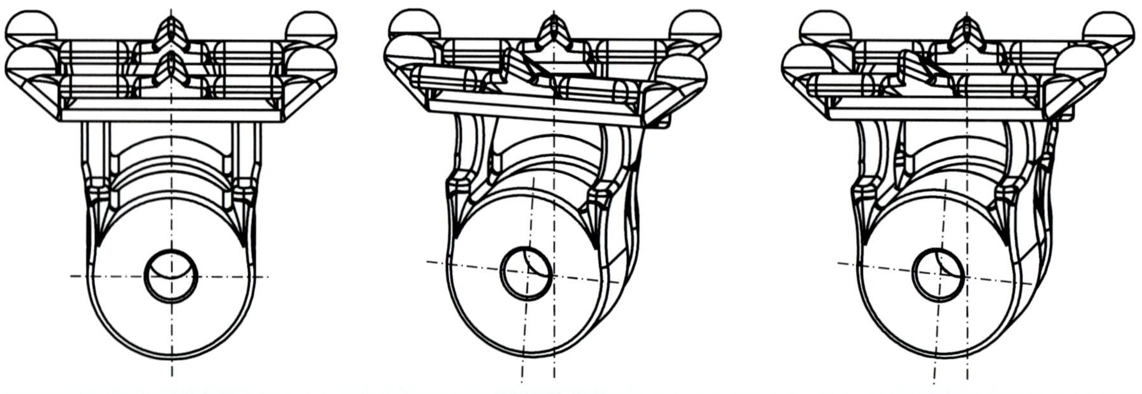

Fig. 3.3.11.
Rotation of vertebrae in bending of the spine

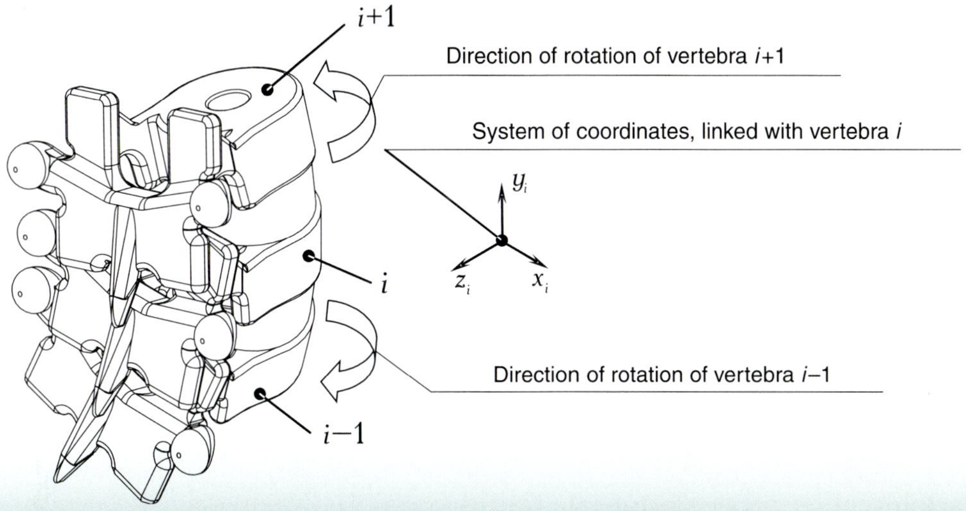

Fig. 3.3.12. Rotation of vertebrae in bending of the spine

vertebra is tilted in the vertical plane (X–Y), whether clockwise or counterclockwise, then this vertebra will rotate in the horizontal plane (X–Z) in the same direction (also clockwise or counterclockwise). This explains how bending of the spine, followed by rotation of the vertebrae about their axis, occurs when the trunk is bent to one side. The intensity of the problem depends on the degree of rotation, strength of the back muscles, elastic properties of the bone and cartilage tissue, co-morbid diseases of the skeleton, endocrine disorders, etc. *In accordance with the laws of mechanics, lateral curvature of the spine will always be accompanied by the rotation of separate vertebrae, and then by torsion of whole segments.*

3.3.1 THE ROLE OF MUTUALLY ANTITHETICAL DISPLACEMENT OF VERTEBRAE, IMPAIRED TROPISM OF ARTICULAR PROCESSES AND LUMBARIZATION OF S_1–S_2 IN FORMATION OF SCOLIOTIC DEFORMITY

The above-described regularity of rotational displacement of the vertebrae was discovered by us in all regions of the spine including the site of maximum curvature, as well as the transitional levels between different regions. On the basis of our accumulated clinical experience, we have drawn several important conclusions.

1. In each region, whether cervical, thoracic or lumbosacral, we constantly observed at the top of the curvature not only a rotational displacement of the vertebrae, but also a mutually antithetical shift of the upper and lower vertebrae (Fig. 3.3.13). These shifts take place to preserve the vertical position of the body, i.e. to ensure

the stability of the vertical structure (the spinal column). The basic laws of mechanics are reflected in this.

Unfortunately, the compensatory ability of the body is limited. Therefore, in the case of a large pelvis tilt, followed by consequent significant lateral curvature of the spine, the mutually antithetical vertebrae do not correct the curvature but only prevent its progression.

2. It is necessary to consider another important fact. We already know that in early childhood and adolescence, the vertebral bodies are deformed in the areas where the spine is curved the maximum, thus becoming wedge-shaped. Later, curvature arcs are formed precisely in these areas (Figs 3.3.14 and 3.3.15). Changes in the shape of the vertebrae affect not only the vertebral bodies but also the processes (*see* Chapter 2.2, Figs 2.2.40–2.2.45). The structure of the articular and transverse processes becomes asymmetrical while developing in the tilt-rotated position. This is especially so in the case of the right and left articular surfaces (facies articularis) (Fig. 3.3.16).

   As a result, *zones of instability arise in each region of the spine.* Describing the causes of lumbosacral facet pain, S.A. Reinberg (1964) paid special attention to this issue (*see* Chapter 2.2, Fig. 2.2.30). However, from our perspective, instability is not limited only to the 5th lumbar and the 1st sacral vertebrae; it is common to all vertebrae in areas where the curvature is maximum.

3. The formation of osseous

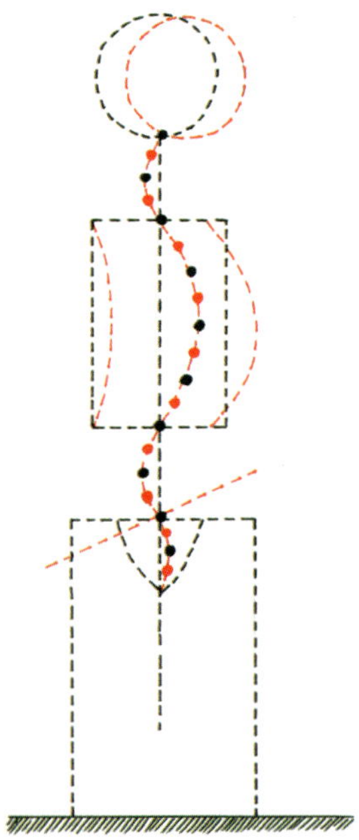

Fig. 3.3.13.
Schematic presentation of changes in body position in lateral bending of the trunk:
- Vertical position of the body in equal length of lower extremities
- Deformation of the body in pelvic tilt due to shortening of the left leg
- Zones of rotational displacement of vertebrae at the top of segment curvature
- Zones of mutually antithetical displacement of vertebrae

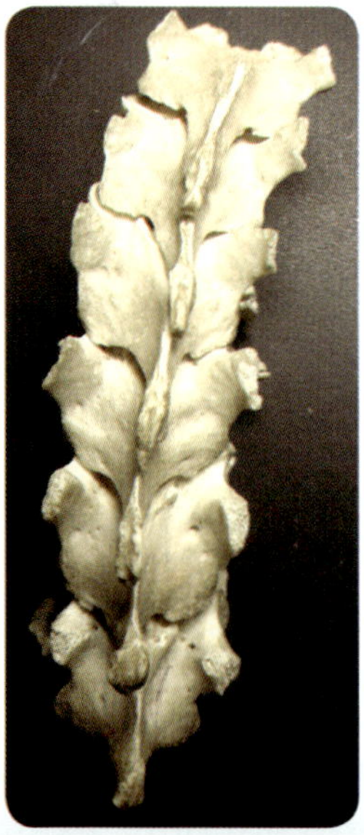

Fig. 3.3.14.
Inclined position of thoracic vertebrae (rear view)

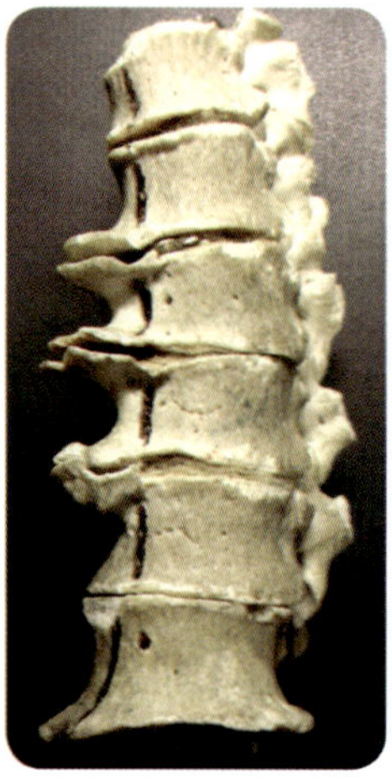

Fig. 3.3.15.
Inclined position of thoracic vertebrae (front view); formation of bony exostoses in sites of segment instability; the wedge-shaped deformity of vertebral bodies

exostoses is also aimed at stabilizing the spine, but their location is not symmetrical. The largest exostosis is located at the centre of curvature of the arc and the smaller ones on the bodies of the overlying and underlying mutually antithetically displaced vertebrae (Fig. 3.3.17).

4. After looking through the radiographs of many patients of different age groups with scoliosis, we found that there were cases in which, in spite of the presence of severe scoliotic deformity of the 2nd, 3rd and even 4th degree, the radiographic picture of the disease was, at first glance, scant. However, in all clinical cases of scoliosis without exception, non-fusion of the first and the second sacral vertebrae, i.e. lumbarization of S_1–S_2 was observed. All patients who visited us to seek help for spinal pain also had unfused sacral vertebrae.
5. During our examination of patients of any age suffering from scoliosis, we found that there was muscular spasm of the spinal extensor on either the right or the left side, and also shortening of one leg. The degree of shortening ranged from a few millimetres to centimetres, regardless of gender or age.

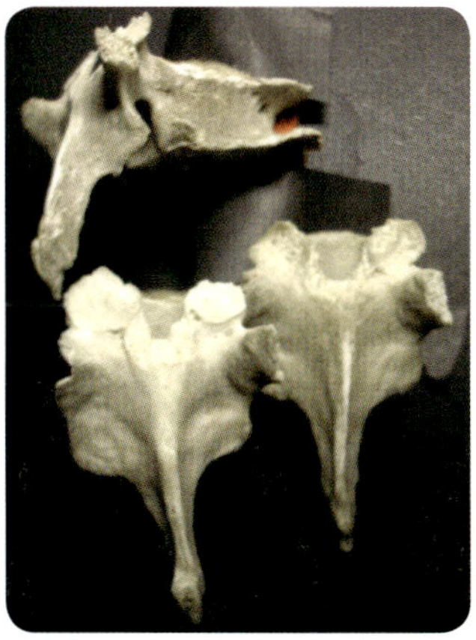

Fig. 3.3.16.
Wedge-shaped deformity of the body of thoracic vertebra combined with an asymmetrical structure of articular processes

Summarizing the material in this chapter, we want to focus your attention on the most important findings that we have established from our theoretical and clinical studies.

1. The simultaneous presence of asymmetry of the trunk muscles and lateral curvature of the spine was observed in all patients without exception.
2. Body asymmetry is caused by certain factors in the functioning of the brain, and its development begins as early as the foetal stage. Lateral curvature of the spine forms from the time a child begins to walk due to varying degrees of spinal muscle tension, which is a sign of 'wrong' conditioned reflex of the vertical position of the body.
3. Various mechanisms of the pathogenesis of scoliosis were studied. It was established that asymmetry of

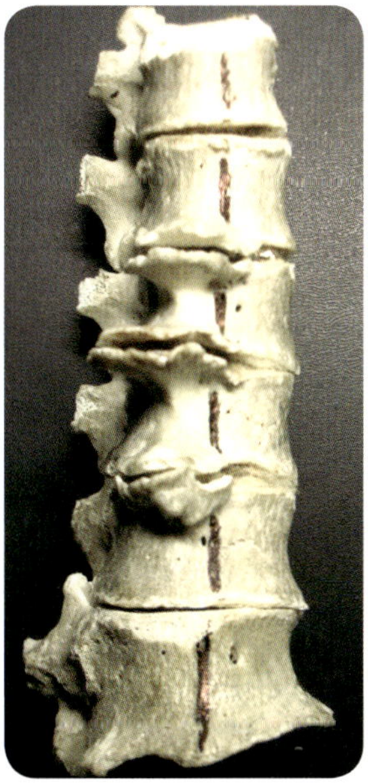

Fig. 3.3.17.
The exostosis of maximum size was formed on the top of segment curvature; it is turned in the opposite direction relative to exostoses of adjacent higher- and lower-lying vertebrae

the spinal extensors is the root cause of deformity. We developed a scheme of the pathogenesis of progressive scoliosis and the stages of its development. The anatomical and physiological features of all regions of the spine in scoliosis were studied in detail.

4. Lateral bending of the spine results in asymmetrical development of the vertebral bodies, arcs, processes, discs, ligaments and other anatomical structures. As a result, zones of instability appear in each segment of the vertebral column. Even a small pelvic tilt is enough to cause rotation of the cervical, thoracic, lumbar and sacral vertebrae about their axes. The leading role belongs to rotation in the lumbosacral spine. Thus, the mechanism of rotation and then of torsion was started.
5. According to the literature, the most frequent form of scoliosis is idiopathic scoliosis (spinal deformity of unknown aetiology). In our view, it is time this term is replaced by 'asymmetrically muscular scoliosis' of conditioned reflex origin. This term not only reflects the essence of the pathological process most completely, but also implies that the existing deformity can be corrected by making a new reflex of the vertical position of the body, with correction of its biomechanics.
6. Spondylosis and osteoarthritis of the large joints develop in accordance with the law that states that such deformities are due to static loading caused by tilt of the body to one side. The formation of osteophytes (exostoses) at an early stage of the disease is not a sign of pathological reorganization of the vertebrae and joints; osteophytes are aimed at providing protection from progression of the disease. If one keeps this law in mind, one can prevent further development of the deformity by restoring the balance of load.
7. Since in lateral bending of the spine the vertebrae always unfold relative to each other in all regions according to areas of instability, the question arises as to what causes this torsion. The answer has been provided by the study of the biomechanics of the spine. It has been proven that this rotation is a natural process, which does not depend on gender, age or ethnicity, and which is based on the laws of classical mechanics. The role of mutually antithetical displacement of vertebrae, impaired tropism of articular processes and lumbarization of S_1–S_2 in the development of scoliotic deformity has also been established.

Finally, we have formulated the following statement to explain the regularity of formation of scoliosis: '*The development of scoliosis is based on zones of instability in all regions of the spine arising as a consequence of unilateral hypertonus of the spinal muscles that is associated with asymmetrical functioning of the cerebral hemispheres.*' This was later recognized as a scientific discovery and awarded a diploma of the Ukrainian Academy of original ideas in February 2008.

3.4 Kyphotic deformity of the spine and its causes

When discussing scoliotic (lateral) spinal deformity, we must include at least a brief description of kyphosis (deformity in the anteroposterior direction). We have not been able to establish a direct relationship between the development of kyphosis and body asymmetry. What is obvious is that there are several mechanisms involved. One of them is associated with the law of curvatures and anticurvatures described by A.M. Schantz in 1933.

Among the conditions that are known to occur are the following:

- Juvenile kyphosis (Scheuermann–Mau disease): The pathogenesis of this condition lies in osteochondropathy of the apophyses of mainly the thoracic vertebrae (Th_{7-10}). This results in the development of persistent thoracic kyphosis, with compensatory hyperlordosis of the cervical and lumbar spine. This condition is sometimes referred to as Schmorl's disease, after the German pathologist who first described the radiological signs of apophyseal inflammation
- Calve's disease: This is characterized by osteochondropathy of the vertebral bodies
- Osteoporotic kyphosis of climacteric origin in women
- Senile kyphosis
- Bechterew's disease (ankylosing spondylitis)
- Wedge-shaped deformity of the vertebrae as a consequence of their destruction due to tumours, trauma, and acute or chronic infection such as tuberculosis (Fig. 3.4.1)
- Congenital wedge-shaped deformity.

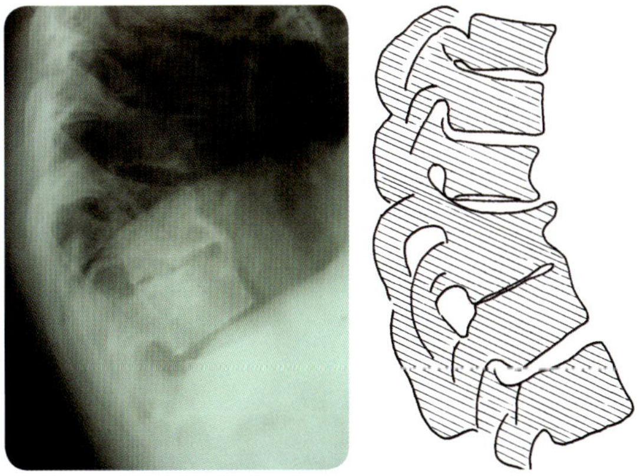

A B

Fig. 3.4.1.
Kyphosis of the thoracic spine, which is a consequence of tuberculous spondylitis; fusion of Th_{10} and Th_{11} vertebral bodies
A - radiograph of the affected area;
B - scheme of the radiograph

In our opinion, which is based on our clinical observations, in a significant number of cases, kyphotic curvature is compensatory in nature. It may be explained by the laws of biomechanics, and is aimed at slowing down the progression of scoliotic curvature. Our hypothesis has been confirmed by our observation that there is a regression of kyphotic deformity in young people after scoliosis has been eliminated.

Although the incidence of kyphosis is lower than that of scoliosis, its aetiology and pathogenesis require special study. However, these issues do not fall within the scope of this book.

In people of all ages, curvature of the spine is accompanied by the development of the spinal pain syndrome. The following chapter contains a detailed description of its mechanisms. The methods of treatment of spinal deformities and spinal pain syndrome will also be discussed.

4 Spinal pain and its origin

IN THE PREVIOUS CHAPTER, WE LEARNT THAT rotary displacement of separate and groups of vertebrae occurs in strictly defined regions of the spine. This is in accordance with the laws of mechanics and can be attributed to the asymmetrical structure of the body and to the presence of various spinal anomalies. The extent of displacement is determined by the inherited anatomical features of the body, as well as the conditions under which a person grows, develops, lives and works. In our view, rotation of individual vertebrae occurs as early as the stage of prenatal development and then the information is stored in the brain of the newborn. Rotation of the vertebrae leads initially to the development of functional scoliosis and then structural scoliosis. The formation of scoliotic deformity is accompanied by the emergence of spinal pain syndrome, which has various clinical manifestations. The main purpose of this book is to elucidate the causes of spinal pain among the patients who visited us, and to find effective methods of treating such pain.

While studying the literature, we found that a colossal number of publications (books, dissertations, articles in journals, etc.) is devoted to the issue of spinal pain. The causes of spinal pain are extremely diverse and even a competent expert can get easily confused while studying them. Thus, we felt it would be useful to systematize the information available. This chapter gives a clear description of the pain syndrome and analyses its origin. For these purposes, we have drawn upon the literature studied by us, as well as our significant volume of clinical observations.

People have suffered from spinal pain since time immemorial. Both the ancient manuscripts and numerous scientific publications by modern-day specialists testify to this. Most people will say that in the course of their lives, there have been times when back pain has hindered their ability to live and work normally. In fact, spinal pain ranks third in frequency, following headaches and acute respiratory diseases.

On any given day, approximately 6.5 million Americans are losing the ability to move due to back pain. Every month, about 1.5 million people in the USA join the ranks of patients with spinal problems, and annual disability due to back pain accounts for more than 90 million working days. The annual expenditure on the diagnosis and treatment of these patients is over $5 billion. In developed European countries such as

Sweden, spinal diseases cause disability in 15%–20% of cases. Every year, more than 20,000 people of working age (40–50 years) need to be given disability pension. Thus, disabilities caused by spinal problems place a significant financial burden on society.

Statistics show that spinal diseases are an important issue worldwide

Patients with radiculitis, sciatica, lumbago, plexitis, etc. form a good proportion of those visiting outpatient clinics, while they constitute the majority of patients visiting neurologists. These diseases are relatively evenly distributed across all age groups and there is hardly any increase in their prevalence with increase in age. In other words, spinal diseases are nearly as common among young people as among the elderly. The frequency of the occurrence of back pain among men is almost twice that among women. This can probably be explained by the fact that more men are employed in manual labour.

Unfortunately, the diagnoses of lumbago and radiculitis are unspecific. It is important to discover the root cause. For example, spinal pain may be a manifestation of destructive processes, such as tuberculosis, benign or malignant tumours, syphilis, osteomyelitis, leishmaniasis, chlamydiasis and multiple myeloma, or the consequence of an injury to the vertebral bodies, their processes, muscles, ligaments, etc.

In 10%–15% of neurosurgical conditions, both the intervertebral disc and its nucleus are damaged. The displacement of these structures towards the spinal canal or the root causes persistent pain, due to which the patient is often forced to undergo surgery. Congenital anomalies (about 50 types), which include unfused arches, and transitional, additional and wedge-shaped vertebrae, should not be forgotten.

However, in only 15%–18% of cases is the nature of the pain clearly spinal pain. More often, patients do not experience any back pain, and marked signs of degenerative disc disease and spondylosis deformans are observed on radiographs taken in another context, e.g. during excretory urography. On the other hand, in many people suffering from back pain, radiography does not reveal any abnormalities. Thus, degenerative changes of the vertebral bodies that are visible on radiographs do not always have a direct correlation with the degree of dysfunction of the spine. In 1936, Professor M.I. Sitenko discussed this issue in a report presented to the fourth Ukrainian Congress of Surgeons on 'Low back pain from orthopaedic perspective'.

The causes of back pain may be divided into two groups—vertebrogenic and non-vertebrogenic. The first group may be subdivided into cases of spinal pain associated with osteochondrosis (degenerative disc disease) and spondylosis deformans, and cases not associated with these conditions.

4.1 Spinal pain of vertebrogenic nature associated with osteochondrosis and spondylosis deformans

A. Hildebrandt (1933) was the first to introduce the term 'osteochondrosis' in the clinical literature. Osteochondrosis (OS) refers to a dystrophic process in the bone and cartilaginous tissue, and was initially used to describe pathological processes not limited to the spine. These include osteochondrosis of the calcaneal apophysis (Haglund–Schinz disease), osteochondrosis dissecans (Koenig disease) and tibial osteochondrosis with proximal varus deformity (Blunt disease). These diseases, which are not directly related to the spine, are now known as osteochondropathies.

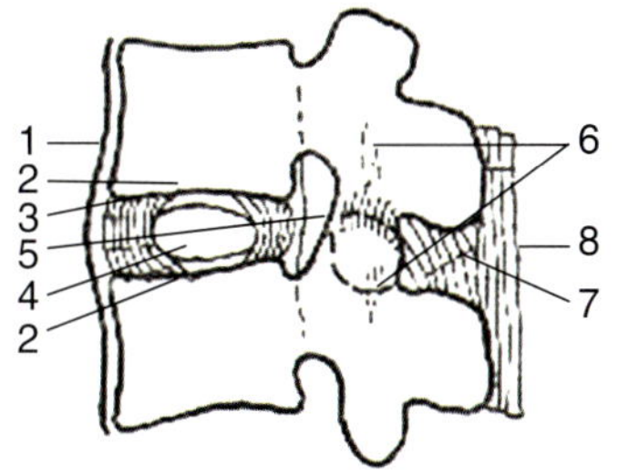

Fig. 4.1.1.
Spinal motion segment:
1 - anterior longitudinal ligament; 2 - hyaline endplate; 3 - fibrous ring; 4 - nucleus pulposus; 5 - facet joint; 6 - yellow ligament; 7 - interspinous ligament; 8 - supraspinous ligament

When we speak of OS today, we understand it as a chronic disease that occurs typically among middle-aged and older individuals, although many vertebrologists believe that it begins gradually at the age of 20–25 years. The frequency of OS ranges from 3.5% to 54.2%. The width of this range can be attributed to factors such as gender differences, age and localization of the process. The pathological changes in OS extend from the nucleus pulposus to the fibrous ring, facet (or intervertebral) joints and the ligament–muscular apparatus of the spinal motion segment (SMS) (Fig. 4.1.1).

The most threatening complication of OS is disc herniation, in which the spinal cord and spinal nerve roots become compressed, giving rise to a variety of orthopaedic, neurological and visceral disorders. The development of a herniated disc takes place in two stages: (i) the disc bulges out and (ii) the nucleus pulposus falls out through the dystrophically changed or damaged annulus. Typically, such herniation is located posteriorly or posterolaterally (Fig. 4.1.2).

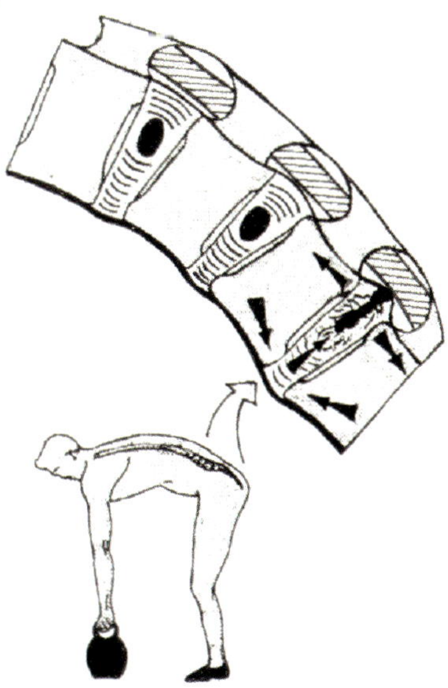

Fig. 4.1.2.
Mechanism of formation of intervertebral disc herniation; incorrect position of the trunk and extremities when lifting load

In severe cases, OS is associated with deforming spondylosis. This is characterized by marked degenerative changes of the discs, joints and ligaments of the spine, with the formation of coracoid and spicular osteophytes along the upper and lower margins of the vertebral bodies (Figs 4.1.3 A–C).

Osteochondrosis and spondylosis can manifest as back and limb pain, stiffness and restricted mobility of the spine.

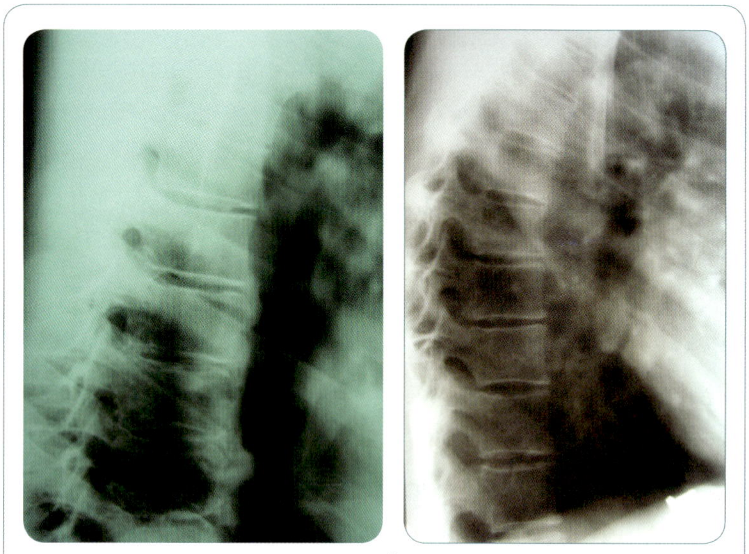

A

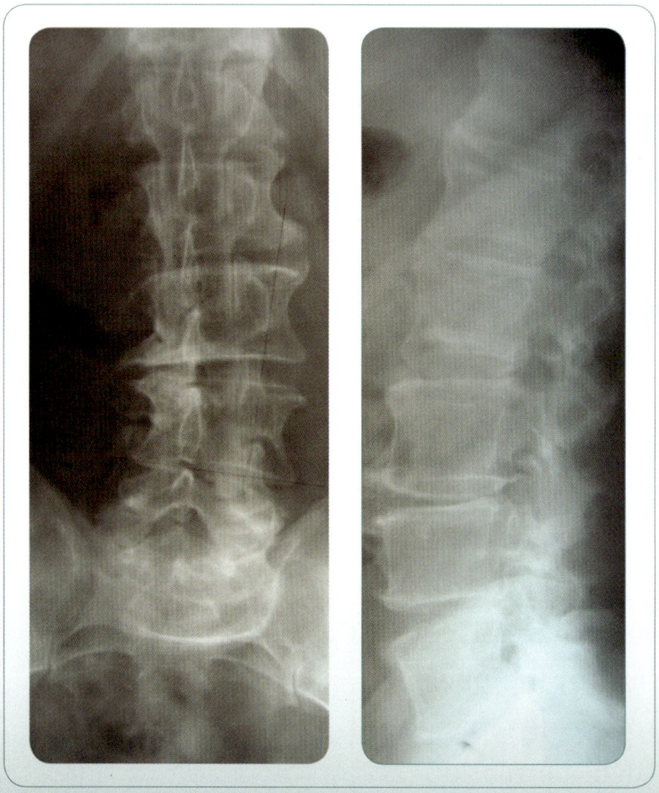

B

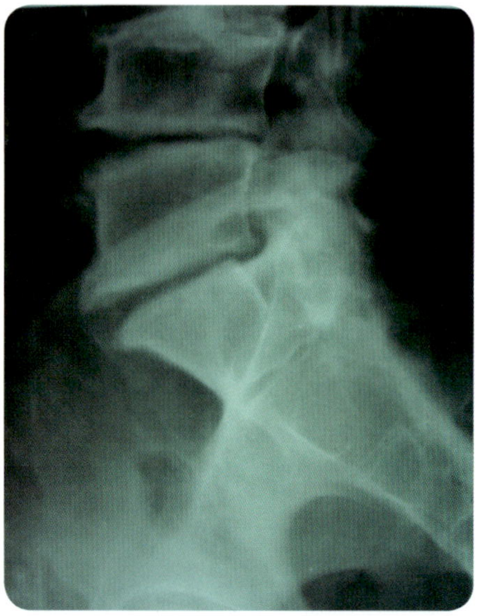

C

Fig. 4.1.3.
Radiographic picture of degenerative disc disease and spondylosis deformans:
A - thoracic spine; **B** - lumbar spine;
C - lumbosacral spine

Due to the enormous health and social significance of OS, deforming spondylosis and spinal pain, more than 200 doctoral and candidate dissertations were published in the USSR during 1965–1991 on the aetiology, clinical picture, pathogenesis, prevention and treatment of these conditions. Republican and all-union conferences and congresses devoted to this subject were held regularly. Moreover, thousands of articles have been published in journals, to say nothing of the numerous monographs that have been written. Interest in this issue has not waned since the collapse of the Soviet Union and the formation of new countries (from the former USSR), with about a hundred doctoral and candidate theses having been written from 1992 up till now.

One would think that such an enormous amount of research would finally throw enough light on the problem of spinal pain that is closely linked with degenerative disc disease and spondylosis. Unfortunately, this did not happen and some very important questions remained unresolved. This prompted us to begin studying the problem and forced us to look at it another way, so that we could uncover what actually happens.

On the basis of our review of the literature, we were able to make a number of generalizations on the aetiology and pathogenesis of OS, deforming spondylosis and other spinal diseases. These will be discussed in the following pages.

We suggest that all professional vertebrologists, as well as neurologists and neurosurgeons, make a detailed study of the seminal work of Y.Y. Popelyansky, *Orthopedic Neurology (Vertebroneurology)* (2003). This manual for physicians contains a detailed description of the clinical picture of and treatment methods for vertebral pain syndromes of the cervical, thoracic and lumbar spine, whether or not associated with OS. This 670-page book includes an analysis of more than 3000 sources of domestic and foreign literature, and contains information that is extremely important and necessary for specialized study.

Aetiology of osteochondrosis of the spine

For many years, the idea that OS was most often of an infectious (tuberculosis, rheumatic fever, influenza) or toxic nature dominated the field of vertebrology. Mixer and Barr (1934) were the first to write on diseases of the intervertebral discs. In the USSR, M.N. Shapiro (1931) and V.I. Lazarev (1935) have proven the concept of the discogenic nature of sciatica. Their ideas received the general acceptance of experts. An infectious-intoxication theory that had preceded this concept was deemed to be incorrect.

The causes of OS are diverse and to facilitate the reader's understanding of them, we have combined them into groups of different factors.

Musculoskeletal anomalies: In 60% of patients with clinical signs of OS, one musculoskeletal anomaly or the other is present. The anomaly increases the load on the spine and sets off a degenerative dystrophic process in the SMS.

In his book, Y.Y. Popelyansky (2003) discusses the role of the cervical spine in patients with OS. Variations in the development of the intervertebral foramina, the diameter of which decreases with age even in apparently healthy people, are mentioned among the most frequent anomalies. These most often occur at the level of C_3–C_6.

While describing anomalies of the transverse processes of the cervical vertebrae, the author has not paid enough attention to differences in the diameter of the foramina located within these processes. According to our findings (Fig. 4.1.4), anatomical variations of these processes such as stenosis, complete atresia and frontal septum, along with pathological changes of the uncovertebral joints, occur quite frequently and can create conditions that can lead to compression of the vertebral arteries, veins and roots of the spinal cord.

According to I.L. Tager and V.F. Kupriyanov (1937), impaired tropism of the articular processes and one-sided hypoplasia of the processes at the level of L_5–S_1 (Figs 4.1.5 and 4.1.6) are the most frequent malformations of the lumbar spine. In their words: 'The lumbosacral region is just as individual as the human face.'

Among the other anomalies of the lumbosacral region, the most frequent mention is made of unfused vertebral arches (Fig. 4.1.7). Splitting of the arches is often associated with a decrease in the diameter of the spinal canal. Among patients with OS, this anomaly occurs, on an average, in every fourth patient.

Transitional vertebrae (sacralization of S_1 and lumbarization of L_5), as well as additional ribs, etc. are also of great importance, occurring on an average in every third person (Figs 4.1.8 A–B).

Anomalies of the pelvis, sacroiliac joints and limbs play a significant role in the subsequent development of degenerative disc disease. For example, shortening of one leg leads to unilateral pelvic imbalance, the disruption of normal locomotor function, static and dynamic overload of different parts of the spine and, eventually, degenerative disc disease.

Traumatic factors: This refers, first of all, to microtraumatization of structures of the musculoskeletal system due to physical overload, long-lasting, non-physiological postures and impaired movement stereotype. These problems are largely a result of professional activity. However, degenerative dystrophic changes of the disc and the nucleus can also occur as complications of major injuries, such as vertebral fractures in various locations.

Endocrine and hormonal factors: Endocrine diseases and conditions associated with disruption of tissue nutrition and a tendency to oedema play an important role in OS. These include acromegaly, myxoedema, diabetes mellitus, sub-optimal functioning of

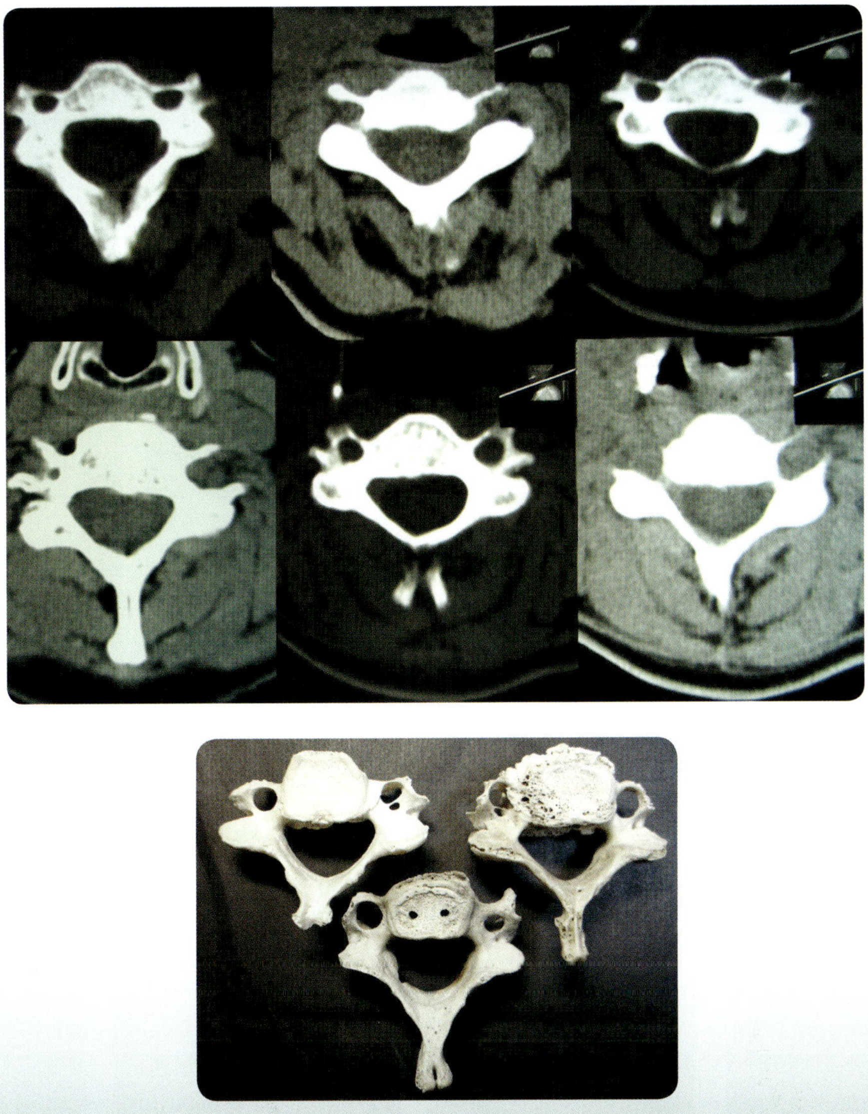

Fig. 4.1.4.
Differences in diameter of vertebral foramina of the cervical vertebrae

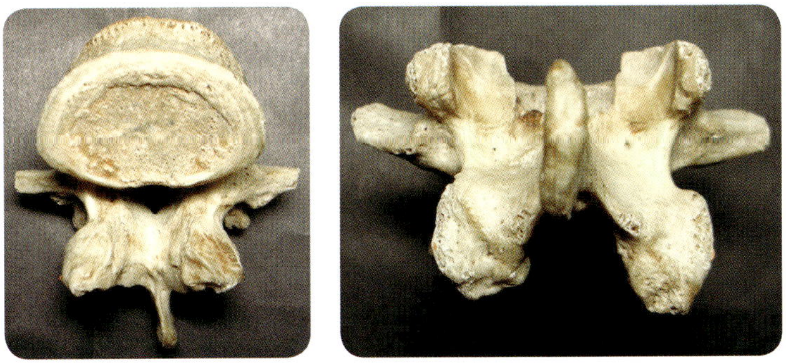

Fig. 4.1.5.
Unilateral hypoplasia of articular processes of lumbar vertebrae

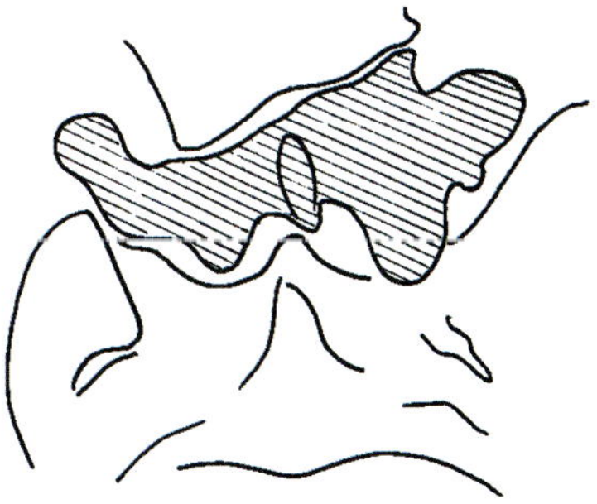

Fig. 4.1.6.
Schematic representation of hypoplasia of articular processes of spinal motion segment L_5–S_1

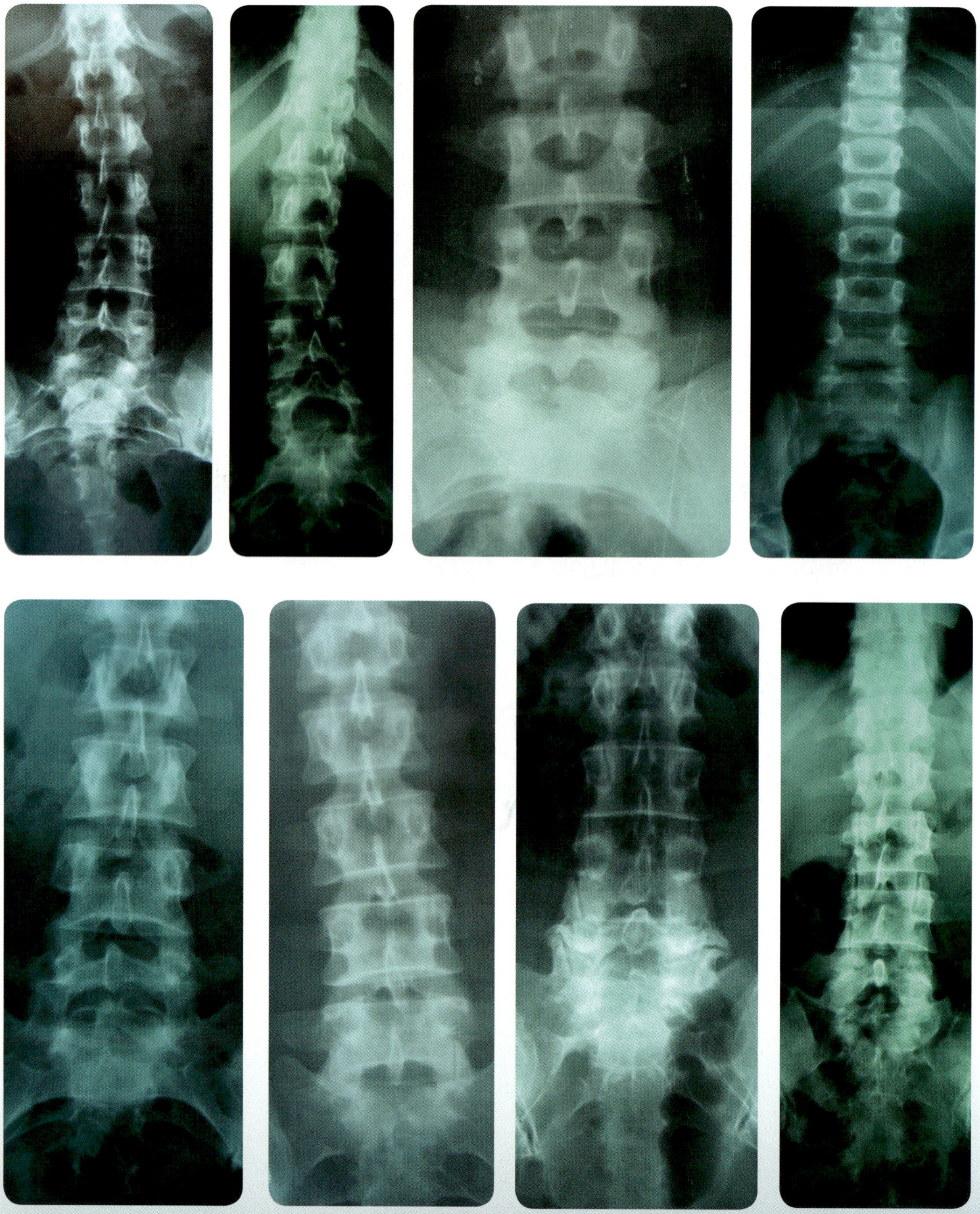

Fig. 4.1.7.
Non-fusion of vertebral arches

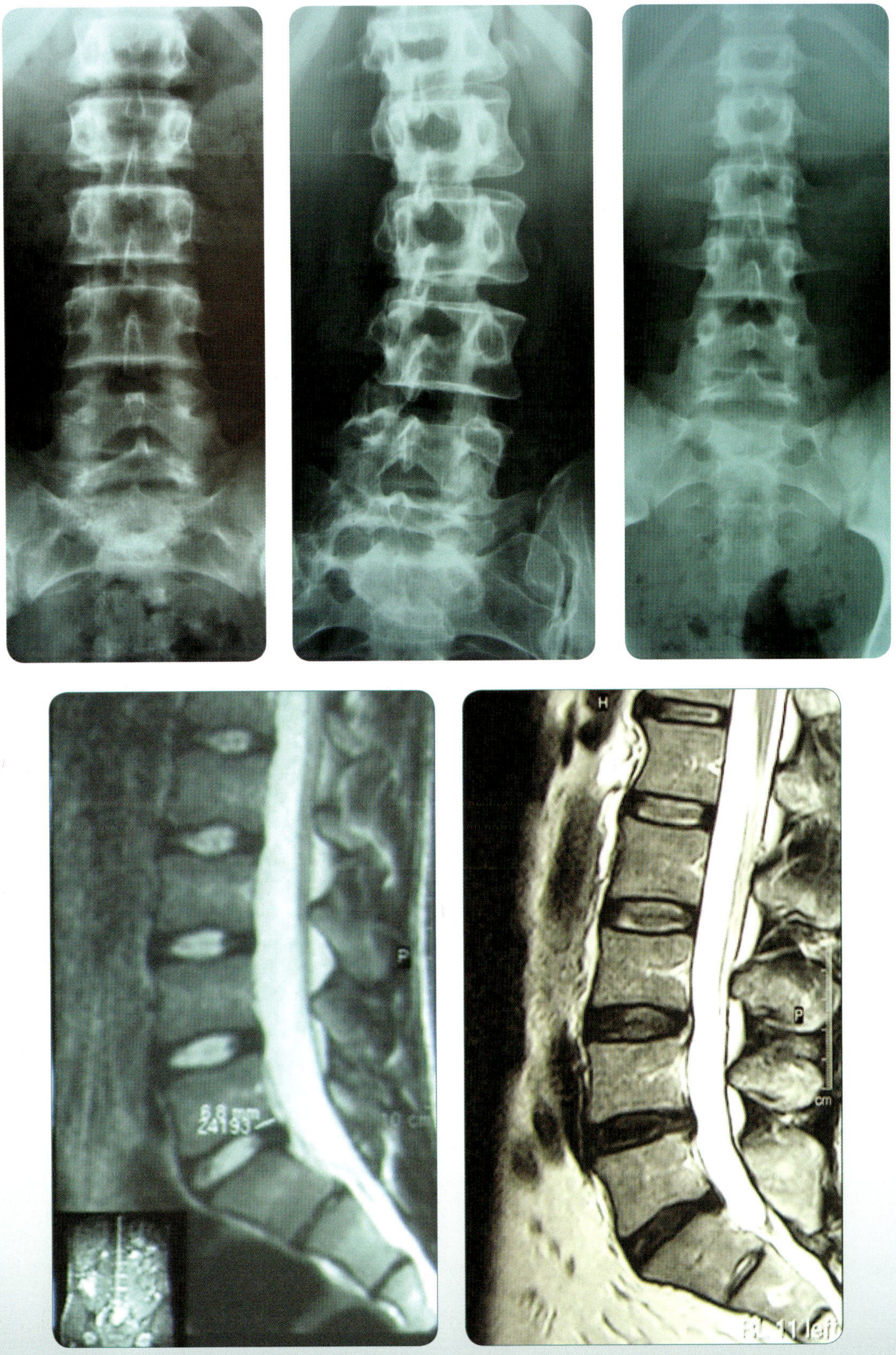

Fig. 4.1.8.
A - Transitional vertebrae (lumbarization of S_1)

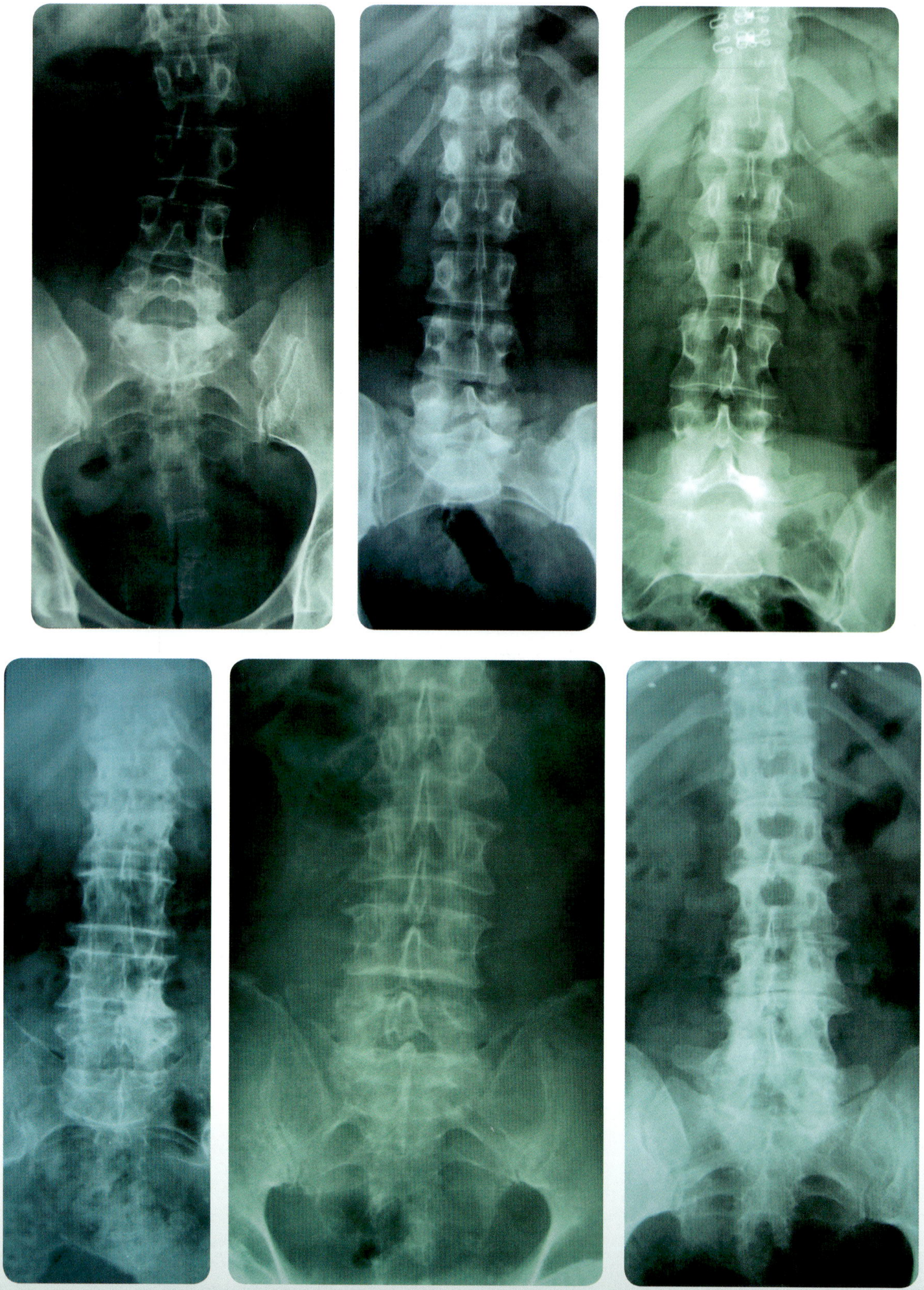

Fig. 4.1.8.
B - Transitional vertebrae (sacralization of L_5)

the sexual glands, disorders of water and salt balance in idiopathic oedema, obesity and pregnancy.

Hereditary factors: Direct inheritance of OS has not been proven. However, it has been established that there is an increased incidence of the clinical manifestations of the condition among members of a family. According to N.I. Hvisyuk *et al.* (1985), in 94.2% of cases, OS of the lumbar spine could be traced back to three generations, and in up to 5.8%, one generation.

Functional factors: Hypokinesia and physical inactivity may be factors that contribute to the disruption of metabolism and functioning of the osseous and cartilaginous tissues of the spine. Leading causes of degenerative changes in the SMS are reduced function of the muscles and consequently reduced blood flow.

Immunological factors: During the penetration of the nucleus pulposus through the cracks of the intervertebral discs, fragments of the nucleus can enter the bloodstream and become autoantigens, to which autoantibodies are produced. Due to the formation of this antigen–antibody complex, biologically active substances are released that, first, promote the degradation of the intervertebral disc and, second, irritate the pain receptors of the sinuvertebral nerve of Luschka, generating pain. Increased activity of lysosomal enzyme also plays an important role in degenerative processes in SMS (citation from N.I. Hvistyuk *et al.*, *Osteochondrosis of the Spine in Children*, Kiev, 1985).

In our opinion, these autoimmune processes may be a cause of ankylosing spondylitis.

Biochemical and vascular factors: Many authors have carried out biochemical studies in the field of vertebrology. For example, A.I. Kazmin and V.A. Kozlov (1973) found that among the mechanisms that trigger profound biochemical changes in the discs are circulatory disorders of the spine (arterial and venous insufficiency). However, the authors were unable to pinpoint the causes of this phenomenon.

Later in 1976, N.I. Hvisyuk studied the biochemical composition of the disc tissues and found that a marked depletion of hyaluronic acid in the tissues is responsible for the progression of OS. This is particularly the case in adolescence, possibly because of inadequate physical activity. Due to the resultant decrease in the hydrophilic properties of the disc, it loses its elasticity followed by a reduction in its height. Normal biochemical processes are disrupted not only in the intervertebral discs, but also in the endplates of the vertebral bodies. Preferential destruction of chondroitin sulphates leads to a decrease in the amount of glycosaminoglycans and, as a consequence, loss of strength in the plates. For children, adolescents and young adults, the values of maximum permissible stress on the endplates are lower than those for adults, so the endplates may be more easily damaged in this group.

Under normal conditions, the endplates ensure active transport of nutrients and oxygen from the blood of the vascular lacunae of the vertebral bodies to the tissue of the intervertebral discs. Thus, injury to the endplates dramatically decreases nutrition to the discs. This leads to further biochemical and structural changes later on. Thus, there is a vicious circle: biochemical and structural changes in the endplates lead to impairment of nutrition to the SMS elements, and impairment of nutrition leads to further biochemical and structural changes of the hyaline plates, etc.

Biomechanical factors: This theory has the largest number of supporters. Excessive mechanical stress can damage the discs, particularly in areas of *heterogeneous tissues:* bone tissue—endplates, fibrous ring—nucleus pulposus. In their pathomorphological studies, A.A. Korzh *et al.* (1974) have shown that the above can lead to the development of a degenerative dystrophic process in the spinal segment.

The joint work of Professor V.Y. Fischenko, G.F. Martynenko, V.S. Shargorodsky and V.A. Shvets (1989) is of great scientific and practical interest and relevance to the study of the role of biomechanics of the spine in OS. We shall briefly describe this study, as we feel that it would help the reader to understand the pathogenesis of degenerative disc disease.

Biomechanics and degenerative disc disease

The observations made over recent years have shown that the aetiology and pathogenesis of this disease are determined by the relationship between the features of the functioning of the musculoskeletal system under constant exposure to the gravitational field, on the one hand, and by the development of adaptive mechanisms in the bone and cartilage tissue of the spine, on the other. The supporting and shock-absorbing function of the spine is associated primarily with the asymmetrical location of the body's centre of gravity in relation to the vertebral bodies.

According to the authors, when the body is in the vertical position, the vertebrae at the SMS level turn around two axes (supporting points). One of them passes through the centres of the intervertebral joints and the other, through the centre of the nuclei pulposus (Fig. 4.1.9). The spine maintains a vertical position as long as the extensor muscles contract with a force equal to 0.45–2.2 p. During their contraction, the body bends forward or backward to a greater or lesser extent. Forward bending of the trunk occurs due to mutual rotation of adjacent vertebrae around the nucleus pulposus, and backward bending due to the rotation of paired intervertebral joints. Studies of the degree of tension of the muscles under the described conditions have shown that during bending of the body, the force of contraction of the spinal extensor muscles is 13 times higher than that in the standing position. This causes significant deformation of the annulus fibrosus and nucleus pulposus.

It is only due to the complex of adaptive mechanisms developed in the course of ontogenesis and phylogenesis that the spine can function fully, without significant pathological disorders. *These mechanisms of adaptation include, in particular, the ability of the trunk muscles to redistribute and reduce the load on elements of the spine.*

Curvatures of the spine are also of important biomechanical significance. Cervical and lumbar lordosis, as well as thoracic and sacrococcygeal kyphosis help to mitigate the load on the spine during walking, running and jumping. The presence of curvatures of the spine, which changes its curve during loading, allows the back muscles to redistribute contact pressure on the intervertebral discs and the stress on the vertebral bodies more effectively. In OS, these protective mechanisms are impaired.

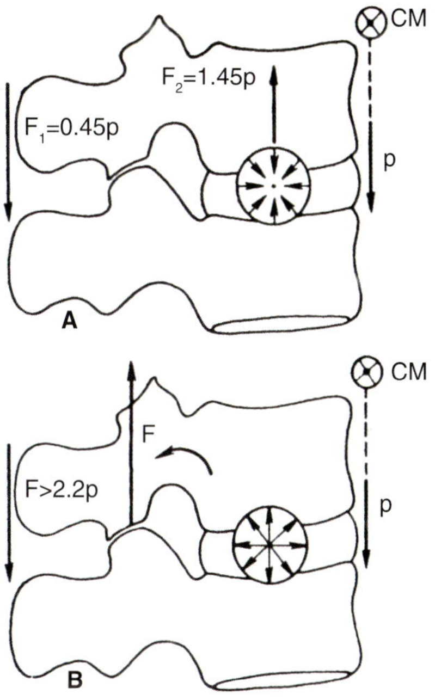

Fig. 4.1.9.
Schematic representation of forces in elements of spinal motion segment (CM - centre of body mass; F_1 - supporting reaction in the intervertebral joint; F_2 - supporting reaction in nucleus pulposus): **A** - in low activity of back muscles; **B** - in significant activity of back muscles (F> 2.2 p)

According to V.Y. Fischenko and his co-authors, from a biomechanical perspective, OS of the spine accompanied with back pain should be regarded as a disease in which, owing to degenerative changes in the intervertebral discs, harmonic correspondence between the effects of mechanical factors and the body's ability to resist those changes is impaired. This creates new compensatory mechanisms for the prevention, to a greater or lesser extent, of the onset of neurological complications.

Osteochondrosis is also characterized by significant changes in the mechanical properties of the intervertebral discs. They become more deformed and their modulus of elasticity decreases. The severity of these changes depends on the extent of the degenerative changes in the SMS. From the biomechanical point of view, the intervertebral disc should be regarded as a hydrodynamic system, the properties of which are linked with metabolic processes in the tissues and the conditions under which it functions. When there is compression of the vertebral annulus, pressure is transmitted through the nucleus pulposus since it lies at a level slightly higher than that of the fibrous ring (by 1–1.5 mm).

Under natural conditions, the role of the nucleus pulposus is not limited to reducing the static and dynamic loads on the spine. It facilitates a more equitable distribution of stresses in the fibrous ring. Impairment of the elastic properties of the nucleus pulposus distorts the mechanism of transmission and transformation of stresses.

Anatomical and biomechanical characteristics of different regions of the spine in osteochondrosis

Cervical spine: There are foramina in the transverse processes of the cervical vertebrae. Situated one above the other, they form a canal (Fig. 4.1.10). The canal gives passage to the vertebral artery, which is wrapped in a sympathetic nerve that originates from the lower node of the cervical sympathetic ganglion, and spinal veins. In Chapter 2, we have mentioned that the diameters of the foramina vary significantly, ranging from a few millimetres to 1.5 cm or more.

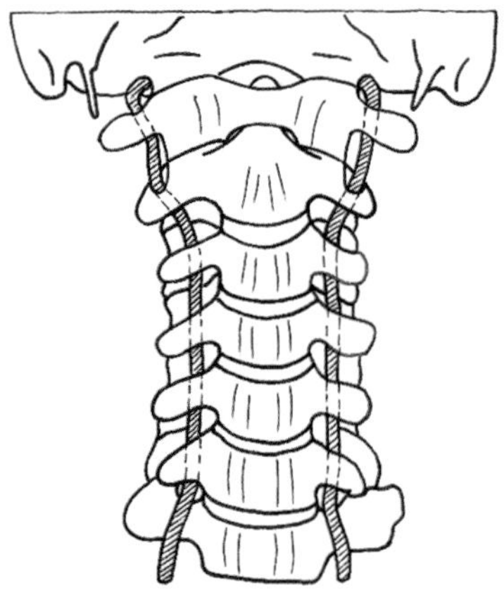

Fig. 4.1.10.
Foramina of transverse processes of the cervical vertebrae form a canal

In cases of weakness of the burso-ligamentous apparatus of different aetiologies, flexion and extension of the cervical spine are accompanied by subluxation of the facet joints. This, in turn, leads to deformation and traumatization of the vertebral artery and sympathetic plexus surrounding it. This is how the so-called vertebral artery syndrome develops.

A knowledge of the interrelation of the above-mentioned anatomical structures with bony outgrowths in uncovertebral arthroses, as well as with pathological changes of the intervertebral discs, is of great importance in understanding circulatory and neurological complications.

Many authors have noted that posterior herniations of the intervertebral discs of the cervical spine are rare. In their view, this is because the density of the posterior longitudinal ligament is sufficient and the size of the discs relatively small. Compression of the roots and blood vessels often develops as a result of rotation of the cervical vertebrae. But it may also be the result of a decrease in the size of the intervertebral foramina due to disc flattening. However, according to V.Y. Fischenko, uncovertebral arthrosis is the main cause of neurological disorders.

Thoracic spine: The fact that the intervertebral discs in this region are of a small height makes for a limited range of motion, which creates relatively favourable biomechanical conditions of functioning and limits the preconditions for the development of degenerative disc disease.

It is comparatively rare to find herniated intervertebral discs in the thoracic spine. Herniation can occur at any level, but most often it occurs in the lower section because of the high mobility of this region. Anterior herniation of the nucleus pulposus (Schmorl's hernia) can occur at multiple vertebrae (Fig. 4.1.11). Most often, it is not manifested clinically and is detected only during radiological evaluation of the spine. Posterior and posterolateral herniations in the thoracic spine are unusual. The thoracic spine is frequently accompanied by deforming arthrosis of the costovertebral joints. If one considers that the paravertebral sympathetic ganglia, which form the sympathetic trunk, are located at the level of these joints (in front of the costal heads), the cause of girdling intercostal neuralgia with vasomotor autonomic reactions in lesions of the corresponding region of the spine becomes clear.

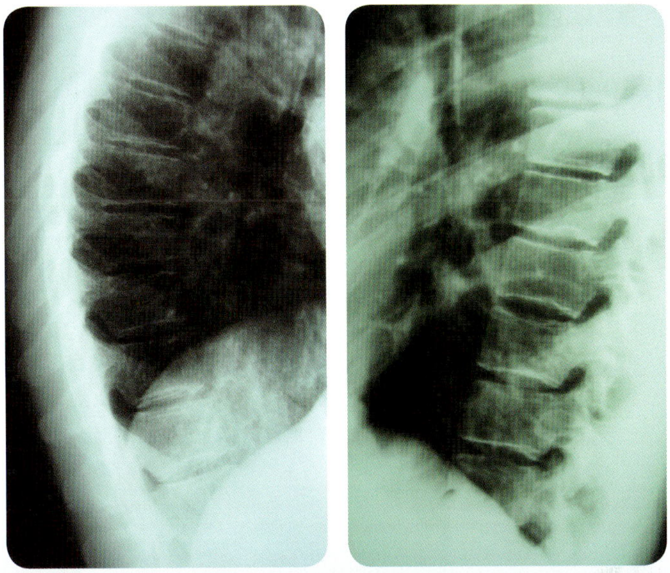

Fig. 4.1.11.
Radiographic picture of Schmorl's hernia

Degenerative dystrophic changes most often affect the lumbar spine. The main sources of the neurological complications of OS of this region, as against the cervical and thoracic spine, are herniated discs and disorders of the intervertebral joints. The posterior longitudinal ligament plays an important role in providing protection against hernial protrusion over the entire spine. At the level of the upper lumbar vertebrae, this ligament is strong enough and its width is 8–15 mm. At the level of L_3, its width decreases to 3–10 mm, and it becomes especially weak at the level of L_5, where its width is 1–4 mm. Most frequently, hernial protrusion develops in the lower lumbar region, where the posterior longitudinal ligament does not provide sufficient resistance to shifting tissues (Fig. 4.1.12).

Pathogenesis of osteochondrosis

Though we have described above various causes of degenerative disc disease, we have still not created a complete picture of the development of the disease in its various stages. We shall now attempt to do so. There are several interpretations of the pathogenesis of degenerative disc disease. Of course, each of these has its own rightful place as it is a reflection of the physicians' long years of experience.

We shall begin with a description of the discogenic-dysplastic model of the pathogenesis of OS. The supporters of this model include leading vertebrologists from around the world, such as the Ukrainian specialists A.A. Korzh, N.I. Hvisyuk, G.H. Gruntovsky and V.Y. Fischenko, and the American vertebrologists, H.A. Keim, W.H. Kirkaldy-Willis, and their colleagues and followers.

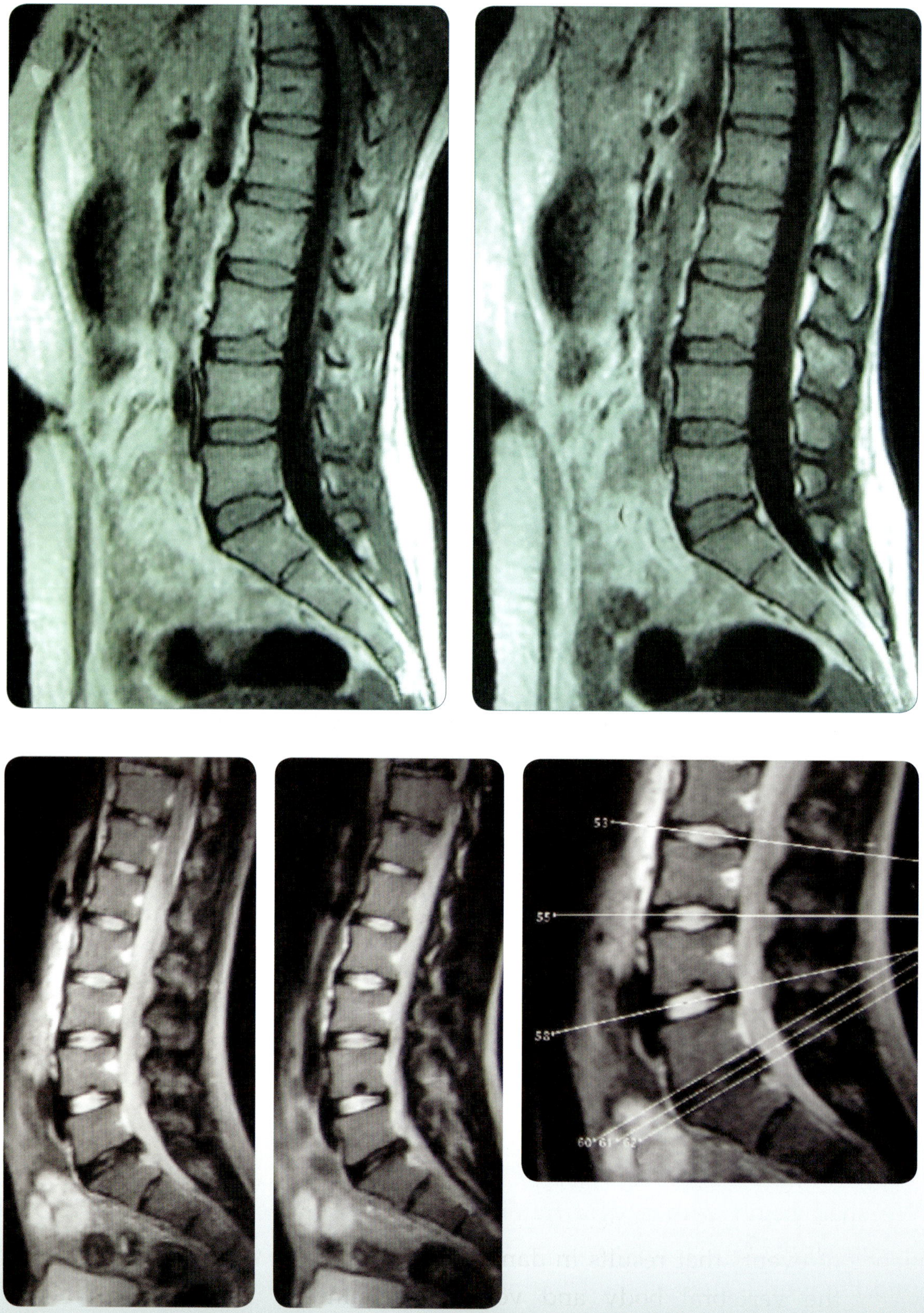

Fig. 4.1.12.
Herniated disc at the level of L_5–S_1 SMS associated with lumbarization of S_1–S_2

Discogenic–dysplastic model of pathogenesis of osteochondrosis

1. Among middle-aged and older patients, degenerative changes in the discs are caused by the following reasons. The first is a genetic predisposition to OS and the other is an influence of unfavourable factors on the intervertebral discs and nuclei, which cause the trophic disorders in these structures.

However, according to V.Y. Fischenko *et al.* (1994), disc dysplasia may be observed even in early childhood. The process begins during the primary formation of the spine, under the influence of harmful factors of exogenous or endogenous origin on the foetus. The authors were unable to definitively establish the nature of these factors. For the record, it should be mentioned that much earlier, in his doctoral dissertation, N.I. Hvisyuk (1976) spoke of the possibility of degenerative changes in the SMS in childhood and adolescence due to congenital anomalies of the spinal structure. He went on to suggest that these anomalies formed the basis for the development of OS later.

Disc degeneration caused by static loading leads to a reduction in its height and consequently, narrowing of the intervertebral foramen (Figs 4.1.13 and 4.1.14). Partly, this also occurs due to impairment of the elastic properties of the nucleus pulposus. Such impairment significantly distorts the mechanisms of transmission and transformation of stresses.

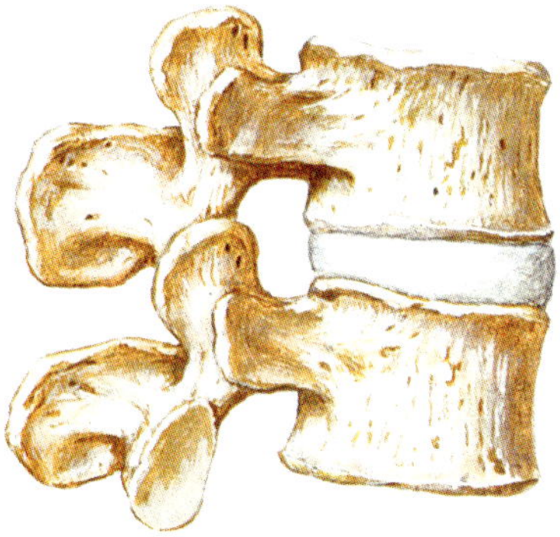

Fig. 4.1.13.
Proper interrelationships of lumbar vertebrae in normal height of intervertebral discs

2. A reduction in the height of the intervertebral discs weakens the attachment between the ligaments and vertebral bodies. It results in approximation of the attachment points of the anterior and posterior longitudinal ligaments, which are woven into the vertebral bodies, as well as the ligaments on the arcs and spinous processes. This leads to instability or 'loosening' of the vertebral segments, which manifests as displacement of the vertebrae in a horizontal plane. The vertebrae may shift 3–5 mm from each other. In addition, there is associated damage of the junctions between the endplates and vertebral bodies. It is this sequence of events that results in damage to the area between the vertebral body and vertebral hyaline cartilaginous tissue, in the form of gaps, cracks and other changes. As a consequence, the delivery of

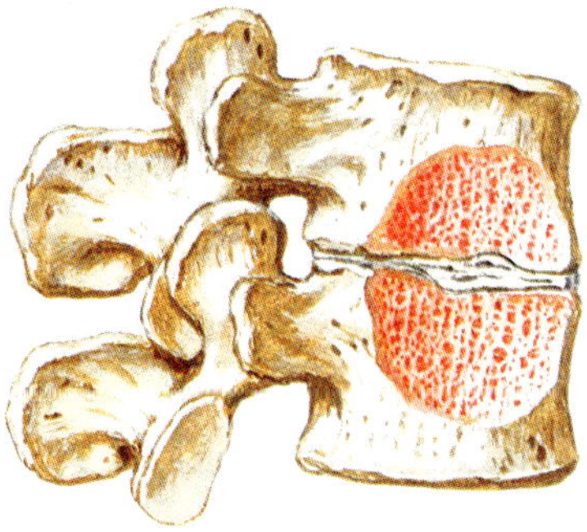

Fig. 4.1.14.
Vertebrae are lying closer to each other due to reduction in disc height; upper articular process of the lower vertebra overlaps the intervertebral foramen

nutrients from the blood vessels of the vertebral bodies to the intervertebral discs, which have no blood vessels, is affected.

Pathological mobility of unstable segments causes continuous destructive and diffuse degenerative changes in all structures of the intervertebral disc. These changes are the most marked in the endplates and sprout plates, as well as in the underlying osseous tissue of the vertebral body. The continuing changes cause a further decrease in the height of the intervertebral disc. This leads to greater instability. Thus, a vicious circle is set up: abnormal segment mobility—destructive and degenerative disc changes—reduction in height—pathological SMS mobility, etc.

3. Excessive mobility of the adjacent vertebral bodies and chronic irritation of the endplates causes sclerosis (Fig. 4.1.15). Marginal bony outgrowths (osteophytes) appear (Fig. 4.1.16) as a compensatory, adaptive reaction, aimed at preventing further displacement of the vertebrae.

As a consequence of subluxation of the intervertebral joints and permanent traumatization of the articular processes, spondylarthrosis occurs (Fig. 4.1.17). It manifests in deforming changes of the facet joints and the formation of marginal bony outgrowths on the vertebral bodies. The osteophytes cause narrowing of the intervertebral foramina. Given the unstable vertebrae syndrome that has already developed due to weakness of the ligaments, compression of the spinal roots and back pain in the vertical position develop.

In the long run, due to the recurring considerable mobility of the SMS, the load on the arch of the vertebral body increases, which can lead to resorption and cause the vertebra to slip anteriorly. So, initially the patient develops degenerative spondylolysis (Fig. 4.1.18), and then spondylolisthesis (Figs 4.1.19 and 4.1.20).

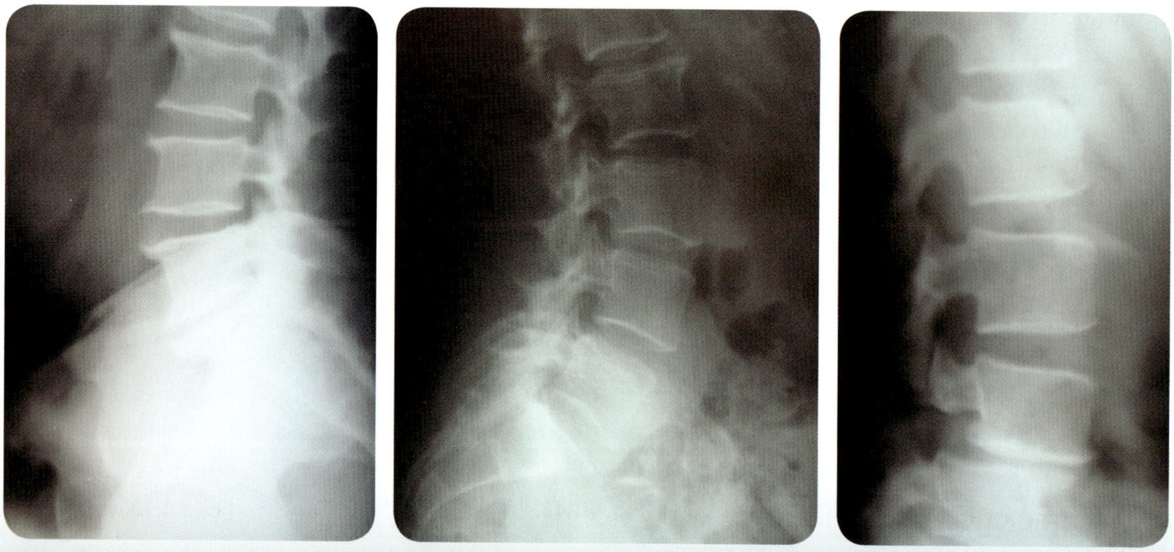

Fig. 4.1.15. Sclerosis of closing plates of vertebral bodies

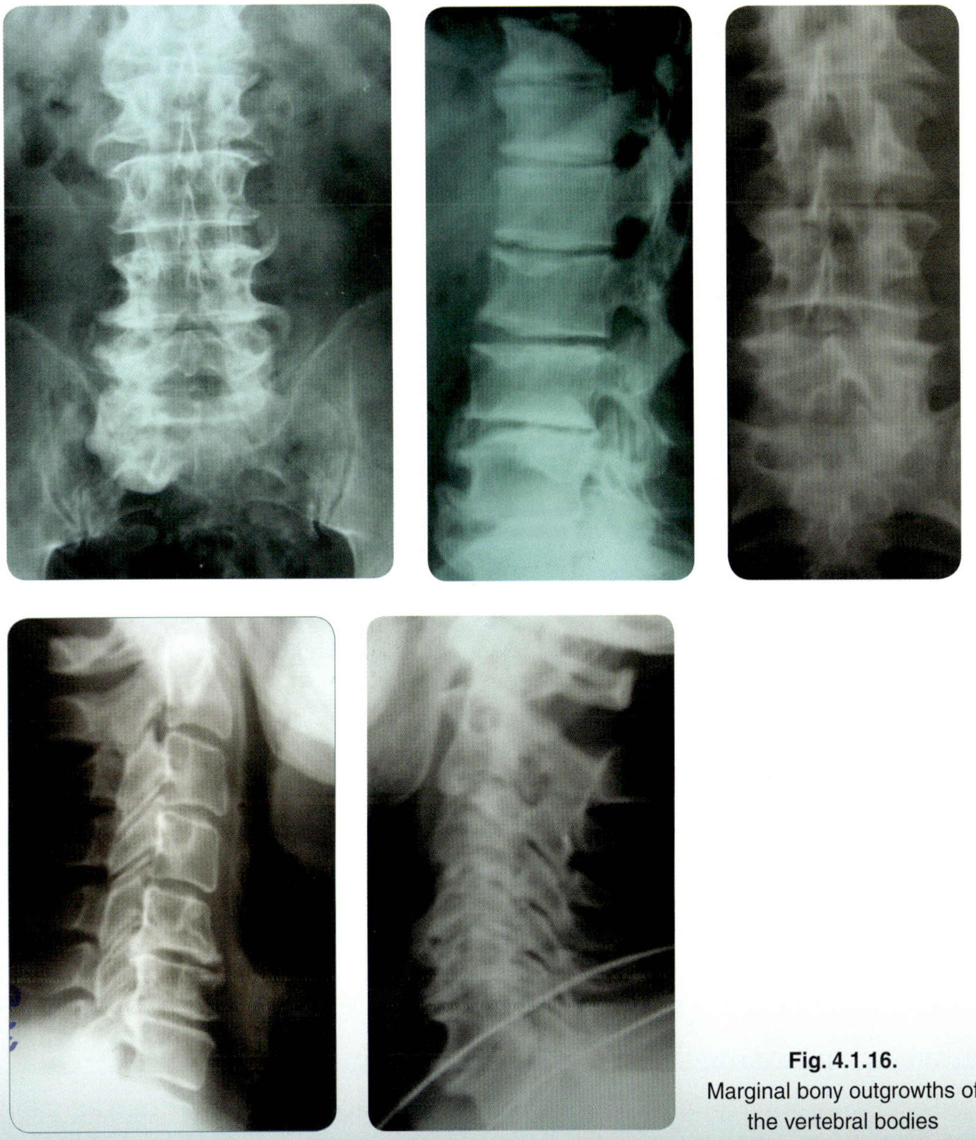

Fig. 4.1.16.
Marginal bony outgrowths of the vertebral bodies

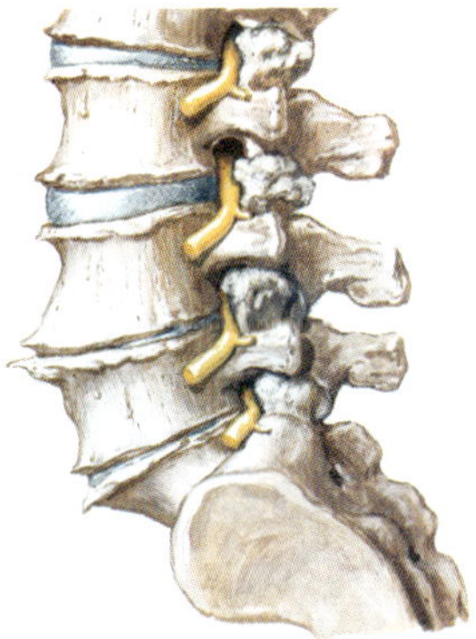

Fig. 4.1.17.
Spondylarthrosis of facet (intervertebral) joints

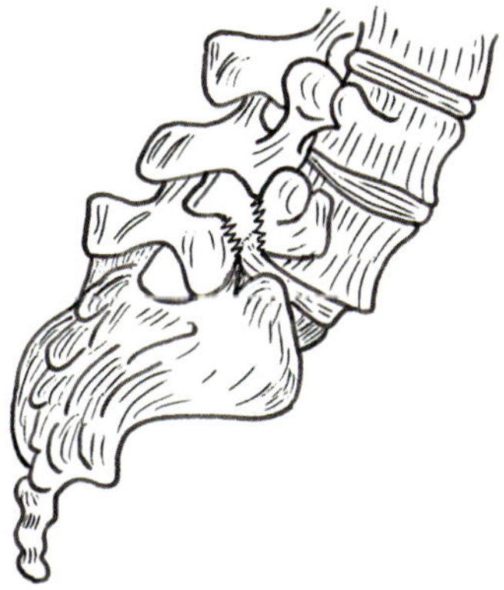

Fig. 4.1.18.
Degenerative spondylolysis; resorption of vertebral arch

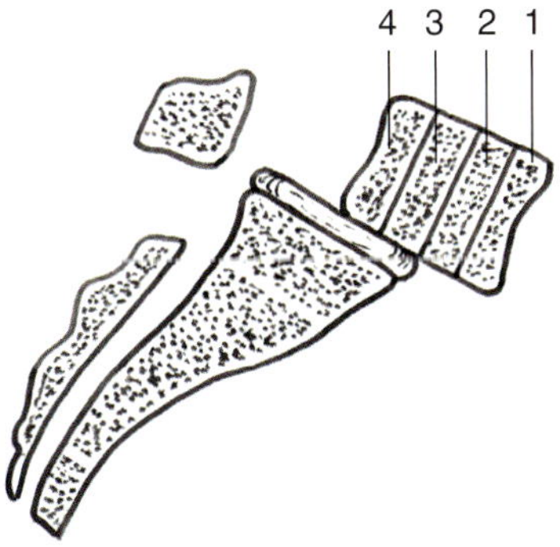

Fig. 4.1.19.
Four stages of degenerative spondylolisthesis

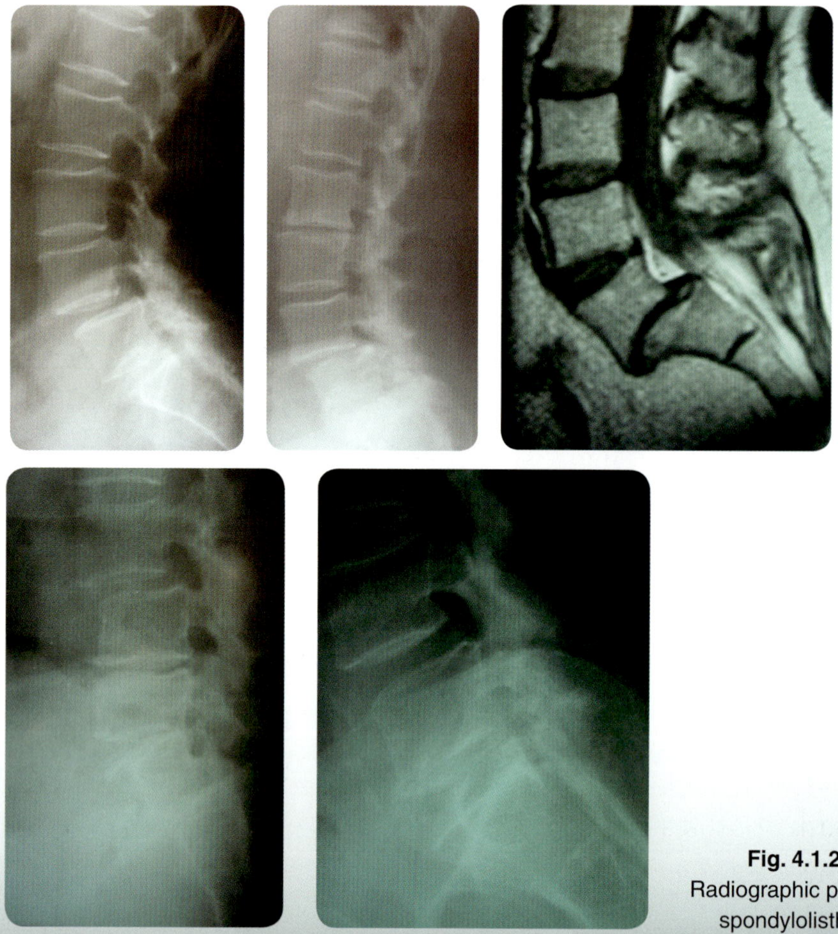

Fig. 4.1.20.
Radiographic picture in spondylolisthesis

4. The deficiency of nutrients and impaired evacuation of metabolites lead to the accumulation of histamine-like biologically active substances. The concentration of hydrogen ions, lactic, fatty and amino acids, ketone bodies, etc. increases. Thus, osmotic and intradiscal pressure increases even more. These processes adversely affect the strength of the nucleus pulposus and disc, with the result that these spread beyond the endplates.

5. Significant deformations of the fibrous ring give rise to cracks and radial tears. Consequently, this process results in the emergence of extensive areas of destruction of the intervertebral discs and endplates to a greater or lesser extent. The penetration of elements of the nucleus pulposus into the disc cracks brings the nucleus in contact with the immunocompetent system. The production of autoantibodies to the antigens of its own nucleus pulposus and the gradual increase in their titre causes an antigen-antibody reaction, which enhances the activity of proteolytic enzymes (as mentioned earlier). As a result, the degenerative dystrophic changes in the SMS continue to progress.

6. As the outer layers of the intervertebral disc contain the sensitive endings of the

spinal nerves, when they are subjected to mechanical irritation by parts of the nucleus pulposus, the result is lumbalgia and the emergence of other clinical features specific to the stage of intradiscal displacement of the nucleus pulposus. Soon, if the nucleus particles remain in cracks of the ring, reactive aseptic inflammation develops in the area.

Exudative phase: In this phase, which is one of inflammation, the products of tissue break-up irritate the sensory endings of the vertebral nerves and cause pain.

Proliferative phase: The proliferative phase of reactive aseptic inflammation is marked by autolysis of dead tissue and the products of cellular break-up, as a result of enzymatic processes and phagocytosis. Exudate is resorbed and the pain gradually subsides. The defect in the damaged nucleus pulposus is replaced by well-vascularized granulation tissue. The nutrition of the disc improves. Transport function of the endplates begins to be restored, as well as active metabolism, although at a lower level.

Phase of regeneration: This is characterized by the regeneration of connective tissue and is followed by the formation of connective scar tissue.

7. Later, in the case of recurrent injuries, sudden movements, lifting of heavy weights or other situations that encourage the recurrence of pathological changes, destructive processes in the fibrous ring increase. A dramatic rise in the intradiscal pressure leads to bulging of the annulus fibrosus. It may rupture in the altered area. At the same time, due to high pressure, the nucleus pulposus shifts (falls out) into the cavity of the spinal canal and forms a disc herniation (Figs 4.1.21 and 4.1.22), or penetrates into the vertebral body to form Schmorl's hernia (Figs 4.1.23 A and B).

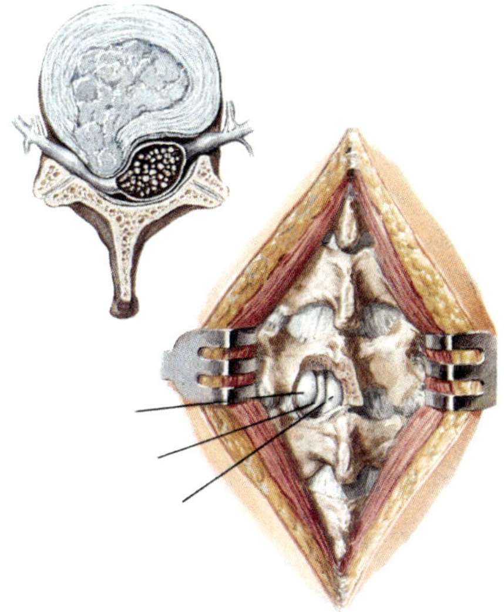

Fig. 4.1.21.
Schematic representation of disc herniation; displaced nucleus pulposus causes nerve root compression

The decreased strength of the fibrous ring leads to a situation in which hernias can be formed even if the load is minimal, not exceeding even the physiological level.

Pathogenesis of osteochondrosis of compensatory and stabilizing genesis

The essence of the discogenic-dysplastic concept of OS, which has replaced the infectious and toxic theory, has been dealt with in the previous section. We shall now present another view on the causes of this disease.

1. A considerable body of clinical material has been accumulated which indicates

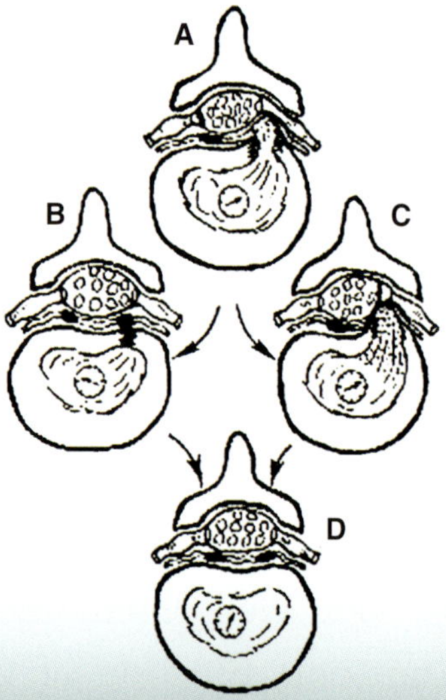

Fig. 4.1.22.
Schematic representation of pathogenesis of clinical symptoms in intervertebral disc herniation (protrusion stage):
A - protrusion of weakened annulus fibrosis beyond normal borders of the disc, mechanical irritation of blood vessels and nerves lying in the spinal canal;
B - self-elimination or reduction of protrusion;
C - reactive aseptic inflammation in an SMS due to penetration of elements of the nucleus pulposus into cracks and crevices of the annulus;
D - substitution of damaged parts of fibrous ring with scar tissue

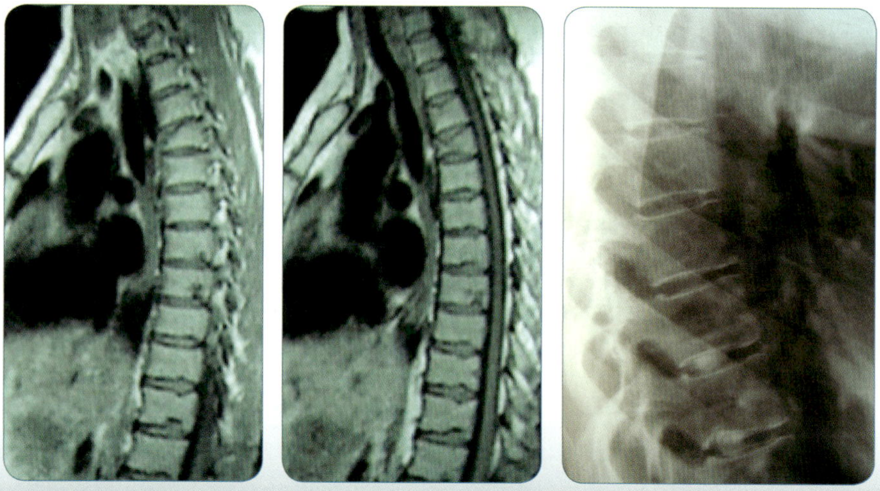

Fig. 4.1.23.
A - Radiographic picture of Schmorl's hernia between bodies of thoracic vertebrae

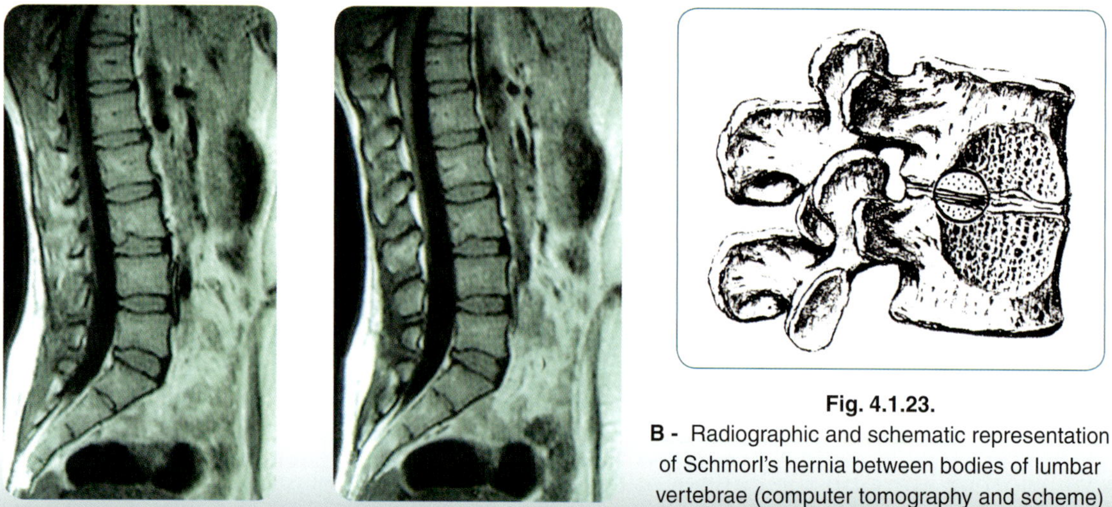

Fig. 4.1.23.
B - Radiographic and schematic representation of Schmorl's hernia between bodies of lumbar vertebrae (computer tomography and scheme)

that OS should not be regarded as premature ageing or weakening of the disc, but as a natural compensatory process that takes place as part of the restructuring of the SMS. This view is supported by neurophysiological and neuroradiological research, as well as neurosurgical experience. The compensatory process is aimed at enhancing the functional supporting capability of the spine in the context of impairment of its dynamic equilibrium due to unilateral muscular hypertonus. It is a natural ongoing process that attempts to compensate for the instability of the SMS through natural spondylodesis.

The results of attempts at artificial fusion have confirmed the correctness of this point of view. Papain injections, which accelerate fibrosis of the intervertebral disc, have been used successfully to eliminate instability of the spinal segments (V.Y. Fischenko *et al.*, 1989).

2. G.A. Ivanichev (1998) takes the example of true spondylolisthesis of L_5–S_1 to explain the idea of the compensating role of degenerative disc disease. Usually, under conditions of severe joint and ligamentous insufficiency, the healthy discs of this segment are unable to keep the affected segment in the normal position. Only rapid disc degeneration, with the subsequent ossification that follows (Fig. 4.1.24), can serve to prevent the imminent possibility of the neurological complications of persistent instability of this SMS. Compensatory blocking of the L_5–S_1 segment occurs not only in spondylolisthesis, but also in instability of the SMS caused by lumbarization of S_1–S_2 (Fig. 4.1.25). In this case, degenerative disc disease and spondylosis deformans (Fig. 4.1.26) are the compensatory orthopaedic factors that are of curative value.

3. We would like to point out that there is no contradiction between the two theories on the pathogenesis of OS (dysplastic and compensatory-stabilizing). Moreover, if we consider the matter in depth, these two theories complement each other or, in other words, they are two stages of the same process.

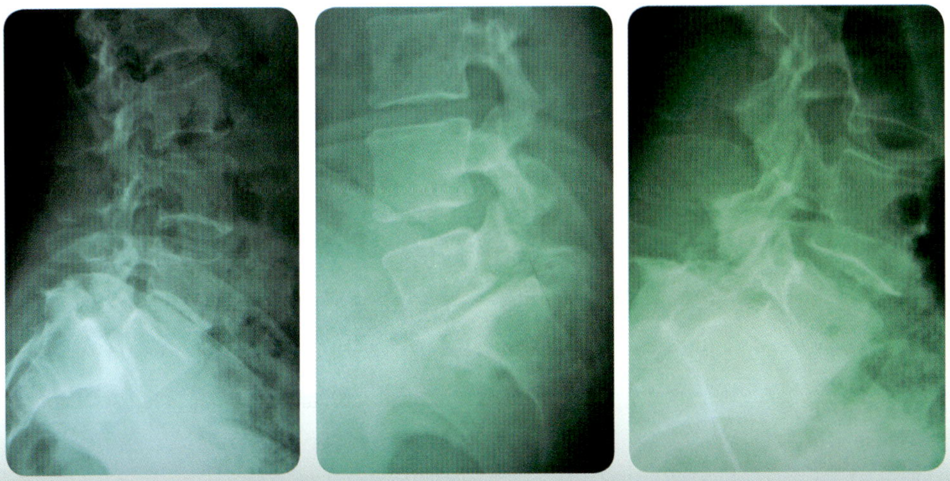

Fig. 4.1.24. Block of L_5-S_1 segment with its instability caused by spondylolisthesis associated with lumbarization of S_1-S_2

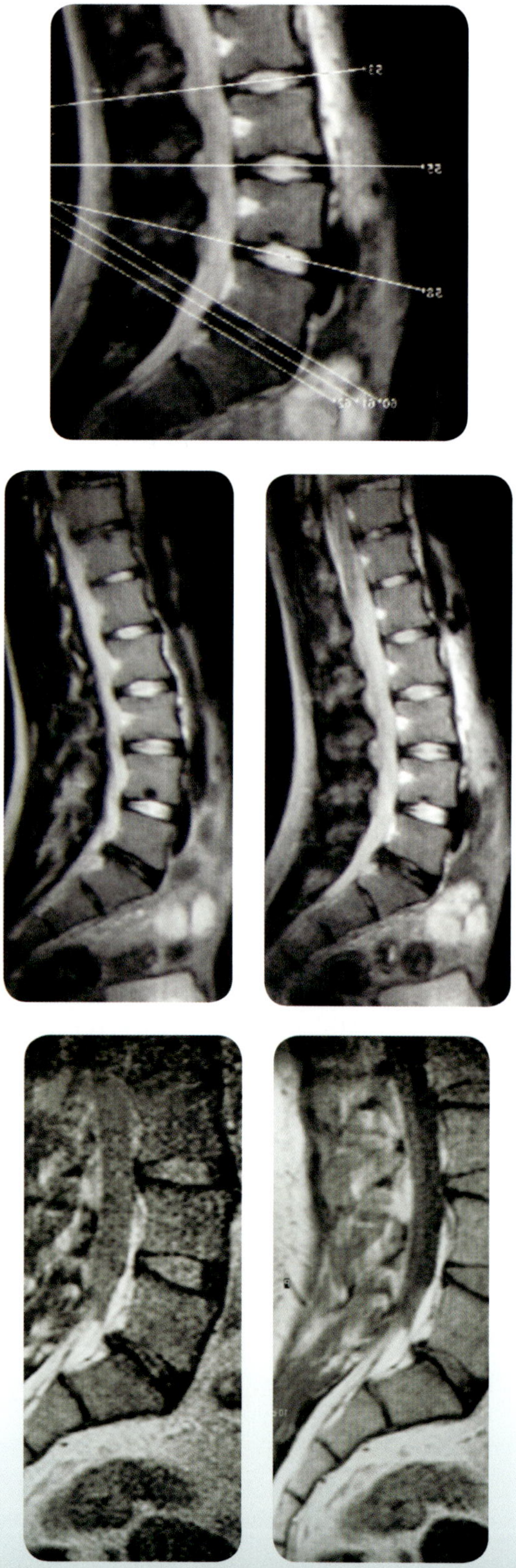

Fig. 4.1.25.
Block of L_5-S_1 segment with its instability caused by lumbarization of S_1-S_2

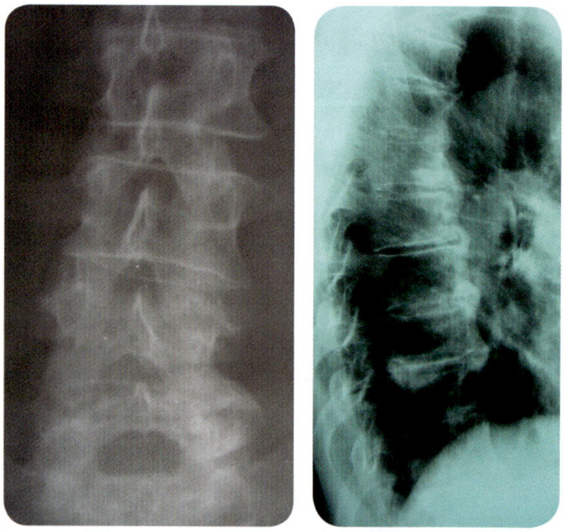

Fig. 4.1.26.
Development of degenerative disc disease and spondylosis deformans of compensatory nature

Everything starts with impairment of the dynamic equilibrium of the spine and its static failure. The result is progressive degeneration of the SMS, which first affects the intervertebral disc and the nucleus pulposus. This leads to the development of chronic fatigue syndrome, as well as degenerative disc disease and spondylosis deformans, which are aimed at stabilizing the SMS with subsequent formation of osteophytes, which fix the boundary areas of the vertebrae. We have already discussed the mechanism of this process.

The pathogenesis of OS lies not only in genetics, but also in the conditions under which the spine is functioning. However, it would be incorrect to deny the role of heredity factors. We already know that the structural features of the human body, particularly the degree of asymmetry of the spinal extensors, are inherited. So once again, we must acknowledge the significance of the consequences of asymmetrical functioning of the trunk muscles, as well as of asymmetry in general. The effective prevention and treatment of OS requires an understanding of the fact that body asymmetry is the origin of dysfunction of the SMS, which leads to degenerative disc disease, spondylosis deformans, pain, etc.

Clinical symptoms of degenerative disc disease

1. The initial stage of the disease is characterized by displacement of the nucleus pulposus, accompanied by local back pain syndrome, i.e. lumbago or lumbalgia.

2. The next stage is marked by sciatica, which is a consequence of protrusion or bulging of the disc. In addition to the pressure put on the spinal nerves and vessels by hernial protrusion, another factor starts acting at the time of formation of the hernia – chemical irritation of the autonomic plexuses by histamine-like substances.

3. The next symptom is pain which radiates to the gluteal region, sacroiliac and hip joints, popliteal fossa, medial femoral condyles and/or tibial bone. Reflexively, such pain manifests in the corresponding dermatome (Fig. 4.1.27). This often causes errors in diagnosis.

In particular, spinal pain due to disorders of the lumbar and/or sacral spine may manifest as deceptive signs of knee meniscus injuries, hip disease, osteochondropathy

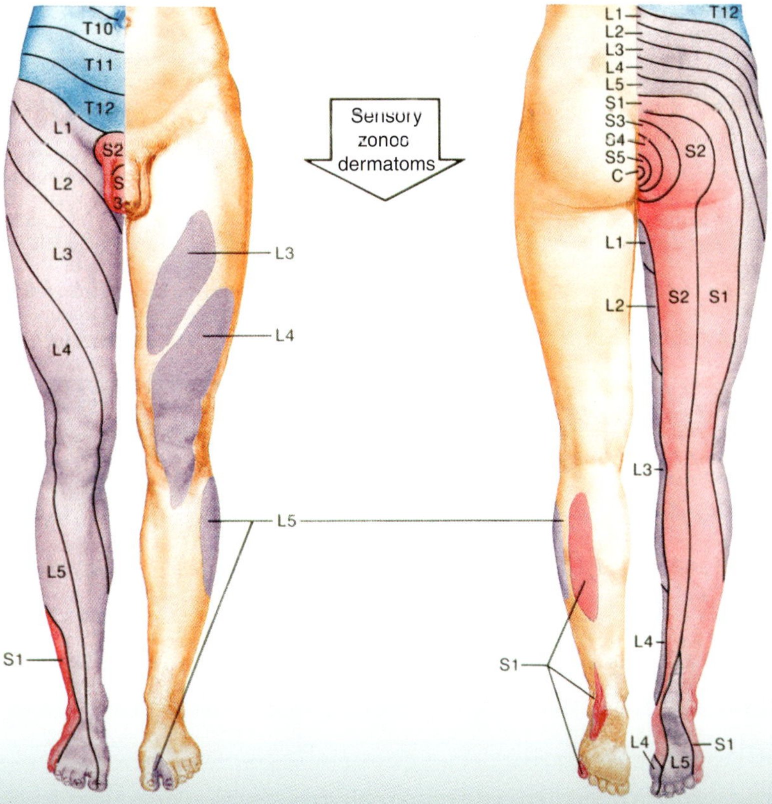

Fig. 4.1.27. Sensory innervation of lower extremities

Level of herniation	Localization of pain	Localization of numbness
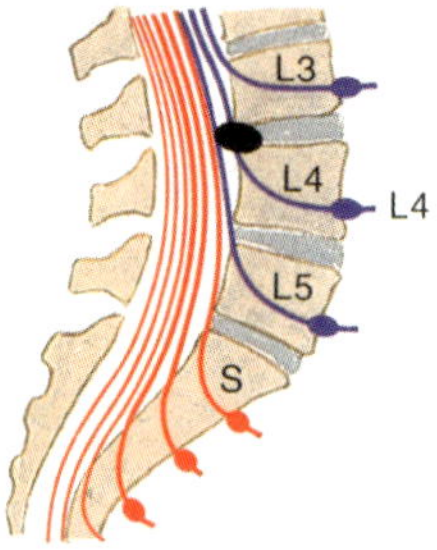	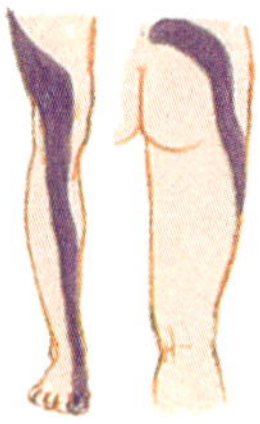	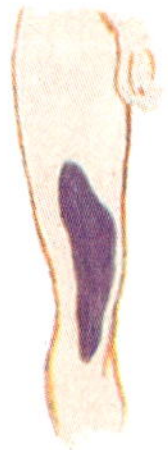
L_3-L_4 – disc, L_4 – nerve root	Lumbosacral region, area of hip joint, posterolateral surface of the thigh, anterior part of lower third of the thigh, tibia and foot	Anteromedial surface of the thigh and knee joint
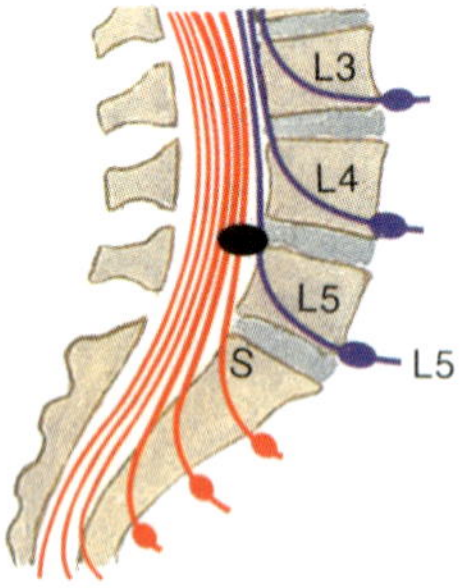	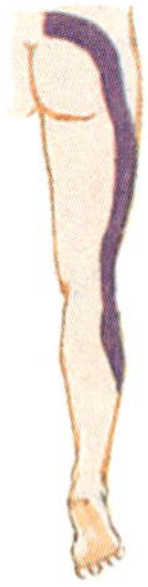	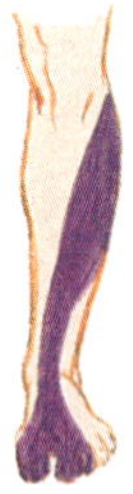
L_4-L_5 – disc, L_5 – nerve root	Area of sacroiliac joint, external surface of the thigh and tibia	External surface of the tibia, 1-3 toes
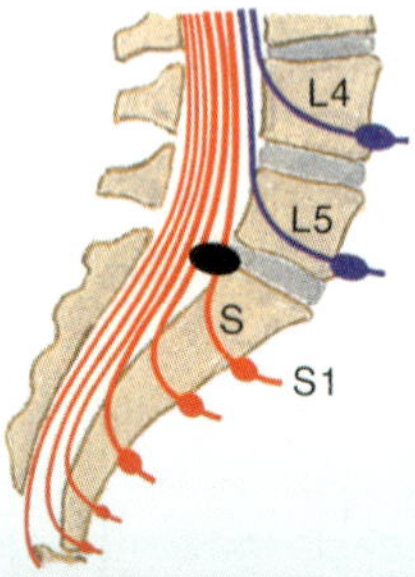	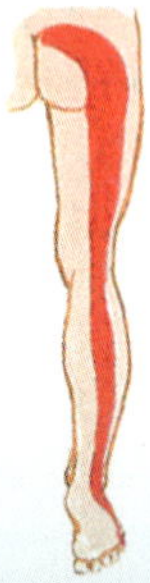	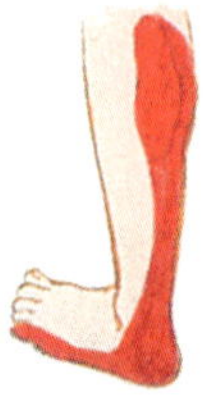
L_5-S_1 – disc, S_1 – nerve root	Area of sacroiliac joint, posterolateral surface of the thigh, tibia and feet	Posterior surface of the tibia, foot and 5th toe

Fig. 4.1.28. Clinical radicular syndromes, depending on the level of disc herniation at the lumbosacral region

of the tibial tuberosity, heel spurs, achillodynia and other conditions (Fig. 4.1.28). According to N.I. Hvisyuk, treatment provided to children and adolescents by neurologists is often ineffective due to misjudgement of the symptoms, and also due to a lack of understanding of the role of early degenerative disc disease as the source of these symptoms.

4. The monoradicular or biradicular symptoms vary according to the location of the disc protrusion or the site at which the nucleus pulposus has fallen out. The symptoms

also depend on the topography of the spinal nerves (Fig. 4.1.29).

5. From the very beginning, nearly all the pathogenetic factors are involved—mechanical, inflammatory and circulatory.

6. However, radicular syndrome may also occur in the absence of disc (nucleus) herniation. A decrease in the height of the disc and the corresponding decrease in the diameter of the intervertebral foramina cause the rootlets to crease and stretch which, given the backdrop of SMS instability, results in impaired liquor circulation, venous stasis and swelling of the rootlets. This can cause pain and disorders of the autonomic-vascular system, an atypical clinical feature of which is the resulting irritation of the spinal nerve roots.

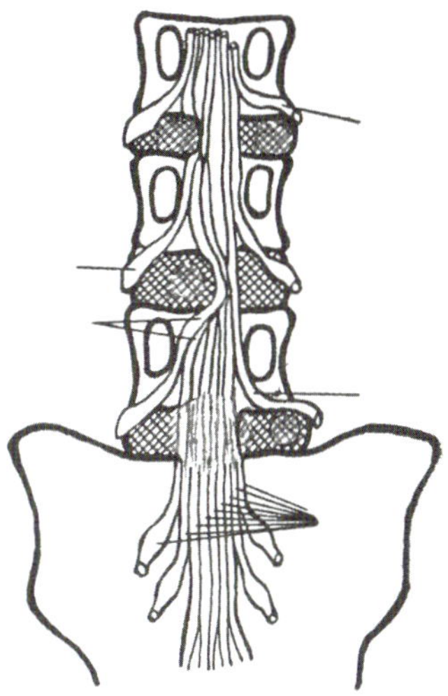

Fig. 4.1.29.
Topographical interrelations of disc herniation of different localization and spinal roots

7. The meniscoids may play an important role in the development of pain in OS (J. Kos and J. Wolf, 1972; J. Wolf, 1975). The joint cavities of the facet (intervertebral) joints are enclosed in a capsule which is internally lined with a synovial membrane and contains synovial fluid. The areas of the synovial membrane that protrude into the joint cavity as an annular cartilage are called meniscoids. They complement the articular surfaces, promote congruence, and strengthen and seal the joint. On the periphery of the facet joint, the meniscoids are intimately connected with the joint capsule. The pressure within the joint is negative in comparison to the atmospheric pressure. As a result of the difference between the internal and external pressures, the articular surfaces adhere to each other, which ensures stability of the joint. Due to this anatomical feature of the meniscoids in various injuries of the intervertebral joints and impaired integrity of these joints, the meniscoids, along with the capsule, are sucked into the joint cavity. This causes irritation of the nerve endings and leads to pain.

8. Patients suffering from OS generally have enhanced thoracic kyphosis, which can be interpreted as a defensive reaction aimed at reducing pain. Bending of the neck and trunk increase the size of the intervertebral foramina, thus releasing the compressed roots of the spinal nerves (Fig. 4.1.30).

9. The acute phase of degenerative disc disease is characterized by functional disorders of posture, with the development of antalgic (reflex pain) scoliosis. The latter, a reflex response of the muscular apparatus, enables the spine to assume positions that will reduce root tension. Occasionally, one can observe alternating scolioses, in which the trunk is bent in different ways. These clinical manifestations are associated primarily with posterior disc hernias, when hernial protrusion is itself mobile.

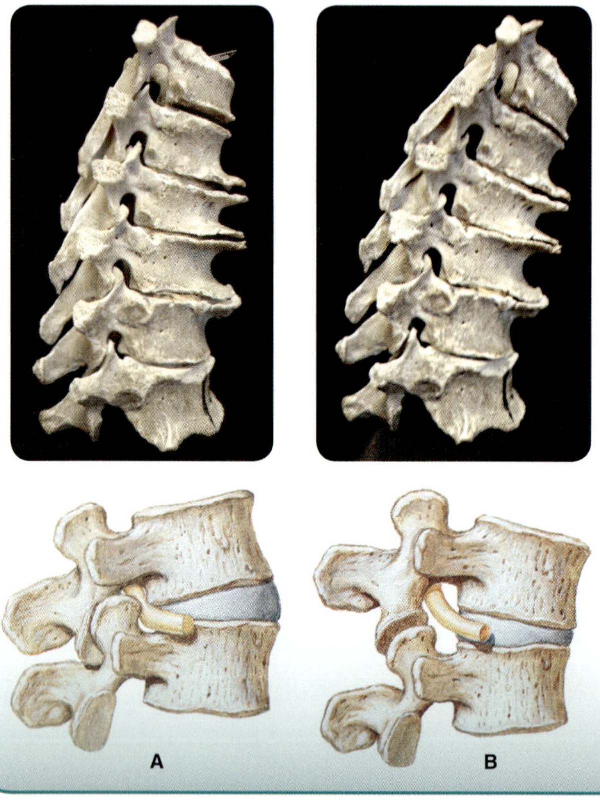

Fig. 4.1.30.
Positions of spinal nerve in hyperextension **(A)** and maximum flexion **(B)** in thoracic spine:
A - intervertebral foramen is narrowed due to the movement of superior articular process of the lower vertebra; the nerve is compressed
B - intervertebral foramen is completely opened and the nerve is free

The final stage in the clinical course of OS may resolve in several ways, such as the following:

A. Formation of a localized fibrous scar at the site of herniation

B. Diffuse scarring at the site of the intervertebral disc (fibrosis of entire disc)

C. Progression of the degenerative process, with diffuse involvement of the fibrous ring and pathological mobility (instability) at the level of the degenerated segment

D. There may be perifocal reactive inflammation and a subsequent adhesive process around a part of the disc that fell out. As a result, the hernial protrusion becomes fixed and irreducible.

The degenerative-dystrophic process is irreversible and resolves with the substitution of the basic elements of an intervertebral disc with connective tissue. This outcome is very favourable in the clinical sense as the patient recovers clinically. From the biomechanical perspective, it can be regarded as a compensatory, adaptive reaction. In such cases, the intervertebral discs, which have lost their property to absorb hydraulic shock, turn into semi-rigid pads that are not capable of performing an antigravitational role. However, clinically, the patient recovers.

4.2 Spinal pain of vertebrogenic origin not associated with osteochondrosis and spondylosis deformans

The largest group of patients suffering from spinal pain that is not directly related to OS and spondylosis deformans consists of those who have sustained various injuries. According to American, Russian and Ukrainian sources, in industrialized countries, the majority of spinal injuries are a result of car accidents. Of the approximately 55,000 people dying on highways in the USA each year, 40,000 die due to head and cervical spine injuries. Injuries are also associated with sports, particularly football, diving, roller skating and riding motorcycles or cycles.

Although much information is available on spinal injuries, this topic is beyond the scope of our work and we shall limit ourselves to drawing the reader's attention to the seminal work by the American scientists, R.L. Gallie, D.W. Speight and R. Simon, *Emergency Orthopedics: The spine* (1995). This book is of major theoretical and practical value to professional traumatologists, and deals with emergency care for patients with various injuries of the spine. The book also provides a wealth of information on spinal tumours, which are divided into two groups: (i) primary, or arising from the tissues of the spine, and (ii) metastatic, or originating in distant organs. Tumours are usually classified according to their origin, which can be bone, cartilage, fibrous tissue, nerves, bone marrow, blood vessels, etc. Since a detailed analysis of tumours of the spine is also not within the scope of this book, we shall focus only on some of those which occur most frequently.

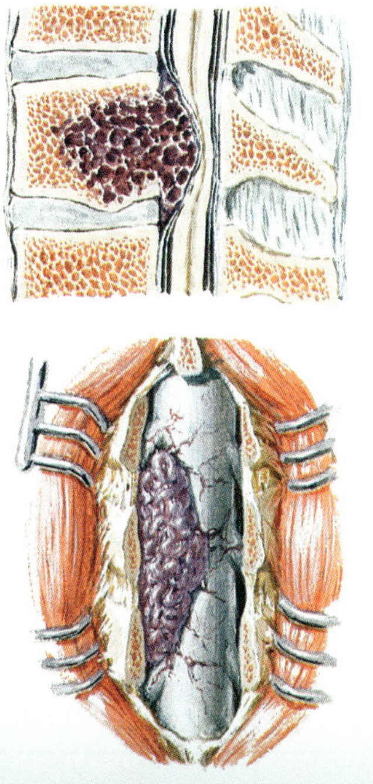

Fig. 4.2.1. Haemangioma

Benign tumours: Osteoid osteoma and haemangioma should be attributed (Fig. 4.2.1) to benign tumours affecting the bone tissue. These tumours cause back pain, mostly at night. Meningioma (Fig. 4.2.2), which arises from the meninges, does not affect the tissue of the spinal cord and manifests itself in muscle weakness, sensory symptoms, and back pain in the areas corresponding to the location of the tumour. Despite their benign nature, these tumours can impair the functioning of the spinal cord due to compression.

Malignant tumours: These may be primary or metastatic. Myeloma is the primary tumour that has been found to occur most frequently (Fig. 4.2.3). It erodes the bony trabeculae, causing intense back pain. The group of malignant secondary or metastatic tumours affecting the spine is considerably large. As for the primary tumour, it can be located in the lungs, breast, prostate gland, thyroid gland or kidneys (Fig. 4.2.4).

Spinal pain unrelated to OS may be triggered by a number of other pathological conditions. These are mentioned next.

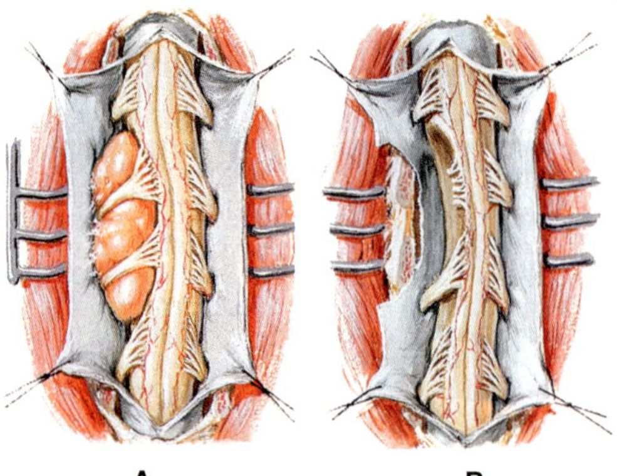

Fig. 4.2.2.
Meningioma; **A** - before surgery;
B - postoperative: on the surface of the spinal cord a depressed zone was formed that corresponds to the location of resected tumour

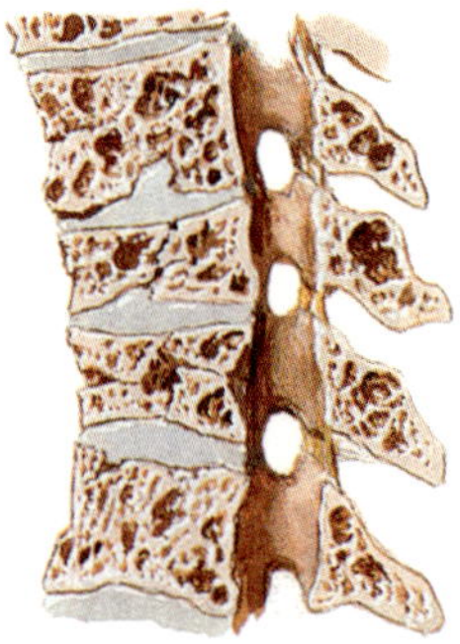

Fig. 4.2.3.
Primary malignant tumour – myeloma

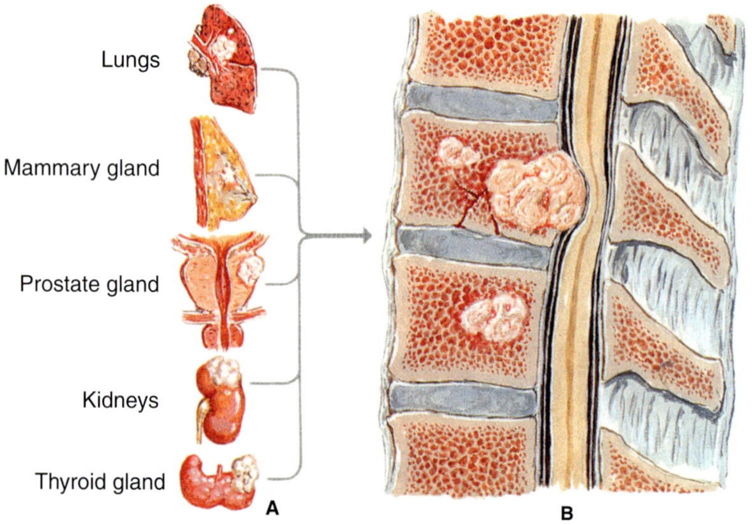

Fig. 4.2.4. Secondary metastatic tumours of the spine
A - primary localization of the tumour;
B - localization of metastases in the spine

Inflammatory diseases

Rheumatoid arthritis: This occurs as a result of damage to the mesenchymal connective tissue of the joints of the arms and legs. It may cause intense spinal pain due to degeneration of the intervertebral discs and the surrounding tissues.

Ankylosing spondylitis: Also known as Bechterew–Strümpell–Marie disease, this occurs predominantly among men (Fig. 4.2.5). Its early signs include iridocyclitis, blue sclera and ossification of the sacroiliac joints. The process of ossification is accompanied by intense sacral pain. Among young men, thoracic kyphosis begins to increase even before changes occur in the sacroiliac joints and ossification of the intervertebral discs and costovertebral joints (Articulatio capitis costae and Articulatio costotransversaria). The final stage of the disease is characterized by ossification of the entire spine, which ultimately acquires the shape of a 'bamboo stick' (Fig. 4.2.6).

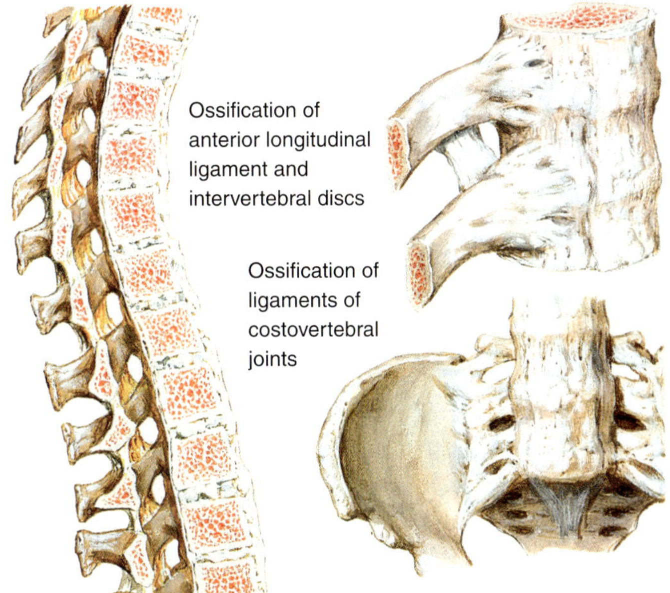

Fig. 4.2.5.
Ankylosing spondylitis (Bechterew–Strümpell–Marie disease)

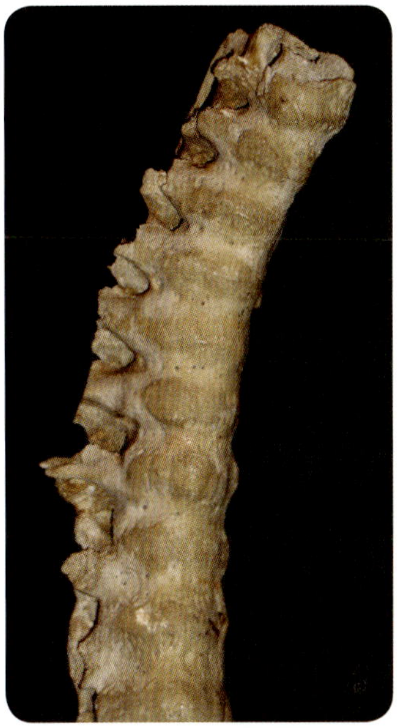

Fig. 4.2.6.
Total ossification of intervertebral discs and ligaments of the spine; macropreparation—a 'bamboo stick' appearance

Acute purulent infections

Among children, these infections are generally of a haematogenous and/or lymphatic origin. They involve mostly the respiratory system, which is the site of localization of staphylococci. In older people, the urinary system may be the site of infection. Acute infection is usually followed by pain in the spine.

Extremely intense back pain may occur 1–8 weeks after surgery on the intervertebral discs due to complications arising from infections. Infection manifests only as pain; the body temperature may be normal. An important method to eliminate pain is to immobilize the patient by using a gypsum bed. Sometimes, incision of an abscess is carried out to remove a local source of infection.

Chronic purulent infections

Chronic osteomyelitis is yet another possible cause of spinal pain. Usually, it occurs due to infractions in aseptic technique, as a purulent complication resulting from paravertebral and other blockades.

Tuberculous spondylitis is quite common in resource-poor countries. However, even in developed countries, this disease may occur in larger settlements due to the accumulation of large masses of people and, consequently, the possibility of the transmission of infection from patients to healthy people. In tuberculosis, the purulent process initially affects the central parts of one vertebral body and then spreads to other SMS. An abscess can spread through the intermuscular and cellular spaces. The treatment is limited to incision of the abscess, directed antimicrobial therapy and complete rest in a gypsum bed.

In *patients with AIDS* who have a purulent focus in the vertebrae, the pattern of the disease is similar to that in tuberculosis.

Those who have studied the problem of spinal pain agree that the largest group of patients suffering from back pain, whether associated with OS or not, consists of those with congenital anomalies of the spine. The main anomaly, as mentioned earlier, is transitional vertebrae (lumbarization of S_1 and sacralization of L_5) which, according to S.A. Reinberg (1964), occurs in 20% or more of all cases of congenital anomalies of the skeleton. Spina bifida, or gaps and defects of the vertebral bodies, particularly the failure of the posterior parts of the bodies and arches of the lumbar and sacral vertebrae to fuse, are somewhat less common (Fig. 4.2.7). The protrusion of the spinal meninges through a split in the posterior wall of the sacral spinal canal is called herniation (meningocele). The entrapment of these meninges causes intense pain, disorders of the pelvic organs, disorders of neural nutrition of the lower extremities and, as a result, development of trophic ulcers of the feet.

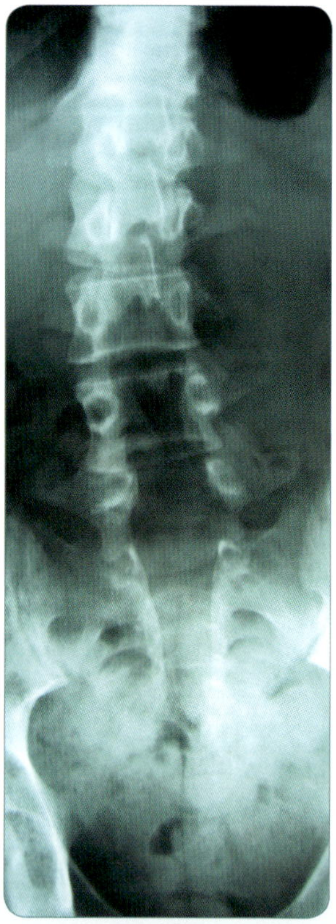

Fig. 4.2.7.
Non-fusion of posterior aspects of the bodies and arches of lumbar and sacral vertebrae

Back pain may also be caused by spinal stenosis. The most frequent cause of this condition is degenerative dystrophic changes in the facet (intervertebral) joints. The formation of osteophytes around the articular processes leads to narrowing of the spinal canal and its lateral recesses (Fig. 4.2.8). Consequently, the spinal roots are compressed, which results in back pain. The radiological picture of chronic spinal hernia, in which there are areas of petrification (ossification) of the hernial protrusion, and the initial manifestations of spinal stenosis have much in common (Fig. 4.2.9). This should be considered in the differential diagnosis.

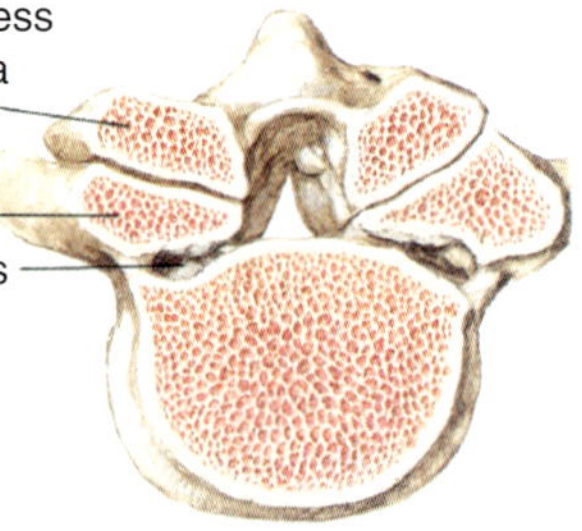

Fig. 4.2.8.
Narrowing of the spinal canal and its lateral recesses

Another group of people with spinal pain are those among whom the structure

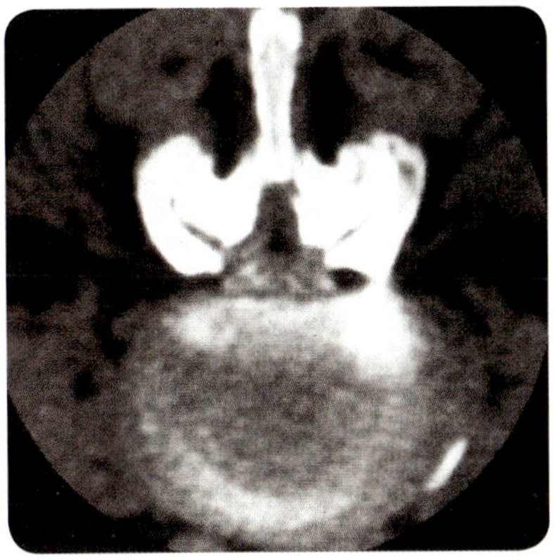

Fig. 4.2.9.
CT scan reveals significant decrease in diameter of the spinal foramina due to formation of internal osteophytes

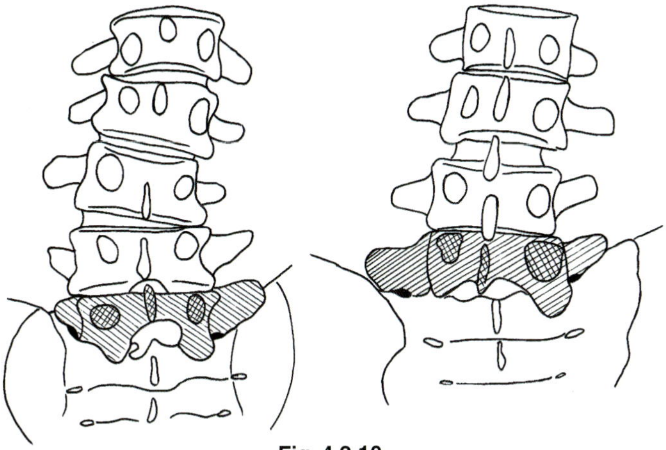

Fig. 4.2.10.
Types of rotational subluxation of vertebrae in areas of asymmetrical structure of articular processes in L_5-S_1 SMS associated with sacralization of L_5, lumbarization and spina bifida of S_1

of the articular and transverse processes, mainly in the lumbosacral spine, is asymmetrical. This gives rise to the facet pain syndrome. The origin of this condition lies in unilateral rotary subluxation of the vertebrae in the anomalous area, due to instability of the SMS at the level of L_5–S_1 and the attendant pelvic tilt towards the shortened lower limb (Fig. 4.2.10).

Due to the displacement of the elements of the joints relative to each other, the nerve 'is taken in pincers'. These and other anomalies have been discussed in Section 2.2.

Back pain need not be directly related to disc and nucleus pathology. It can also be the result of physical overload caused by functionally abnormal postures, as well as spondylolysis or spondylolisthesis, osteoporosis of various origins, including post-menopausal and senile, juvenile kyphosis of the lumbar spine (Scheuermann–Mau disease), osteochondropathy of the vertebral bodies (Calve disease), etc.

Endoscopic and radiological methods, computed tomography, nuclear magnetic resonance imaging, diagnostic myelography, epidurography and vertebral venography are widely used for the differential diagnosis of the above diseases. Morphological, biochemical, serological, immunological, cytological and other methods are also used. It is important to take a thorough medical history and perform a clinical examination. The treatment of patients with low back pain of vertebrogenic origin will be discussed in Chapter 6.

4.3 Back pain of non-vertebrogenic origin

The preceding sections have extensively discussed the role of OS and spondylosis deformans in the origin of spinal pain. Those have dealt with the causes of vertebrogenic pain not associated with these conditions.

According to modern vertebrologists and manual therapists (G.A. Ivanichev, 1998), OS, previously believed to be a universal cause of back pain, is no longer considered the leading factor in the development of this symptom. This is due to the fact that the formation of zones of pain, which has been widely observed in the paravertebral tissues, limbs and distant joints, is often not attributed to pathological changes of the spine. Such symptoms of pain are caused by other aetiological factors, which are often discovered far from the spine.

Also, in numerous cases, patients with radiographic evidence of severe degenerative changes of the spine do not complain of pain. On the other hand, in 'X-ray-negative' OS, the patient may be suffering from pain of considerable intensity. Thus, it is not possible to associate pain syndromes of the limb joints, muscles and ligaments with only dystrophic changes of the spine. This connection can be traced clearly only in some specific syndromes of discogenic lesions of the peripheral nervous system. The introduction of the discogenic concept of spinal pain led to the blossoming of neurosurgery. Extensive spinal surgeries aimed at hernia removal have been performed in cases of lumbar pain. Analysis of this material showed that in some cases, such operations led to functional or static disability of the spine. Of course, it would be wrong to deny or underestimate the need for neurosurgery in abscesses, fractures of the spine and other conditions where urgent surgical intervention is essential. Neurosurgery is also indicated for the removal of irreducible herniated disc (nucleus). Thus, neurosurgical treatment cannot and should not be ignored, but it should be indicated for a limited number of conditions. Both patients who have undergone disc surgery and physicians from commissions of professional medical experts will testify that often after surgery, the intensity of the pain remains unchanged and sometimes even increases. The question that naturally arises is whether the pain is caused by herniation of the annulus fibrosus or something else.

The structure of spinal pain syndrome turned out to be more complex than it appeared when it was believed to be of vertebrogenic origin, or associated only with dysplastic and degenerative-dystrophic disc changes. The observations made over the years and the accumulated objective data formed the basis of the emergence of a new direction in vertebrology—that linking the origin of spinal pain syndrome with compensatory myoadaptative processes in the body.

We have already discussed this. Indeed, the first description of painful muscular syndromes was made in 1843 by the German surgeon and pathologist A. Froriep (cited by Y.Y. Popelyansky, 2003). Subsequently, this line of research was forgotten. Only in the 1970s were the basic provisions of the theory of myoadaptive syndromes described, thanks to the fundamental studies of V.P. Veselovsky. *According to this theory, pain syndromes occur as a tonic response of certain muscle groups to an overload arising from an altered posture.*

Various sources in the literature and publications of the authors mentioned above, as well as a seminal work by A. Vein and M.Y. Avrutsky (1997), provide us with answers to the question of what can cause spinal pain apart from spinal disorders. Once again we would like to draw the reader's attention to the encyclopaedic work of Y.Y. Popelyansky (2003), which provided data on the symptoms and treatment of many spinal pain syndromes that are directly associated with disorders of the spine and also described spinal pain syndromes of myoadaptive origin.

Thus, it became clear that spinal pain could be caused by factors other than vertebral. But which factors? The most common types of pain syndromes caused by factors other than vertebral are outlined below. A knowledge of these is of great practical value for a physician.

Myofascial pain syndrome (MFPS)

(*Synonyms: fibromyalgia, generalized tendomyopathy, muscular rheumatism, myalgia, myofibrositis, chronic fatigue syndrome, a defect of composition and execution of movements, etc.*)

This syndrome is characterized by local tenderness of various muscles, which is accompanied by a number of non-specific clinical manifestations. These include diffuse musculoskeletal pain persisting for more than 3 months, localized in the neck, shoulder girdle, back and lower extremities. There may also be other symptoms characteristic of vegetative and functional disorders: morning stiffness lasting for more than 30 minutes, chronic fatigue syndrome, sleep disorders, headaches, depression, menstrual disorders, female urethral syndrome, oedema, Raynaud and Sjögren syndromes, etc. (F.T. Masi, 1997; H. Menninger, 1997) (cited from G.A. Ivanichev, *Manual Medicine*, 1998, 470 pp.).

(Raynaud syndrome is a disease of unknown aetiology, characterized by paroxysmal spasms of the arteries of the fingers and, rarely, of the feet. Its clinical manifestations are pallor, pain and paraesthesias. Sjögren syndrome, also of unknown aetiology, is characterized by a combination of symptoms of insufficiency of the glands of external secretion—perspiratory, salivary, sebaceous and others.)

Numerous studies have shown that fibromyalgia is not a distinct disease, but only a complex of symptoms. The aetiopathogenesis of fibromyalgia remains unclear in spite of the considerable amount of interest it has evoked among physicians of different specialties, as evidenced by the annual World Congress on Muscle Pain, the World Institute of Pain, as well as by many other congresses and conferences. Thus, in particular, the causes of the conversion of local myofascial pain to a generalized algic (pain) syndrome are poorly understood. We also do not know much about the roles of the autonomic and immune systems and psychiatric factors, and have been unable to establish a reliable link between the possible factors concerned.

After studying the problem in depth, G.A. Ivanichev (1998) proposed his own clinical classification of fibromyalgic syndrome:

1. Mild fibromyalgic syndrome—This is manifested in local pain, local compaction and convulsive response of the myofascicular hypertonuses. Autonomic dysfunction is manifested in local changes such as sweating and decreased electrodermal resistance.
2. Moderate fibromyalgic syndrome—The complaints typical of this syndrome are morning stiffness and aches all over the body that subside after a workout.
3. Severe fibromyalgic syndrome—In addition to the complaints typical of the first two stages, chronic fatigue syndrome develops. Autonomic disorders occur quite frequently.

According to A.M. Vein and M.Y. Avrutsky (1997) who, too, have studied the problem of fibromyalgia in depth, the syndrome manifests itself generally in unilateral muscle spasm (local muscular hypertonus). Depending on the presence of trigger points (TP), which are zones of maximum pain located in the skeletal muscles and/or their fasciae, the unilateral muscle spasms may be active or latent.

Each TP is related to a very specific area of pain, usually located within a single dermatome. In an area of reflected pain, one may also observe autonomic and trophic signs such as skin hypertrichosis and hyperpigmentation, as well as changes in its oiliness and sweating.

A brief mention has been made of local skin hypertrichosis and hyperpigmentation in the lumbosacral region earlier (Section 2.2), in the discussion of spinal anomalies and their association with back pain. In particular, dysplastic scoliosis, which is characterized by symptoms of myelodysplasia and paresis of the lower limbs, manifests externally as skin hypertrichosis and hyperpigmentation at the level of the first sacral vertebra.

However, these symptoms do not appear instantly. They develop over several years, the external manifestations increasing with the progression of the cause or causes that triggered them. If the patient is a child, it means that everything starts from early childhood. And what may appear at this age? The answer is still the same; one-sided muscle contracture or, in other words, local muscular hypertonus caused by already described reasons.

Thus, we can assume that all the symptoms described above are essentially caused by unilateral spasm of the trunk muscles and, therefore, MFPS originates in an anomalous area of the spine.

In this context, it would be relevant to once again mention the opinion of Schantz (1933), who, while describing static insufficiency of the spine, stated that it results from chronic fatigue and is characterized by a feeling of fatigue and back pain radiating to the chest and the abdomen. This description of spinal insufficiency corresponds exactly with the clinical picture of MFPS, which is usually not associated with OS and occurs independently.

The main causes of myofascial pain syndrome (MFPS)

Body asymmetry in the form of unequal length of the legs or reduced size of one half of the pelvis is of crucial importance. Defects of the posterior part of the spinal canal, unfused posterior walls of the lumbar and sacral vertebrae, lumbarization of S_1, sacralization of L_5, platypodia, a long second metatarsal bone with a shortened first metatarsal bone, and short shoulders with an elongated trunk are also important.

Anomalies in the structure of the body change its static and impair the functioning of the trunk muscles. In our opinion, MFPS occurs as a result of constant uneven tension of individual muscle groups.

A.M. Vein and M.Y. Avrutsky (1997) were of the view that a discrepancy in the length of the legs is physiological, since it is found in 92% of young people. According to our investigations, relative shortening of one of the legs is present in 100% of people and is linked with asymmetrical function of the brain's hemispheres. The actual point to be considered is the extent of this difference.

If the difference between the length of the legs exceeds 1 cm, it is a risk factor as this has been found to significantly correlate with low back pain. According to the above-mentioned authors, in such a tilt of the trunk, the common extensor and m. quadratus dorsi contract asymmetrically. If it persists over a period of time, the unilateral muscle spasm increases the body tilt, eventually causing rotation of individual vertebrae and later even torsion of whole segments.

The rotation of vertebrae, because of a decrease in disc height, dramatically minimizes the diameter of the intervertebral foramina, resulting in compression of the spinal roots and dysfunction of the peripheral nervous system.

This stage of the disease is clear enough, but there is some uncertainty regarding the causes of the transformation of local myofascial pain to generalized pain syndrome, with pathological involvement of the peripheral and central nervous systems.

In our view, the most likely cause of this situation is torsion and mutually antithetical rotation of the vertebrae at all levels of the spine. The local syndrome is converted to a generalized process because of almost simultaneous occurrence of compression of the spinal cord, sympathetic and parasympathetic ganglia, and plexuses. This is the basic cause of conversion of a local syndrome to a generalized process.

Of course, the severity of these effects varies and depends on many factors, such as the degree of rotation or torsion of the vertebrae. The latter, in turn, depends on the severity of the spinal deformity, the presence or absence of skeletal abnormalities, age, the degree of asymmetry of the trunk muscles, etc. The clinical diversity of myofascial pain can be explained by these factors.

However, if this were so and everything was associated with asymmetry of the trunk and its consequences, it would mean that elimination of the asymmetry would do away with the leading mechanism of the pathogenesis of MFPS and greatly improve the effectiveness of treatment. Also, it would become possible to prevent this disease.

According to A.M. Vein and M.Y. Avrutsky (1997) and other researchers, there are some more possible causes of MFPS:

- Muscle tension in non-physiological positions
- Long-term immobilization of muscles, after plastering
- Hypothermia and muscle compression by clothes, belts, bags, etc.
- Sprains, bruises and overload of untrained muscles, etc.

While discussing the origins of MFPS, a mention should be made of diseases of the visceral organs and joints. Myofascial pain may accompany almost any somatic disease. This is part of a protective mechanism: pain impulses from the affected internal organ or joint cause protective tension of the corresponding muscles in order to immobilize the joint or create a 'muscular corset' around the diseased organ.

In clinical practice, the presence of cutaneous hyperalgesic areas (CHAs), which were described by G.A. Zakharin (1883) and N. Ged (1889, is well known in diseases of the internal organs (Fig. 4.3.1). These areas acquired special importance in diagnostics in the field of cardiac pathology. The neurophysiological basis of CHAs is a segmental correspondence between afferent inputs from an internal organ and a corresponding dermatome (*see* Section 2.1 on 'Autonomic nervous system').

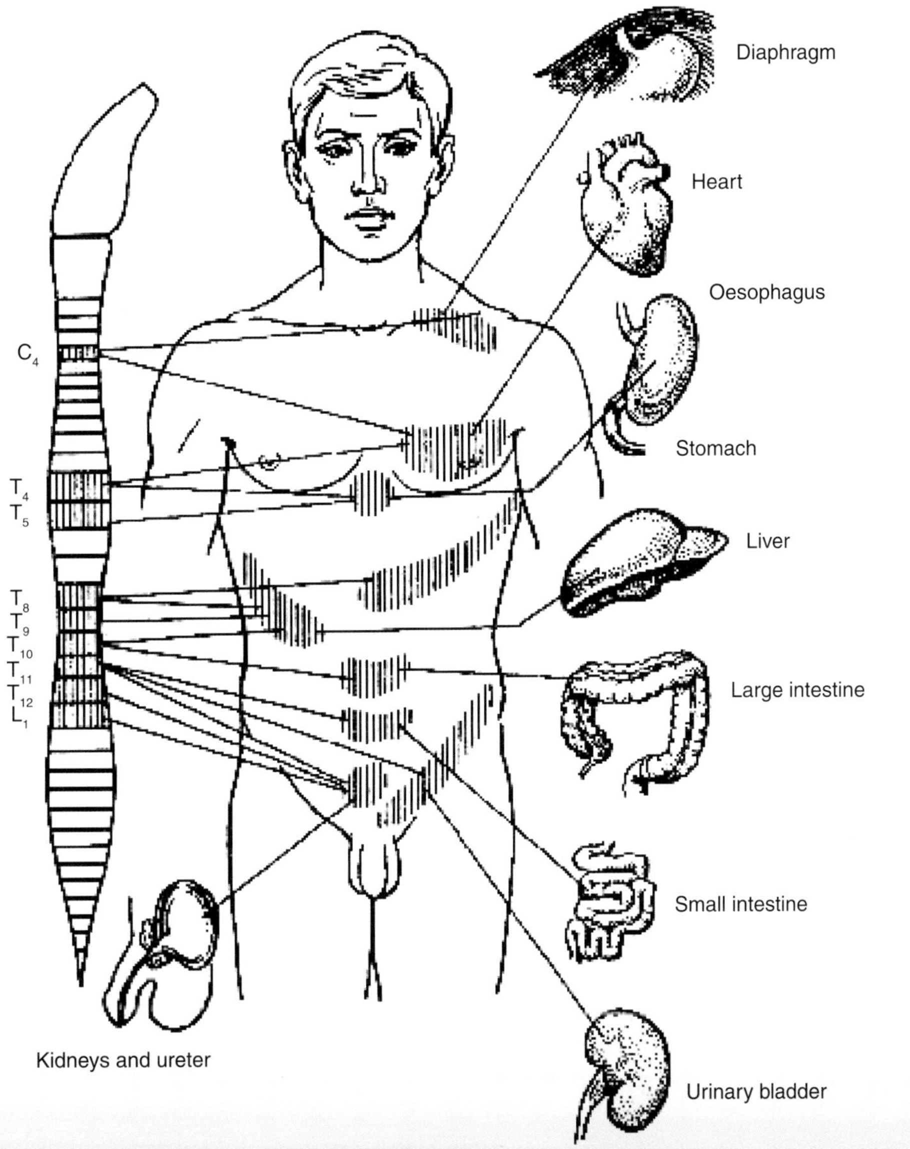

Fig. 4.3.1.
Zones of Zakharin-Ged: interrelations among internal organs and segments of the spinal cord (L.I. Sundrigailo, 1988)

Recent times have seen an increasing interest in CHAs, not so much due to their diagnostic value, but because efficient use has been made of manual therapy to eliminate them. This is achieved by stretching the skin in the CHAs in opposite directions to restore its elasticity. Most often, after this fairly simple procedure, the area of hyperalgesia disappears and the size of the area of myofascicular hypertonus decreases.

Localization of MFPS

Back pain is usually categorized according to the main location of the pain. Thus, neck pain is called *cervicalgia* and in cases in which it radiates to the arm or head, the terms *cervicobrachialgia* and *cervicocranialgia*, respectively, are used. Pain in the thoracic spine is called *thoracalgia*. Low back pain is called *lumbalgia* and pain radiating to the leg, sciatica (*lumboischalgia*). The term lumbago is used to denote acute, abrupt onset of back pain. Recently, the term *dorsalgia* is being used quite widely in clinical practice to refer to any back pain that does not radiate to the limbs. Mention should also be made of *tunnel syndrome*, which refers to acute or chronic nerve compression in the area where it is normally located (i.e. in the musculo-fibrous or musculo-osseous bed or tunnel). These terms are used only to describe pain and are not diagnoses.

Psychogenic back pain

The role of psychological factors in the origin of pain of any location and nosology is large. Psychogenic back pain exists only in the patient's mind and often has no morphological substrate. The pain may occur after emotional stress, or be linked to anxiety, fear, panic or depressed mood. Psychogenic pain is also observed among patients suffering from hysteria, depression, delusions, hallucinations, etc. *Abdominalgic syndrome*, which begins as back pain and then spreads to the abdomen, should also be regarded as psychogenic pain. This type of pain, which is not associated with organic changes, occurs in 90%–95% of children suffering from gastrointestinal disorders.

Reflected back pain

Vertebrologists should know that in addition to fibromyalgia and psychogenic back pain, there are a variety of pathological conditions, including diseases of the internal organs, that manifest themselves in sudden attacks of back pain. This type of pain is described as reflected pain (Fig. 4.3.2). The causes include:

- Aneurysm of the thoracic or abdominal aorta
- Pleural effusion
- Intestinal obstruction
- Bleeding into the retroperitoneal space
- Diseases of the pelvic organs (peritonitis and ectopic pregnancy)
- Prostatitis
- Urinary tract infection

The diseases mentioned above are not discussed in this book. We present this information in order to emphasize the need for a thorough examination of each patient with spinal pain. It is necessary to analyse the patient's history, examine him/her clinically and get the relevant laboratory investigations using instrumental and other evaluation methods.

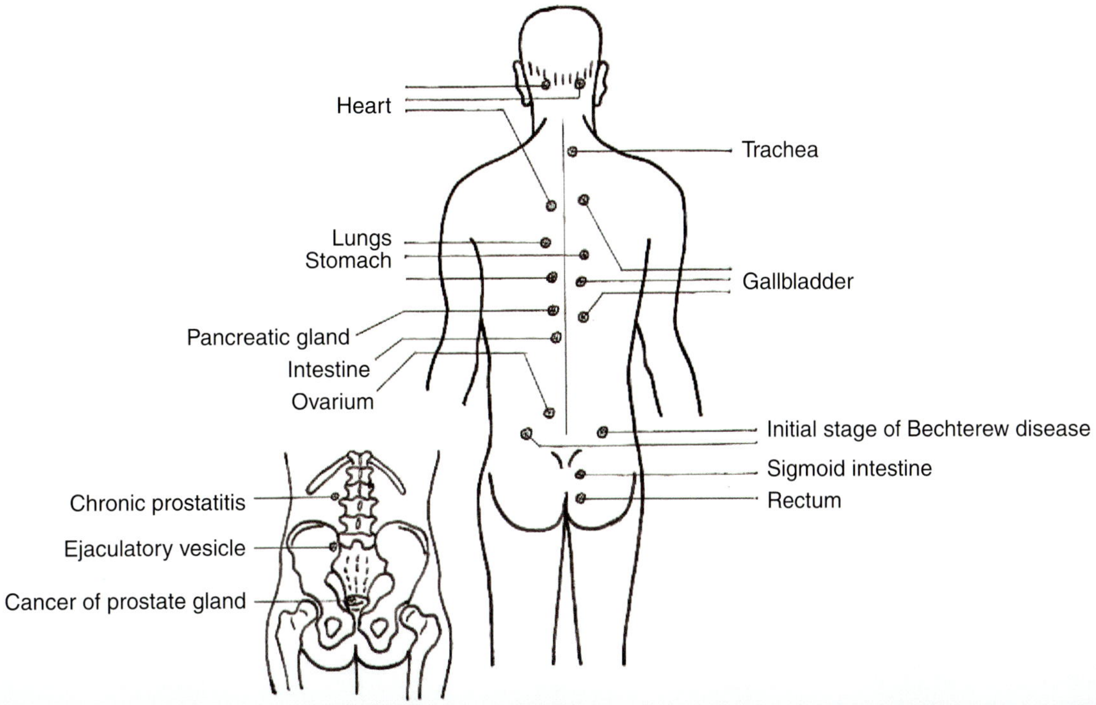

Fig. 4.3.2.
Reflected back pain in diseases of the internal organs

Prevention and treatment of non-vertebrogenic back pain

The main measures that can help prevent non-vertebrogenic back pain are maintaining correct posture, exercising regularly, keeping oneself physically fit and maintaining a normal body weight. The treatment measures that have been shown to yield positive results include detorsional correction, manual therapy, acupuncture, massage, physical therapy, vitamin therapy, and the administration of antidepressants, psychoactive drugs or sleeping pills.

Also, the following measures are recommended: orthopaedic compensation for the shortened lower extremity, infiltration of trigger points with procaine or other anaesthetics, relaxation of the shortened extremities and activation of flaccid muscles, sauna, etc.

The type of treatment depends on the stage of the disease and the localization of the trigger points.

4.4 Pathogenesis of spinal pain

We have reached the end of our brief description of the voluminous and complex material on the origins of spinal pain, the main causes of which are listed below:

1. Osteochondrosis, complicated by disc herniation and falling out of the nucleus pulposus in the thoracic or, more often, lumbar region gives rise to spinal pain.
2. Decrease of disc height causes instability of the SMS. This leads to narrowing of the intervertebral foramina and causes creasing and stretching of the spinal roots, besides impairing microcirculation, which results in venous congestion and oedema. In turn, this results in the typical clinical picture of radicular pain in the absence of disc (nucleus) herniation.
3. If there are cracks in the fibrous ring, fragments of the nucleus pulposus penetrate through them. As a result, reactive aseptic inflammation develops in these areas, leading to irritation of the pain receptors of the sinuvertebral nerves (recurrent nerves of Luschka). Clinically, this process manifests itself in acute lumbalgia.
4. Persistent instability of the SMS gives rise to deforming spondylosis, resulting in destructive and dystrophic changes in all structures of the intervertebral disc, mostly in the endplates and sprouting plates. In the areas where these changes have taken place, compensatory bony outgrowths (osteophytes) are formed to prevent further displacement of the vertebrae from each other. However, the formation of osteophytes also has a negative consequence. They gradually grow larger, thus decreasing the size of the spinal foramina and injuring the spinal nerve roots, the result being chronic spinal pain.

Spinal pain may also be caused by the following:

- Congenital anomalies of the spine (lumbarization of S_1 and sacralization of L_5) can cause spinal pain, as can incomplete fusion of the spinous processes and posterior wall of the vertebrae (spina bifida), in which vertebral rotation may lead to herniation of the spinal meninges (meningocele).
- Rotary subluxation of the vertebrae of the presacral SMS (L_5–S_1) can cause facet pain due to anomalies in the structure of the articular processes of these vertebrae.

- Spinal pain may also be caused by the compression of spinal nerves by the meniscoids when displaced in the cavity of the intervertebral (facet) joints due to injuries.
- Spinal stenosis
- Fractures of the spine in different regions
- Spondylolisthesis
- Osteoporosis of various aetiologies
- Osteochondropathy of the vertebral bodies
- Benign tumours
- Malignant tumours (primary and metastatic)
- Acute and chronic purulent infections and rheumatoid arthritis, ankylosing spondylitis, etc.
- Myofascial pain syndrome
- Psychogenic and reflected back pain
- A combination of several factors.

As is evident from the review of the literature on the causes of spinal pain, there is a large body of information that is extremely important to a practitioner. However, the 18 or more causes of pain described above may lead to a dead end for any physician and/or a highly competent specialist, because it is still not clear where to begin the search for the truth. The question arises: How to make a correct diagnosis and what should be the prescribed treatment?

In our view, a physician trying to determine the causes of spinal pain should first get a clear understanding of which of them are found most often. Thus, we decided to analyse our own clinical material. This consists of data on the evaluation and ambulatory treatment of more than 8000 patients, who were of various ages and were united by the same problem—spinal pain in its various manifestations. We also felt it was necessary to look for a link between spinal deformities and spinal pain, as well as between spinal pain and various diseases that can afflict people from childhood to old age.

Before we present our analysis, let us reflect on the information given in the previous chapter on the origin of body asymmetry, scoliosis and regularities of rotational (torsional) displacement of the vertebrae, as well as the information on the origin of spinal pain given in this chapter. The following conclusions can be drawn on the basis of the information available till now:

1. In our view, the root of all the causes that have been described is asymmetrical functioning of the cerebral hemispheres, which causes unilateral spasm of the spinal

extensors. The resulting lateral tilt of the body has two effects. The first is torsion of the vertebrae relative to each other, in accordance with the laws of biomechanics. The second is asymmetrical growth of the vertebral bodies and discs, leading to the development of a wedge-shaped deformity. This is in accordance with the law of Hueter–Volkmann, and takes place due to varying degrees of pressure on the discs and nuclei on the concave and convex sides of the deformed spine.

These are major factors in the development of initial functional scoliosis, which is followed by structural scoliosis. Asymmetrical load on the spine results in the formation of a lateral curvature which inevitably leads to torsion of the vertebrae.

Among the causes of such lateral curvature, a difference in the length of the lower extremities, as well as the condition of muscular corset of the body, the person's living conditions and nature of work, level of nutrition, etc. play a significant role in the formation of the curvature (*see* Chapter 3, Scheme 3.2.1).

2. Asymmetrical axial load on the intervertebral disc and the nucleus pulposus causes displacement of the nucleus towards the convex side of the curved spine, and of the annulus, towards the concave side (*see* Chapter 3, Fig. 3.2.46). Simultaneously, in all regions of the spine (cervical, thoracic and lumbosacral), one can observe not just rotation of the vertebrae at the top of the curved segment but also of mutually opposite displacements of the upper and lower vertebrae (*see* Chapter 3, Fig. 3.3.14). As mentioned by V.Y. Fischenko *et al.* (1994) in their description of the nature of dysplastic scoliosis, these processes begin *in utero,* i.e. a child is born with initial changes in the discs and nuclei. Thus, N.I. Hvisyuk *et al.* (1985) were right when in their monograph *Osteochondrosis of the Spine in Children* (1985) they pointed out the existence of early forms of this disorder in children and adolescents.

   Growth of vertebral bodies and discs in the position of trunk bending leads not only to further development of wedge-shaped deformity, but also to subsequent impairment of the dynamic equilibrium of the spine. The result is static insufficiency which, on the one hand, leads to the progression of scoliosis, and on the other to the development of degenerative disc disease and spondylosis deformans.

   One of the signs of functional insufficiency of the spine is spondylosis deformans, which serves to protect the spine from damage during its overloading. This illustrates the law of deformation due to static loading, as described by A. Shantz (1933).

4. The initial manifestations of OS in early childhood are caused by dysplasia due to uneven loading, but later in life OS develops as a consequence of impairment of the supportive and amortizative functions of the spine. At this stage, as we already know, OS and spondylosis deformans begin to act as stabilizing factors,

the purpose of which is to immobilize the affected SMS and thereby restore the dynamic equilibrium.

5. Thus, our original supposition that the process begins with muscle spasm, which leads to the development of a lateral curvature of the spine, is correct. In turn, the lateral curvature leads to the rotation (torsion) of the deformed, wedge-shaped vertebral bodies and discs, and then to impairment of their growth, through the development of compensatory OS and spondylosis.

All the above causes of degenerative disc disease are, of course, important in the progression of OS.

Lateral curvature of the spine, which is the factor primarily associated with the origin of the disease, begins to form during the stage of foetal development and the first few months of life. If it is not eliminated in early childhood, it persists into adolescence and adulthood, becoming the basis for a variety of diseases of the organs and systems of the human body.

We hope that the information in this chapter has been useful both for curious readers without a medical background as well as for health professionals. The association of spinal deformities with human diseases will be discussed in the next chapter.

5 Effect of spinal deformities on the origin of various human diseases (analysis of author's observations)

BESIDES CLARIFYING THE CAUSES OF SPINAL PAIN, we also attempted to establish an association between spinal deformities and a variety of diseases (disorders of the internal organs, peripheral and central nervous systems, etc.) that were present in our patients.

The basic question that we, as well as our colleagues and predecessors, wanted to answer was how and why diseases emerge? Additional questions also appeared. If the patient is elderly, the disease can be linked with age, but what if the patient is a child, that too, only in his early childhood? Why is it that hospitals, including paediatric ones, are not empty even in the richest and most highly developed countries, where healthcare receives all the necessary support? How and why do children, who have only the initial manifestations of various diseases, grow up to become a reservoir of illnesses?

We found that the literature available contained different answers to these questions. They pertained to nutrition, water supply, environmental factors, etc. These factors do operate in modern times and probably did so, to some extent, in the past as well. However, most of the diseases afflicting modern humans have been known for thousands of years, as is evident from the tractates of the physicians of antiquity, the early and late middle ages, and later periods of human development. Thus, there are probably some other factors that caused diseases in the previous millennia and continue to act today. The challenge facing us was to identify them.

While focusing on the issue of spinal pain, we examined thousands of patients who were suffering from pain along the extremities as well as in the spine, and who complained of the malfunctioning of various organs and even systems. *Thus, the following question arose: Is there a connection between spinal disorders and internal diseases?* Which conditions lead to their development and what causes their progression?

In the previous chapter, we discussed reflected pain, i.e. a condition in which disease in an organ causes pain in a corresponding segment of the spine. Now we will deal with the interrelationship between the spine and the internal organs. Through an analysis of our clinical material, we will try to answer all the questions that have been raised and describe our understanding of the nature of the problem.

From February 1996 to February 2013, we examined more than 8000 patients, whose ages ranged from several months to 90 years and who were receiving outpatient treatment for spinal pain and various neurological disorders associated with spinal deformities. The patients were admitted in the City Trauma Centre (Department of Traumatology and Orthopaedics of Odessa National Medical University; the chairman of which is Professor Y.V. Sukhin), as well as in the outpatient department of the 8th Odessa Hospital (the chief medical officer of which is M.E. Babkova).

Children and adolescents had been referred to the hospital for spinal deformities (scoliosis, kyphosis, kyphoscoliosis), as well as pain in any region of the spine. Older patients and those of advanced age had been referred for various types of pain in the cervical, thoracic or lumbar spine. This section contains a detailed description of the patients' complaints and the relationship of these with particular spinal deformities.

Lateral curvature of the spine, predominantly caused by unilateral spasm of the spinal extensors, was observed in all patients, i.e. infants, children, adolescents and adults. In 80%–85% of cases, the spasm, which has its origin in the functioning of the cerebral hemispheres, was right-sided, while in the rest, it was left-sided. The tilt of the body was responsible for the vertebral–pelvic imbalance. Lowering of the right or left half of the pelvis led to shortening of the corresponding leg. This shortening should be called relative, since the anatomical (absolute) length of the bones was the same.

In 10%–15% of cases, relative shortening was combined with an absolute reduction in the length of one of the lower extremities. In adults, this was due to anomalies of the hip joints, including dysplasia, congenital dislocation and aseptic necrosis of the femoral head, and in children, it was due to Perthes disease. A loss in the absolute length of the leg may also be caused by traumatic injuries which, for example, result in a shortened femur or tibia, flat-valgus or flat-varus foot. Some other causes of a loss in the absolute length of the leg are destructive processes in the bones of the lower extremities, poliomyelitis, and congenital deformities of the hips, legs and feet.

Various deformities of the spine had developed among the patients, depending on the side of shortening (Figs 5.1, 5.2). Thus, in cases of shortening of the left leg, left-sided lateral curvature had formed in the cervical region, right-sided curvature in the thoracic region and left-sided curvature in the lumbar region, and finally, right-sided curvature had formed in the sacrum in the unfused S_1–S_2. In shortening of the right leg, all these deformities had developed in the opposite direction.

Further, during the tilting of vertebrae, the laws of mechanics come into force in each segment. According to these laws, initially, mutually antithetical rotational displacement of individual vertebrae occurs above the arc of the curvature and this is followed by the displacement of groups of vertebrae. The severity of the curvature among our patients depended on the degree of shortening of the left or right leg.

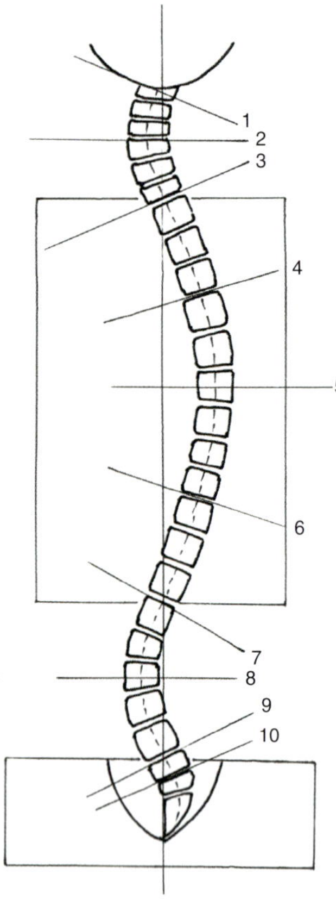

Fig. 5.1.
Location of rotational displacements of vertebrae in cervical, thoracic, lumbar and sacral regions in shortening of the left leg
1–10 - zones of typical location

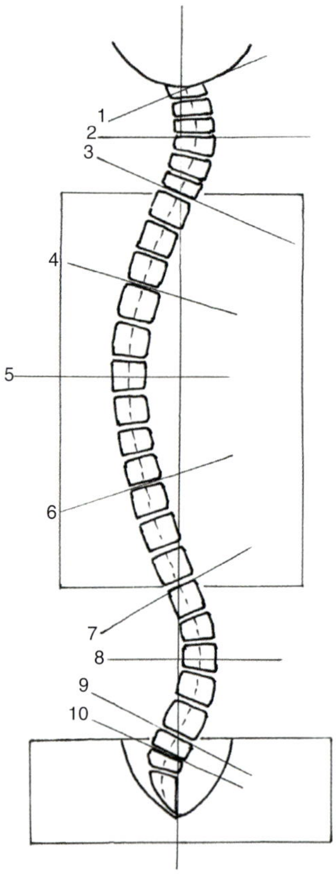

Fig. 5.2.
Location of rotational displacement of vertebrae in cervical, thoracic, lumbar and sacral regions in shortening of the right leg
1–10 - zones of typical location

The difference in length ranged from a few millimetres to five centimetres or more. The severity of the curvature was also related to the presence or absence of structural anomalies in the vertebral bodies, their processes and other anatomical structures.

Among patients with rotation of the vertebrae, compression of the spinal roots in the spinal apertures by the articular processes of these vertebrae occurred in each segment of the spine. Among individuals in the earlier years of life, when the height of the intervertebral discs is considerable, such displacement either did not cause compression of the nerve roots or was accompanied by slight pain. Children often do not complain of pain along the neural plexuses because while growing up, they get used to constant pain, which they believe is the order of things. Usually their neurological and functional disorders were detected only during prophylactic examinations.

Radicular pain could be caused by herniation of the intervertebral disc and its nucleus, stenosis (of various origins) of the intervertebral foramina, and spinal canal meningeal herniation due to posterior non-fusion of the lower lumbar and/or sacral vertebrae, a variety of specific and non-specific inflammatory diseases of the spinal tissues, benign or malignant tumours, etc.

Our research focused only on those cases, both among children and adults, in which different diseases of the internal organs and systems were associated with various spinal deformities. We have to say that such situations were observed in most cases. Each patient was examined thoroughly to exclude specific and neurosurgical conditions, tumours and undiagnosed injuries. The diagnostic methods included radiological and laboratory tests, ultrasound transcranial Doppler and

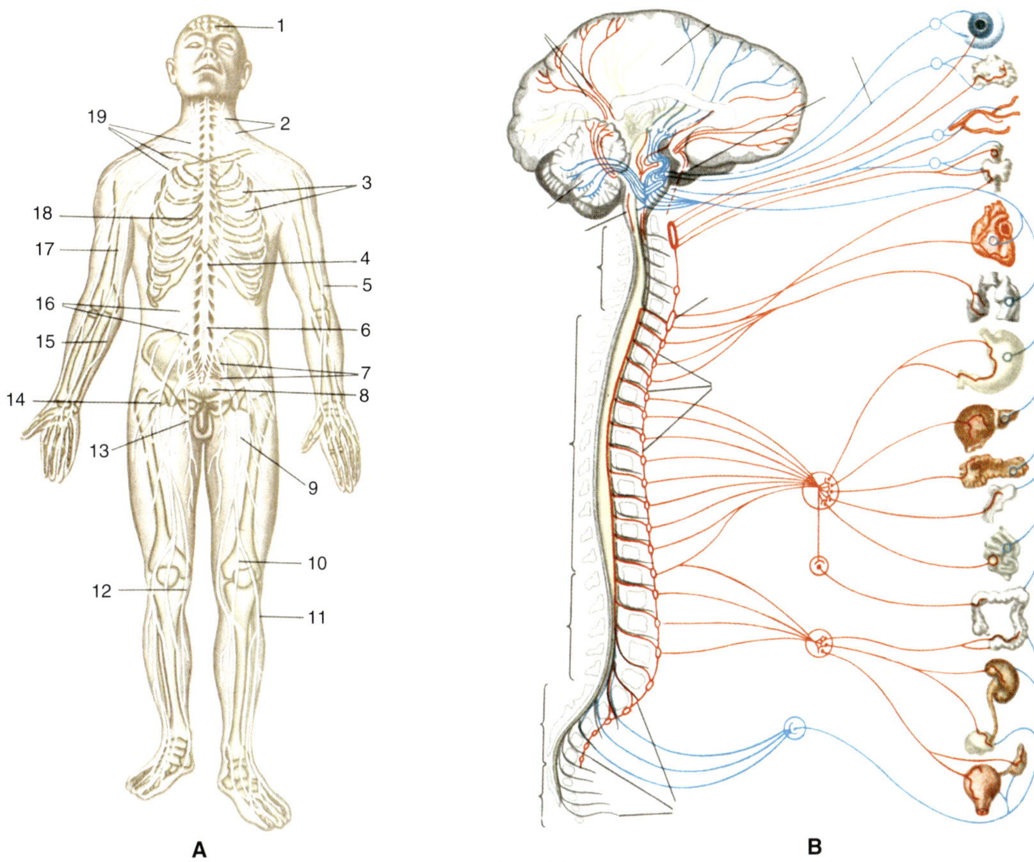

Fig. 5.3.
The nervous system
A - general scheme: 1 - brain; 2 - cervical plexus; 3 - intercostal nerves (anterior branches); 4 - spinal cord; 5 - radial nerve; 6 - cauda equina; 7 - sacral plexus; 8 - coccygeal nerves; 9 - sciatic nerve; 10 - tibial nerve; 11 - peroneal nerve; 12 - internal cutaneous nerve of the lower extremity; 13 - obturator nerve; 14 - femoral nerve; 15 - ulnar nerve; 16 - lumbar plexus; 17 - median nerve; 18 - sympathetic nerve trunk; 19 - brachial plexus
B - the brain, spinal cord and the autonomic nervous system (semi-schematic)

echoencephalography. After an accurate diagnosis was established, the patients received controlled outpatient treatment. In some cases of severe pain, the patient was hospitalized for treatment, which will be described in Chapter 6.

In Chapter 2, we have mentioned that the central and peripheral nervous systems play a role in controlling the functioning of the various organs, as well as the vasomotor, respiratory, digestive, urinary and other systems as a whole. This is confirmed by other sources of information (Fig. 5.3). A considerably smaller volume of information is devoted to elucidating the relationship between dysfunctioning of organs and systems and the corresponding deformities (anomalies) of individual vertebrae or groups of vertebrae. However, we have come across such information and will acquaint the reader with what we learnt from L.I. Sandrigailo's *Anatomo-clinical Atlas on Neuropathogy* (Fig. 5.4) [Minsk, 1988, 320 p.].

We shall start the presentation of our clinical material with a description of the

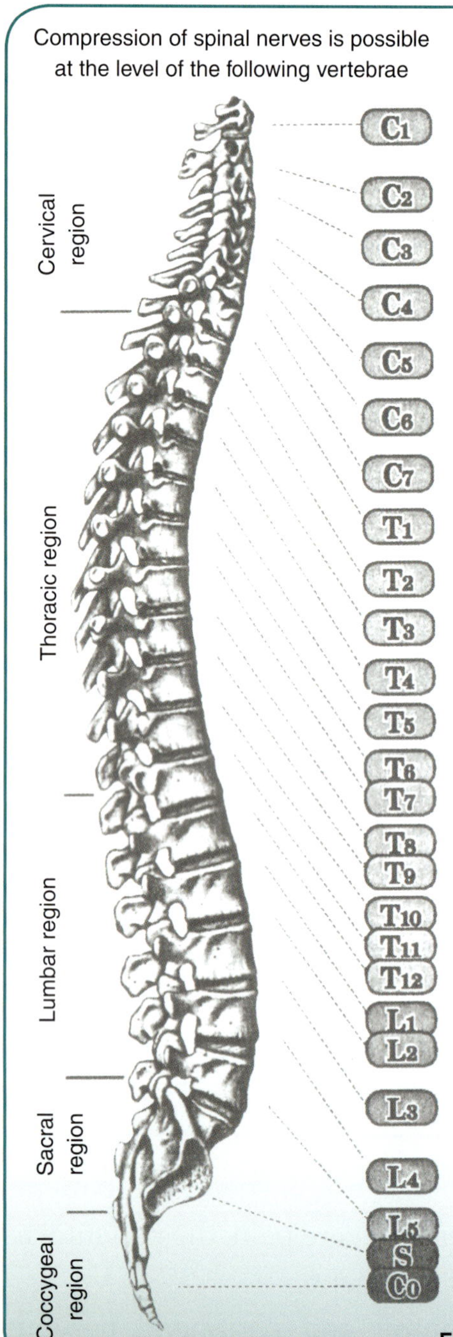

Consequences of spinal nerve compression

C_1, C_2 – psychosis, neurasthenia, hysteria, headache, dizziness, insomnia, cerebral haemorrhage, hydrocephalus, trismus, hemiplegia, amnesia, epilepsy, sweating of the head, torticollis, paranasal sinusitis, hormonal disorders, strabismus

C_3 – amaurosis, hyposmia, deafness, blindness, conjunctivitis, trismus, diseases of the eye, nose, ears

C_4, C_5 – neurasthenia, hysteria, hypochondria, loss of taste, trigeminal neuralgia, adenoiditis, cerebral haemorrhage, amblyopia, headache, trismus, tonsillitis, vomiting, nose and ear diseases

C_6 – eye diseases, diseases of the oral cavity, throat, laryngitis, tonsillitis, angina, loss of taste

C_7 – shortness of breath, asthma, chronic bronchitis, shoulder-scapular periarthritis, parotitis, diseases of the thyroid gland

T_1 – shortness of breath, cough, asthma, broncho-pulmonary haemorrhage, graphospasm, allergies

T_2 – myocarditis, endocarditis, pericarditis, cardiomegaly, oligogalactia, bronchitis, arteriosclerosis

T_3 – pleuritis, pneumonia, pulmonary oedema, bronchospasm, emphysema, pulmonary tuberculosis

T_4, T_5 – acholia, hepatomegaly, jaundice, hepatitis, liver cirrhosis, heart disease, neurasthenia, hysteria, hypochondria, fever, gout

T_6, T_7 – gastric cancer, indigestion (dyspepsia), gastrectasis, pyloric stenosis, gastric and/or duodenal ulcers, gastroptosis, anorexia, intercostal neuralgia

T_8, T_9 – liver disease, pancreatolithiasis, splenomegaly, diaphragmatic hernia, nausea

T_{10}, T_{11}, T_{12} – kidney disease, aciduria, haematuria, diabetes insipidus, dyspepsia, diarrhoea, cholelithiasis, a tendency towards constipation

L_1, L_2 – hepatomegaly, prostatomegaly, chronic constipation, diarrhoea, colitis, intestinal tuberculosis, cancer of abdominal organs

L_3, L_4 – menstrual disorders, oophoritis, cystoma, uterine cancer, retro- and anteflexed uterus, urethritis, infertility, testicular disease, haemorrhoids, inguinal hernia, cystitis, cystolithiasis, anal fistula, prostatomegaly, enuresis, abasia, sciatica

L_5, $S_{1–2}$ – sciatica, paraplegia, rheumatism, diseases of the bladder, lower limb joint disease, gout, abasia, coccyalgia

Fig. 5.4. Spine—the support of life

patients, according to sex, age and the side of relative shortening of the lower extremity (Tables 5.1–5.3). The data presented in the tables show that among patients with spinal deformities and pain, the largest group (32.88%) consisted of people in the prime of their lives (28–50 years). Sixty per cent of the patients were females and 40% males. Relative shortening of the lower limb was observed predominantly on the left side (89.3%), the corresponding percentage for the right side being only 10.7%.

Our patients included not only citizens of Ukraine, Belarus and Russia, but also people from Asia, Africa, Latin America, the USA, Canada, India and Australia.

Despite the differences in nationality and race, all of them shared identical spinal deformities, as well as similar clinical manifestations of spinal pain. Our interactions with these patients revealed that most of them had certain common standard complaints.

Children were usually brought for consultation by their parents. The parents reported growing deformation of the spine, frequent headaches, dizziness, partial or complete loss of the field of vision, and even loss of consciousness when turning the head sharply. Reduced visual acuity and/or loss of hearing, different speech disorders, ptosis (incomplete raising of the eyelids), torticollis, strabismus and facial asymmetry of a greater or lesser extent were among the other complaints.

The conditions usually affecting children and adults, to varying degrees of severity, were as follows:

- Numbness and/or spasm of the fingers or entire hand, especially at night when sleeping with the hands raised
- Sweaty hands, coldness of the skin, usually accompanied by emotional lability and features of vascular dystonia
- Frequent diseases of the lungs, bronchial asthma, sudden breath delay
- Allergies
- Heart pain
- Heartburn, eructations, gastric or duodenal ulcer, gastritis (both in adults and children of different ages, including pre-school age)
- Diseases of the gallbladder, such as dyskinesia and cholelithiasis
- Diseases of the pancreas, including diabetes
- Pain in the region of the kidney, nephroptosis
- Pain in the region of the ovaries and/or uterus, cramping pain in the lower abdomen (with various manifestations)

Table 5.1 Characteristics of patients by age

Age	No. of patients	Ratio
<1 year	83	1.02
1–3	175	2.15
4–6	410	5.03
7–10	615	7.55
11–13	536	6.58
14–16	586	7.20
17–19	382	4.69
20–23	479	5.9
24–27	495	6.08
28–30	465	5.7
31–40	1159	14.2
41–50	1054	12.94
51–63	928	11.40
64–70	470	5.77
71–74	118	1.45
75–79	104	1.27
80–90	85	1.04
Total no. of patients	**8144**	**100%**

Table 5.2 Characteristics of patients by gender

Gender	Total no. of patients	Ratio
Male	3258	40%
Female	4886	60%
Total	8144	100%

Table 5.3 Characteristics of patients by the side of limb shortening

Side of shortening	Total no. of patients	Ratio
Left	7273	89.3%
Right	871	10.7%
Total	8144	100%

- Painful or irregular periods. Tendency to constipation or frequent urge to defaecate
- Nocturnal urinary incontinence (mostly among children)
- Weakening of male potency
- Male and female infertility
- Localized pain in the lumbosacral spine, possibly radiating to one leg or sometimes both legs
- Cramps in the calf muscles and toes
- Sensitivity disorders of the skin, mainly on the outer surface of the foot
- Sweaty feet, coldness of the skin
- Varicose veins in the lower extremities, more pronounced on one side.

The severity and pattern of these symptoms depended on the duration of the disease, the patient's age and the location of the rotational displacement of the vertebrae (cervical, thoracic, lumbar and sacral segments). In the case of children, the complaints were mostly localized to a single area. The spinal curvature increased with age.

The older the patient became, the more the spinal curvature increased with formation of various deformities of the spine and increased severity of pain in all its regions. There was also an increase in dysfunction of the various organs and systems with age.

In our opinion, the pathogenesis of a variety of human diseases is based on or related to compression of the cranial and spinal nerves, spinal cord, ganglia, and sympathetic and parasympathetic nerves. The compression results in impairment of their conducting and organ-controlling function. This causes pain, as well as symptoms of various diseases of the heart, lungs, liver, gallbladder and other organs, even in the absence of pathological changes in these organs. Studies using special instruments and laboratory tests have confirmed this. Prolonged dysfunction of various parts of the neuroregulatory system and of the organs which are under the control of these gradually leads to persistent changes in the anatomical structure of the tissues and the development of true disease.

Thus, rotational displacement of the vertebrae, which starts in early childhood, forms the pathological foundation for the development of a variety of diseases in the later years of life. Children form a reserve army of adult patients. This regularity of *'the development of diseases in adults depending on the deformities of spine they have as children'* has been recognized as a scientific discovery by the Ukrainian Academy of Original Ideas (UAOI), which awarded a diploma to the author Professor Valentyn Serdyuk in 1995.

To help the reader gain a better understanding of our clinical material and analysis, we decided to categorize our observations into three main groups, according to the predominant location of the problem—cervical, thoracic and lumbosacral.

5.1 Cervical spine

Although for a number of years we attempted to deal with patients complaining of headache, blurred vision, stiffness of the neck, discomfort, dizziness and even loss of consciousness, it was after our meeting with the eminent paediatric ophthalmologist and physician, Komashko Alexandra, that we gained an insight into the matter. Knowing about our fascination with the problem of spinal pathology, she asked us to look into the causes of strabismus, one of the most common diseases afflicting children and adults. This condition is characterized by the deviation of one eye from a joint point of fixation (and inability of both eyes to focus on the same point in space). Due to various reasons, ophthalmologists consider strabismus a serious problem: it leads to decreased acuteness and depth perception of vision, mars the person's appearance and is thus a cause of mental suffering. It also limits the occupational eligibility of the patient, and the existing treatments, especially those for children, are not very effective (I.I. Merkulov, 1962; E.M. Belostotsky, 1964; M.M. Zolotareva, 1964; S.F. Zubarev, 1988; M. Schapero, 1971; V.J. Revell, 1971).

A study of the available literature did not provide us with a direct answer to the causes of strabismus. However, our research did throw some light on the disease and played a part in helping us arrive at certain conclusions.

Despite the existence of many theories on the aetiology and pathogenesis of strabismus (muscular, accommodative, fusional, functional, conditioned-reflexive, infectious, neurogenic, hereditary), there were no clear answers regarding its origin.

The main type of strabismus is the concomitant form, which is manifested by the obvious deviation of one eye or both eyes, i.e. alternation from the symmetrical position relative to one another. Normal vision with both eyes is possible only if all the constituent elements of the sensory apparatus (visual acuity, or the ability of the brain to fuse the images formed on the two retinas, and coordinated functioning of the eye muscles) function coherently. If any of them becomes disrupted, the visual lines of one or both eyes, alternately, continuously or periodically, deviate from the correct position, causing disturbance of binocular vision and strabismus.

It is known that normal binocular vision is of a conditioned reflexive nature and develops gradually. The period of the maximum development of binocular vision and depth perception among children is between 7 and 15 years of age. The cortical analyser of horizontal eye movements is located on the base of the second frontal gyrus and that of vertical movements, on the base of the third frontal gyrus. These areas control spontaneous eye movements and the cortical reflex regulated by the analyser is located on the outer surface of the occipital lobe.

E.M. Belostotsky (1964), one of the supporters of the conditioned reflexive theory of strabismus, believed that impairment of the dynamic stereotype of binocular vision leads to the deviation of one of the eyes from the common point of fixation. Such deviation occurs most frequently in early childhood, when conditioned reflexive associations are not yet consolidated. The author believes that the external and internal factors that hinder the consolidation of normal reflexive associations are the direct causes of concomitant strabismus. This has been confirmed by electroencephalographic findings, which have shown the existence of disrupted cortical connections of binocular vision in patients with strabismus.

The goal of treatment for concomitant strabismus is to restore binocular vision. Usually, the therapy starts with the prescription of corrective glasses for permanent wear. In a significant number of cases (36.7%, according to A.V. Chvatova; cited by M.M. Zolotariova, *Eye Diseases,* Minsk, 1963, 253 p.), the angle of deviation may disappear after a period of wearing glasses (up to two years). If this line of treatment is not effective, one may initiate orthoptic treatment, which consists of performing special training exercises to improve various functions of the eye, including mobility, using special instruments. If wearing of the right glasses for 1.5–2 years fails to restore the symmetrical eye position, then surgery is indicated. Surgeries may be weakening (partial tenotomy with simultaneous amplification of the antagonist) or amplifying (shortening of muscle and suturing it to the anatomical site of attachment). The treatment for children of 6–10 years of age is generally limited to a single surgery. Often, it needs to involve both the horizontal and vertical muscles. The treatment for paralytic strabismus is similar.

However, the existing conservative and surgical methods of treatment for strabismus are known for their low efficacy and frequent relapses. This explains the ongoing search for new, more optimal solutions. Our goal is not to underestimate the value of these treatments, but to gain a thorough understanding of the mechanism of the development of strabismus in children and develop a non-invasive treatment method on the basis of our understanding of the aetiopathogenesis of the disease.

In our daily work, we had to provide outpatient care to patients of different ages and with pain localized in different regions. We noticed that the vast majority of children and adults who complained of headache and dizziness also had varying degrees of some other visual impairment (myopia, hyperopia, astigmatism, amblyopia, convergent or divergent strabismus, etc.). While examining patients, we observed that rotary subluxation of the 2nd cervical vertebra (C_2) relative to the 1st (C_1) was always accompanied by one of the wide variety of manifestations of strabismus. Detorsional correction of the subluxation not only eliminated the headaches and dizziness, but also led to normalization of the eyes' position. Such rotary subluxation of the cervical spine occurred mainly in paediatric patients with scoliotic deformity. In these patients, rotation of the vertebrae around their axes in accordance with the laws of biomechanics occurred not only in the cervical, but also in the thoracic and lumbosacral spine. This process occurred in specific parts of the curvature and anticurvature—the beginning of the arc, the site of maximal curvature and the base of the arc (*see* Chapter 3, Section 3.3).

In the majority of cases, scoliosis is a hereditary disease. This fits well with the position of ophthalmologists, who believe that strabismus is a hereditary condition. *Thus, it may be said that every child with scoliosis has a predisposition to hereditary strabismus if he has disorders of refraction*. If the scoliosis is not significant, the refractive anomalies are not accompanied by strabismus and the child has stable binocular vision.

In order to clarify the causal relationship between rotary subluxation of the cervical vertebrae and strabismus, we conducted some special anatomical research. A study of textbooks, atlases, as well as gross anatomical specimens, carried out under the guidance of Professor Romanenko Vladimir Nikolaevich of the department of normal anatomy of Odessa National Medical University, helped us to establish the following.

Binocular vision is based on normal convergence of the eyes, i.e. on the convergence of the visual axes of both eyes on a given object. This is accompanied by a combined reflexive contraction of the striated muscles of the eyeball (rectus medial and lateral as well as superior and inferior, superior and inferior oblique, levator palpebrae superioris). The muscles are innervated by three nerves: oculomotor (n. oculomotorius), or the third pair of cranial nerves (CN); trochlear (n. trochlearis), or the fourth pair of CN; and abducent (n. abducens), or the sixth pair of CN (Figs 5.1.1–5.1.3).

The lateral rectus muscle (m. rectus lateralis) is innervated by the n. abducens. Its motor nucleus is located in the pons Varolii, which is supplied by the a. basilaris. This artery is formed by the confluence of two vertebral arteries (a. vertebralis) (Scheme 5.1.1 and Fig. 5.1.4). The motor nuclei of the n. trochlearis and n. oculomotorius are located in the cerebral peduncles, which are also supplied by the a. basilaris (Scheme 5.1.2). In our view, rotational displacement of the cervical vertebrae, especially C_1–C_2–C_3 (zone of the medulla oblongata) (Figs 5.1.5, 5.1.6) causes compression of this structure, which leads to the impairment of the functioning of the nuclei of the CN, pituitary and pineal glands, olives, reticular formation, and centres of respiration and circulation. Moreover, it causes damage to the pathways located in the medulla oblongata. It is

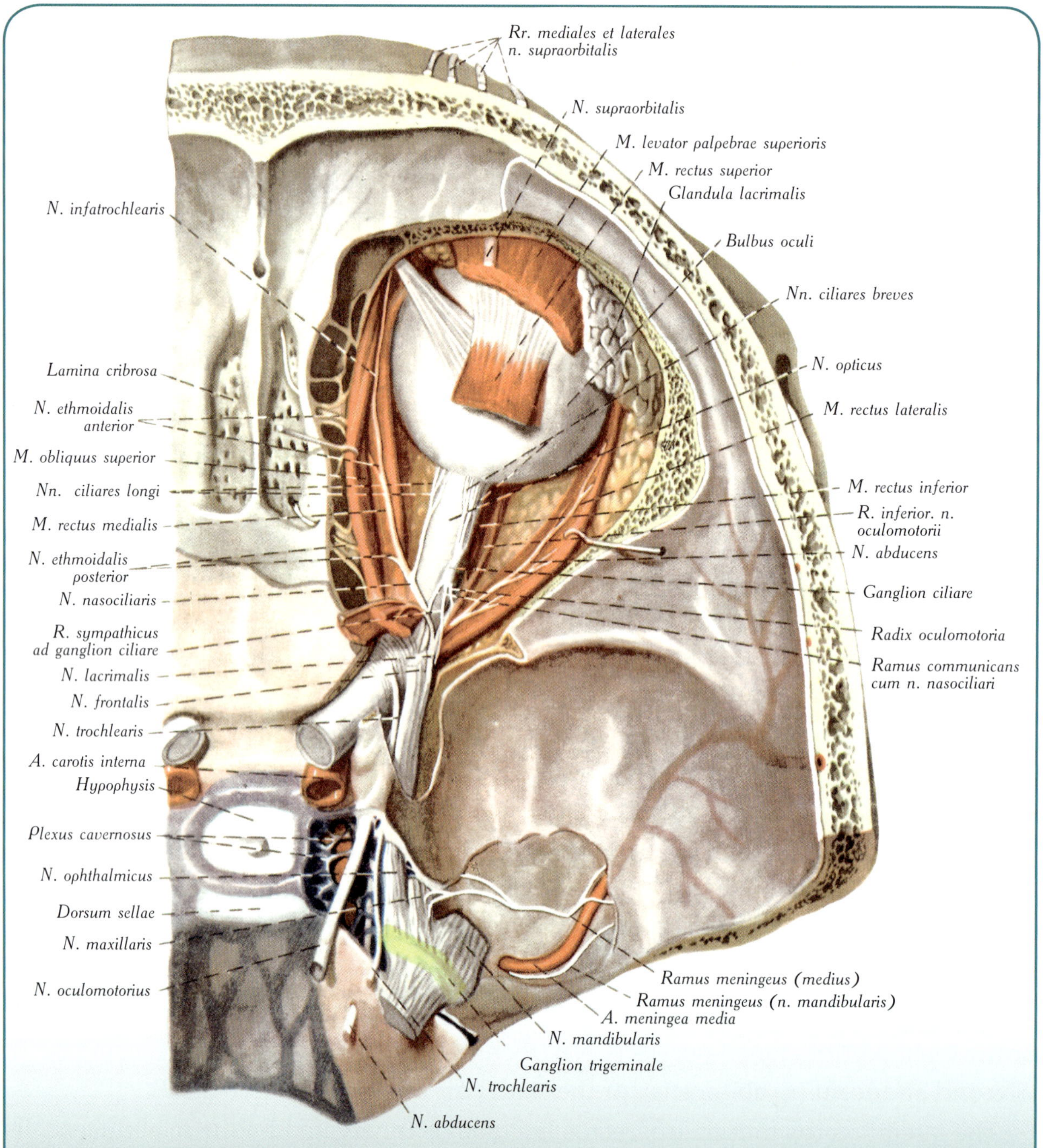

Fig. 5.1.1.
Nerves of the right orbit

not necessary to bore the reader with a detailed description of the functions of the medulla, as such descriptions are available in several textbooks on normal anatomy. Suffice it to say that the medulla oblongata is responsible for everything that occurs in our body. (Andreas Vesaly [1514–1564], the greatest anatomist of the Middle Ages in his fundamental treatise in 7 volumes entitled *About the Structure of Human Body*, pointed out the vital importance of medulla oblongata and said that in this anatomical structure resides the soul.)

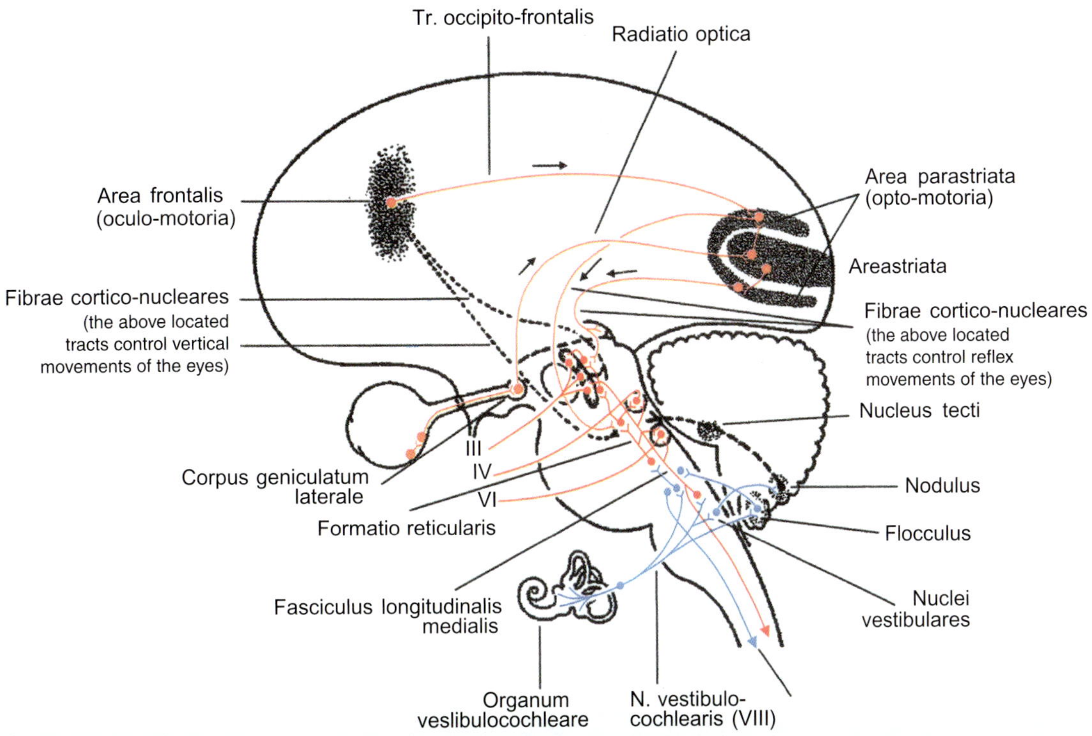

Fig. 5.1.2.

Topographic diagram of the centres and pathways of the opticovestibular system of a human (according to R. Jung [1953], modified)

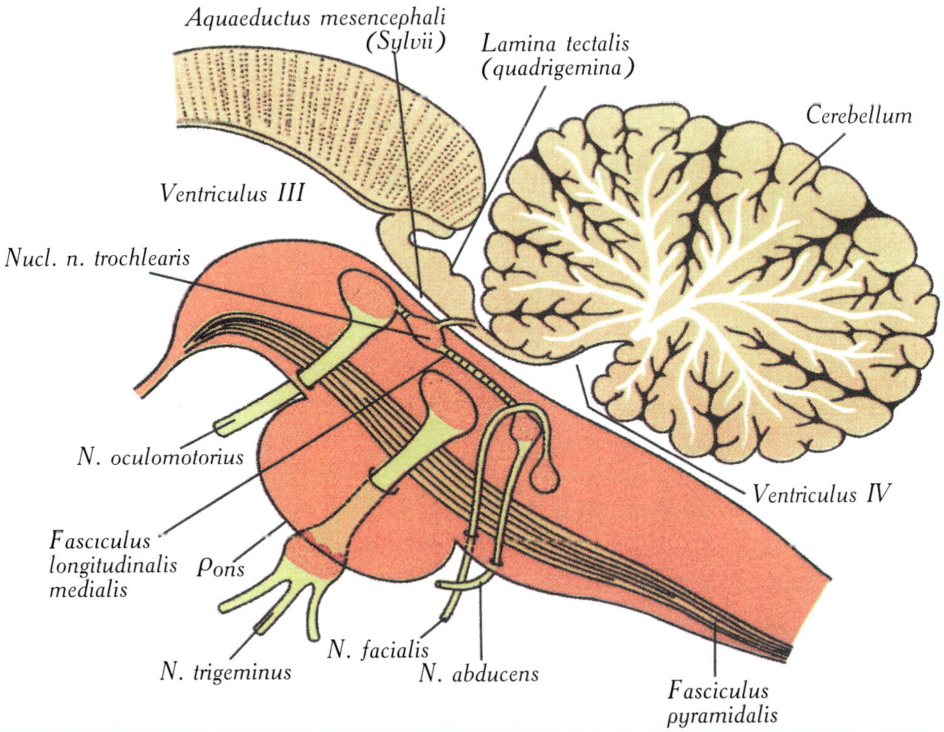

Fig. 5.1.3.

The scheme of location of the nuclei of cranial nerves in the brainstem, which provide motor and sensory innervation of the organ of vision

Scheme 5.1.1.

Blood supply and innervation of the anatomical structures of the eye

Lateral rectus muscle (M. rectus lateralis)

Innervated by abducens nerve (N. abducens)

Motor nucleus of this nerve in located in the pons

Pons and the motor nucleus of

abducent nerve are supplied from the basal artery (A. basilaris)

The basal artery is formed by the confluence of two
(right and left) vertebral arteries (A.a. vertebrales)

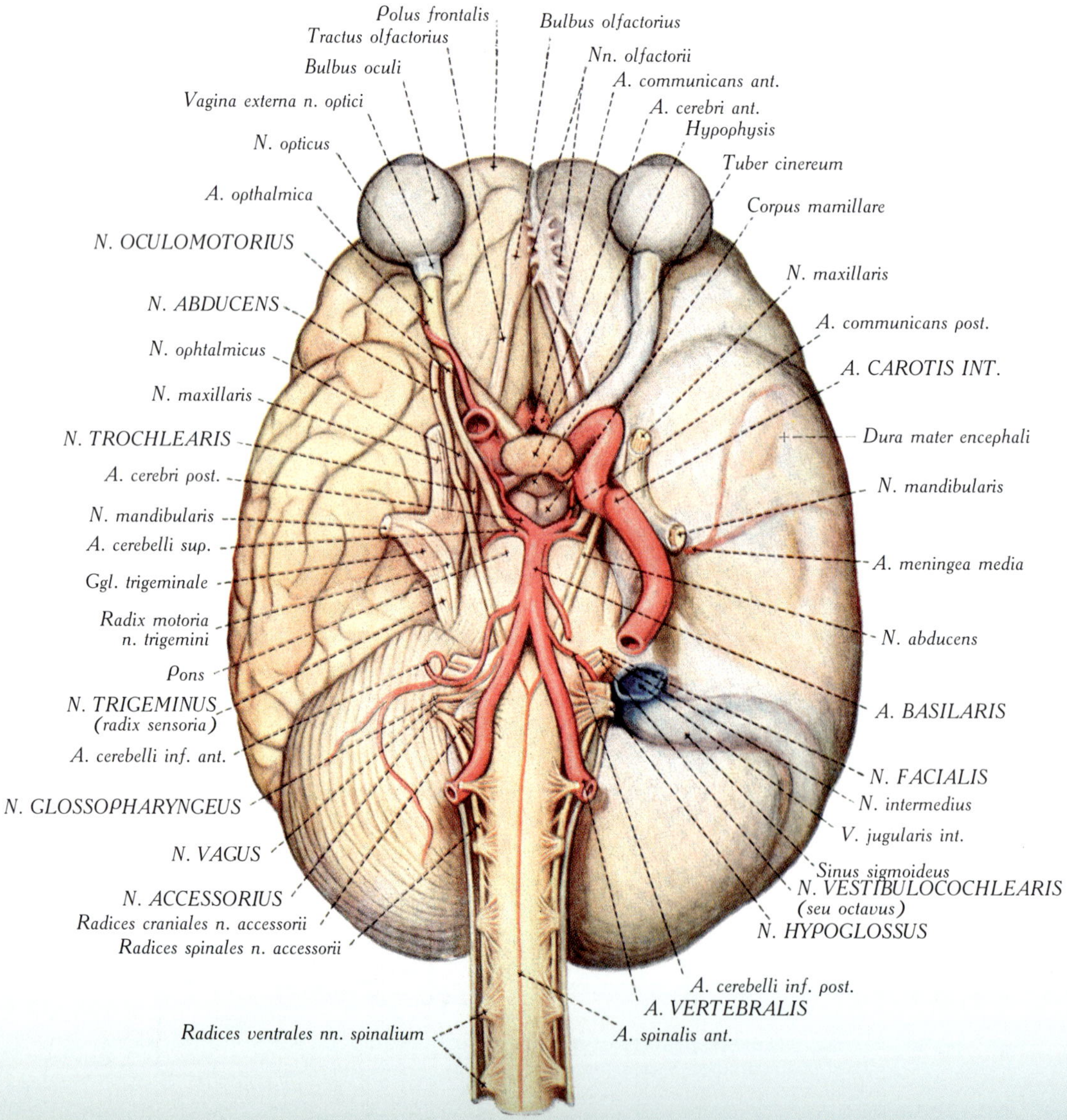

Fig. 5.1.4.
Arteries of the base of the brain and cranial nerves

Scheme 5.1.2.

Blood supply and innervation of the anatomical structures of the eye

Medial rectus muscle (M. rectus medialis), superior and inferior rectus muscles (M. rectus superior et inferior), superior and inferior oblique muscles (M. obliquis superior et inferior), elevating muscle of the upper eyelid (M. Levator palpebrae superioris)

These anatomical structures are innervated by the oculomotor nerve (N. oculomotorius) and trochlear nerve (N. trochlearis)

Motor nuclei of these nerves are located in the brainstem (pedunculi cerebri)

Pedicles of the brain are supplied by the basal artery (A. basilaris)

The basal artery is formed by the confluence of two (right and left) vertebral arteries (A.a. vertebrales)

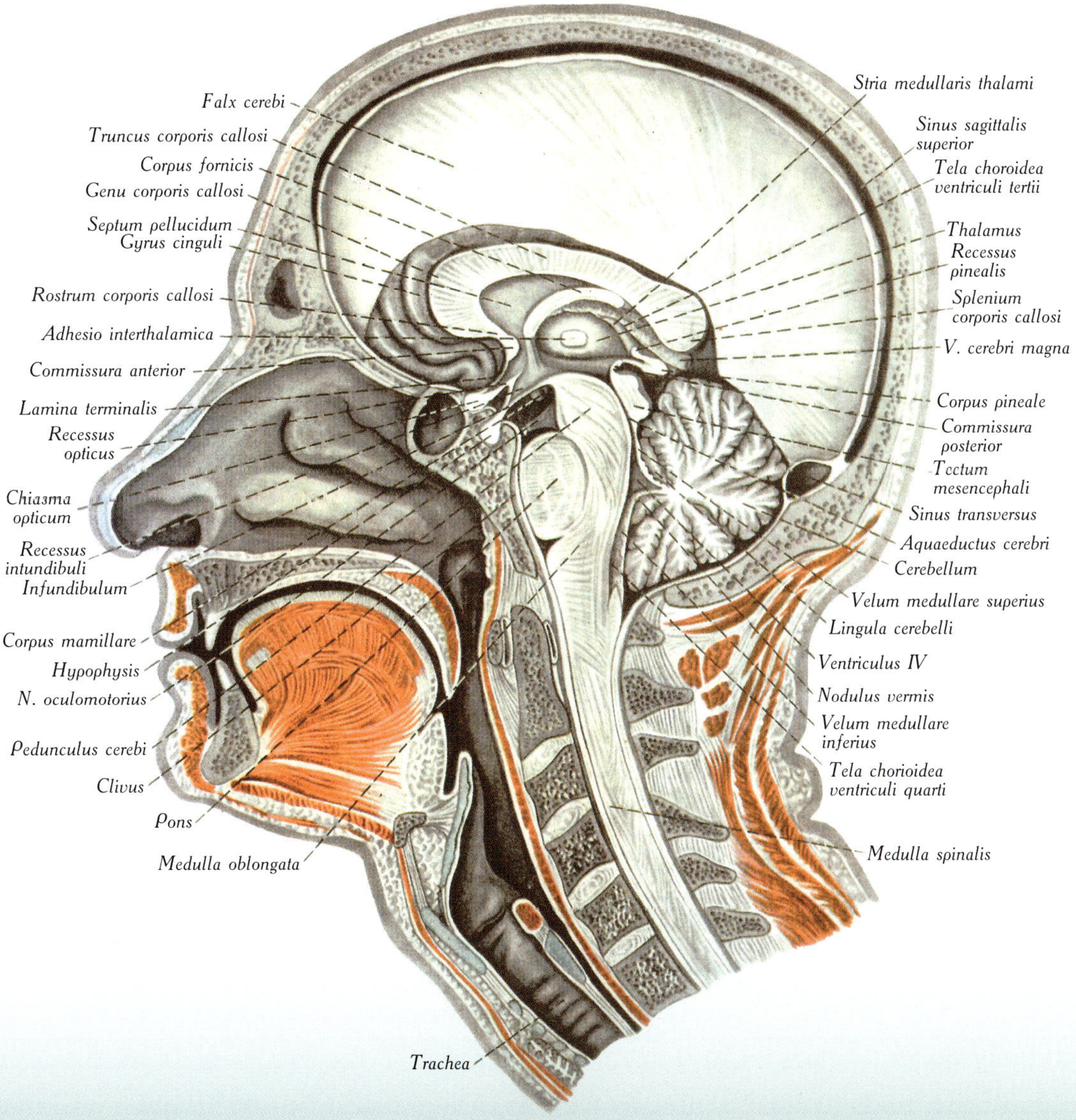

Fig. 5.1.5.
Interrelationship between the location of the thalamus, pons, medulla oblongata and upper cervical vertebrae

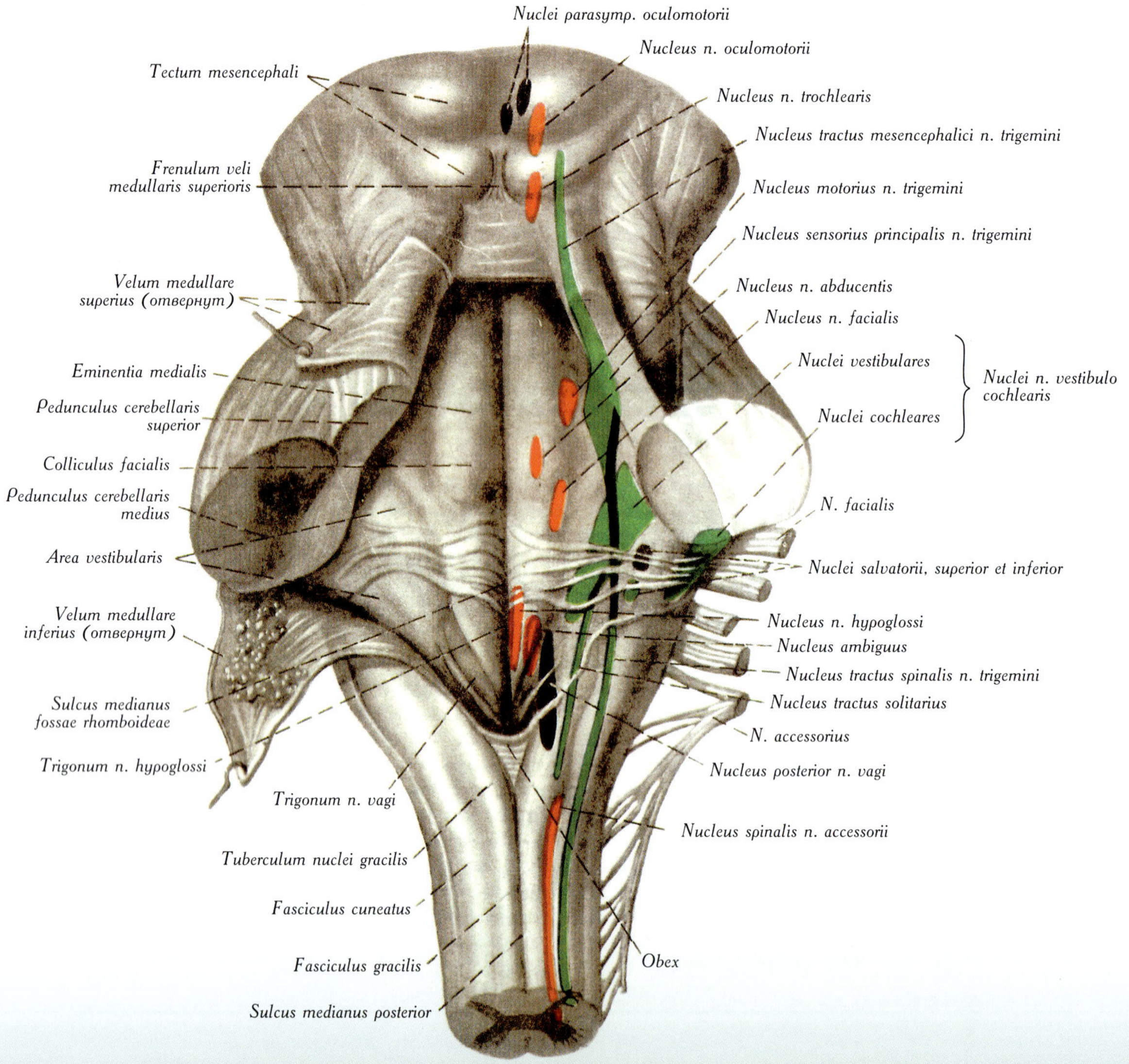

Fig. 5.1.6.
Nuclei of cranial nerves (nuclei nervorum cerebralium) located in the midbrain and rhombencephalon (semi-schematic) — projection of the nuclei, rear view

Rotational displacement of the cervical vertebrae also leads to the compression of the anatomical structures located in the transverse foramina (vertebral arteries, sympathetic fibres of the n. spinalis, which surround them and vertebral veins) (Fig. 5.1.7). This results in a decrease in the blood supply not only to the medulla oblongata, but also to the cerebellum and occipital region of the brain, where the visual centre is located. Such ischaemia, when prolonged (often having lasted the entire course of the patient's life prior to consultation), causes predominantly unilateral hypoplasia of the occipital region and leads to unilateral impairment of the reflex of binocular vision. This eventually leads to strabismus, as well as other conditions, which we will discuss further.

In the case of congenital strabismus, subluxation of C_1–C_2 probably occurs *in utero.*

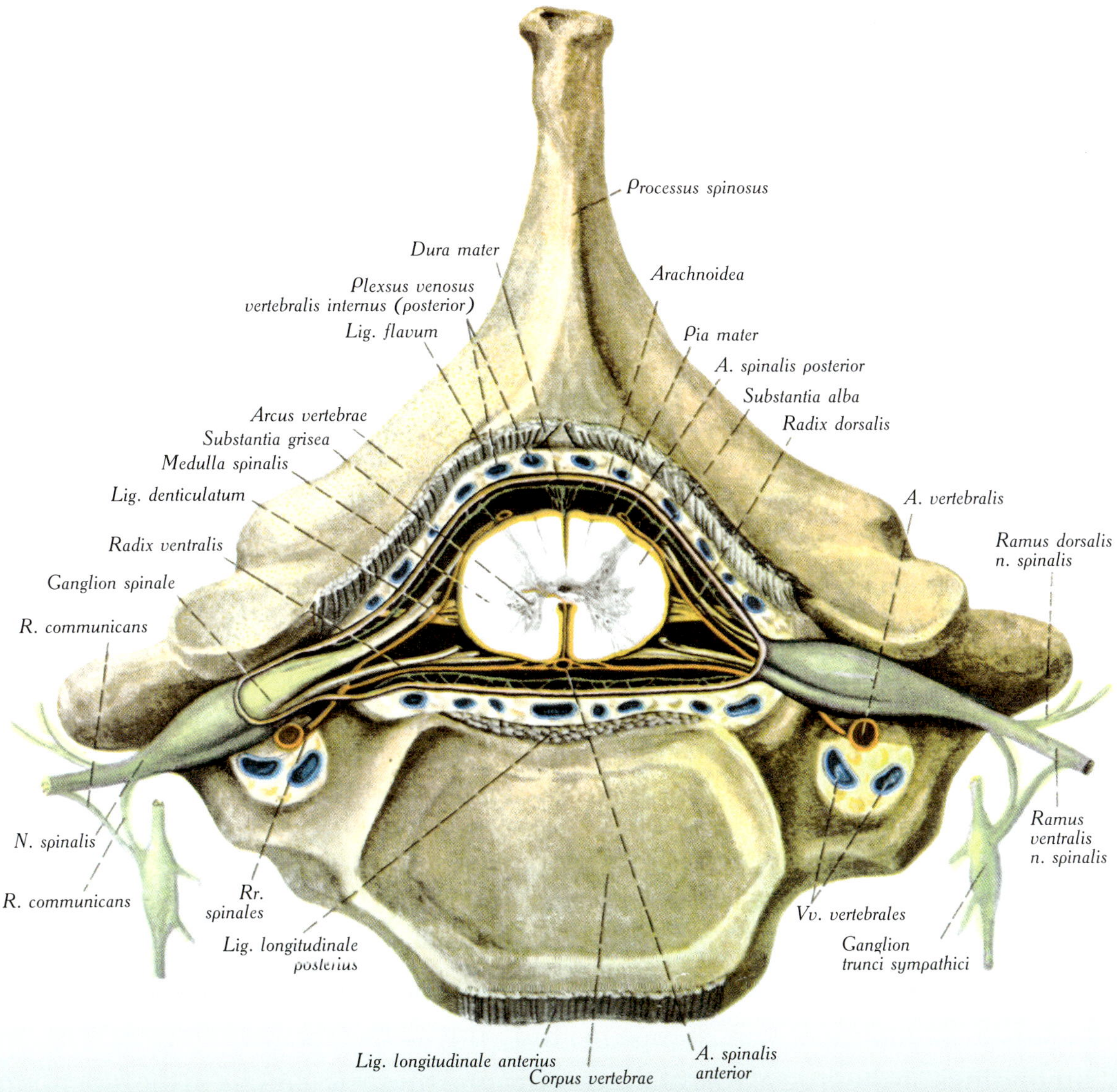

Fig. 5.1.7.
Location of the vertebral arteries, veins and sympathetic fibres of the spinal nerve in transverse holes of the cervical vertebrae

The causes may be oligohydramnios and polyhydramnios, in which the umbilical cord twists around the head and neck of the foetus, creating preconditions for the occurrence of subluxation both at particular and other levels. Injuries of the upper cervical spine occur often during childbirth, when the head of the foetus is pulled out, during extraction of the foetus using forceps or during vacuum extraction.

The results of ultrasound dopplerography, echoencephalography and rheoencephalography of the brain vessels in children and adults with strabismus indicate disorders of circulation in the brainstem (medulla oblongata, pons and cerebral peduncles), caused by extravasal compression of the vertebral arteries in the backdrop of instability of the cervical spine. These cerebral circulatory disorders are manifested as vasospasm and an increased intracranial pressure due to obstructed venous outflow.

We are of the opinion that there is another parallel mechanism in the pathogenesis of strabismus. This mechanism is neurogenic (Fig. 5.1.8, Scheme 5.1.3), and its essence is follows.

The right and left upper cervical ganglia (ganglion cervicale superior dexter et sinister) are located at the level of the 1st (C_1), 2nd (C_2) and 3rd (C_3) cervical vertebrae. The post-ganglionic sympathetic fibres contained in these ganglia form the periarterial plexus of the left and right a. carotis interna and spread over its branches, including a. ophtalmica. The periarterial sympathetic fibres run to the plexus ophthalmicus (plexus ocular). This anatomical structure controls the skeletal muscles of the eyes in particular. Compression by the upper cervical vertebrae (C_1–C_3) of the upper cervical ganglion on one or both sides causes disorders of the nerves of the eye muscle which, in turn, disturbs their normal functioning.

The details of eye innervation, blood supply to the brainstem, motor nuclei and ophthalmic nerves have been described in several recently published textbooks of anatomy (M.P. Sapin, G.L. Bilich, *Human Anatomy* in two volumes, Moscow, 2000, 463 p. and 432 p.; E.E. Somov, *Clinical Anatomy of the Human Organ of Vision*, Moscow, 2005, 136 p.).

Our findings have shown that the upper, middle and lower cervical ganglia, as well as the spinal ganglia located at the level of the 1st–4th thoracic vertebrae, play a significant role in the aetiopathogenesis of strabismus. Considering that our review of the literature available on anatomy yielded no such information, anatomists and other professionals might find it worthwhile to study the matter further.

Our findings on the crucial role of the cervical and thoracic ganglia in the functioning of the eye muscles and, consequently, the presence or absence of strabismus were repeatedly validated by our experience with our patients. Since the elimination of the rotational displacement of C_1–C_3 in projection of the medulla and upper cervical ganglions did not always succeed in correcting the position of the eyes, we later corrected the position not only of all the cervical, but additionally upper thoracic vertebrae. In most cases, we were able to achieve positive results.

Our collaboration with Professor V.N. Romanenko and physician A.N. Komashko resulted in the publication of *Method of Treatment of Strabismus* for which the Ukraine Government awarded a patent (No. 48900) from 15 August 2002 (*see* Chapter 6 for a detailed description). Sustained collaboration with ophthalmologist Dr A.N. Komashko and certain anatomists allowed us to establish other facts.

Virtually all patients suffering from strabismus had associated pain in the eyeballs. They also suffered from acute pain in the exit zones of nn. infratrochlearis,

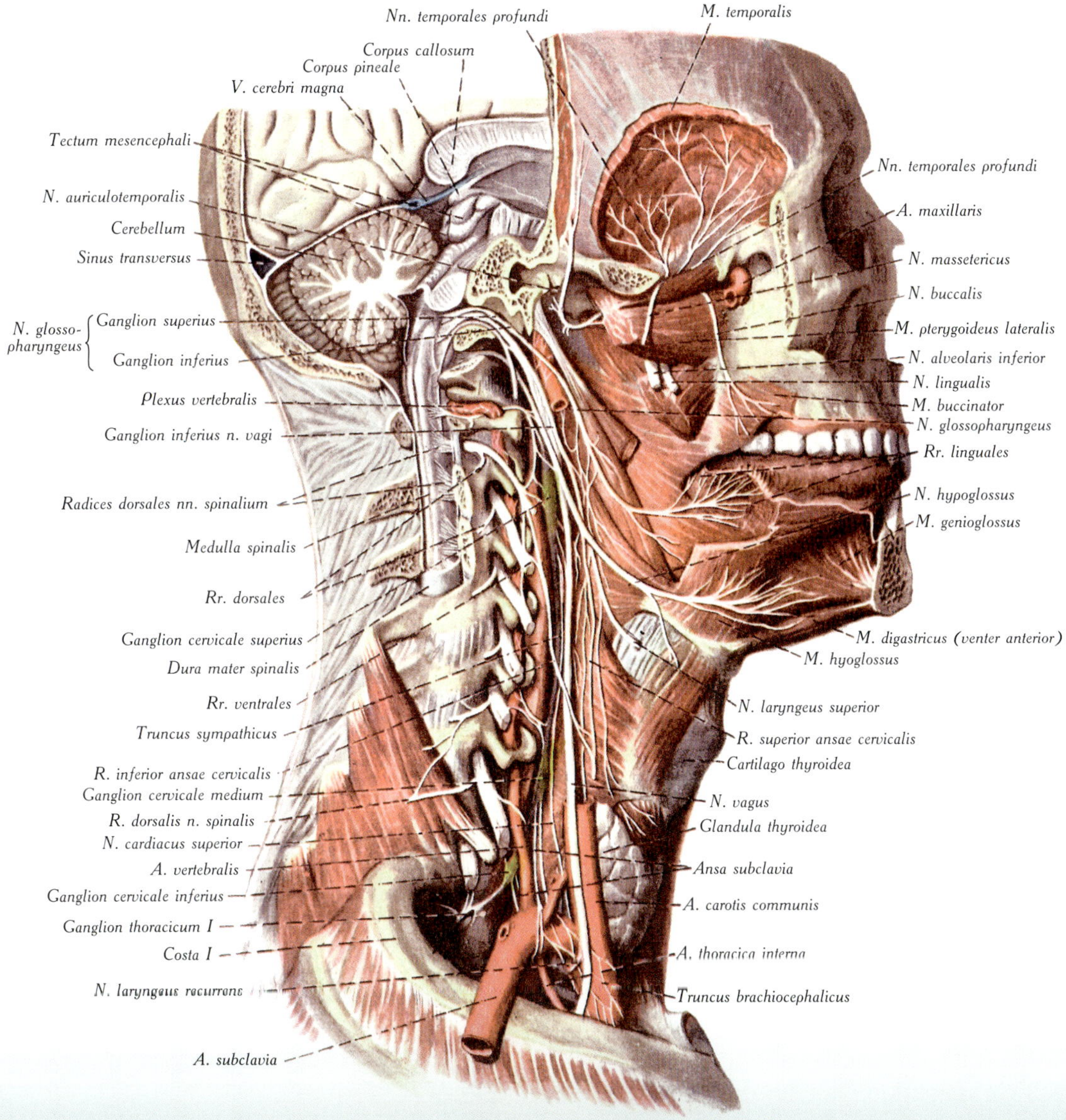

Fig. 5.1.8.
Nerves of the head and neck

Scheme 5.1.3.

Blood supply and innervation of the anatomical structures of the eye

At the level of the first, second and third cervical vertebrae, the right and left upper cervical ganglions (Ganglion cervicale superior dexter et sinister) are located

Sympathetic postganglionic fibres form a periarterial plexus of the right and left internal carotid arteries (A. carotis interna)

These sympathetic fibres form the n. carotis internus and then the nerve plexus of internal carotid artery (Plexus carotis internus)

Sympathetic fibres are involved in formation of the ocular plexus (Plexus ophthalmicus)

The ocular plexus provides the nerve supply to skeletal muscles of the eye supratrochlearis and supraorbitalis, that is, in the orbital, maxillary and mandibular regions. The pain caused by compression of the branches of the trigeminal nerve (n. trigeminus)—nn. maxillaris, mandibularis and ophthalmicus—was so intense that patients were forced to seek help, take strong analgesics and even undergo radiotherapy. The latter essentially entails denervation of the sensory nerve endings with the help of X-rays.

In our view, the cause of inflammation of the trigeminal nerve (trigeminitis) is the compression of this nerve in the zone of the trigeminal ganglion (Fig. 5.1.9), and of its nuclei at the level of the pons near the 1st and 2nd cervical vertebrae (C_1–C_2). We believe that in scoliotic deformity of the cervical spine, the rotation of these vertebrae leads to compression of the pyramidal part of the medulla. Thus, to put an end to compression of the trigeminal ganglion, its nuclei at the level of the pons and the medulla, it is necessary to eliminate rotation of the cervical vertebrae and scoliotic spinal deformity, which is the main reason for the rotation. Detorsional correction, combined with a

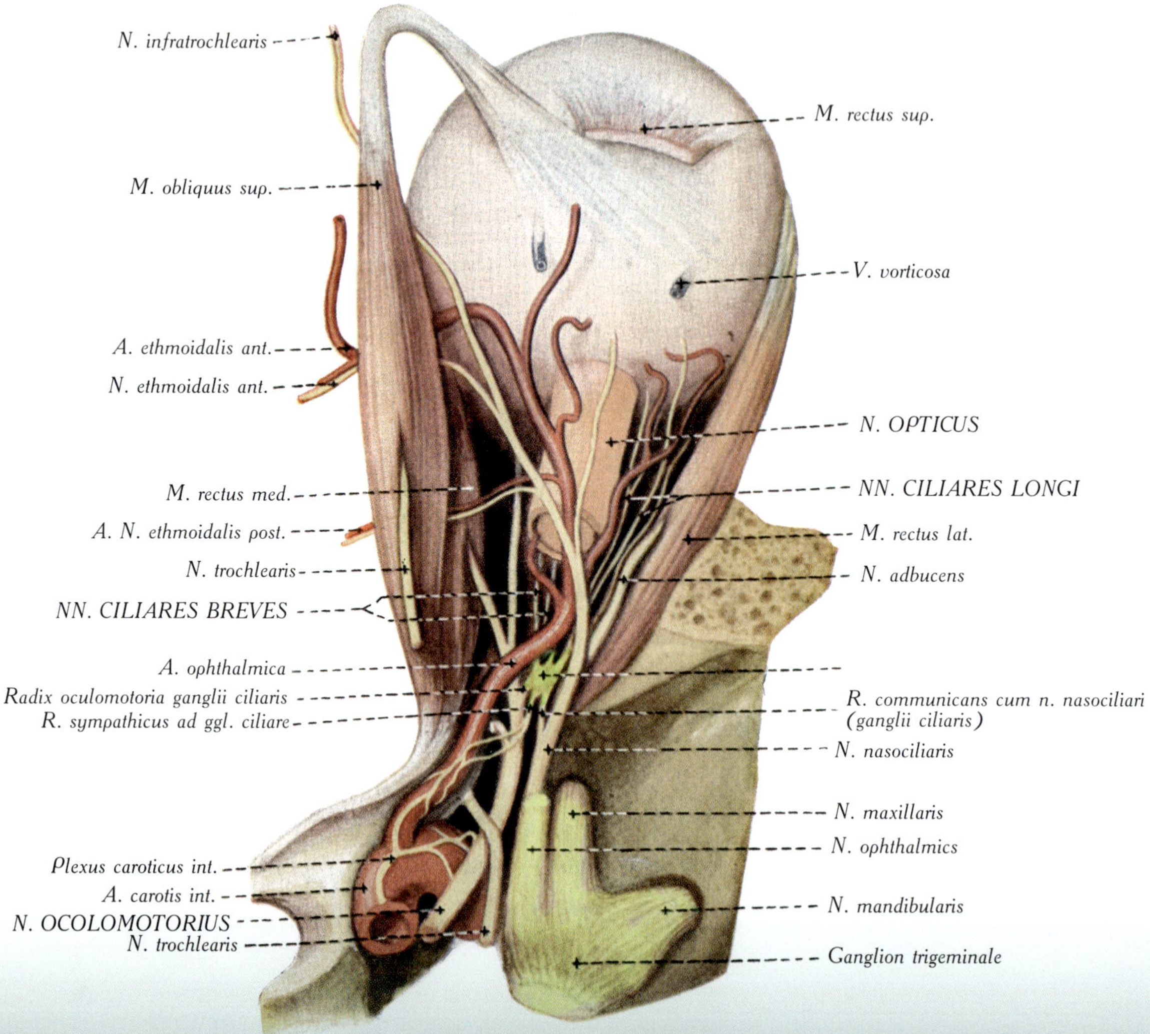

Fig. 5.1.9. Anatomy of the orbit

specially designed scheme of physical therapy, the use of an orthopaedic insole under the heel of the shortened leg, as well as the application of magneto-acoustic therapy on the cervico-collar zone and on the exit sites of nerves have proved to be of high therapeutic efficacy, as shown by our clinical experience. This 'Treatment method of inflammation of the trigeminal nerve (trigeminitis)' was recognized as an invention by the Ukrainian Academy of Original Ideas (024HX) on 28 March 2005 and we were awarded a 'know-how' certificate for the invention. A detailed description of the treatment is given in Chapter 6.

In addition to patients with convergent or divergent strabismus and those with trigeminitis, we also examined patients, mostly children, suffering from other eye diseases.

These included:

- Progressive myopia and hyperopia
- Amblyopia (functional dysfunction of the visual analyser)
- Different types of astigmatism (refractive anomalies, in which there is no convergence on the retina of the focal image)
- Glaucoma
- Accommodation spasm (impairment of visual perception of objects at different distances)
- Functional scotoma (alteration of image perception, related to the central zone of the retina of one eye)
- Heterophoria (latent strabismus)
- Accommodation spasm, etc.

In 1994, the ophthalmologist Dr M.A. Kuznetsova (cited by G.A. Ivanichev, *Manual Therapy*, Moscow, 1996, 470 p.) reported that functional blockade of the craniovertebral junction, which corresponds to the level of C_1–C_2, is of great importance in the origin of myopia in children. According to the author, manual therapy improved accommodation in 97.7% of children, normalized this function in 87% and stabilized myopia in 80.4% of cases. Moreover, the positive effect was maintained over the next 3–5 years. It should be noted that this treatment had no such outstanding effect among adults. Although many patients reported an improvement in vision ('eyes brightened', 'became brighter'), there was no objective evidence of an improvement in vision. The positive effect, according to the author, was associated with improved haemodynamics in the vertebrobasilar circulation.

It was heartening that Dr M.A. Kuznetsova's conclusions coincided completely with our own findings, which were that local muscular hypertonus and functional blockades of the cervical SMS play a leading role in the development of various eye diseases. We also found that the older the patient, the less effective the treatment and the more time required for treatment. In our opinion, this fact has an explanation. Positioning of the head in a spastic torticollis for a prolonged period has a significant effect on the condition of the cervical SMS, causing persistent blockades and hypertonus of the rotators. Moreover, as we already know, if the SMS is in an unstable state for a prolonged period, the result is compensatory degenerative disc disease and spondylosis, which restrict the mobility of the cervical vertebrae. Thus, a vicious circle is formed: torticollis—persistent blockade of the SMS—spondylosis deformans and osteochondrosis—more pronounced torticollis, etc.

The largest group of patients with changes of the cervical spine consisted of individuals who complained of prolonged and persistent headaches, dizziness, transient loss of consciousness, and alterations in the visual field when suddenly turning or tilting the head. There was a significant variation in the age of the patients, who ranged from children to adolescents and adults. Quite often, the complaints of the young and older patients were similar.

To exclude specific and oncological diseases, radiography and computed tomography of the brain, cervical spine and, if necessary, other regions of the spine were performed. Transcranial ultrasonic dopplerography of the head and neck vessels, rheoencephalography and other tests were also performed. Among children of 6–7 years of age, radiography was carried out only in exceptional cases. On most of the dopplerograms, extravasal vertebral artery compression was detected at the level of C_3–C_4 on either side, with a deficiency of blood flow ranging from 20%–60% or more. Unilateral or bilateral reduction of the flow of blood in the internal carotid arteries, abnormal tortuosity of the a. basilaris, problems related to venous outflow, hypertonicity of the jugular veins, etc. were also observed. Clinically, these findings corresponded to constant headaches, increased blood and intracranial pressure.

Comparing the data from the examination of our patients with the results of laboratory and instrumental (radiography, dopplerography and computed tomography, etc.) studies, we found that in most cases, disorders of the cerebral circulation had the same causes. The primary cause was compression of the blood vessels in the vertebral foramina due to rotatory displacement of the cervical vertebrae. Frequently, CT scans of the cervical spine clearly revealed asymmetry of the diameter of the vertebral foramina. Thus, significant compression of the vertebral arteries, veins and sympathetic nerves was caused by a combination of the reduced diameter of the foramina and rotation of the vertebrae. Compression of these nerves, in turn, resulted in the activation of the central mechanism of angiospasm.

Among all patients (young, middle-aged and old), there were cases of fixation of the vertebrae in a position of subluxation in a background of degenerative disc disease and spondylosis deformans. Consolidated fractures of the vertebral bodies and diverse deformities were also observed. The latter were combined with rotational displacements, which usually occurred at the site of maximum curvature of the cervical spinal segment, corresponding to the zone of C_3–C_4.

In all cases, there was relative shortening of one leg due to pronounced spasm of the right or left common back extensor. It may be remembered that spasm of the extensor muscles causes pelvic tilt and leads to the development of scoliotic spinal deformity, with subsequent rotary subluxation of the vertebrae at the sites specified earlier.

An analysis of our clinical material showed that deformations of the cervical spine were also associated with endocrine disorders (excessive or reduced body weight). In our view, this process involves the pituitary and pineal glands in the thalamic region and pons. In several of our cases, the patient's weight was restored to normal and obesity was eliminated when he/she was treated for strabismus, persistent headache and vertigo, when the rotational displacement of C_1–C_3 was corrected, and he/she was given physical therapy and magnetotherapy in the region of the neck and collar area. In young girls with high pilosity of the face and a body with masculine features, the treatment gradually neutralized the symptoms.

However, this line of research requires specialized, focused study involving neurologists, endocrinologists and other specialists. Any advances in this area could be very promising for the thousands of patients who are overweight or underweight, and who suffer from other hormonal disorders.

Among our patients, there were children suffering from various ophthalmological conditions associated with weakened hearing. As shown in Fig. 5.1.2, the centre of n. vestibulocochlearis is located close to that of n. abducens and, therefore, it could be assumed that vestibular and acoustic disorders have the same origin as visual disorders. We believe that the key mechanism of the pathogenesis of these disorders is compression of the medulla, its pathways and centres.

The data from numerous cases indicated that there was an association between a combination of headaches and a tendency towards increased or reduced blood pressure, on the one hand, and impaired functioning of the sympathetic ganglia and medulla oblongata and its vasomotor centre, on the other. The nature of the medical care that we administered included correction of rotational displacement of the cervical vertebrae with the help of an inflatable rubber collar, physical therapy, magnetotherapy in the region of the neck and collar area and restoration of the correct biomechanics of the body's muscles using insoles. We called this scheme a standard therapy. Of course, the patients were treated in close collaboration with physicians from other relevant disciplines.

Our clinical observations coincided completely with those of L.I. Sandrigailo (1988) (Fig. 5.4), who studied the consequences of compression of the anatomical structures of the brain, as well as the spinal nerves and cervical ganglia at the level of C_1–C_4 (Fig. 5.1.10). The variety of pathological conditions that may occur as a result include torticollis, eye diseases, trigeminal neuralgia, headache, dizziness, sleep disorders, weakening of the memory, neurasthenia, and nose and ear diseases (including deafness). We also found that compression of the anatomical structures of the spinal nerves and cervical ganglia at the level of C_5 caused eye diseases, tonsillitis, sore throat (angina), hoarseness and loss of taste. In patients with neurological disorders at the level of C_6, the conditions observed included asthma, pharyngitis, laryngitis, breathlessness, chronic cough, psoriasis of the head, neck and upper limbs, and signs of plexitis (more pronounced on the side of the pelvic and cervical tilt). When the

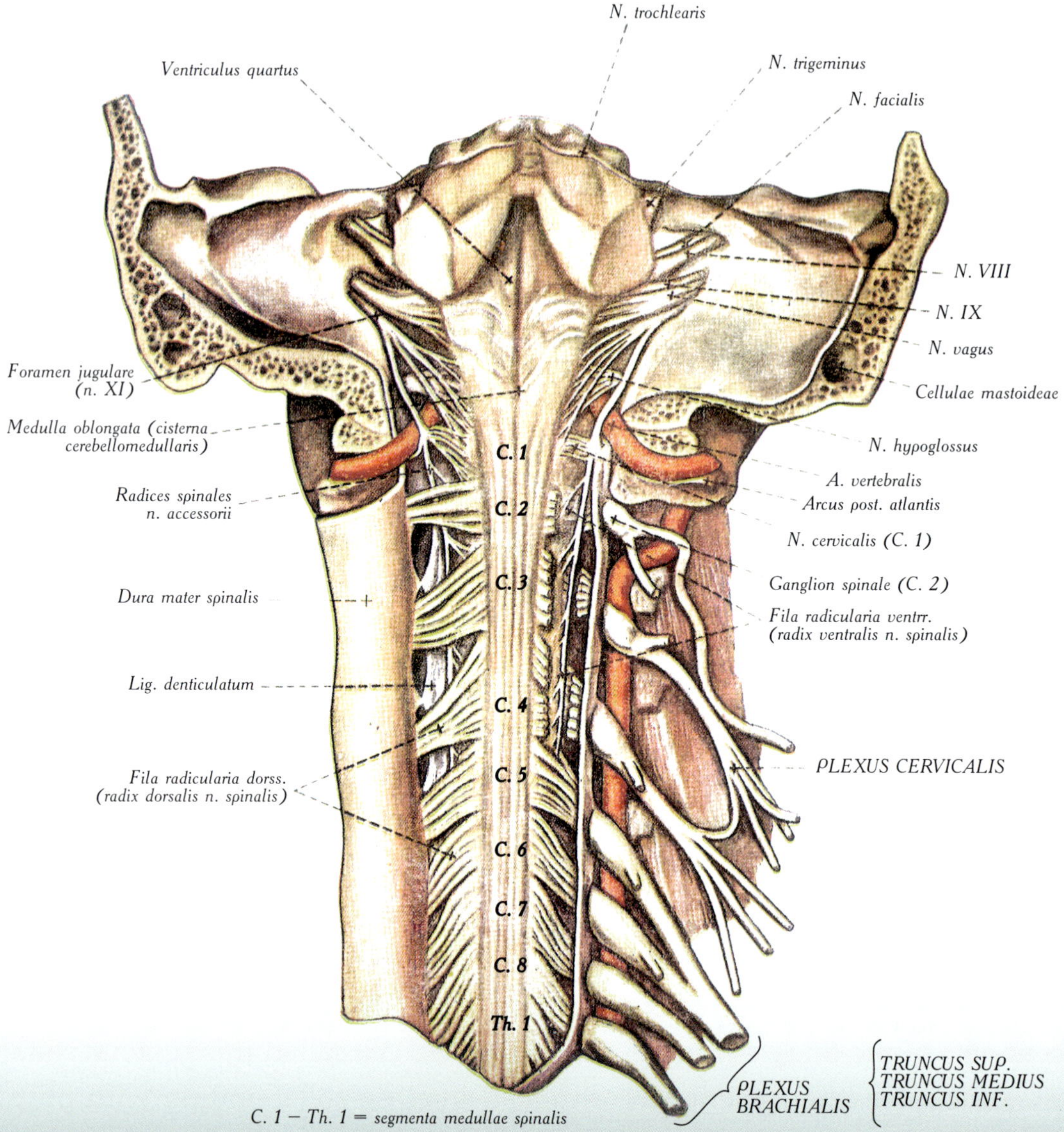

Fig. 5.1.10. Cervical and brachial plexus

compression was localized at the level of C_7–Th_1, the major symptoms were unilateral shoulder–scapular periarthritis, chronic bronchitis, asthma, allergy and various types of thyroid dysfunction.

We shall now give some examples of the conditions mentioned above by drawing on our case material. We will start with cases in which visual impairment was the leading symptom.

We would first like to draw the reader's attention to the fact that base therapy was administered to all patients, regardless of gender, age and type of spinal deformity, and concomitant pathology of the internal organs. This therapy included getting the patient to wear an orthopaedic insole on the side of the shortened lower limb, corrective detorsional exercises and local magnetotherapy. A significant proportion of patients also used an inflatable rubber collar, which ensured dosed traction of the cervical and upper thoracic vertebrae and atraumatic repositioning of these vertebrae.

Assessments of the results of treatment were made as early as 6–8 months and the latest within 12 months of treatment.

1. Patient G., a 3-year-old boy. According to the diagnosis of the ophthalmologist, he had a high degree of congenital myopia, astigmatism, hypoplasia of the visual analyser, convergent strabismus and a high degree of amblyopia.

Ultrasound dopplerography of the cerebral vessels showed signs of extravasal compression in the vertebral artery (VA) system at the level of C_3 on the left and C_4 on the right. This had caused a reduction of up to 40% in the blood flow in these vessels, and decreased the vertebral venous outflow by 30%.

G. had a scoliotic posture, with relative shortening of the left leg. This was compensated for with an insole of a height of **20 mm**. There was significant rotational displacement of the vertebrae at all levels (cervical, thoracic and lumbar). Palpation was acutely painful.

G. was put on the standard treatment, which yielded positive results. During the follow-up examination 6 months later, his vision was seen to have improved. Palpation of the spine was painless and its axis was correct.

2. Patient P., a 4.5-year-old boy, had been diagnosed with convergent strabismus by the ophthalmologist. His main complaint was persistent headaches. Medical therapy had proved ineffective. A rheoencephalography showed that blood flow was reduced by 30% in the zone of the left internal carotid artery. Venous drainage was impaired.

P. had a right-sided scoliotic posture, with relative shortening of the left leg. This was compensated for with an insole of a height of **7 mm**. On examination, marked rotational displacement of the cervical vertebrae (C_1–C_7) was observed. This led to a significant reduction in the angle of rotation of the head to either side. Palpation in the areas of rotational displacement was acutely painful to the patient.

We trained P.'s mother to perform physical therapy (detorsional gymnastics). Other than wearing a shoe insole, the patient underwent magnetotherapy. During the follow-up examination 6 months later, it was found that the treatment had had a positive effect. The headaches had resolved completely and there was a marked improvement in vision. The axis of the spine was correct. The patient had no complaints.

3. Patient M., a 5-year-old boy, had been diagnosed with convergent strabismus and spasm of accommodation by the ophthalmologist.

Ultrasound dopplerography of the cerebral vessels showed signs of extravasal compression in the vascular territory of the VA, at the level of C_3 on the left and C_4 on the right. This had led to a reduction of up to 40% in the blood supply.

M. had a scoliotic posture, with relative shortening of the left leg. This was compensated for with an insole of a height of **10 mm**. There was significant rotational displacement of the vertebrae at all levels (cervical, thoracic and lumbar). Palpation of these areas caused the patient acute pain.

M. was put on the standard treatment. Positive results were observed during the follow-up examination 6 months later. The patient's vision had improved and the spinal deformity had been corrected. M. had no complaints.

4. Patient K., a 7.5-year-old girl, had been diagnosed with convergent strabismus by the ophthalmologist. For four years, she had been suffering from chronic bronchitis and asthma, and was allergic to flowers. She also had vegetovascular dystonia. Her hands and feet were sweaty.

K. had a scoliotic posture, with relative shortening of the left leg. This was compensated for with an insole of a height of **3 mm**. There was significant rotational displacement of the vertebrae at all levels (cervical, thoracic and lumbar). Palpation in these areas gave rise to acute pain. The patient also had plano-valgus feet.

Radiographs of the cervical and upper thoracic spine revealed abnormalities of the structure of the vertebral body of the 1st thoracic vertebra (spina bifida) (Fig. 5.1.11).

While analysing the causes of chronic bronchitis, asthma and allergy, we noticed that the anomalous area corresponded to the location of the upper right and left spinal ganglia. Hernial protrusion of the spinal meninges in the area of the vertebral defect had led to compression of the meninges. This had resulted in impairment of the functioning of the spinal cord and ganglia, and this, in our opinion, was the cause of the vegetovascular dystonia and its consequences. Shortening of the left leg was an additional negative factor, resulting in rotation of the vertebrae and increasing compression of the spinal cord meninges.

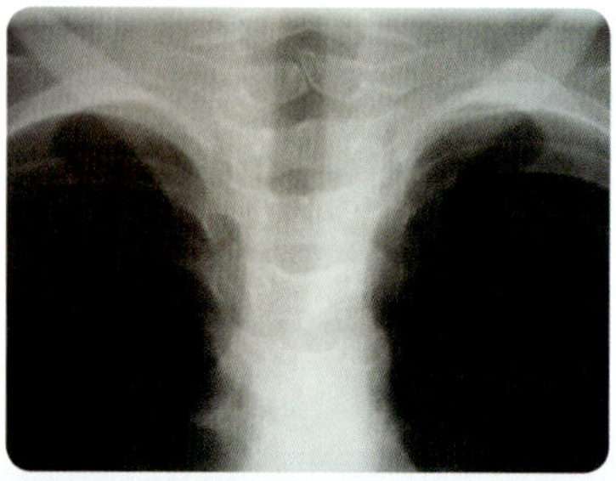

Fig. 5.1.11.

K. was put on the standard treatment. The follow-up examination 5 months later showed good progress. There was a significant improvement in the patient's vision and respiratory function. The spinal deformity had been corrected.

5. Patient K., an 11-year-old girl, had been diagnosed with divergent alternating strabismus and spasm of accommodation by the ophthalmologist. The patient looked as if she was 16–17 years old and all the secondary signs of sexual maturity were present. In our opinion, this situation could be explained by dysfunction of the pituitary gland.

K. had a scoliotic posture, with relative shortening of the left leg. This was compensated for with an insole of a height of **15 mm**. Significant rotational displacement of the cervical vertebrae was observed (Fig. 5.1.12). Palpation of these areas was acutely painful. Displacement of the thoracic and lumbar vertebrae was also observed. The patient had bilateral lumboischialgia.

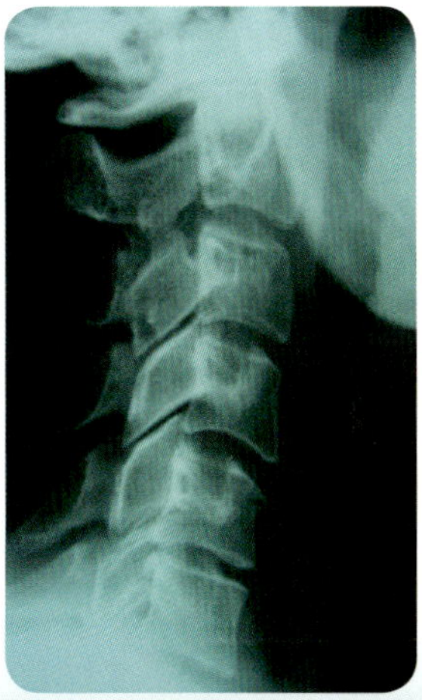

Fig. 5.1.12.

The standard treatment (insole, physiotherapy, local magneto-acoustic therapy) was initiated. At follow-up examination 9 months later, the difference between the length of the legs was found to have decreased to 3 mm. She had no complaints. There was a significant improvement in the patient's vision and the position of the eyes was correct. Signs of mild gigantism remained. The axis of the spine had become correct.

6. Patient V., a 10-year-old girl, had been diagnosed with hypermetropic astigmatism, spasm of accommodation and divergent strabismus by the ophthalmologist. She suffered from persistent headaches and dizziness and the functioning of the vestibular apparatus was impaired (she fell down when she closed her eyes).

V. had a scoliotic posture, with relative shortening of the left leg. This was compensated for with an insole of a height of **3 mm**. There was rotational displacement of the vertebrae at all levels. This was particularly marked in the cervical region (Fig. 5.1.13). The patient also had signs of bilateral femoral nerve neuritis and bilateral sciatica.

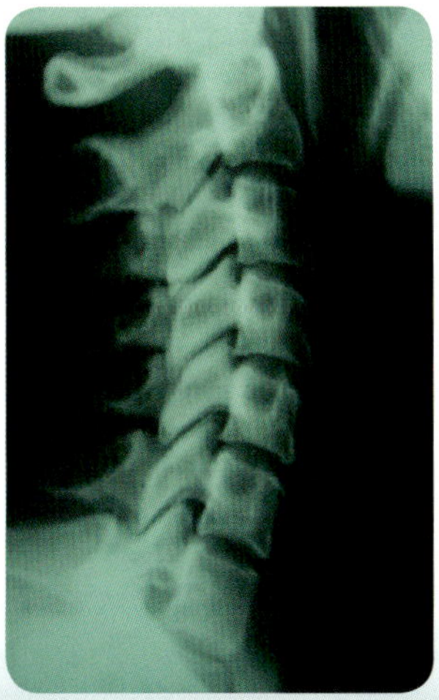

Fig. 5.1.13.

V.'s parents were trained to perform exercises for detorsional correction. She was put on the basic course of treatment (orthopaedic insole, physiotherapy, local magneto-acoustic therapy).

A follow-up examination was carried out after 6

months. The position of the eyes had returned to normal and the axis of the spine was correct. The patient had no complaints.

7. Patient T., an 11-year-old boy, had been diagnosed by the ophthalmologist with complex myopic astigmatism and divergent strabismus. He had suffered an injury to the cervical spine at birth. In his mother's words, 'the large size of the foetus had complicated the delivery'. The obstetrician had had to make a great effort to extract the head.

The patient complained of headaches, dizziness, poor memory and loss of concentration. He looked much older than his age and had all the secondary signs of sexual maturity, resembling a young man of 17–19 years of age.

Transcranial dopplerography of the cerebral vessels showed extravasal compression of the vertebral arteries in the C_3–C_4 segment. There was a symmetrical deficit of up to 30% in the blood flow Venous outflow in the vertebral veins was impaired.

Our examination of the patient revealed that there was a marked decrease in the range of movement of the head in the cervical spine (it did not exceed 80% of the total range of movement of 180 degrees).

T. had a scoliotic posture, with relative shortening of the left leg. This was compensated for with an insole of a height of **15 mm**. He also had bilateral plexitis, lumboischialgia and femoral nerve neuritis.

Radiographs of the cervical spine (Fig. 5.1.14) showed marked signs of deforming spondylosis at the level of C_3–C_6, which are characteristic of adult male patients. In anteroposterior projection at the level of C_5, the arch of the vertebral body was observed to be defective (spina bifida). This was presumed to be of post-traumatic origin. We assumed that during delivery, abrupt turns of the foetus's head caused injury to the vertebral bodies and subsequently impaired the process of ossification.

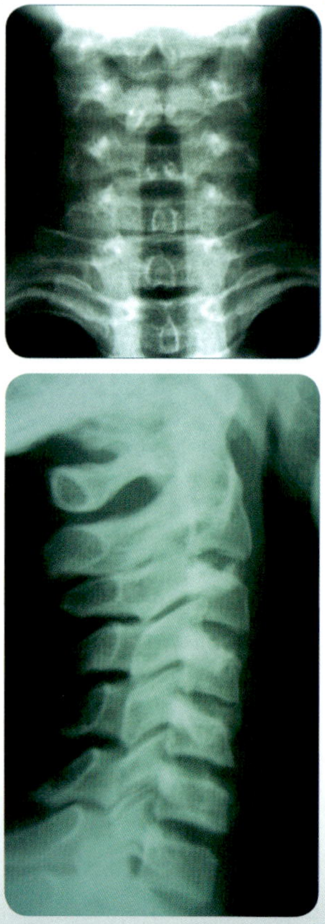

Fig. 5.1.14.

Due to instability the C_3–C_5 segment and deforming spondylosis, there was disruption of the flow of blood at the same level. In our opinion, rotary subluxation at the level of C_1–C_3 had led to compression of the thalamic structures and, in particular, had indirectly impaired pituitary function, causing excessive production of growth hormone.

T. was put on the standard treatment. The follow-up examination performed 6 months later showed that the treatment had had a positive effect. The patient's vision had improved, and the pain and dizziness had disappeared. The axis of the spine was correct. T. had no complaints.

8. Patient S., a 14-year-old girl, had been diagnosed by the ophthalmologist with convergent concomitant alternating strabismus (after surgery), as well as complex hypermetropic astigmatism.

S. complained of frequent headaches and progressive weakening of her vision. Her neck movements had become markedly limited, as confirmed by the radiograph (Fig. 5.1.15). We observed rotational displacement of the cervical vertebrae on the upper point of the curvature (C_4-C_5-C_6). The patient also had bilateral plexitis, femoral nerve neuritis and bilateral lumboischialgia.

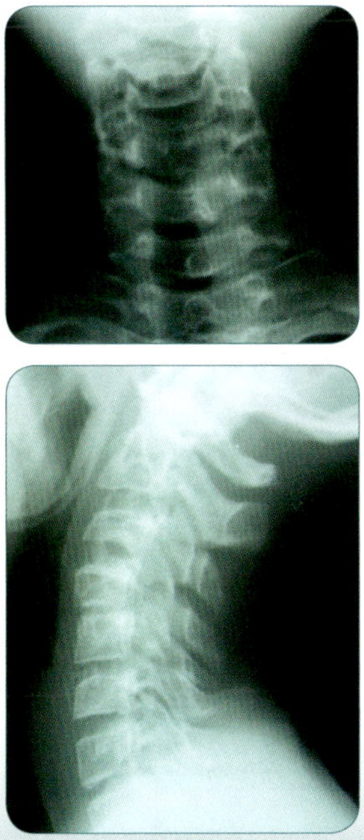

Fig. 5.1.15.

Ultrasound dopplerography of the cerebral vessels revealed extravasal compression of the vertebral arteries at the level of the C_4-C_5, and asymmetrical deficiency of blood flow of up to 40%. The other findings were cerebral vasospasm and impaired outflow in the jugular veins.

S. had a scoliotic posture, with relative shortening of the left leg. This was compensated for with an insole of a height of **7 mm**.

S. was put on the standard treatment. The follow-up examination 6 months later showed good progress. There was an improvement in the patient's vision. She had no complaints. There were no more headaches. The axis of the spine was corrected.

9. Patient Y., a 15-year-old girl, had been diagnosed by the ophthalmologist with hypermetropic astigmatism and external strabismus. Her complaints were impairment of memory, recurrent intense headaches, blurred vision, loss of consciousness when suddenly raising the head, emotional lability and sweaty hands. Her sleep was disturbed. She complained of pain in the pancreas and gallbladder, as well as low back pain and pain in the knees. Her feet were constantly cold. Y. had sustained a neck injury at the age of 7.

Y. had severe kyphoscoliosis of the thoracic spine, with relative shortening of the left leg. This was compensated for with an insole of a height of **10 mm**.

On ultrasound dopplerography of the cerebral vessels, a deficit in blood flow was observed at the level of the C_3-C_4 segment. The deficit, of up to 40%, was mainly right-sided. The vertebral venous outflow was impaired.

The radiograph of the cervical spine (Fig. 5.1.16) showed evidence of deforming spondylosis at the level of C_4-C_7. This was probably a result of the injury sustained by the patient eight years earlier. There was clear evidence of rotational displacement of the vertebrae at this level. Y. had Schmorl's hernia at the level of Th_{12}–L_1–L_3. There was a consolidated fracture of the L_1 body.

Y. was put on the standard treatment, which was seen to have had positive results at 6 months. There was no pain in the parenchymatous organs, large joints or lower back. The headaches had almost resolved and there was an improvement in the patient's vision. The axis of the spine was correct.

10. Patient G., an 18-year-old young woman, had been diagnosed with moderate myopia and astigmatism by the ophthalmologist. Among her complaints was that her vision became almost lost when she suddenly stood up. Rotation of her head to the left was limited by up to 50% of the total range of 180°, as confirmed by the radiograph (Fig. 5.1.17). The radiograph clearly showed rotational displacement of the cervical vertebrae at the level of C_4.

G. had a scoliotic posture, with relative shortening of the left leg. This was compensated for with an insole of a height of **3 mm**.

The patient's symptoms included 'tingling' of the heart and irritability. In addition, she had clinical signs of left-sided plexitis, bilateral neuritis of the femoral and obturator nerves, and bilateral lumboischialgia.

Ultrasound dopplerography of the cerebral vessels showed signs of bilateral extravasal compression of the vertebral artery at the level of the C_4 segment. The blood supply was reduced by up to 50%.

G. was put on the standard treatment. When she was assessed a year later, she and her parents reported that there were no more complaints. The axis of the spine was found to be correct.

11. Patient R., an 18-year-old young man, had been diagnosed by the ophthalmologist with high-grade congenital myopia with changes of the fundus, as well as astigmatism. According to his mother, a caesarean section had been performed because of complications during birth (asphyxia). R. also sustained a head injury at the age of 6, and suffered

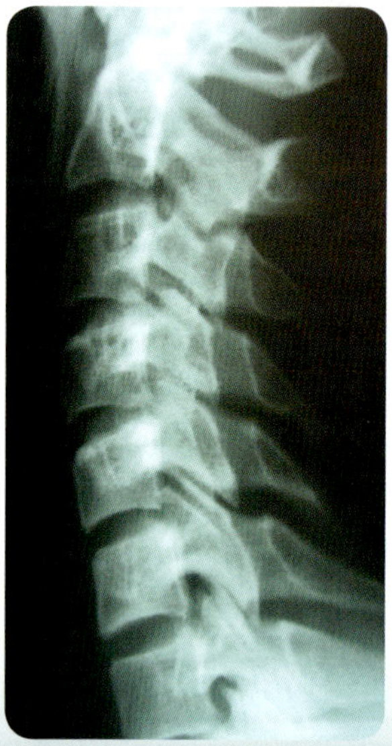

Fig. 5.1.16.

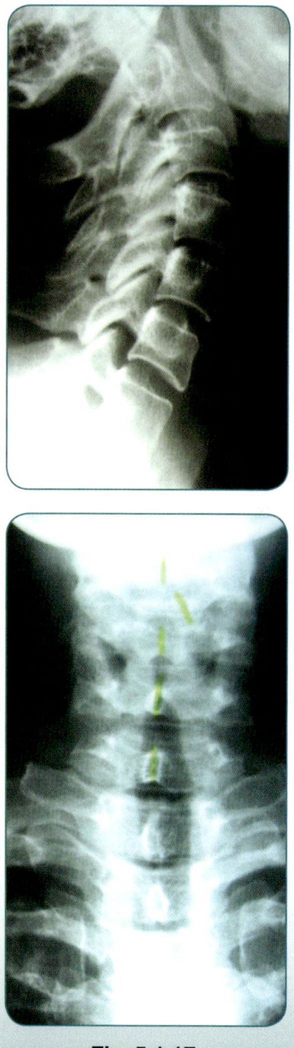

Fig. 5.1.17.

from epileptiform convulsions of the whole body a day after the injury. Such seizures, accompanied by an increase in the body temperature, recurred every 3 months. The patient was often admitted to the intensive care unit.

Ultrasound dopplerography of the cerebral vessels showed signs of extravasal compression of the vertebral artery at the level of the C_1–C_2 segment. The blood supply was reduced by 50%. It was observed that there was a deficiency of blood supply of up to 30% in the vascular territory of the right middle cerebral artery. A CT scan of the head revealed slightly marked cortical hypotrophy.

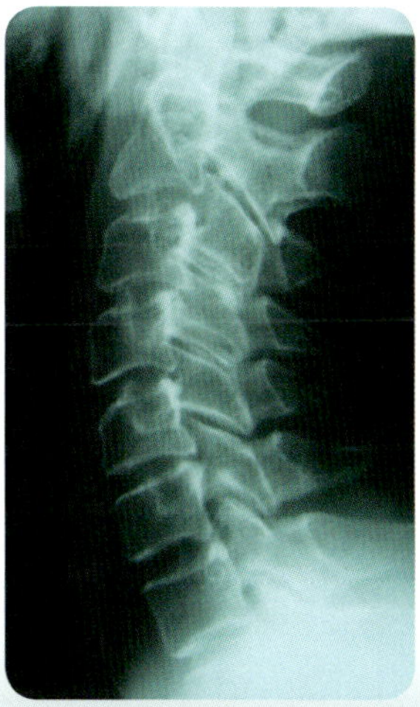
Fig. 5.1.18.

R. had a scoliotic posture, with relative shortening of the left leg. This was compensated for with an insole of a height of **3 mm**. Marked rotary displacement of the cervical vertebrae (Fig. 5.1.18) had caused bilateral plexitis. There was also rotational displacement of the thoracic and lumbar vertebrae. This was manifested clinically in bilateral obturator and femoral nerve neuritis, as well as bilateral lumboischialgia.

R. was put on the standard treatment and his progress assessed after 6 months. The episodes of headaches and seizures had stopped, and his vision had improved. The axis of the spine was found to be correct.

12. Patient G., a young woman of 18 years of age, had been diagnosed with hypermetropic astigmatism and external strabismus by the ophthalmologist. Her complaints included frequent headaches, signs of right-sided trigeminitis, and congenital spastic contractions of the muscles of the limbs. Her hands and feet were usually sweaty and cold, and her periods were very painful. G. also suffered from biliary dyskinesia.

Ultrasound dopplerography of the cerebral vessels showed that the blood supply in the vascular territory of the right vertebral artery in the C_4 segment was asymmetrical (insufficiency of up to 50%). The venous outflow was significantly impaired.

G. had a scoliotic posture, with relative shortening of the left leg. This was compensated for with an insole of a height of **10 mm**. Marked rotary displacement of the vertebrae could be observed in the cervical, thoracic and lumbar regions, manifesting clinically as bilateral plexitis, femoral nerve neuritis and lumboischialgia. Clinical signs of subluxation of the cervical vertebrae were confirmed by a radiograph (Fig. 5.1.19).

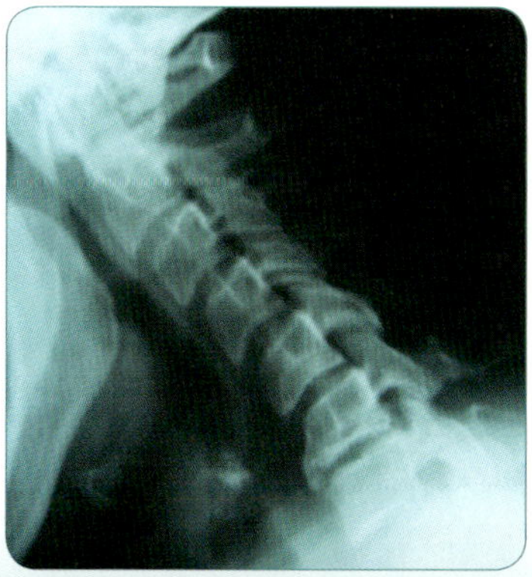
Fig. 5.1.19.

G. was put on the standard treatment and was followed up within 6 months. She had made good progress, with the headaches and seizures having resolved. There was an improvement in her vision and the axis of the spine was correct.

13. Patient T., an 18-year-old woman, had been diagnosed with progressive myopia, astigmatism and divergent strabismus by the ophthalmologist. T. complained of impaired vision, general weakness, cold hands and feet, low blood pressure and frequent nosebleeds. She reported that she collapsed when she suddenly turned her head. She had earlier suffered a head injury while practising judo. T. said that she got a backache in the lumbar region when she straightened her body. Her hands and feet were cold. The angle of rotation of the head to either side was limited. The neurologist had diagnosed her with vegetovascular dystonia.

Doppler ultrasound of the cerebral vessels showed extravasal compression of the vertebral arteries at the level of the C_3–C_4 segments, and symmetrical insufficiency of blood flow of up to 25%. The tone of the ophthalmic veins was increased.

T. had a scoliotic posture, with relative shortening of the left leg. This was compensated for with an insole of a height of **15 mm**. The radiograph of the cervical spine (Fig. 5.1.20) revealed moderate rotary displacement of the vertebrae in the C_4–C_7 segment, osteochondrosis and spondylosis deformans.

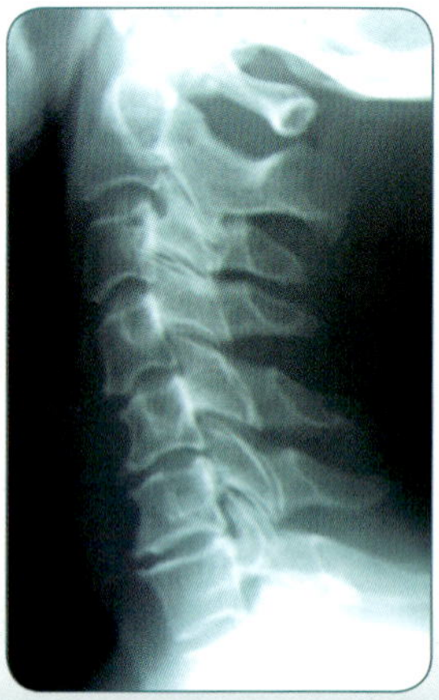

Fig. 5.1.20.

T. received the standard treatment, which was seen to have a positive effect during follow-up 6 months later. Her blood pressure had stabilized, her vision had improved and there were no more nose bleeds. She had no complaints. The axis of the spine was correct.

14. Patient Ch., a 22-year-old woman, had been diagnosed with marked spasm of accommodation by the ophthalmologist. One-and-a-half years earlier, Ch. had sustained a cervical spine injury as a result of a motor vehicle accident. Thereafter, her vision had worsened progressively and she had become prone to episodes of headaches.

Ultrasound dopplerography of the cerebral vessels showed extravasal compression and symmetrical insufficiency of blood flow of up to 35% in the vertebral arteries in the C_3 and C_4 segments. Vasospasm of a. basilaris, causing insufficiency of up to 40%, was also observed. In addition, there was asymmetrical insufficiency of blood flow of up to 30% in the posterior cerebral arteries.

Ch. had a scoliotic posture, with relative shortening of the left leg. This was compensated for with an insole of a height of **20 mm**.

According to the patient, her hands and feet were always 'cold as ice'. The angles to which Ch. could rotate her head to either side were significantly limited. She complained of back pain, especially in the lumbar region. The radiograph of the cervical spine (Fig. 5.1.21) showed rotational displacement of the cervical vertebrae. In the lumbar region (Fig. 5.1.22), lumbarization of S_1 (the presence of a sixth lumbar vertebra) was observed, as were impaired tropism of the articular processes of the SMS (spinal motion segment) L_5–S_1 and spina bifida at the S_1 level.

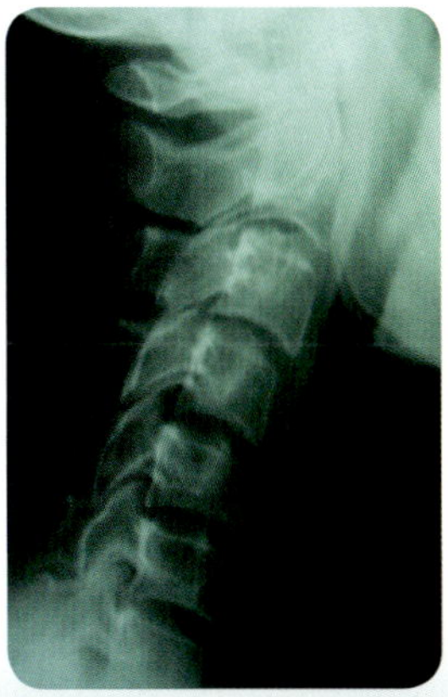
Fig. 5.1.21.

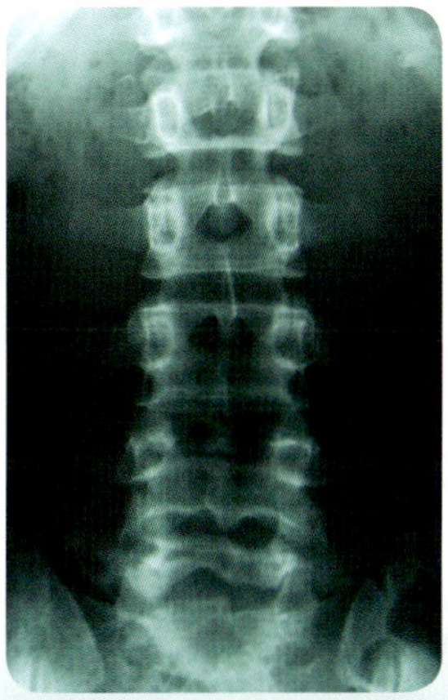
Fig. 5.1.22.

Ch. was put on the standard treatment and a follow-up examination performed 5 months later showed positive results. Her vision had improved, and her hands and feet no longer felt cold. The difference between the length of the two legs had decreased to **7 mm**. She had no complaints. The patient was encouraged to continue with the recommended treatment.

15. Patient K., a 33-year-old woman, had been diagnosed with convergent strabismus by the ophthalmologist. Her complaints included headaches, dizziness, limited angles of rotation of the head, pain between the shoulder blades, numbness of the hands, and cramps in the arms and legs. She also had diabetes type 1 (blood sugar 13 mmol/L). Her periods were painful and she had a tendency to constipation.

K. had a scoliotic posture, with relative shortening of the left leg. This was compensated for with an insole of a height of **18 mm**. We observed marked signs of degenerative disc disease and spondylosis deformans at the C_5–C_6 level (Fig. 5.1.23).

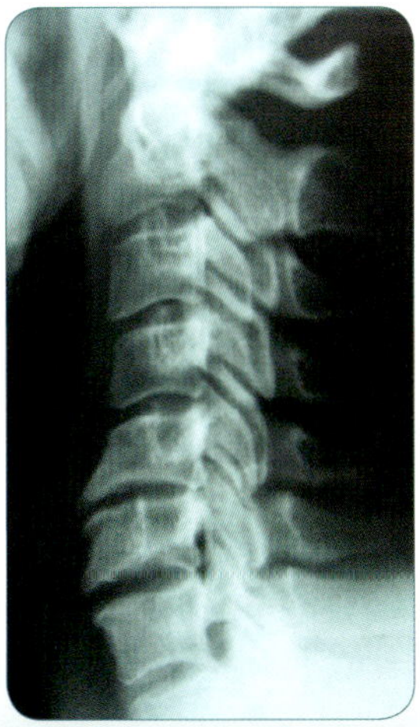
Fig. 5.1.23.

The standard treatment (insole, physiotherapy, local magneto-acoustic therapy) was initiated. On follow-up examination 8 months later, it was found that the length of the two legs had become equal. The patient's bowel function was normal and the blood glucose level was 8.7 mmol/L. The axis of the spine was correct. K. was advised to continue the treatment until one year from the time of its initiation.

16. Patient K., a 35-year-old woman, had been diagnosed with moderate myopia by the ophthalmologist. She complained of frequent headaches, radiating to the occiput and temples, and pain in the eyes. Medications had proved ineffective. Twelve years earlier, the first reduction of cervical vertebrae was done and her symptoms had resolved. However, she later fell from a bicycle and injured her neck, which led to a recurrence of all the symptoms.

K. had a scoliotic posture, with relative shortening of the left leg. This was compensated for with an insole of a height of **18 mm**. The patient had marked signs of bilateral plexitis, lumboischialgia and femoral nerve neuritis. The range of rotation of the head was limited. The radiograph of the cervical spine showed rotary subluxation of the vertebrae in the C_3–C_6 segments (Fig. 5.1.24).

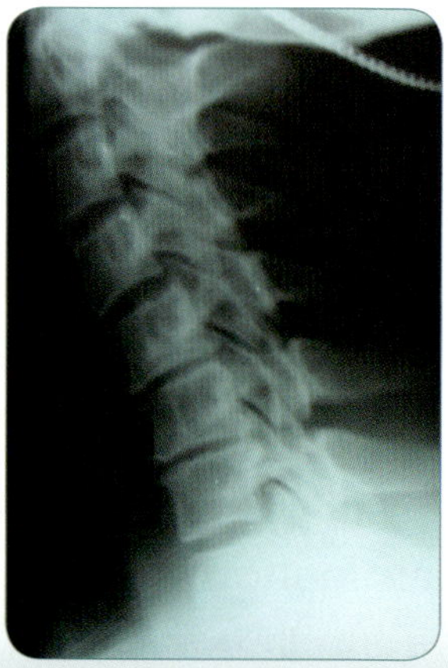

Fig. 5.1.24.

The standard treatment was initiated and there was a follow-up examination 6 months later. K. had made good progress. She no longer suffered from headaches and her vision had improved. The difference between the length of her legs had decreased to **7 mm**. The patient was advised to continue with the treatment for one year more from the time of its initiation.

17. Patient R., a 43-year-old woman, had been diagnosed with mixed congenital astigmatism and convergent strabismus by the ophthalmologist. She complained that her vision and hearing had become weaker. In addition, she had frequent headaches and felt dizzy when she moved her head suddenly. The mobility of her neck was restricted.

Ultrasound dopplerography of the cerebral vessels showed a symmetrical circulatory insufficiency of up to 20% in the vertebral arteries in the right C_3 segment, and of more than 50% in the left C_4 segment.

R. had a scoliotic posture with relative shortening of the left leg. This was compensated for with an insole of a height of **18 mm**. There were marked clinical signs of bilateral plexitis, femoral nerve neuritis and lumboischialgia. The radiograph of the cervical region (Fig. 5.1.25) showed signs of degenerative disc disease and spondylosis deformans at the level of C_5–C_7. The plexitis was probably a result of compression of elements of the brachial plexus at this level.

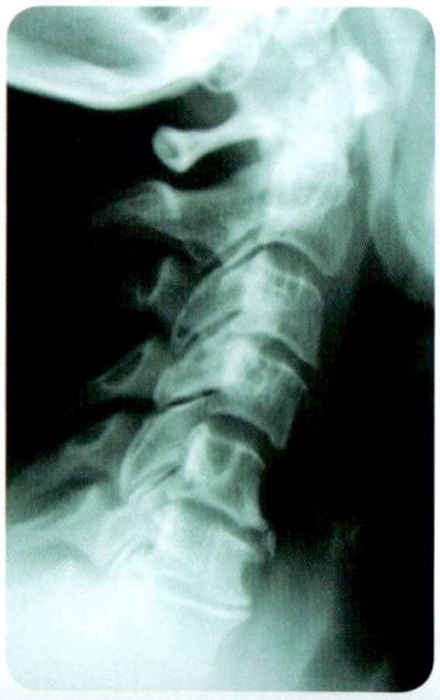

Fig. 5.1.25.

The standard treatment was initiated and the follow-up examination, carried out 6 months later, showed good progress. Her vision had improved, and she no longer suffered from dizziness and headaches. There were no neurological symptoms. The difference between the length of the legs had decreased to **7 mm**.

18. Patient K., a 51-year-old woman, had been diagnosed with hypermetropic astigmatism and right-sided trigeminal neuralgia (trigeminitis) by the ophthalmologist. Her complaints included persistent headaches and discomfort in the neck, which had begun 10 years earlier. Recently, there had been a slight increase in her arterial blood pressure. Transcranial ultrasonic dopplerography of the cerebral vessels showed pathological tortuosity of a. basilaris. In the right C_4 segment, one could observe extravasal compression of both arteries and veins, causing circulatory insufficiency of up to 30%.

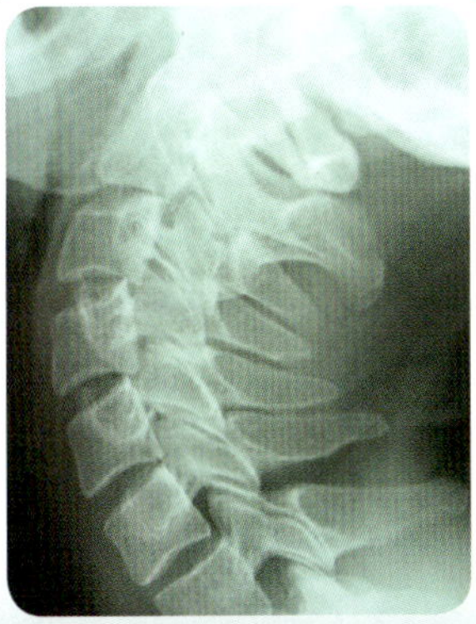

Fig. 5.1.26.

K. had a scoliotic posture, with relative shortening of the left leg. This was compensated for with an insole of a height of **17 mm**. There were signs of bilateral plexitis, lumboischialgia and femoral nerve neuritis. In addition, there was clinically marked rotational displacement of the vertebrae in the cervical, thoracic and lumbar regions. Rotational displacement of the vertebrae at the level of C_3–C_4–C_5, as seen on the radiograph of the cervical spine, is shown in Fig. 5.1.26.

The standard treatment was initiated. At follow-up 6 months later, the results seemed to be encouraging. The effect was positive. K. no longer complained of headaches and her blood pressure was normal. She had no complaints. The axis of the spine was correct.

19. Patient K., a 63-year-old woman, had been diagnosed with marked signs of bilateral trigeminitis and spasm of accommodation by the ophthalmologist. The patient's complaints were pain in the eyes, dizziness and frequent headaches.

Ultrasound dopplerography of the cerebral vessels showed a reduction in blood flow of up to 30% in the C_3 segment of the right vertebral artery and of up to 35% in the C_4 segment of the left vertebral artery.

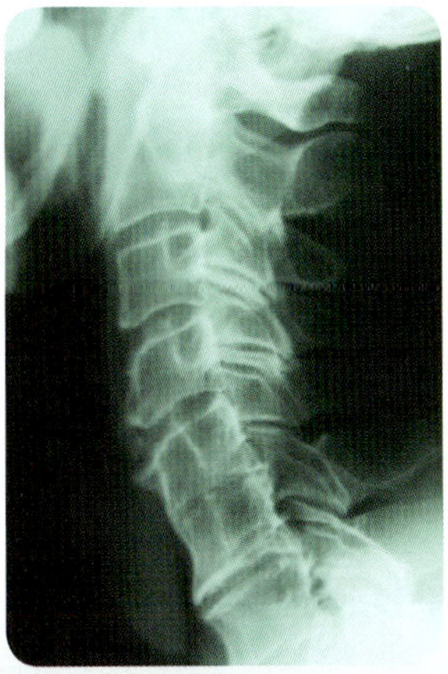

Fig. 5.1.27.

K. had a kyphoscoliotic posture, with relative shortening of the left leg. This was compensated for with an insole of a height of **3 mm**. She had clinical signs of bilateral plexitis (more marked on the left side), femoral nerve neuritis and bilateral lumboischialgia. In addition, there were rotational displacements in the spine, the most marked ones being located in the cervical spine (Fig. 5.1.27). The bodies of C_5–C_6 were blocked.

The standard treatment was initiated. The follow-up examination performed 6 months later showed an improvement in her condition. The headaches, signs of trigeminitis and dizziness had resolved. There were no symptoms of neurological disorders. The patient was satisfied with the results of the treatment. The axis of the spine was correct.

20. Patient B., a 71-year-old man, had been diagnosed with astigmatism by the ophthalmologist. His complaints included intense headaches and dizziness. He was unable to walk due to severe pain in the lumbar spine.

Radiographs of the spine showed rotational displacements of the vertebrae in all regions. The most pronounced signs of degenerative disc disease and spondylosis deformans were seen at the level of C_5–C_7 (Fig. 5.1.28). In the lumbar region (Fig. 5.1.29), dysplasia of the lumbosacral vertebrae was observed (sacralization of L_5 and lumbarization of S_1).

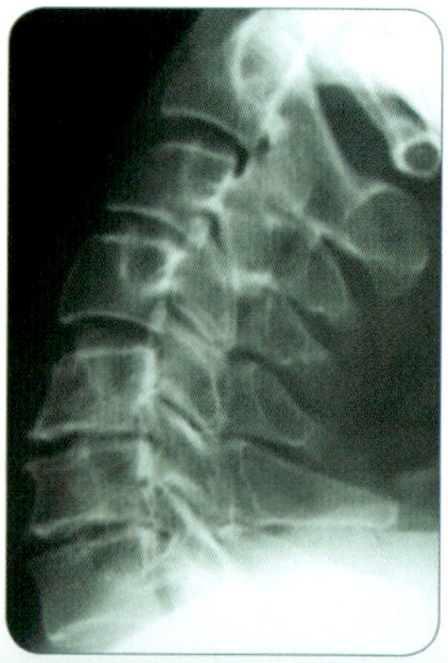

Fig. 5.1.28.

B. had a kyphoscoliotic posture, with relative shortening of the left leg. This was compensated for with an insole of a height of **15 mm**.

The standard treatment was initiated and the outcome was assessed after 10 months. The clinical signs of trigeminitis, as well as the headaches and dizziness had resolved. The pain along the femoral and sciatic nerves was now negligible. The patient was satisfied with the results of the treatment. He was advised to wear an insole of a height of **7 mm** for another year.

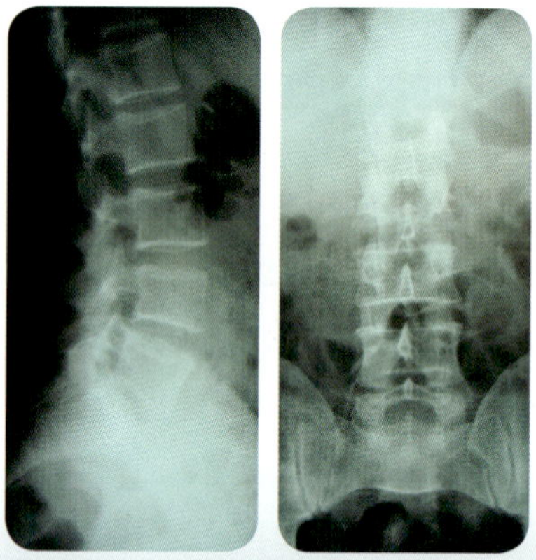

Fig. 5.1.29.

21. Patient G., a 75-year-old man, had been diagnosed with glaucoma and severe myopia by the ophthalmologist. The patient had been short-sighted since childhood. His complaints were constant headaches and significant dizziness.

Transcranial ultrasonic dopplerography of the cerebral vessels showed extravasal compression of the vertebral arteries at the level of C_3–C_4. The deficiency in blood flow of the vertebral artery was the most pronounced at the level of C_3, being above 50%. In the diastolic phase, the deficit reached 100%.

G. had a kyphoscoliotic posture, with relative shortening of the left leg. This was compensated for with an insole of a height of **20 mm**. The movements of the cervical spine were significantly restricted, and there was sclerosis of the right and left trunks of the vertebral arteries. The patient had marked signs of degenerative disc disease and spondylosis deformans (Fig. 5.1.30).

G. was put on the standard treatment, which included the use of an inflatable rubber collar. The follow-up examination performed 6 months later showed that the treatment had had a positive effect. There were no more spells of dizziness and the intensity of the headaches had decreased significantly. The vision had improved slightly. The difference between the length of the legs had decreased to **10 mm**. The patient was advised to continue with the recommended treatment for another 2 years.

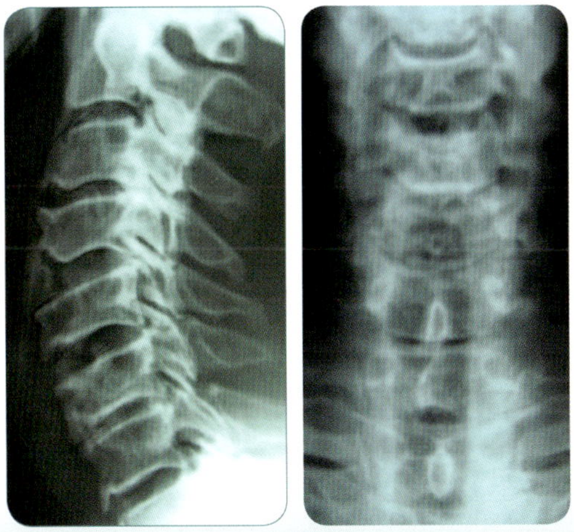

Fig. 5.1.30.

The following patients were people whose predominant complaint was cervical spine disorders, but dopplerography of the cerebral and cervical vessels was not performed.

1. Patient F., a 3-month-old boy who was being breastfed, was brought to us by his parents because he cried day and night. We found that he had increased intracranial pressure. The child could not lie flat on his back due to episthotonus of the head. He had a rash, which was apparently an allergic reaction.

On examination, marked asymmetry of the *trunk muscles, particularly of the back extensors, was observed*. The back extensors were much wider on the right side than the left. This asymmetry had caused a lateral spinal curvature. In the thoracic region, the arc of the curvature turned to the right.

F.'s mother was taught certain techniques of detorsional gymnastics. Several absolutely non-traumatic movements were sufficient to eliminate the muscular asymmetry and align the spinal axis. During the follow-up examination 3 months later, F. was seen to have no signs of allergy. His parents reported that he had become calm and slept well. The extensor muscles were now symmetrical and the axis of the spine was correct. During the next follow up in 6 months, the child no longer had a spinal deformity, and the volume of the back extensor muscles on the right and left sides was the same. He slept well and had no problems with feeding. The mother continued to perform detorsional gymnastics for the child.

2. Patient L., a 3.5-month-old girl who was being breastfed. While examining her, the paediatrician discovered a deformity, i.e. the right common extensor was much wider than the left. A lateral curvature of the spine was also observed. In addition, L.'s capacity to rotate her head to the left was significantly limited. The child was restless. She did not sleep well and was problematic during feeding at night.

Radiography of the cervical spine (Fig. 5.1.31) showed rotary displacement of the vertebrae at the level of C_5–C_6.

After several non-traumatic detorsional movements in the cervical and thoracolumbar regions of the spine, the spinal axis became correct, symmetry of the spinal erectors was restored and the complete range of neck movements was restored. The mother was trained to administer the scheme of physical therapy to the child.

Three weeks after the commencement of the therapy, the baby was able to sleep well and was calm, and there were no problems in her breastfeeding. The mother continued with the detorsional gymnastics. After 3 months, there were no complaints and L.'s development was normal.

3. The parents of Patient S., a 4.5-month-old boy who was being breastfed, noticed that the length of one of his legs was different from that of the other, and the gluteal folds were asymmetrical. Moreover, there was a limitation of head movements to both sides.

The pelvic radiograph showed no signs of hip dysplasia. The physical examination of the child revealed that his right common back extensor was twice as wide as the left. His parents were trained to perform physical therapy (turns of the body and head, hip rotation, massage of the gluteal muscles, etc.).

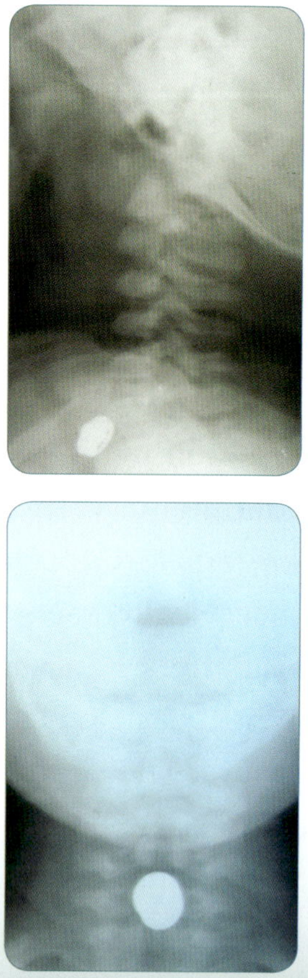

Fig. 5.1.31.

During the follow-up examination 2 months later, it was seen that the patient could rotate his head normally, the gluteal folds were symmetrical, the legs were equal in length, and the volume of the back extensors on the right and left sides was the same.

4. Patient B., a 14-year-old girl, complained of frequent headaches and dizziness. Her neck movements were restricted, mostly on the left. Her palms were wet and cold. Her other complaints were emotional lability, 'tingling' of the heart, frequent episodes of bronchitis, numbness of the hands and freezing feet. B. had clinical signs of bilateral plexitis, lumboischialgia and femoral nerve neuritis.

B. had a scoliotic posture, with relative shortening of the left leg. This was compensated for with an insole of a height of **30 mm**.

The standard therapy, i.e. insole and the scheme of physiotherapy, local magneto-acoustic therapy, was initiated. B. was examined 9 months later. There was no relative shortening and she had virtually no complaints. Her father continued helping the girl to perform the scheme of detorsional gymnastics. Magnetic therapy was also continued.

5. Patient G., a 33-year-old woman, first started suffering from dizziness, headaches and tinnitus (ringing in the ears) 2 years earlier. She could not maintain her balance during sudden movements of the head and would fall down. She had vegetovascular dystonia and severe swelling of the face. G.'s neck movements were significantly limited, mainly on the left.

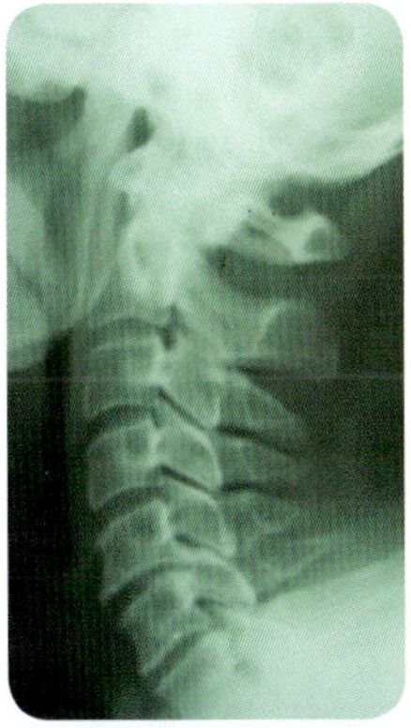

Fig. 5.1.32.

There were clinical signs of bilateral plexitis and lumboischialgia. The patient also had low back pain radiating downwards to the abdomen (towards the ovaries) and was unable to sit due to this pain. Her periods were very painful.

The radiograph of the cervical spine (Fig. 5.1.32) showed deforming spondylosis at the level of C_5–C_7, caused by rotary displacement of these vertebrae and resultant instability. The radiograph of the lumbosacral region (Fig. 5.1.33) showed lumbarization of S_1–S_2. G. had a scoliotic posture, with relative shortening of the left leg. This was compensated for with an insole of a length of **27 mm**.

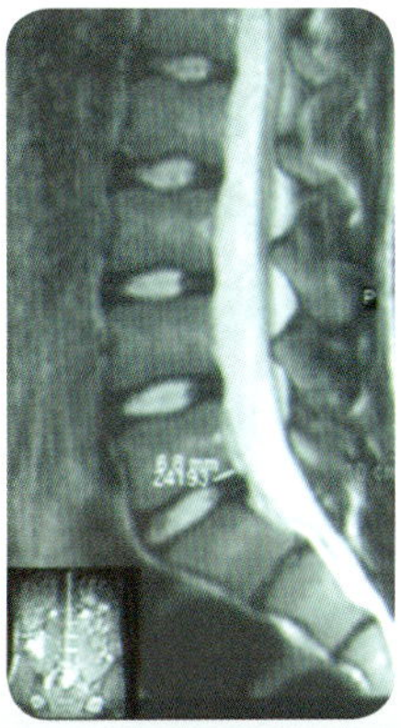

Fig. 5.1.33.

The standard therapy, i.e. insole and the scheme of physiotherapy and magnetotherapy, was initiated. After 8 months, it was observed that there was no difference in the length of the two legs, as well as no complaints. The facial oedema had subsided and the axis of the spine was correct.

6. Patient K., a 34-year-old man, had first developed pain in the neck and lower back 6 years before contacting us, after he had lifted a heavy physical load. He had earlier sought the help of a neurologist and then traditional healers, but their treatment did not have the desired effect and the pain persisted.

K. reported that he lost consciousness when he turned his head suddenly. He had significant limitation of neck movements on both sides. Due to back pain, he could not get up once he had sat down.

He noticed that the pain disappeared when he quickly climbed the ladder of the merchant ship he worked on. In ordinary life, outside the ship, the back pain came back. K. also complained that his memory had become weak. Further, he had hypertrichosis in the lumbosacral region (Fig. 5.1.34).

The radiograph of the cervical spine (Fig. 5.1.35) showed rotary displacement at the level of C_4–C_6. Computed tomography of the brain yielded some important

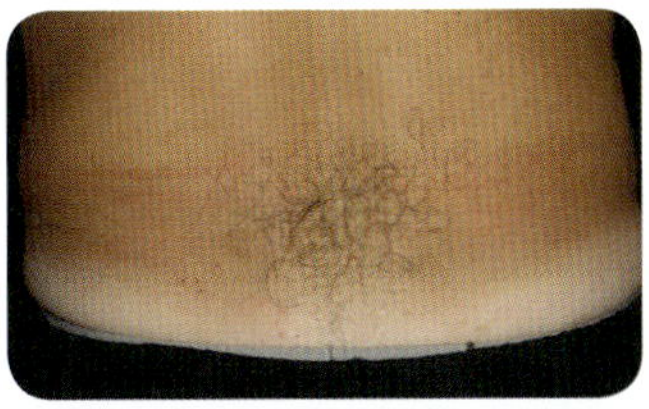

Fig. 5.1.34.

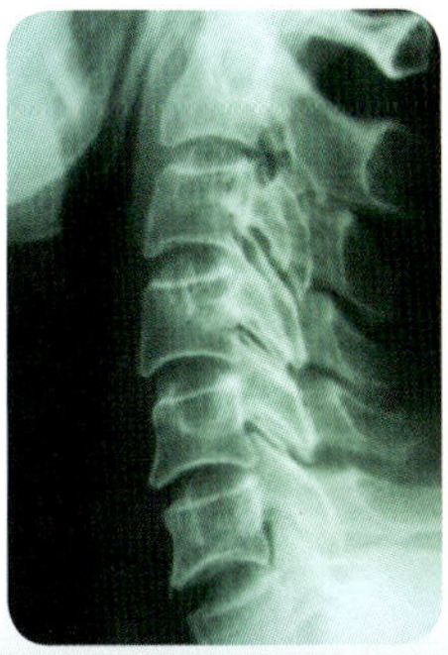

Fig. 5.1.35.

information (Fig. 5.1.36). There were initial signs of atrophy of the cerebral cortex. This was probably related to the weakening of the patient's memory. The radiograph of the lumbosacral region (Fig. 5.1.37) showed lumbarization of S_1 and sacralization of L_5.

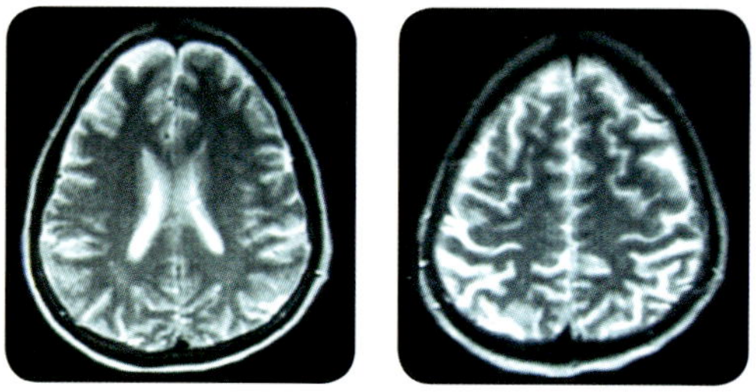

Fig. 5.1.36.
CT of the brain; signs of atrophy and sclerosis of the cerebral cortex

K. had a scoliotic posture, with relative shortening of the left leg. This was compensated for with an insole of a height of **15 mm**.

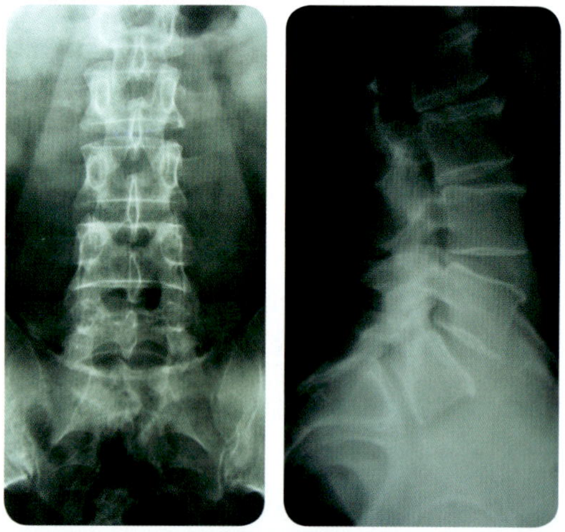

Fig. 5.1.37.
Lumbo-sacral region; lumbarization of S_1; sacralization of L_5

The standard therapy, i.e. the scheme of physical therapy, local magneto-acoustic therapy, use of an insole and inflatable rubber collar, was initiated. The patient was examined regularly for some time. After 3 months of treatment, he noted complete absence of complaints, both legs had become equal in length and his memory had improved. Even though K. had no more complaints, we recommended that he continue with all the treatment measures for the next 6–8 months for preventive purposes.

7. Patient M., a 39-year-old man, consulted us with the complaint of mainly right-sided headaches that had first appeared 15 years earlier. At the age of 10 years, he had sustained a head injury while diving. He had lost consciousness and had suffered from nausea, and had also vomited. Since then, the headache would appear when he exerted or was fatigued, or with exposure to strong odours. M.'s hands and fingers were constantly numb. He suffered from pain in the cervico-collar region of the spine. His other complaints included arrhythmia, heartburn and low back pain, which appeared after lifting loads. Since childhood, he had suffered from cramps in the calf muscles at night. In addition, there was sensory impairment in his right foot (numbness of the big toe). From the manual therapist he received practical skills on how to help himself in reducing dislocation of the lumbar vertebrae, after which the pain would disappear for a long period of time. He did not recover completely.

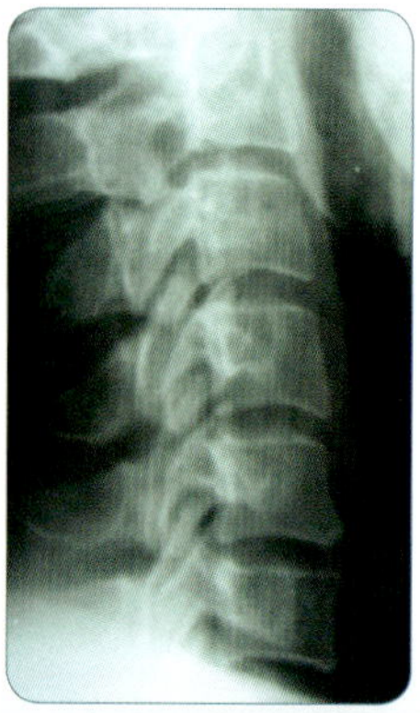

Fig. 5.1.38.

The radiograph of the cervical spine (Fig. 5.1.38) showed that in the lateral plane, there were signs of moderate degenerative disc disease and spondylosis deformans. In addition, there was rotational displacement of the vertebrae at the level of C_4–C_6. Lateral curvature of the spine could be observed in the upper thoracic region (Fig. 5.1.39). M. had a scoliotic posture, with relative shortening of the left leg. This was compensated for with an insole of the height of **3 mm**. The standard therapy, i.e. orthopaedic insole under the left heel, and the scheme of detorsional exercises, local magneto-acoustic therapy, inflatable rubber collar, was initiated. The patient was asked to come for regular monthly check-ups.

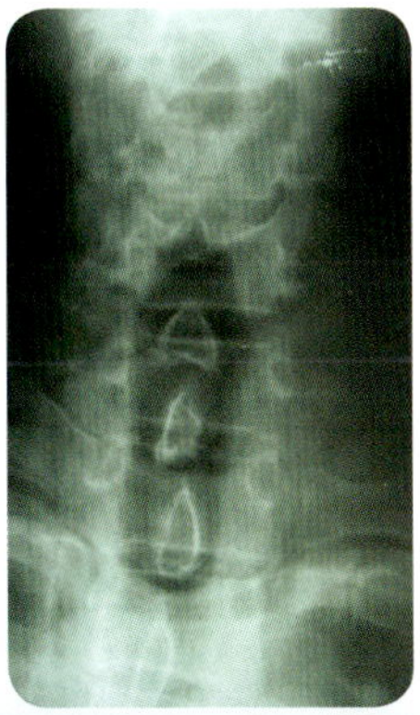

Fig. 5.1.39.

The last check-up was carried out a year after the initiation of the treatment. The pain had resolved in all regions of the spine. Extrasystoles and heartburn occurred periodically. The patient no longer suffered from cramps in the calf muscles. There were no other complaints. He was satisfied with the results of the treatment. M. was advised to repeat the whole course of treatment every 6 months.

8. Patient P., a 39-year-old woman, complained that she lost consciousness or fell when she made slight movements of the head, e.g. while washing her hands or raising her arms after eating. She could not walk independently because she repeatedly lost consciousness. The syncopal condition could last from several minutes to several hours. P. also complained of recurrent headaches, low blood pressure and 'tingling' in the heart. Her face was hyperaemic and oedematous. Her hearing and vision were normal.

P. could not stand, walk or sit for too long and thus always stayed at home. She had 1st stage of neurological disability. At the age of 10, she had undergone surgery for muscular torticollis. She had been under continuous treatment by neurologists and neurosurgeons. She had received treatment in different medical centres, including the Evminov centre, as well as in a psychiatric clinic.

On examining the patient, we observed signs of bilateral plexitis, lumboischialgia and femoral nerve neuritis. Her head movements, both to the right and left sides, were substantially limited.

The radiograph of the cervical spine (Fig. 5.1.40) showed rotary displacement of the vertebrae at the level of C_5–C_6, with no advanced signs of degenerative disc disease and spondylosis. The radiographs of the lumbosacral region (Fig. 5.1.41) showed sacralization of L_5 (wide transverse processes), lumbarization of S_1 and spondylosis deformans.

P. had a scoliotic posture, with relative shortening of the left leg. This was compensated for with an insole of a height of **30 mm**.

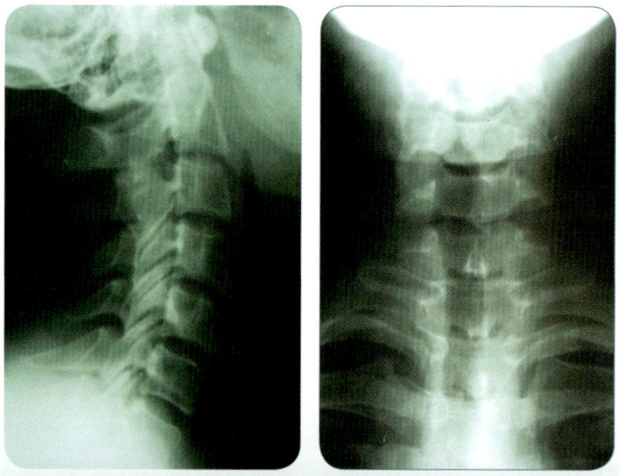

Fig. 5.1.40.

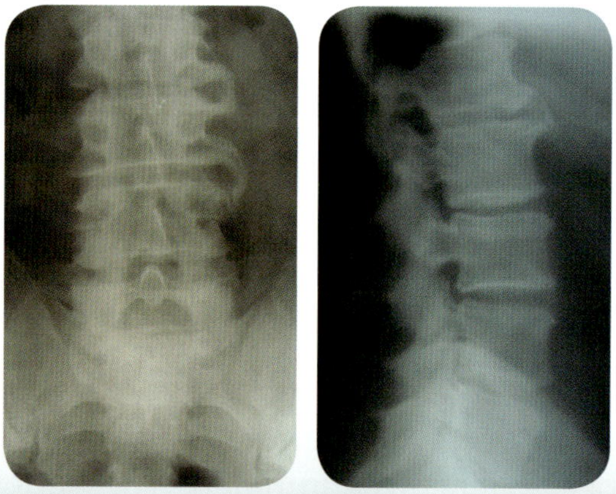

Fig. 5.1.41.

The standard treatment, which included the use of an orthopaedic insole and inflatable rubber collar, besides a set of detorsional exercises, was prescribed. The patient was asked to come for regular monthly check-ups. The last follow-up examination was conducted 4-and-a-half months after the initiation of the treatment. The left leg was still **3 mm** shorter than the right, but there were no more episodes of dizziness and loss of consciousness. P. reported that there had been a significant improvement in her overall condition. She continues with the recommended course of treatment.

9. Patient B., a 40-year-old woman, visited us complaining of constant headaches, vertigo, fluctuations in blood pressure and numbness of the fingers of both hands. She also complained of pain and crackling in the ears when swallowing. There were clinical signs of left-sided plexitis. Heart pain, tachycardia, shortness of breath, heartburn and a tendency to constipation were among her other problems. The patient had a constant pain in the lower back and bilateral lumboischialgia.

B. had a scoliotic posture, with relative shortening of the left leg. This was compensated for with an insole of a height of **10 mm**. Radiography of the cervical spine (Fig. 5.1.42) showed instability and rotational displacement of the vertebrae at the level of C_5–C_6. Radiography of the lumbosacral spine (Fig. 5.1.43) showed lumbarization of S_1, and an intervertebral disc could be observed between the bodies of S_1 and S_2.

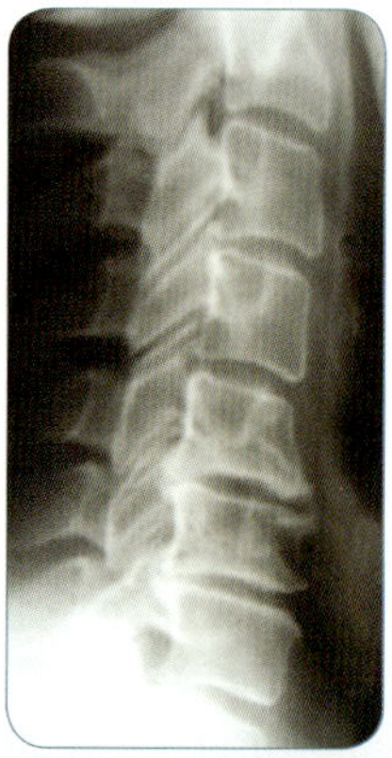

Fig. 5.1.42.

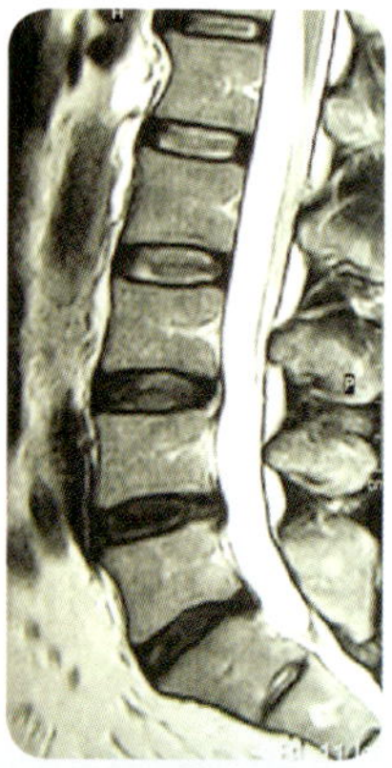

Fig. 5.1.43.

The standard therapy, i.e. insole and the scheme of physical therapy, inflatable collar, local magneto-acoustic therapy, was initiated. A follow-up examination 6 months later showed that the treatment had had a stabilizing, positive effect. The headaches and dizziness had resolved, and the blood pressure had stabilized. The functioning of the intestine had normalized and B. no longer complained of numbness in the fingers. She was satisfied with the outcome of the treatment.

10. Patient M., a 40-year-old woman, complained of persistent headaches, dizziness and discomfort while suddenly turning the head. She said she felt as if a 'stake has been hammered into the neck'. Two years before consulting us, she had had a motor vehicle accident, which had resulted in a cervical injury. She had received ambulatory treatment.

M.'s major complaint was that her body temperature was always raised in the evenings (up to 37.3–37.6 degrees). The fever was accompanied by general weakness. The doctors had suspected various diseases and for quite some time, the patient had been put on various antibiotics, but did not get better.

In addition, M. had 'shooting' pain that radiated to both her legs. She also had chronic tonsillitis. Further, the patient mentioned numbness of the hands and feet, cramps in the calf muscles, 'tingling' in the heart, heartburn and belching.

M. had a scoliotic posture, with relative shortening of the left leg. This was compensated for with an insole of a height of **25 mm**.

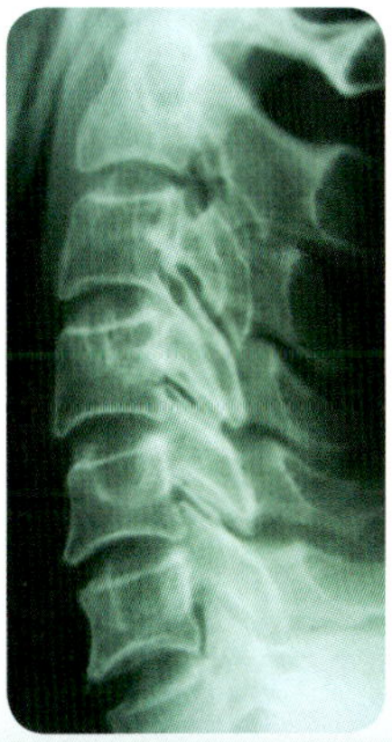
Fig. 5.1.44.

The radiograph of the cervical region (Fig. 5.1.44) showed signs of advanced degenerative disc disease and spondylosis deformans. In addition, segments of C_5–C_6 were rotated and blocked; there were osteophytes on their anterior surface and lordosis was reduced.

The standard therapy, i.e. insole under the left heel and the scheme of physical therapy, local magneto-acoustic therapy, inflatable rubber collar, was initiated. The patient was asked to report for monthly follow-ups. During the assessment 4 months after the initiation of the treatment, M. reported that she had no complaints. There was no more evening fever. The shortening of the left leg was reduced to **3 mm**. M. constantly wore the insole. The patient had made a clinical recovery.

11. Patient O., a 49-year-old woman, complained of frequent headaches, dizziness, hypertensive blood pressure fluctuations and spasms of the cerebral vessels. There were clinical signs of bilateral plexitis and the patient had bilateral femoral nerve neuritis. She complained of numbness of the arms, especially the left one. O. also suffered from recurrent pain in the heart area. Her other complaints included chronic cholecystitis, atrophic gastritis and painful periods. She reported that when she walked for a prolonged period of time, she felt pain along the right and left sciatic nerves.

O. had a scoliotic posture, with relative shortening of the left leg. This was compensated for with an insole of a height of **23 mm**.

The radiograph of the cervical spine (Fig. 5.1.45): showed rotational displacement of the vertebrae at the level of C_4–C_5, while the lumbosacral CT scan (Fig. 5.1.46) showed lumbarization of S_1–S_2.

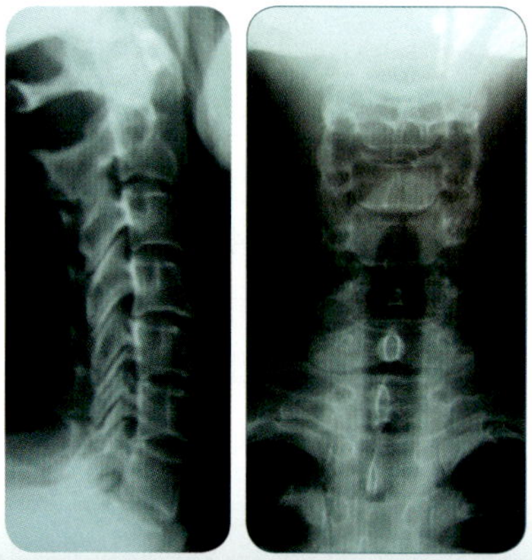

Fig. 5.1.45.

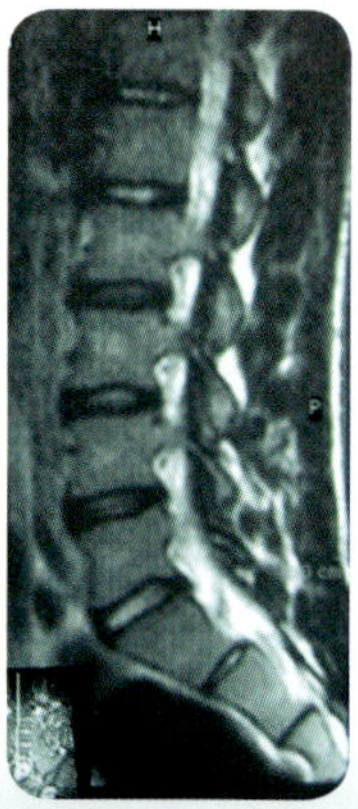

Fig. 5.1.46.

The standard therapy, i.e. insole and the scheme of therapeutic detorsional gymnastics, local magneto-acoustic therapy, was initiated. When the patient was examined 7 months later, shortening of the left leg was no longer observed. She had no complaints. Clinical recovery was apparent, with the headaches, dizziness and numbness of the fingers having subsided. O. no longer complained of numbness of the fingers. Her periods had become painless. Nevertheless, we recommended that she continue with the prescribed treatment and wear an orthopaedic insole of a height of **3 mm** for the next 6–8 months.

12. Patient M., a 50-year-old woman, complained of headaches that involved half her head and tinnitus aurium of 5 years' duration. According to the patient, 'My head is like a drunkard's.' She reported that there had been a marked decline in her memory. M. also complained of pain under her left shoulder blade, 'tingling' in the heart and occasional shortness of breath. It was seen that palpation of her cervical vertebrae caused severe pain. M. also had low back pain that radiated to both legs. Her feet were very cold.

M. had a scoliotic posture, with relative shortening of the left leg. This was compensated for with an insole of a height of **20 mm**. The CT scan of the brain showed signs of partial atrophy of the frontal lobe cortex (Fig. 5.1.47). The radiograph of the cervical spine (Fig. 5.1.48) revealed that there was advanced deforming spondylosis at the site of rotary displacement of the vertebrae in the C_5–C_6 segment. It was blocked by exostoses on the anterior and posterior surfaces. At the level of C_4–C_7, there was kyphotic curvature instead of physiological lordosis.

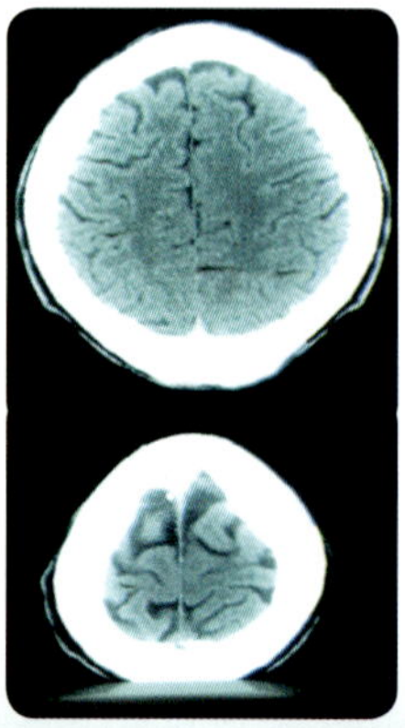

Fig. 5.1.47.

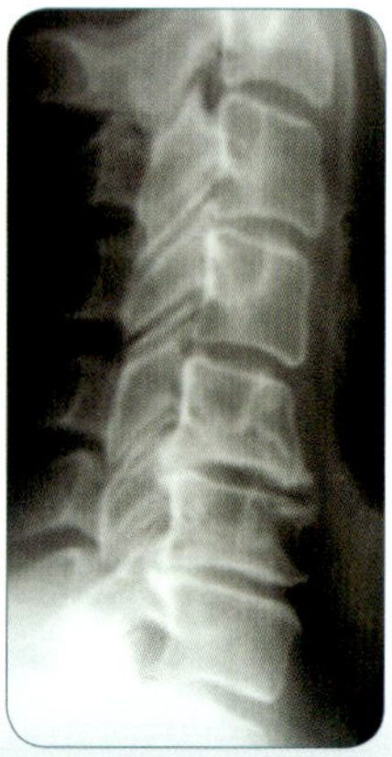

Fig. 5.1.48.

The standard therapy, i.e. insole and the scheme of physiotherapy, local magneto-acoustic therapy, inflatable rubber collar, was initiated. During the follow-up examination 9 months later, M. reported that she did not suffer from headaches any longer and had no other complaints. There was no shortening of the left leg.

13. Patient K., a 50-year-old woman, complained of dizziness and 'ringing' in the left ear. These problems had begun 4–5 months earlier. She had sustained a cervical spine injury 2 years before consulting us and had received treatment in the neurological department of the city hospital. The consequences of the trauma (rotating displacement of C_4–C_6, flattening of lordosis) were evident on the radiograph of the cervical region (Fig. 5.1.49). K. had a scoliotic posture, with relative shortening of the left leg. This was compensated for with an insole of a height of **10 mm**.

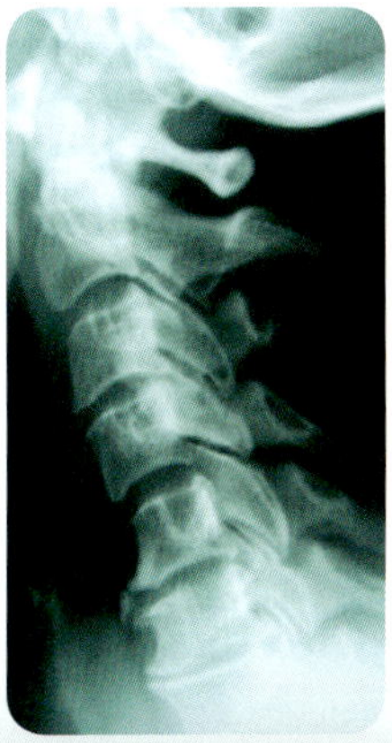

Fig. 5.1.49.

The standard therapy, i.e. insole and the scheme of therapeutic detorsional gymnastics, local magneto-acoustic therapy, inflatable rubber collar, was initiated. The follow-up examination 9 months later showed that the two legs were now equal in length. The patient reported that there had been a significant improvement in her overall condition and she had no complaints.

14. Patient O., a 50-year-old man, came to us complaining of persisting shoulder pain of several years' duration. It appeared at night and was more pronounced on the right. In his adolescence, he had sustained a cervical spine injury while exercising. The radiograph of the cervical spine (Fig. 5.1.50) showed signs of rotational displacement of the vertebrae at the level of the C_5–C_6 segment, followed by osteochondrosis and spondylosis deformans.

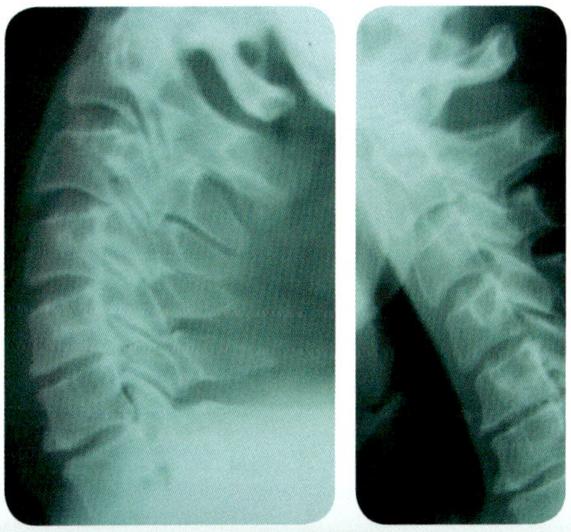

Fig. 5.1.50.

The patient also complained of lumbosacral pain radiating to both hip joints. The radiograph of this region (Fig. 5.1.51) revealed sacralization of L_5, lumbarization of S_1 and asymmetry of the articular processes in the L_5–S_1 segment.

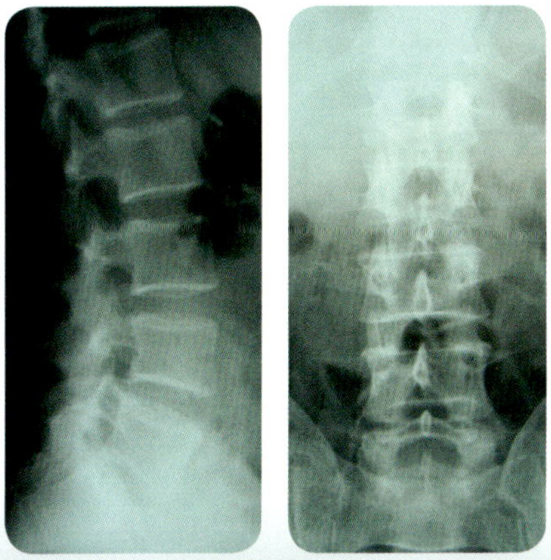

Fig. 5.1.51.

O. had a scoliotic posture, with relative shortening of the left leg. This was compensated for with an insole of a height of **20 mm**. The standard therapy, i.e. insole and the scheme of therapeutic detorsional gymnastics, local magneto-acoustic therapy, inflatable rubber collar, was initiated. Follow-up examination was performed 8 months after the treatment. O. had no complaints. The left leg was of the same height as the right. Clinical improvement was observed in the patient's condition. He was advised to further his recovery at a sanatorium and resort.

15. Patient G., a 50-year-old woman, complained of frequent headaches and numbness of the hands, especially at night. About 8 years before she consulted us, she used to suffer from very intense pain in the lumbar spine and had cramps in the legs. She had been treated by neurologists and traditional healers, but had not recovered.

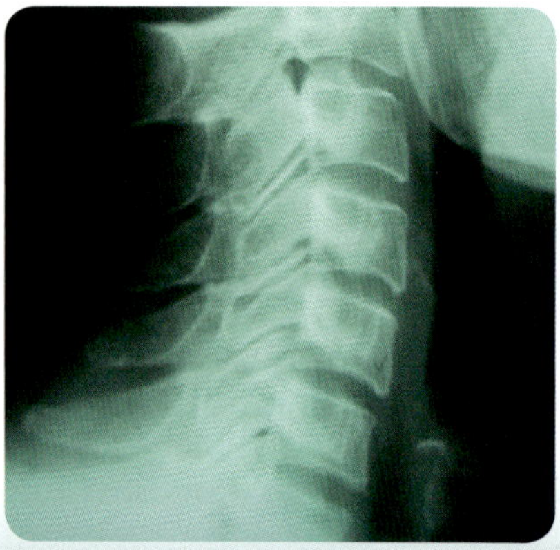

Fig. 5.1.52.

G. had a scoliotic posture, with relative shortening of the left leg. This was compensated for with an insole of a height of **23 mm**. The radiograph of the cervical region (Fig. 5.1.52) showed rotational subluxation of the vertebrae in the C_4–C_6 segment. The radiograph of the lumbar region (Fig. 5.1.53) showed lumbarization of S_1, spina bifida S_1 and sacralization of L_5.

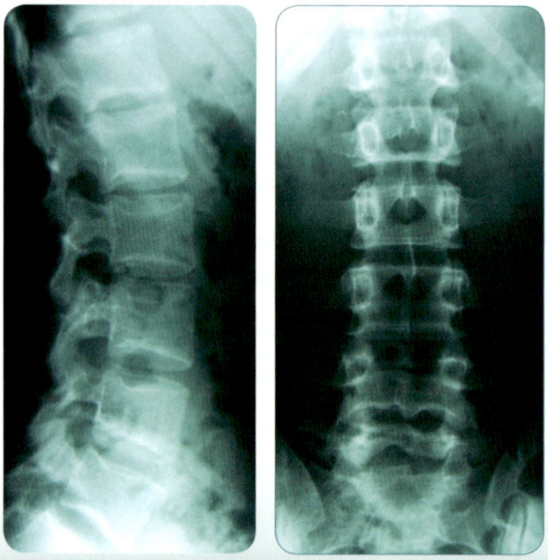

Fig. 5.1.53.

The standard therapy, i.e. orthopaedic insole under the left heel and the scheme of detorsional exercises and local magneto-acoustic therapy, was initiated. Treatment at a sanatorium and resort, including underwater traction, was recommended. When G. was examined 8 months later, it was seen that the left leg was shorter than the right by **3 mm**. The numbness of the hands, leg cramps and pain had subsided. The patient had made a clinical recovery.

16. Patient P., a 52-year-old man, was referred to our clinic with the complaints of persistent headache, hypertensive fluctuations in blood pressure and periodic breathlessness. The range of head movements of the cervical spine was limited. From the history, we knew that the patient had sustained a cervical spine injury at the age of 45.

The radiograph of the cervical region (Fig. 5.1.54) showed marked signs of degenerative disc disease and spondylosis deformans at the level of the C_5–C_7 segments with their rotational displacement. Ossification of the anterior longitudinal ligament could also be observed.

P. had a scoliotic posture, with relative shortening of the left leg. This was compensated for with an insole of a height of **17 mm**.

The standard treatment, i.e. orthopaedic insole under the left heel and the scheme of physical therapy, local magneto-acoustic therapy, inflatable rubber collar, was initiated. The results of the treatment, as assessed a year and 2 months after initiation, were encouraging. The left leg was no longer shorter than the right and P.'s blood pressure was within the range appropriate for his age. The patient had no complaints and had recovered clinically.

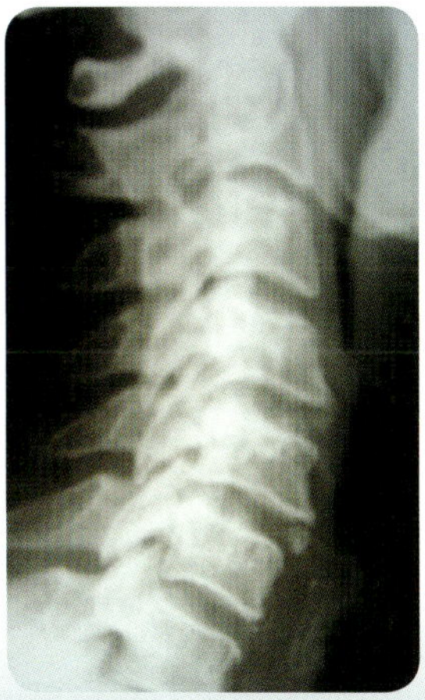

Fig. 5.1.54.

17. Patient L., a 55-year-old man, complained of numbness of the fingers of the right hand, bilateral plexitis (more pronounced on the right side), coldness of the hands and bilateral lumboischialgia. Nine years before consulting us, L. had sustained a traumatic brain injury in a motor vehicle accident and had been unconscious for a few hours. Both his hands were paralysed by severe pain. Then a psychic had reduced the cervical vertebrae, after which he had had no complaints for the next nine years. However, the pain had appeared again several weeks before he contacted us, due to lifting of loads (together with rotation of the body).

The radiograph of the cervical spine (Fig. 5.1.55) showed rotational displacement of C_4–C_6. The resulting instability of these injured segments led to their blockade. There were advanced signs of post-traumatic deforming spondylosis.

L. had a scoliotic posture, with relative shortening of the right leg. This was compensated for with an insole of a height of **20 mm**.

The standard treatment, i.e. orthopaedic insole under the right heel and the scheme of detorsional physiotherapy, local magneto-acoustic therapy, inflatable rubber collar, was initiated. During the follow-up examination 6 months later, it was found that the reduction in height of the right leg had decreased to **3 mm**. There was virtually no pain and the patient was satisfied with the results of the treatment. He was advised to continue with the same treatment for one year more.

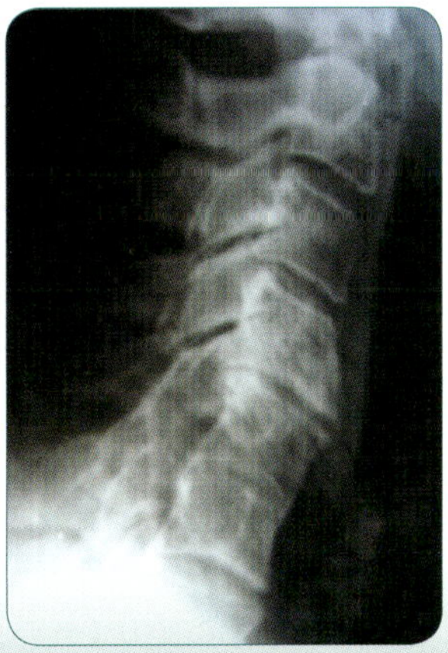

Fig. 5.1.55.

18. Patient G., a 64-year-old woman, complained of dizziness, headaches, tinnitus (ringing in the ears), buzzing in the head and low blood pressure. She reported that she could not walk independently or maintain a vertical body position—'she skids off'. She suffered from persistent pain in the heart and legs, as well as severe cramps in the calf muscles.

G. had a scoliotic posture, with relative shortening of the right leg. This was compensated for with an insole of a height of **18 mm**.

The radiograph of the cervical spine (Fig. 5.1.56) showed advanced signs of deforming spondylosis at the level of C_5–C_7. One could also observe ossification of the anterior longitudinal ligament and bony exostoses. Segment C_4–C_6 was blocked, being rotated around its axes.

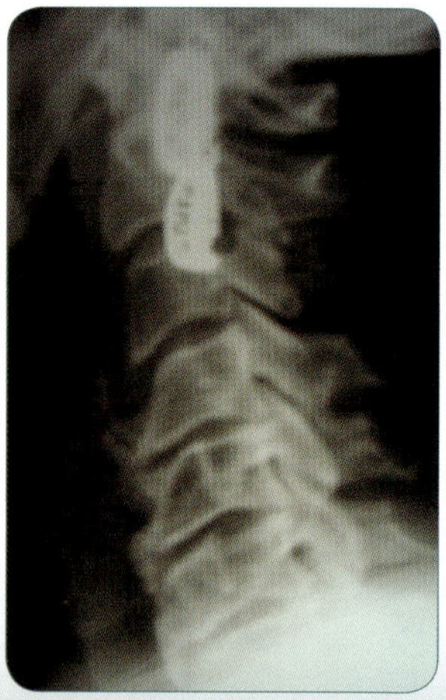

Fig. 5.1.56.

The standard treatment, i.e. orthopaedic insole under the left foot and the scheme of physical therapy, local magneto-acoustic therapy, inflatable rubber collar, was initiated. During the follow-up visit 6 months later, the patient reported that the treatment had had a very beneficial effect. Her blood pressure had returned to normal, she could walk along the street alone, and there was no dizziness or headaches. The cramps in the calf muscles had also resolved. The right leg was still **7 mm** shorter than the left. G. was advised to continue with the treatment for one year from the time of its initiation.

19. Patient G., a 68-year-old man, complained of dizziness, constant headaches and hypertensive fluctuations in blood pressure. His fingers felt numb and his hands sweaty and cold. About 15 years earlier, he had sustained a cervical spine injury in a car accident. On examining him, we found that the range of movement of his neck was severely limited. G. had a scoliotic posture, with relative shortening of the right leg. This was compensated for with an insole of a height of **15 mm**.

The radiograph of the cervical spine (Fig. 5.1.57) showed signs of advanced degenerative disc disease and spondylosis deformans. Rotation of the vertebrae at the level of C_5–C_7 had resulted in instability leading, in turn, to ossification of the anterior and posterior longitudinal ligaments, as well as the formation of bony exostoses, mainly in the area of C_5–C_6. Further, segment C_5–C_7 was blocked.

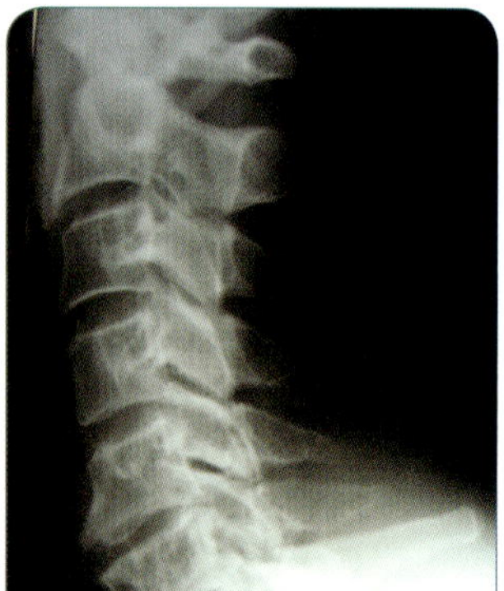

Fig. 5.1.57.

The standard treatment, i.e. orthopaedic insole under the right heel and the scheme of physical therapy, local magneto-acoustic therapy, inflatable rubber collar, was initiated. The long-term outcome of the treatment was assessed in one year: The blood pressure had become normal, and the headaches and dizziness had resolved. The patient considered himself healthy. As a preventive measure, he was advised to permanently wear an insole of a thickness of **3 mm**.

Our analysis of cases from clinical practice highlighted the following conclusions.

1. Rotational displacement of the cervical vertebrae was observed in all patients. It always occurred in certain typical locations: C_1–C_2, in addition to the physiological curvature; C_3–C_5; at the level of C_6–C_7; and at the level of the transition to the upper thoracic region. These types of displacements are determined by the laws of biomechanics of the musculoskeletal system, as mentioned in Chapter 3.
2. Rotational displacements of the vertebrae in these areas led to compression of the medulla oblongata and its centres and pathways, as well as of the spinal cord, ganglia, cervical plexuses of the vagus nerve, sympathetic and parasympathetic trunks, spinal nerves, etc. As a result, the symptoms of various pathological conditions appeared. The subsequent prolonged dysfunction of parts of different neuroregulatory systems and the organs and tissues which functioned under their control eventually led to changes in the anatomical structure and development of true pathology.
3. The severity of the complaints as well as the deficiency in blood flow through the vertebral arteries were not directly related to the degree of relative shortening of one leg. The deficit in blood supply could reach 40%–50% or more in patients with a minimum degree of shortening of 3 mm, as well as in those with the maximum degree of shortening of 20 mm. It was the diameter of the transverse foramina that was of crucial importance. The smaller the diameter and the greater the degree of rotation of the vertebrae, the more vertebral arteries, veins and nerves were compressed.
4. In all patients, the use of an orthopaedic insole led to correction of the scoliotic posture. It seems natural to ask why and how.

We consider it useful to elaborate on some of the observations made above.

In the cases discussed above, scoliotic (lateral) curvature of the spine was of a compensatory–adaptive nature and of a conditioned reflexive origin. In essence, this process consisted of the following: unilateral spasm of the spinal extensors resulted in a pelvic tilt towards the right or left side and, accordingly, development of deformation of the spine. The entire process was the result of asymmetrical functioning of the cerebral hemispheres. This body position was fixed in the cerebellum as a conditioned reflex. We call it a reflex of 'wrong' vertical body position.

The prolonged use of an insole of the appropriate height led to the gradual formation of the 'correct' reflex and consequently correction of the spinal deformity. This new body position came to be fixed in the brain and preserved in later life.

5. When the vertebral axis was corrected so as to be made perpendicular to the pelvic

plane, it led to reduction in the lateral curvature and release of all the anatomical structures mentioned earlier from compression. The pathological symptoms subsided due to dosed traction of the cervical vertebrae with the help of an inflatable collar and detorsional gymnastics, as well as local magneto-acoustic-therapy, which has pronounced anti-inflammatory, anti-oedematous and analgesic effects. Thus, clinical recovery occurred.

6. The reader might be interested in knowing how we explain the fact that in the same location of displacement of vertebrae in a single region (cervical localization) such a diversity of clinical symptoms were observed. This situation can probably be attributed to the fact that the anatomical structures of the vertebral bodies, their processes, arches, etc. have many variants.

Besides the displacement of the cervical vertebrae relative to each other, compression of the anatomical structures of the medulla oblongata, blood vessels and nuclei of the cranial nerves, as well as pathways of the brain and spinal cord could be a result of reduction in the height of the intervertebral discs and consequently of the diameter of intervertebral foramina. The reason for this is degenerative disc disease and spondylosis of varying degrees of severity.

Such a variety of symptoms can be likened to musical compositions that are built on endless combinations of seven notes, which sound different because of the manner in which the notes have been arranged. One can also compare it to the way we can obtain a myriad colours by mixing just three basic colours.

Although at first glance our conclusions and findings did not give us cause for optimism, we could say on the basis of our clinical experience that, given a deep understanding of the aetiopathogenesis of the diseases discussed above, the doctor can prescribe extremely effective preventive measures and even treatment of these diseases. With the help of a active therapeutic physical training (detorsional gymnastics), combined with physiotherapy (magneto-acoustic therapy), use of an inflatable rubber collar and orthopaedic insoles, which will be discussed in the concluding chapter of this book, we were able to provide effective treatment to a large number of the patients who consulted us.

5.2 Thoracic spine

When we started working on this section, we faced a dilemma as how to choose several dozens of the most interesting cases from the thousands of available observations. We wanted to show that we had been able to help even in very difficult cases, when a patient had been suffering from one or more diseases for a long time, sometimes for years. We tried to select those cases in which the patient complained of pain predominantly in the thoracic region of the spine. However, if you take a look at Fig. 5.2.1, it becomes clear that the incredibly complex system of innervation of our body exists only as an organic whole. All parts of the central and peripheral nervous systems are interrelated and, therefore, the allocation of patients to a separate group (e.g. thoracic spine) should be considered rather conditional, although it is necessary to facilitate an understanding of our material.

Patients who complained of pain predominantly in the thoracic region of the spine often had one or more of the following conditions:

- Osteochondrosis and spondylosis deformans
- Spinal hernias, including Schmorl's hernia
- Scoliosis and kyphoscoliosis
- Compression of vertebral bodies as a result of injury, osteoporosis, bone tissue destruction in multiple myeloma, tumours, tuberculosis, etc.

These pathological conditions were usually accompanied by pain in the interscapular region, retrosternal pain radiating to the heart, pain in the stomach and abdomen (in women towards the ovaries), and the signs of various diseases. They included:

- Hypothyroidism
- Vegetovascular dystonia
- Chronic maxillary sinusitis
- Vasomotor rhinitis
- Hypertension liquorodynamic syndrome
- Plexitis
- Bronchial asthma

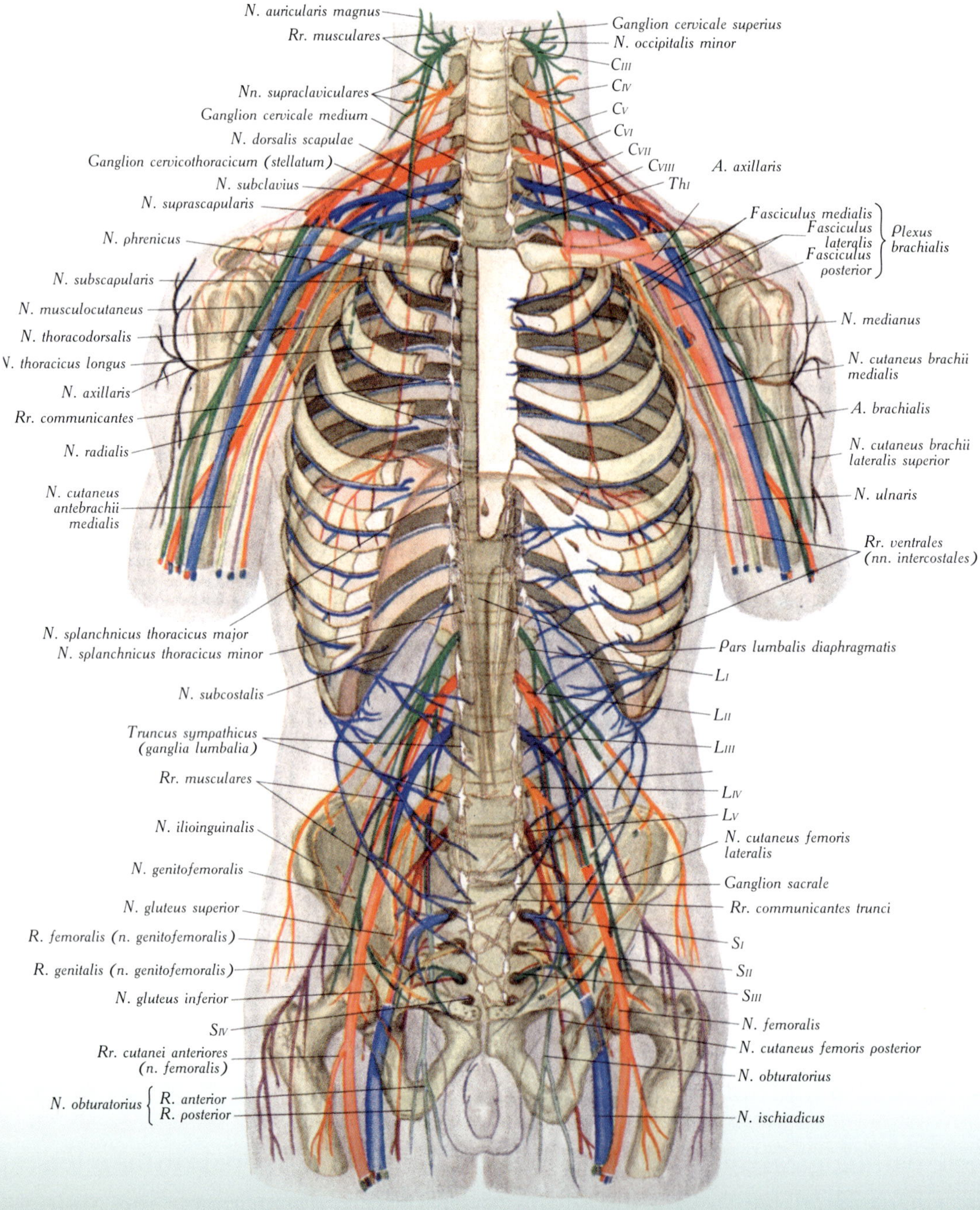

Fig. 5.2.1.
Spinal nerves, nn. spinales; front view (diagram)

- Breath-holding, shortness of breath
- Breathlessness, chronic bronchitis
- Extrasystoles, tachycardia, arrhythmias
- Coronary artery disease
- Unstable angina
- Belching, flatulence
- Hyperacid gastritis with a tendency to constipation

- Cramps in the stomach and intestines
- Gastric and/or duodenal ulcers
- Cholecystitis, chronic pancreatitis
- Constipation or diarrhoea (or alternation of the two)
- Frequent urge to urinate
- Sudden weight loss or obesity
- Psoriasis with lesions of the scalp and upper extremities.

The reader is probably wondering what these diseases have in common and may be speculating that perhaps they have the same or similar aetiological origin. We immediately explain—yes, they do.

The loss of height of the thoracic intervertebral discs led to the formation of wedge-shaped and other deformations of the vertebral bodies, rotational displacements of vertebrae about their axes, and compression of the spinal cord and its meninges (*see* Figs 2.29, 2.30), the blood vessels supplying it, spinal nerves, ganglia, plexuses, as well as sympathetic and parasympathetic nerve fibres (Figs 5.2.2–5.2.5). This caused not only spinal pain, but also deregulation of the functioning of the ascending and descending pathways of the cerebrum, medulla oblongata and cerebellum which, in turn, led to

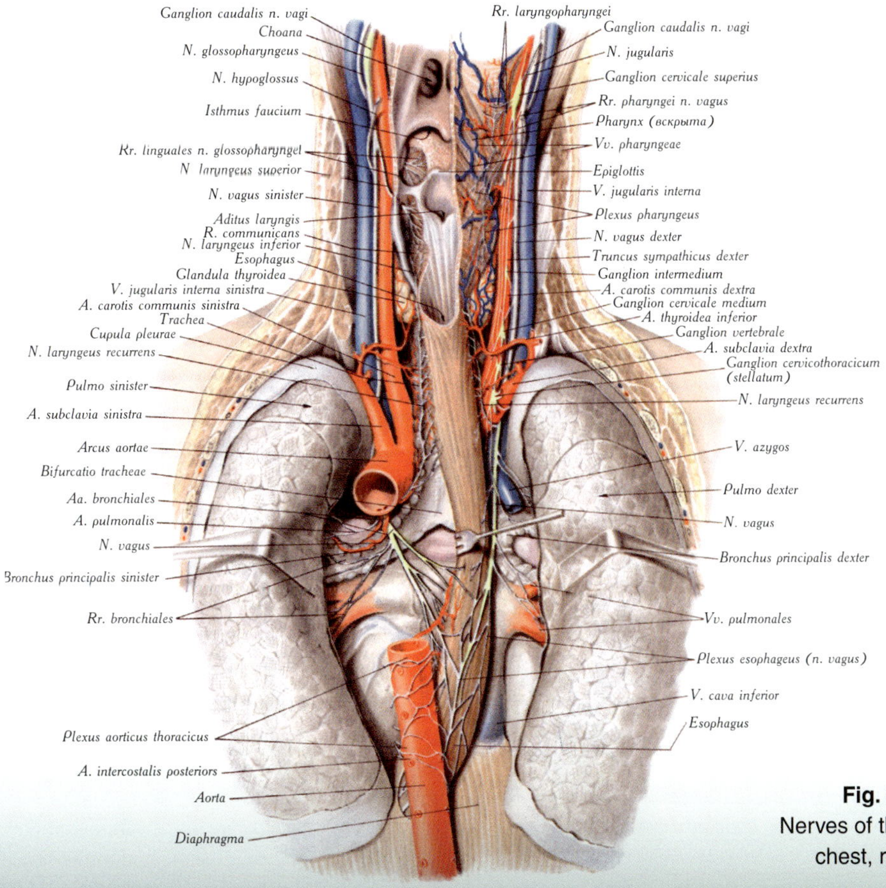

Fig. 5.2.2.
Nerves of the neck and chest, rear view

Fig. 5.2.3.
Nerves of the heart, view from the left (2/5)

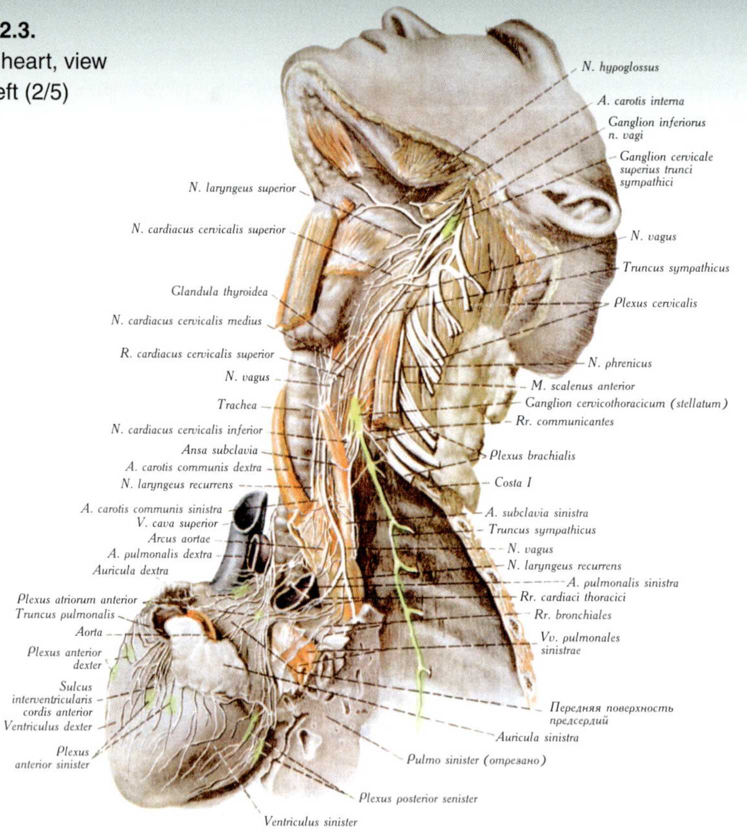

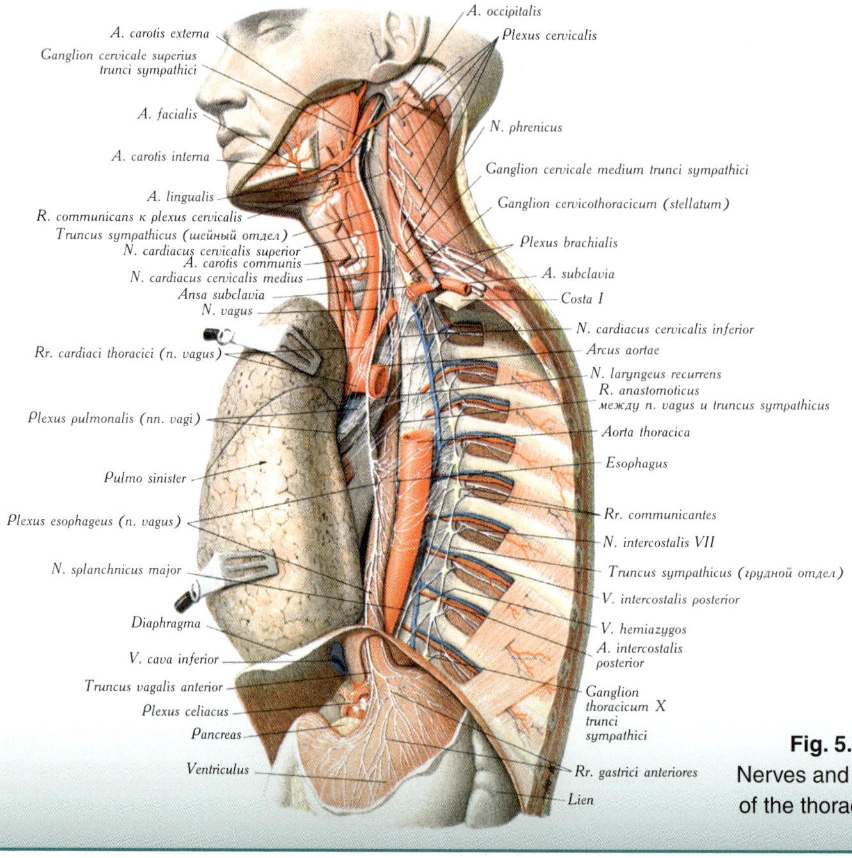

Fig. 5.2.4.
Nerves and plexuses of the thoracic cavity

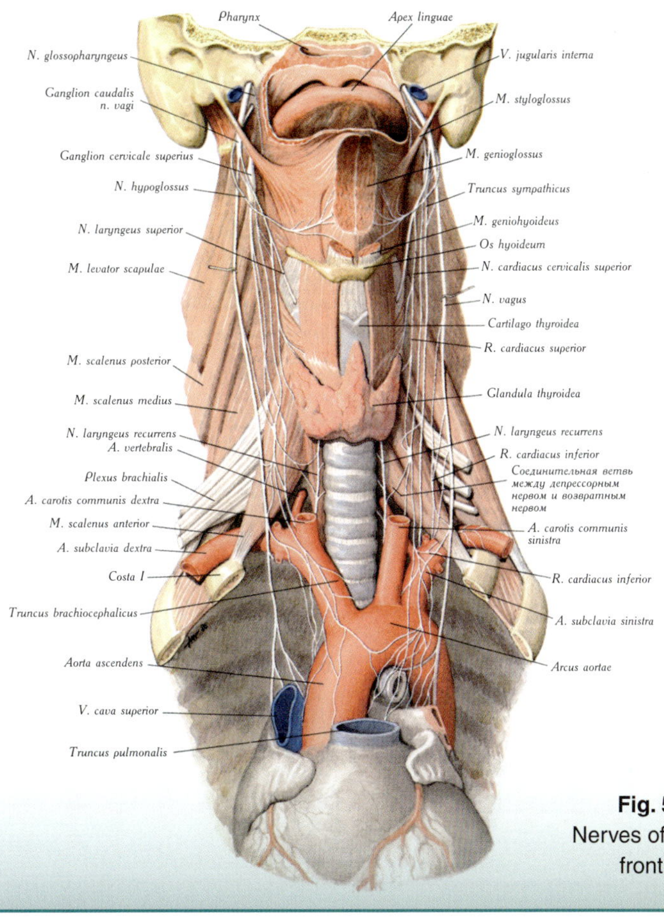

Fig. 5.2.5.
Nerves of the neck, front view

malfunctioning of the heart, lungs, stomach, liver, pancreas, kidneys, adrenal glands, intestines, bladder, organs of the large and small pelvis, etc. Compression of the above-mentioned structures of the spinal cord and other surrounding anatomical formations at different levels of the thoracic spine caused symptoms of various diseases.

Thus, when the process of compression occurred at the level of C_6–Th_3, we often found signs of vegetovascular dystonia (coldness of the hands and sweaty hands, usually accompanied by emotional lability and exophthalmos). Arrhythmias with extrasystoles were characteristic in such cases. Often, symptoms of asthma, pharyngitis, laryngitis, breathlessness and chronic cough were also present.

Rotational displacements of vertebrae at the level of Th_1–Th_4 may be accompanied by allergies (including in infants), cardiac pain, asthma or emphysema, chronic bronchitis, sudden breath-holding, pneumonia, tuberculosis, frequent colds, etc.

As for compression of the spinal cord, nerves and ganglia at the level of Th_4–Th_5, the patient may have symptoms of a wide variety of diseases, including acholia, hepatomegaly, jaundice, hepatitis, cirrhosis of the liver. Compression at the level of Th_6–Th_7 may give rise to gastric cancer and gastric and/or duodenal ulcers, both among adults and children of different ages, including those in pre-school. When the site of compression is at the level of Th_8–Th_9, the patient may suffer from liver disease, pancreatolithiasis, cholelithiasis, splenomegaly or diaphragmatic hernia.

If compression of the spinal structures mentioned above occurs at the level of Th_9–Th_{12}, the main symptoms are pain in the region of the liver and gallbladder, associated with biliary dyskinesia and cholelithiasis, as well as heartburn, belching and gastritis. These patients can also have symptoms of diabetes mellitus and diabetes insipidus, kidney disease with prolapse of one kidney, haematuria, aciduria, diarrhoea, indigestion, and a tendency to constipation or a frequent urge to defaecate and urinate.

Our everyday experience with patients who had spinal deformities showed us how the various diseases listed in Fig. 5.4 actually occurred. In the initial stages of the disease, the patient had only vertebrogenic symptoms, with no disruption in the anatomical structure of the organ concerned. However, there were significant morphological changes subsequently that led to the development of true pathological processes. Thus, early detection of thoracalgia allows one to initiate treatment in good time and avoid progression of disease in the organs of the chest and abdomen.

It is important to note that in all our patients, irrespective of age, pathological conditions involving the internal organs were necessarily associated with spinal deformities. Among young people, the correction of these deformities led to the elimination of the symptoms of certain diseases fairly quickly, while among those who were middle-aged or older, the healing process did take place but its pace depended on the overall duration of the illness.

Of course, the effectiveness of our treatment varied if the patient was a 2- year-old or a 90-year-old, but nonetheless it was seen to have a positive effect, which brought us more and more new patients. However, as in the case of the group of patients with changes predominantly in the cervical spine, among the group with changes predominantly in the thoracic spine, it was extremely rare for the pain to be confined only to the thoracic region. Even among children, scoliotic and kyphotic deformities that posed a challenge, predisposition for rotational displacement of the vertebrae in all regions of the spine (Chapter 3) led to functional impairments both of the chest and abdominal organs and other body parts (neck, lower back, sacrum and the extremities). This issue will be discussed further later.

We present a number of clinical cases from our observations, in which the outcomes of treatment were assessed both in the short term and long term (up to 18 months).

1. Patient M., a 56-year-old woman, had been diagnosed with vegetovascular dystonia and had been under the treatment of a neurologist for the past 15 years. She suffered from dizziness and could not get out of bed. She received inpatient treatment in the neurological department twice a year, but the treatment had proved to be ineffective. For the one-and-a-half months before she consulted us, the dizziness had become continuous. Her vision had deteriorated drastically. At night, M. suffered from seizures and her hands went numb. Her other complaints included heart pain, breathlessness, arrhythmias, gastritis, constant belching and cramps in the calf muscles, especially at night. In addition, the patient reported pain in the lumbar region, radiating to both legs. She said that she 'screamed like crazy' because of pain.

The dopplerography of the cerebral and cervical blood vessels revealed that there was extravasal compression of the vertebral artery at the level of C_3. There was a deficiency in blood flow on the left side of up to 35% and on the right side of 25%. A CT scan of the head showed areas of cortical sclerosis caused by chronic ischaemia (Fig. 5.2.6).

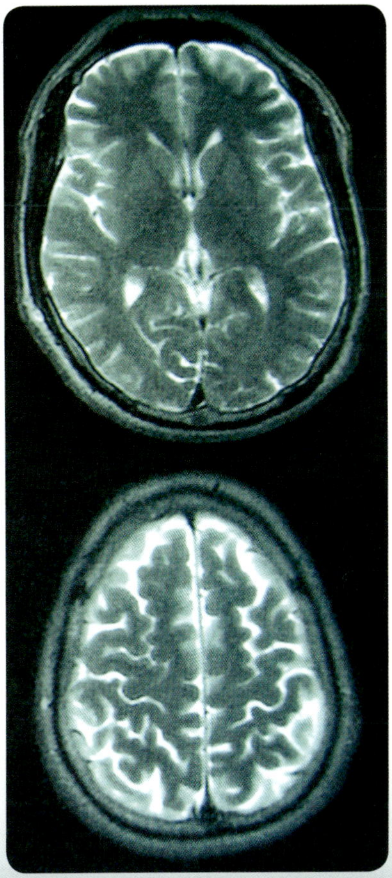

Fig. 5.2.6.

On examination of the patient, we found that she had a severe scoliotic deformity of the chest (2nd–3rd degree), with a right-sided rib hump. Pressure on the cervical, thoracic and lumbar vertebrae was causing severe pain. Movement of her head was severely limited. She had clinical signs of bilateral plexitis, as well as femoral and sciatic nerve neuritis. Relative shortening of the left leg (**15 mm**) was observed.

The standard treatment, i.e. orthopaedic insole, detorsional gymnastics, local transcranial and paravertebral magneto-acoustic therapy, inflatable rubber collar, was initiated. The patient was followed up regularly every 1.5–2 months. When she was examined after 2 months, the relative shortening of the left leg was found to have decreased to **10 mm**. The pain in the lumbar region had resolved almost completely, and there was no pain in the heart or breathlessness. At 6 months' follow-up, the patient reported that she suffered only slight dizziness and her vision had stabilized. She had no other complaints. The axis of the spine was correct and there was no asymmetry of the spinal muscles. The relative shortening of the leg was reduced to **3 mm**. The patient continued to wear an orthopaedic insole. Though she considered herself healthy, we recommended that she continue to perform detorsional corrective exercises during the coming year.

2. Patient B., a 45-year-old woman, complained of burning pain in the chest and spine (interscapular region). She said that her hands turned numb when she raised them. Her other complaints included asthma attacks and deterioration in her hearing and vision. All these symptoms had been intensifying over the past 5 years. B. had been diagnosed with 'chronic bronchitis' and was under the treatment of an internist. She periodically received treatment as an inpatient in the therapeutic department.

Radiographs of the thoracic spine revealed signs of degenerative disc disease and spondylosis deformans (Fig. 5.2.7), as well as lateral curvature of the spine (Fig. 5.2.8).

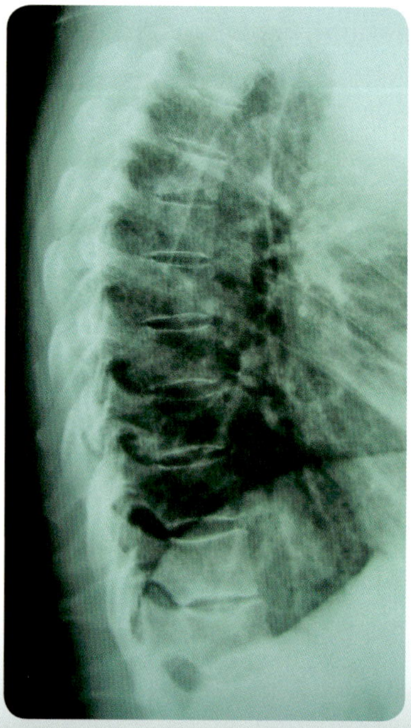

Fig. 5.2.7.

Examination of the patient showed that she had a scoliotic deformity of the thoracic spine. There was a significant pelvic inclination towards the left side, which was compensated for with an insole of a height of **20 mm**. The rotation of the neck was severely limited. The pressure on the spinous processes of the cervical and thoracic vertebrae caused severe pain to the patient.

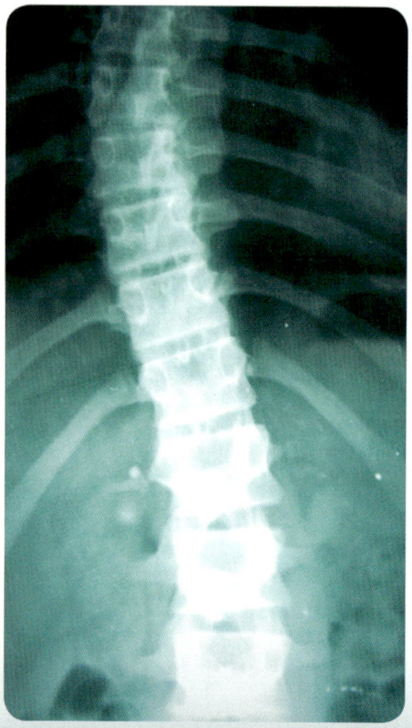

Fig. 5.2.8.

The standard treatment, i.e. orthopaedic insole, detorsional exercises, local transcranial and paravertebral magneto-acoustic therapy, inflatable rubber collar, was initiated. When B. was examined in two-and-a-half months, her hearing and vision had stabilized. The pain in the interscapular region had resolved. She reported that there had been a significant improvement in respiratory function and she had had no asthma attacks. At 8 months' follow-up, the axis of the spine was found to have become correct and there was no asymmetry of the spinal muscles. There were residual signs of chronic bronchitis. The patient no longer suffered from pain in the chest or numbness of the hands. The relative shortening of the left leg had been reduced to **3 mm**. B. was satisfied with the results of the treatment, and considers herself healthy. She was advised to perform detorsional exercises on a regular basis.

3. Patient B., a 36-year-old man, who had sustained a spinal injury during his childhood, visited us with the complaint of persistent pain throughout the spine, especially in the neck and lower back. His other complaints included deafness, chronic sinusitis, numbness of the fingers, extrasystoles, and cramps in the calf muscles and toes. The treatment he had received so far had been ineffective.

A radiograph of the cervical area revealed rotational displacement of C_3–C_5 (above the curvature), osteochondrosis and spondylosis deformans, the severity of which was not significant (Fig. 5.2.9). Radiographs of the lumbosacral spine revealed spondylosis deformans, sacralization of L_5, lumbarization of S_1 and asymmetry of the articular processes of the L_5–S_1 SMS (Fig. 5.2.10).

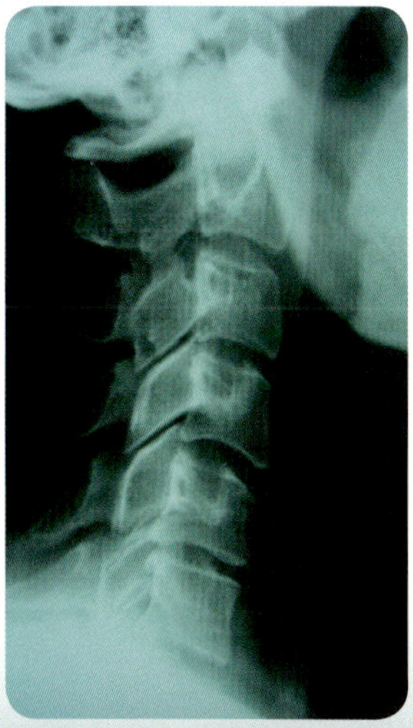

Fig. 5.2.9.

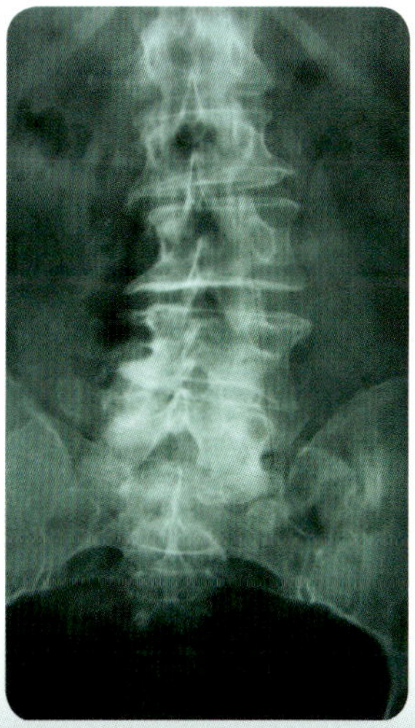

Fig. 5.2.10.

On examination of the patient, we observed signs of relative shortening of the left leg by **20 mm**. He had scoliotic deformation of 2–3 degrees. The movements of his head were severely restricted. There were rotary displacements of the vertebrae in the cervical, thoracic and lumbosacral regions. Clinically, this was manifested as bilateral plexitis, lumbar ischialgia and neuritis of the femoral nerves. At all levels, palpation of the spinous processes gave rise to severe pain.

The standard treatment, i.e. orthopaedic insole, physiotherapy, local paravertebral and transcranial magneto-acoustic therapy, inflatable rubber collar, was initiated. During an examination 3 months later, the patient reported that the pain had more or less retreated in all the regions of the back. There was no numbness or cramping of the fingers, and no extrasystoles. The signs of plexitis and lumbar ischialgia were now minor. At 9 months' follow-up, B. had no complaints and considered himself healthy. The axis of the spine was in the process of being corrected and the back muscles were no longer asymmetrical. However, since the left leg was still **3 mm** shorter than the right, the patient was advised to continue with detorsional gymnastics for another 6–7 months.

4. Patient Z., a 54-year-old woman, complained of arrhythmia, extrasystoles, heartburn, belching, stomachache before meals, hyperacidity and hyperacid gastritis. She had been suffering from severe headaches for more than 20 years. She had been treated by a neurologist, neurosurgeon and gastroenterologist, but nothing had helped. Her medical history revealed that at the age of 12 years, she had fallen from the upper berth of a train and suffered a brain concussion. She had learnt how to reduce rotational dislocation of cervical vertebrae herself and the pain would resolve after she performed this manoeuvre. Z. also suffered from vegetovascular dystonia

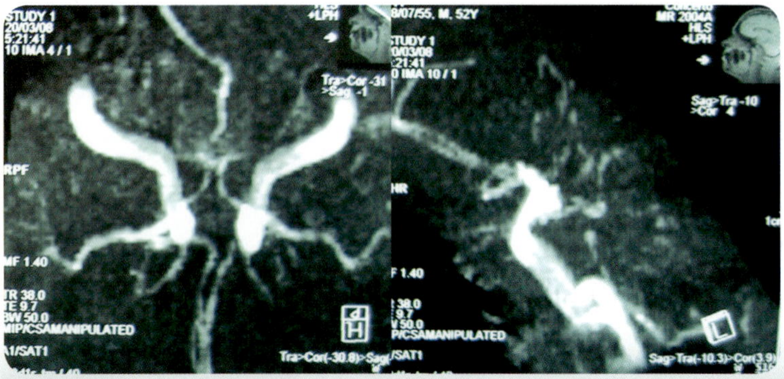

Fig. 5.2.11.

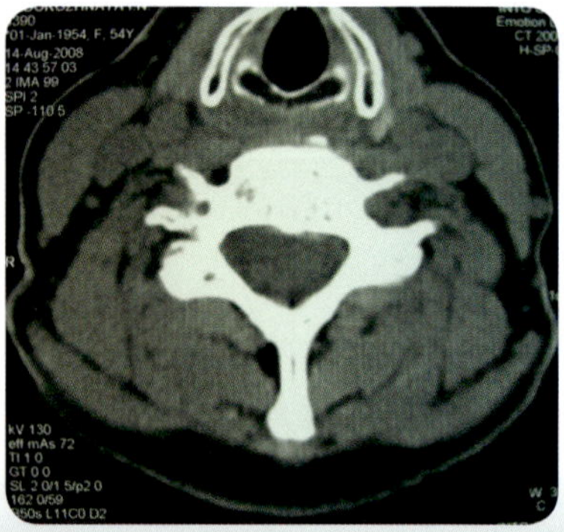

Fig. 5.2.12.

(sweaty hands, emotional lability).

CT scan of the brain showed signs of cerebral atherosclerosis (Fig. 5.2.11). Transcranial dopplerography revealed that the linear velocity of the blood flow in the common carotid arteries was reduced by 40% on the right side and 12% on the left. Due to decreased visual acuity, the patient was evaluated in the Filatov Ophthalmological Institute, where a diagnosis of maculodystrophy was made: Marked asymmetry of the diameters of the vertebral foramina was observed on the CT scan of the cervical spine (Fig. 5.2.12). The radiograph of the cervical spine showed rotational displacement of the vertebrae at the level of C_3–C_5, signs of advanced deforming spondylosis and osteochondrosis (Fig. 5.2.13).

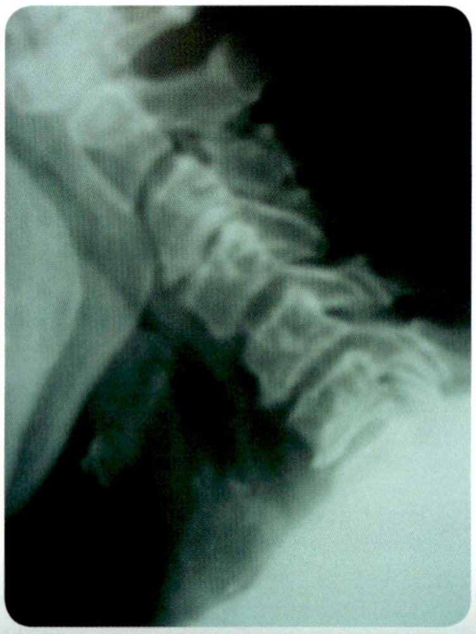

Fig. 5.2.13.

During examination of the patient, it was observed that she had a scoliotic deformity of the thoracic spine (2nd–3rd degree). To correct the left-sided tilt of the body, Z. was asked to wear an insole of a height of **10 mm**. The movements of her head were severely restricted. It was noted that there was rotational displacement of vertebrae in the cervical, thoracic and lumbosacral regions. The patient also had bilateral plexitis. The application of pressure on the spinous processes of the vertebrae gave rise to severe pain.

The standard treatment, i.e. constant wearing of 10 mm height orthopaedic insole under left heel, detorsional gymnastics, local paravertebral and transcranial magneto-acoustic therapy, inflatable rubber collar, was initiated. When Z. was examined 3 months later, the relative shortening of the left leg had reduced to **3 mm**. The frequency of the arrhythmias and extrasystoles had decreased significantly, and heartburn and regurgitation had become rare. There was also a decrease in the intensity of the back pain when pressure was applied to the vertebrae. The long-term results of treatment were assessed in one year. The axis of the spine was found to be correct and the back muscles were no longer asymmetrical. The height of the left leg was now the same as that of the right. Z. considered herself healthy because all her prior problems had been resolved. We recommended that she perform detorsional exercises on a regular basis.

5. Patient S., a 33-year-old woman, complained of pain in the heart and stomach, as well as occasional breath-holding, tachycardia, arrhythmias and extrasystoles. She also suffered from nausea and allergies to odours, besides persistent constipation. Despite these complaints, no cardiac or gastrointestinal diseases had been diagnosed during evaluation by different specialists.

Examination of the patient revealed a scoliotic deformity of the 2nd degree in the thoracic region. We attempted to correct this with an orthopaedic insole of a height of **10 mm**, to be placed under the left heel. There were significant rotational displacements of vertebrae in the cervical, thoracic and lumbar regions. Clinically, they manifested as bilateral plexitis, femoral nerve neuritis and bilateral lumbar ischialgia. Palpation along the thoracic spine caused severe pain.

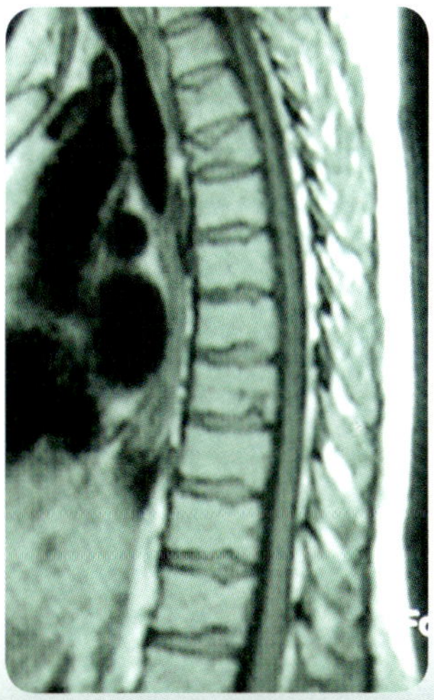

Fig. 5.2.14.

CT scans of the thoracic spine revealed multiple Schmorl's hernias; deforming spondylosis and osteochondrosis; a consolidated compression fracture of Th_4 (Fig. 5.2.14); and deforming arthrosis of the costo-vertebral joints. The diameter of the spinal canal was greater than that of the spinal cord (Fig. 5.2.15).

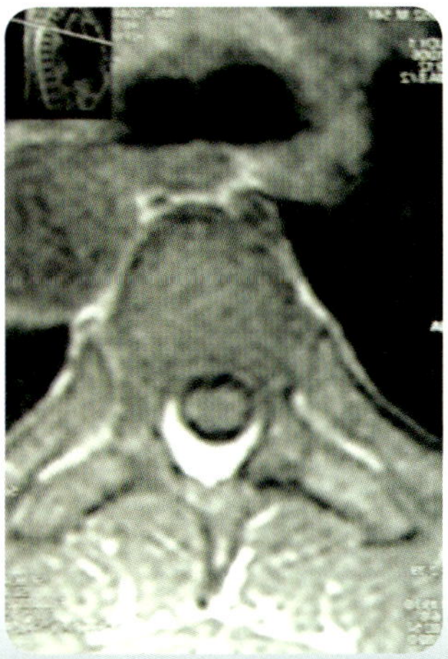

Fig. 5.2.15.

The standard treatment, i.e. constant wearing of orthopaedic insole, detorsional gymnastics, inflatable rubber collar, transcranial and paravertebral magneto-acoustic therapy, was initiated. When examined after 3 months, the patient reported a significant improvement in her general condition. The shortening of the left leg had decreased to **3 mm**. The neurological signs of plexitis, femoral nerve neuritis and lumbar ischialgia had become mild. Palpation of the vertebrae no longer caused pain. There was no nausea and the allergy had become less intense. S. actively followed the given recommendations.

During an assessment 1 year after the initiation of treatment, it was found that the left leg was no longer shorter than the right. The axis of the spine was correct and the back muscles were symmetrical. Intestinal functioning had normalized completely. The patient no longer had tachycardia, arrhythmias and extrasystoles. She considered herself practically healthy and was very pleased with the results of the treatment.

6. Patient Sh., a 39-year-old woman, complained of pain in the interscapular area of 8 years' duration. She suffered from extrasystoles, arrhythmias, periodic pain in the heart and breath-holding. An examination by a cardiologist revealed no abnormalities. Sh. also complained of headaches and dizziness, and said that several times a month, she lost consciousness when suddenly turning her head. In the patient's words, her 'head was spinning'. In addition, she experienced numbness of the fingers. During her childhood, Sh. had fallen from a height of 1.5 metres.

The radiograph of the cervical spine revealed rotational displacement of C_5 relative to C_6, minor signs of osteochondrosis and spondylosis deformans, as well as a consolidated compression fracture of C_5 (Fig. 5.2.16). The radiograph of the thoracic region showed a consolidated fracture of Th_8 and multiple Schmorl's hernias (Fig. 5.2.17).

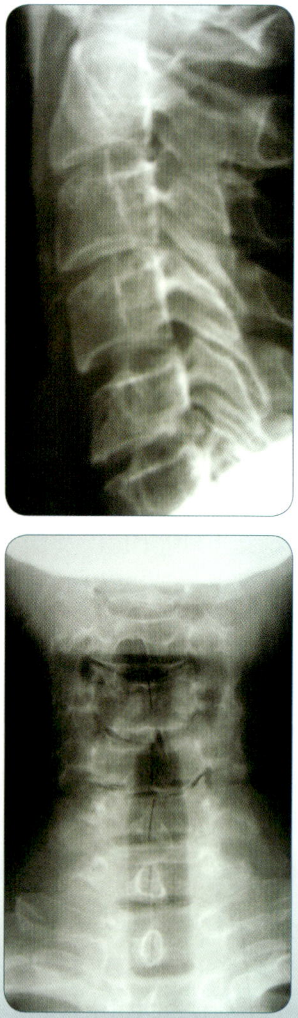

Fig. 5.2.16.

Examination of the patient showed that she had a scoliotic deformity of the 2nd–3rd degree in the thoracic region. We attempted to correct the left-sided pelvic tilt with an insole of a height of **15 mm**. Sh.'s head movements were severely limited. We noted that there were rotational displacements of vertebrae in the cervical, thoracic and lumbosacral regions. Clinically, they manifested as bilateral plexitis. Palpation of the thoracic vertebrae at the level of Th_2–Th_7 caused the patient severe pain.

The standard treatment, i.e. orthopaedic insole, detorsional gymnastics, inflatable rubber collar, transcranial and paravertebral local magneto-acoustic therapy, was initiated.

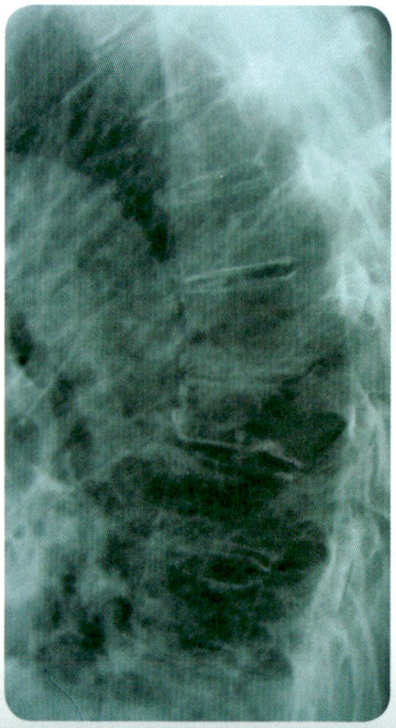

Fig. 5.2.17.

When examined 3 months later, Sh. reported that the frequency of the episodes of dizziness and headaches had decreased substantially. She no longer lost consciousness and the pain in the heart was negligible. She had been regularly adhering to the prescribed treatment. At 1 year's follow-up, the pain in the heart, arrhythmias, extrasystoles and dizziness had resolved. The axis of the spine was in the process of being corrected and the back muscles had become symmetrical. The patient was satisfied with the results of the treatment.

7. Patient K., a 47-year-old woman, complained of episodes of breathlessness that were associated with anxiety and fear. She also complained of flatulence, constant burping and numbness of the fingers of the right hand. She occasionally experienced pain in the heart and extrasystoles. K.'s muscles were well developed as she had earlier been actively involved in sports. Her problems had begun after she suffered a contusion of the spine as a result of a road traffic accident in 2005. She had been treated by a neurologist, internist and cardiologist, but without relief. Radiographs of the cervical spine revealed signs of osteochondrosis and spondylosis deformans, predominantly in the area of C_3–C_5 (Fig. 5.2.18), as well as lateral curvature of the spine (Fig. 5.2.19).

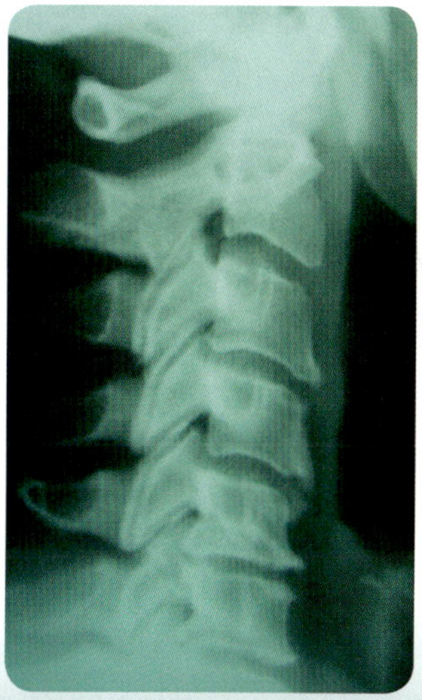

Fig. 5.2.18.

On examination, the patient was found to have a scoliotic deformity of 2–3 degrees of the thoracic spine. Severe hypotrophy of the gluteal muscles on the left half of the pelvis was observed. There was relative shortening of the left leg, which was compensated for with an insole of a height of **15 mm**. There were marked rotary subluxations of vertebrae in the cervical, thoracic and lumbar regions. Palpation of these areas, particularly at the level of Th_3–Th_5, caused severe pain. There was a marked limitation in the patient's capacity to turn her head. The other findings were the presence of right-sided plexitis, bilateral femoral nerve neuritis and lumbar ischialgia.

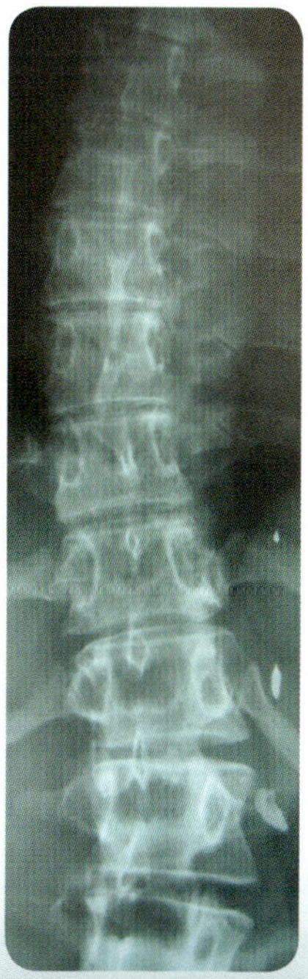

Fig. 5.2.19.

The standard treatment, i.e. orthopaedic insole, inflatable collar, local transcranial and paravertebral magneto-acoustic therapy, detorsional gymnastics, was initiated.

During an examination 3 months later, it was found that the left leg was still **7 mm** shorter than the right. There were no neurological signs of plexitis and lumbar ischialgia. Intestinal functioning had normalized, and K. no longer complained of flatulence and regurgitation. In addition, she was now free of the pain in the heart and extrasystoles, and the episodes of breathlessness had ceased. The patient had been systematically adhering to the treatment regimen. The long-term results of treatment were assessed a year and a half after its initiation. The axis of the spine was found to be correct (Fig. 5.2.20) and the back muscles were symmetrical. The left leg was shorter than the right by only **3 mm**. The patient had no complaints. We recommended continuation of the treatment, with another follow-up examination 6 months later.

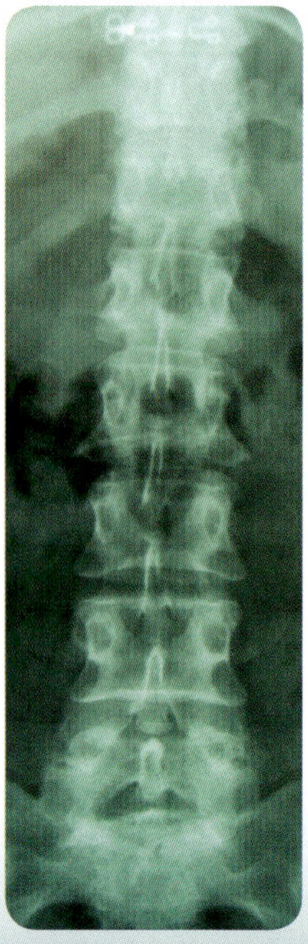

Fig. 5.2.20.

8. Patient B., a 25-year-old man who was strong and well built, consulted us to seek help for vasomotor rhinitis (constant nasal stuffiness, breathing through the mouth). He had occasional episodes of pricking pain in the heart, breathlessness and choking. These lasted an average of 25–30 seconds, after which the pain would resolve and his breathing would normalize. B.'s memory was worsening progressively.

Radiographs of the cervical spine revealed rotational subluxation of vertebrae at the level of C_3–C_6 and ossification of the posterior longitudinal ligament at the same level (Fig. 5.2.21). In the thoracic region, Schmorl's hernias and haemangioma of Th_8 were observed (Fig. 5.2.22).

On examination, the patient was found to have a scoliotic deformity of the 2nd–3rd degree, as well as a moderate right-sided rib hump. There was relative shortening of the left leg, which was compensated for with an insole of a height of **15 mm**. Marked rotational displacements of vertebrae in the cervical, thoracic and lumbar regions were observed. These manifested clinically as bilateral plexitis, neuritis of the femoral and obturator nerves, and bilateral lumbar ischialgia. Palpation of the spinous processes of the vertebrae at the level of Th_3–Th_5 was severely painful.

The standard treatment, i.e. orthopaedic insole, physical therapy—detorsional gymnastics, local transcranial and paravertebral magneto-acoustic therapy, was initiated.

When the patient was examined 2 months later, it was found that the difference between the lengths of the legs had decreased to **10 mm**. He still had mild neurological signs of plexitis and lumboischialgia. The episodes of pain in the heart, breath-holding and breathlessness were now sporadic, while

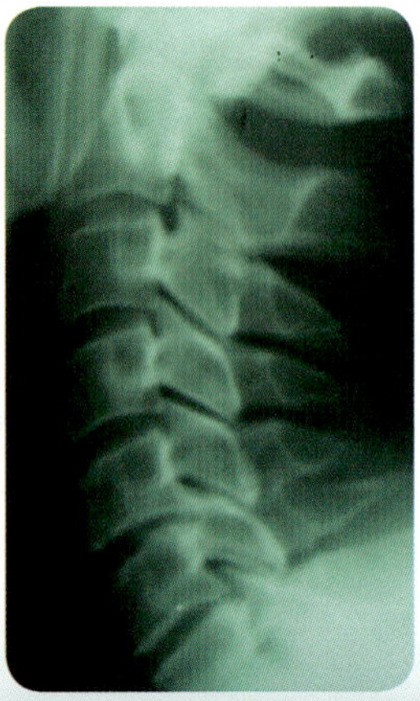

Fig. 5.2.21.

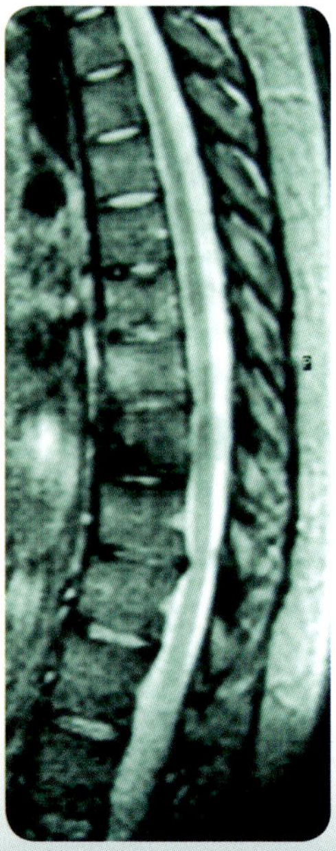

Fig. 5.2.22.

his memory was slowly recovering. At 6 months' follow-up, the patient reported that his nasal breathing was normal, and the episodes of breathlessness and heart pain had resolved. The difference between the lengths of the legs had decreased to **7 mm**.

The long-term outcome of treatment was assessed 1 year after its initiation. The axis of the spine was in the process of being corrected and the back muscles had become symmetrical. There was a significant reduction in the rib hump. The patient had no complaints. The left leg was shorter than the right by only 3 mm. We advised B. to continue with the therapeutic measures for the next 6 months.

9. Patient K., a 29-year-old woman, 8 months before consulting us had felt an acute pain in the sacrum when getting up from the bed suddenly. She had consulted a neurologist and manual therapist for this problem, and had been receiving hormonal therapy for autoimmune hypothyroidism over the past 2 years. However, she had not recovered from her problems.

Moreover, K. suffered from constant pain in all regions of the spine, dizziness and tinnitus, severe headache when turning the head, loss of consciousness and double vision. She also felt a 'tingling' in the heart and breathlessness. K.'s other complaints were irregular menstruation, constipation alternating with diarrhoea, a frequent urge to urinate, cramps in the calves and constant coldness of the feet.

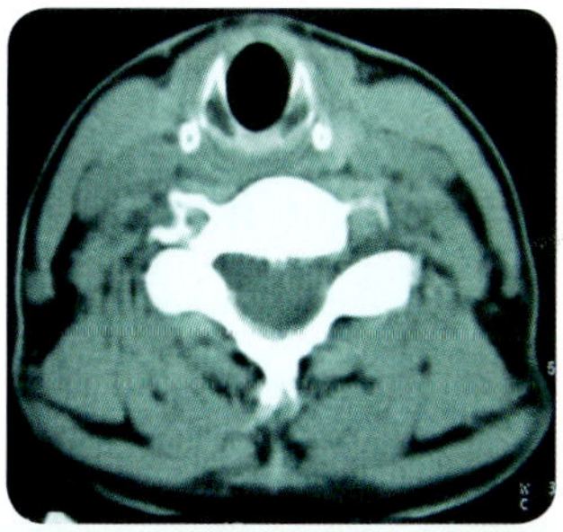
Fig. 5.2.23.

CT scan of the neck revealed marked asymmetry of the vertebral foramina (Fig. 5.2.23). Radiographs showed rotational displacement of the cervical vertebrae above the curvature and flattening of lordosis (Fig. 5.2.24). In the thoracic region, osteochondrosis and spondylosis deformans were observed (Fig. 5.2.25).

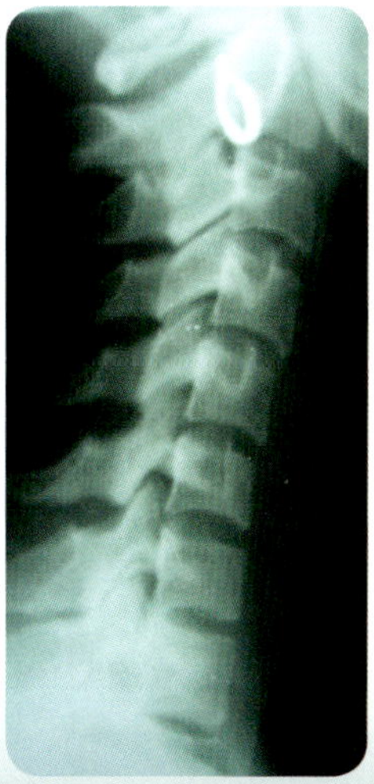
Fig. 5.2.24.

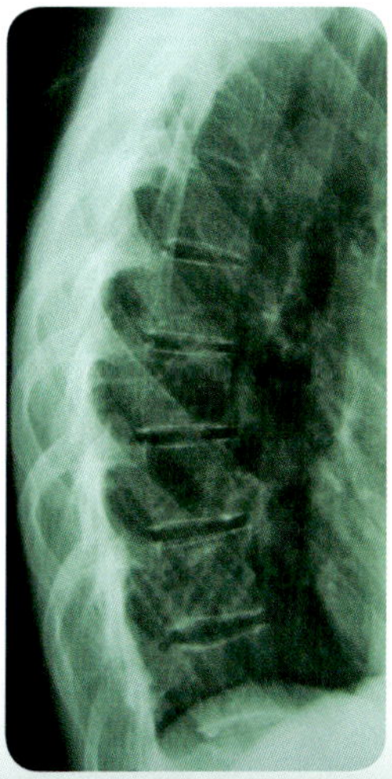
Fig. 5.2.25.

On examination, the patient was found to have a severe scoliotic deformity of the 2nd to 3rd degree, with a right-sided rib hump. Putting pressure on the vertebrae in the cervical, thoracic and lumbar regions caused pain. She had clinical signs of bilateral plexitis, neuritis of the obturator and femoral nerves, and bilateral lumbar ischialgia. There was a significant left-sided pelvic tilt, which was compensated for with an orthopaedic insole of a height of **55 mm**. During the first examination, we prescribed the use of an insole of a height of **15 mm** and the plan was to gradually increase its height. During the first consultation with the help of an inflatable collar we corrected the position of the cervical vertebrae. As a result, the signs of plexitis and the headaches resolved a short time later.

The standard treatment, i.e. orthopaedic insole, local paravertebral and transcranial magneto-acoustic therapy, detorsional gymnastics, inflatable rubber collar, was initiated.

The patient was assessed 3 months later. Thanks to the fact that she had worn the insole regularly and had followed the other advice faithfully, relative shortening of the left leg had been reduced to **30 mm**. There were no headaches, tinnitus and dizziness. The low back pain was hardly a source of trouble any more. When K. was examined 10 months after the initiation of the treatment, the left leg remained relatively shorter than the right by **7 mm**. Her menstrual cycle and the functioning of the intestines had become normal. At 1 year's follow-up, the left leg was shorter than the right by **3 mm**, the axis of the spine was normalizing and the back muscles had become symmetrical. The patient had no complaints. She considers herself healthy. However, we encouraged her to continue with the prescribed therapy for the next 6–8 months.

10. Patient K, a 14-year-old girl, was brought to us by her mother because an orthopaedic surgeon had told them that she had a scoliotic deformity. It turned out that the girl suffered from vasomotor rhinitis and vegetovascular dystonia. She complained of occasional cramps in the calf muscles and could not walk for too long because of severe fatigue in the legs. Radiographs of the cervical spine revealed rotational displacement of the vertebrae at the level of C_3–C_4 (Fig. 5.2.26). As for the lumbar region, there was lumbarization of S_1 and spina bifida S_1 (Fig. 5.2.27).

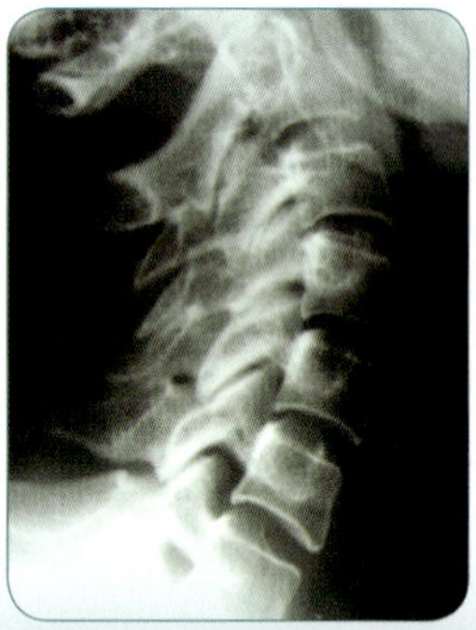

Fig. 5.2.26.

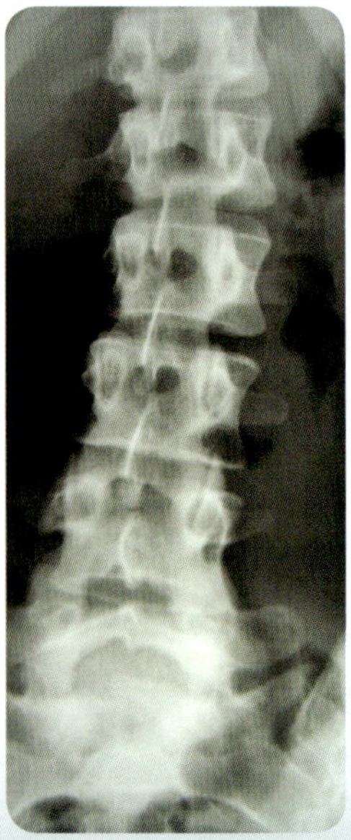

Fig. 5.2.27.

On examination, the patient was found to have a scoliotic posture and hypotrophy of the gluteal muscles of the left half of the pelvis. We attempted to eliminate the left-sided tilt of the pelvis with the use of an insole of a height of **3 mm**, placed under the left heel.

The standard treatment, i.e. training the mother to perform detorsional maneouvres, orthopaedic insole, local transcranial and paravertebral magneto-acoustic therapy, was initiated.

At 3 months' follow-up, the spinal erectors were found to be symmetrical and the axis of the spine had more or less normalized (Fig. 5.2.28). It was now easy for the patient to breathe nasally. She continued to adhere to the prescribed treatment. At 6 months' follow-up, K.'s hands were noticeably warmer and she was emotionally calm. The fatigue and leg cramps had resolved. We advised her to continue with the treatment for the next 6 months.

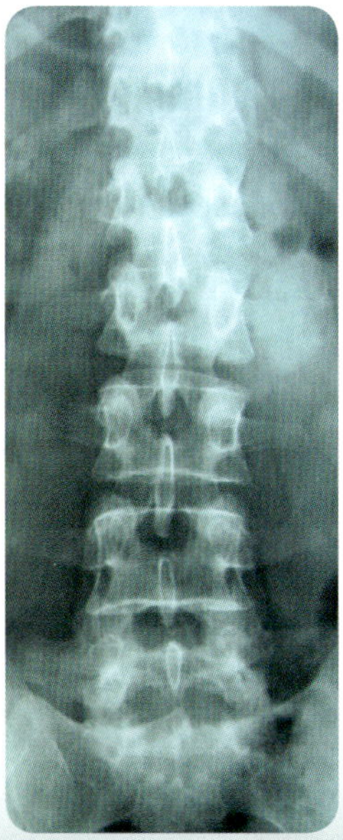

Fig. 5.2.28.

11. Patient P., a 51-year-old woman, complained of chest pain that had been persisting for over 4 years. She found it difficult to breathe and had numbness of the head. The patient's hands and feet periodically became numb and cold.

In addition, the patient suffered from severe pain in the legs and cramps in the calf muscles. She had been diagnosed with vegetovascular dystonia and often been treated by therapists and neurologists, but to no avail.

Examination revealed relative shortening of the left leg (**15 mm**). P. had a scoliotic deformity of the 2nd degree. The movements of her head were severely limited. Rotational displacements of vertebrae in all regions of the spine were observed. There were clinical signs of bilateral plexitis, lumbar ischialgia, and neuritis of the obturator and femoral nerves. Hypotrophy of the gluteal muscles of the left half of the pelvis was also noted.

Radiographs of the thoracic region showed advanced signs of osteochondrosis and spondylosis deformans (Fig. 5.2.29). The lumbosacral radiographs revealed lumbarization of S_1 and sacralization of L_5 (Fig. 5.2.30).

The standard treatment, i.e. orthopaedic insole, detorsional gymnastics and local magneto-acoustic therapy—transcranial and along the spine, inflatable rubber collar, was initiated.

During the follow-up examination 3 months later, the patient reported that the chest pain had become insignificant, there was no pain in the upper and lower extremities, and the leg cramps had subsided. Relative shortening of the left leg had decreased to **7 mm**. Another follow-up examination 8 months after the initiation of the treatment revealed that the axis of the spine was normalizing and the back extensors had become

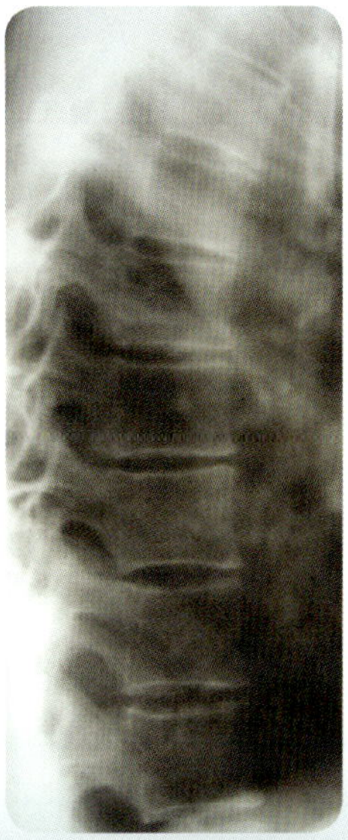

Fig. 5.2.29.

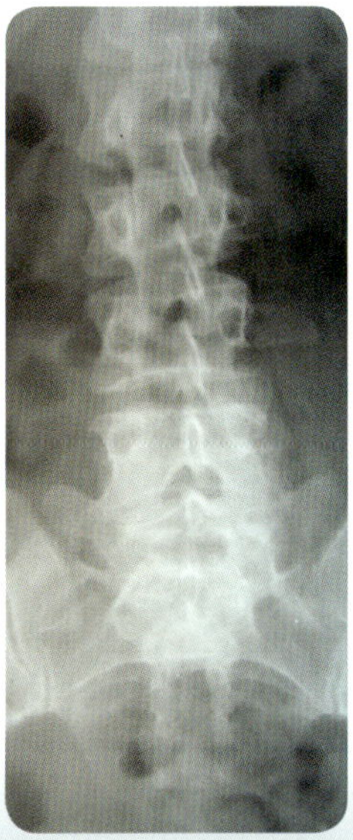

Fig. 5.2.30.

symmetrical. There was no retrosternal pain and no neurological signs of plexitis, lumbar ischialgia, and neuritis of the femoral and obturator nerves. Though the patient had no complaints, she still had relative shortening of the left leg (by **3 mm**). She was satisfied with the results of treatment. Nevertheless, she was advised to continue with the treatment for another 6–8 months.

12. Patient R., a 32-year-old man, came to us with the complaint of spinal pain. However, his major problem was bronchial asthma, from which he had been suffering from the age of 3 years. The asthma attacks occurred regularly every 10–14 days. He had continuously been under the treatment of pulmonologists, but with no improvement. He had been referred to our clinic by his father, who had received treatment at our clinic for spinal pain.

Examination of the patient revealed significant kyphoscoliotic deformation of the thoracic spine (2nd–3rd degree), with a right-sided rib hump. There was rotational displacement of the vertebrae in all regions of the spine. Pressure on the thoracic vertebrae revealed tenderness. There was relative shortening of the left leg of **25 mm**.

Radiographs of the thoracic region revealed signs of advanced degenerative disc disease, spondylosis deformans and multiple Schmorl's hernias (Fig. 5.2.31).

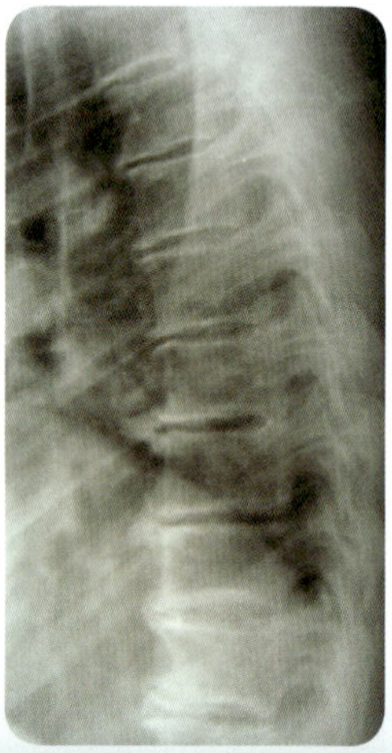
Fig. 5.2.31.

The standard treatment, i.e. orthopaedic insole, detorsional gymnastics and local magneto-acoustic therapy, was initiated. When examined after 2 months, the patient reported that the attacks of bronchial asthma had become much less frequent. Palpation of the spinous processes along the thoracic region was now painless. When he wore the insole, the scoliotic deformity disappeared. During the follow-up examination 1 year after the initiation of the treatment, the left leg was still relatively shorter than the right by **3 mm**. The axis of the spine was normalizing. The patient was adhering strictly to the prescribed therapy. He felt there had been a significant improvement in his overall condition and was pleased with the results of the treatment. When R. was examined 15 months after the start of the treatment, the asthma attacks had stopped altogether.

13. Patient B., a 15-year-old girl, complained of dizziness and blurred vision, in addition to the fact that she would collapse every time she suddenly turned her head. She also said she felt a 'tingling' in the heart and had sudden episodes of breath-holding, which were accompanied by fear. Her other complaints included occasional numbness of the hands, frequent pain in the lower abdomen towards the ovaries and a tendency to constipation. B. was concerned about pain and limitation of movements in the joints.

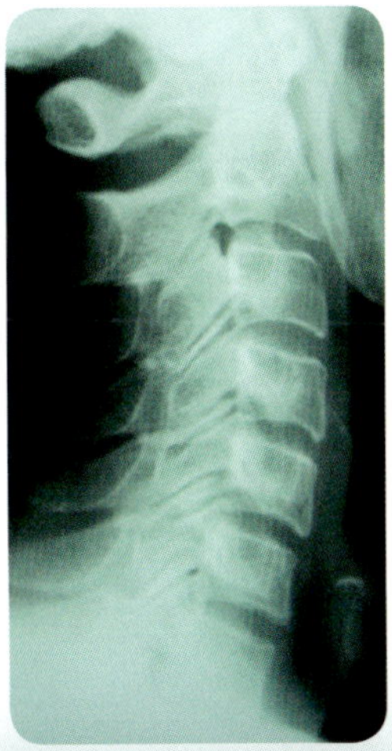
Fig. 5.2.32.

Radiographs of the cervical spine revealed slight rotational displacement of the vertebrae at the level of C_4–C_6, with virtually no signs of degenerative disc disease and spondylosis (Fig. 5.2.32). In the thoracic region, an S-shaped curvature was observed. There were no signs of dysplasia and structural anomalies (Fig. 5.2.33).

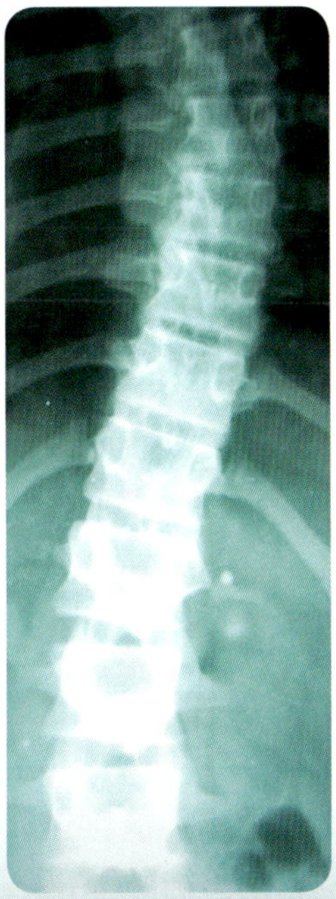
Fig. 5.2.33.

Examination revealed a scoliotic deformity of the 2nd–3rd degree in the thoracic region with left-sided rib hump. There was also hypotrophy of the gluteal muscles of the right half of the pelvis. We attempted to correct the pelvic tilt with an insole of a height of **15 mm**. Palpation revealed rotational displacement of vertebrae in the cervical, thoracic and lumbosacral regions. The patient had signs of bilateral plexitis, neuritis of the obturator and femoral nerves, and lumbar ischialgia.

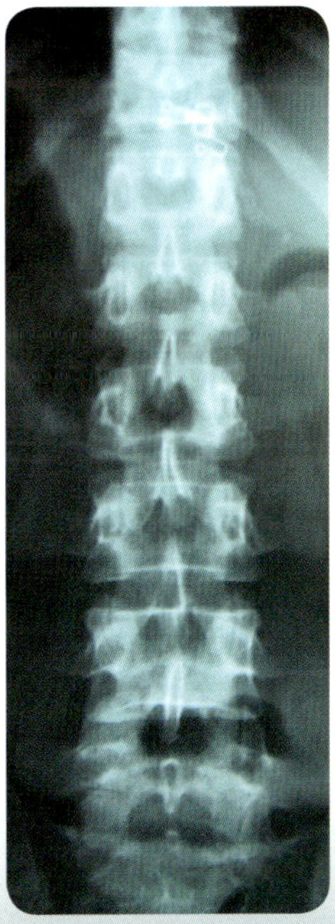
Fig. 5.2.34.

The standard treatment, i.e. orthopaedic insole, detorsional gymnastics, local transcranial and paravertebral magneto-acoustic therapy, inflatable rubber collar, was initiated. B. was asked to report for follow-up visits once a month. The last of these was one year after the initiation of the treatment. There was no difference in the length of the legs, and B. had no more episodes of dizziness and loss of consciousness. The axis of the spine was correct (Fig. 5.2.34) and the back muscles were now symmetrical. All the pain syndromes had resolved. The intestines were functioning properly. Though the patient considered herself healthy, we advised her to continue regularly with the physical therapy.

14. Patient S., a 17-year-old young woman, had a severe kyphoscoliotic deformity. Earlier, an orthopaedic surgeon had diagnosed juvenile kyphosis. S. complained of severe retrosternal pain, frequent episodes of breath-holding and lack of appetite. She suffered from hyperacid gastritis and had a tendency to constipation. There was severe hypotrophy of the gluteal muscles on the right side. We attempted to compensate for the right-sided pelvic tilt with an insole of a height of **7 mm**.

Radiographs of the thoracic spine (Fig. 5.2.35) revealed an advanced kyphotic deformity, osteochondrosis, wedge-shaped deformity of Th_5 and Schmorl's hernia. The radiograph of the lumbar spine (Fig. 5.2.36) revealed scoliotic deformity, spina bifida of S_1 and physiological lumbarization of S_1.

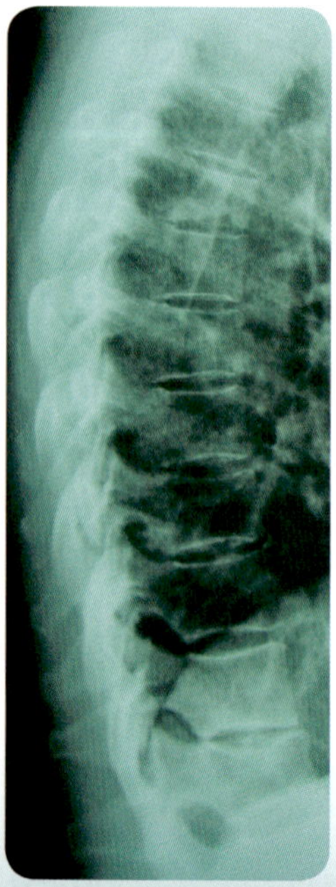

Fig. 5.2.35.

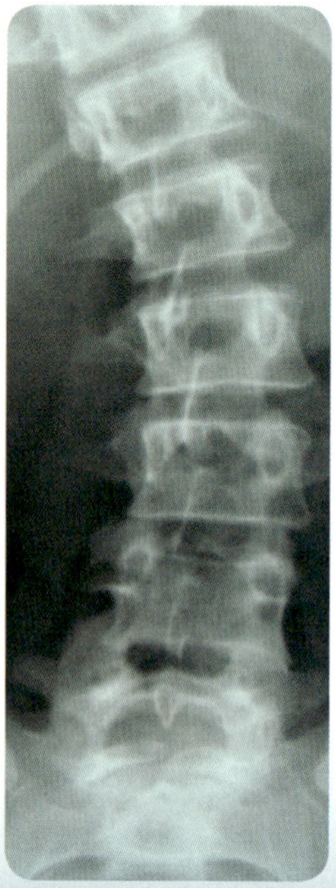

Fig. 5.2.36.

The standard treatment, i.e. orthopaedic insole, local paravertebral and transcranial magneto-acoustic therapy, detorsional gymnastics, inflatable rubber collar, was initiated. When examined after 3 months, the patient reported that the intensity of the spinal pain had decreased significantly. The difference in the length of the legs was only **3 mm**. The kyphotic deformity persisted and, therefore, S. and her parents were advised to contact the Kharkov Research Institute of Traumatology and Orthopedics so that they could provide her with a corrective corset and determine whether surgical treatment would be appropriate.

15. Patient K., a 33-year-old woman, complained of a deterioration in her memory, increased blood pressure, periods of blurred vision, frequent attacks of pain in the heart and breath-holding. The cardiologist found no pathology and the electrocardiogram was normal. Vegetovascular dystonia (sweaty hands, emotional lability) and vasomotor rhinitis (breathing through the mouth, stuffy nose) were diagnosed. Despite normal nutrition (in terms of volume and caloric intake), the patient was very thin. Her stomach hurt on palpation and she had a constant low-grade fever. The phthisiologist found no specific pathology.

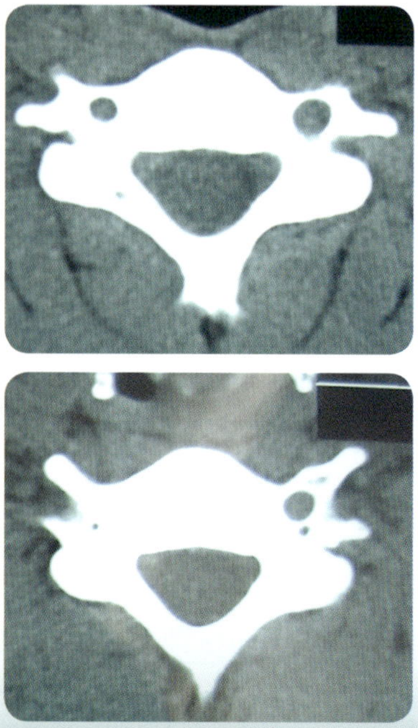

Fig. 5.2.37.

On CT scans of the cervical spine, the transverse foramina were observed to have an anomalous structure (Fig. 5.2.37). Radiograph of the thoracic spine showed kyphoscoliotic deformation, in addition to Schmorl's hernias (Fig. 5.2.38). Radiograph of the lumbosacral spine revealed sacralization of L_5 and spina bifida of S_1 (Fig. 5.2.39).

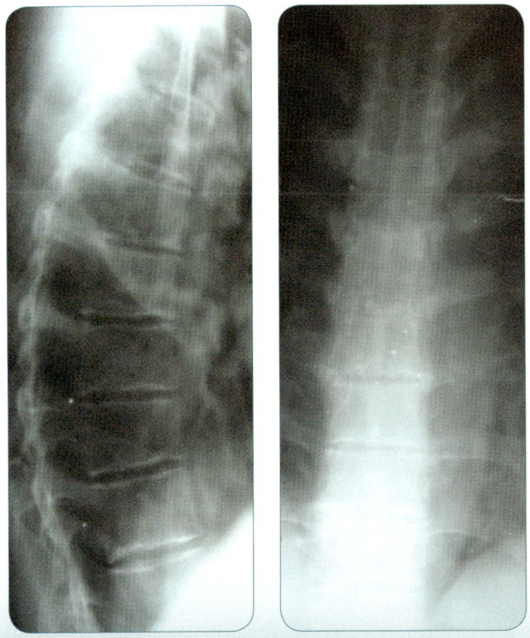

Fig. 5.2.38.

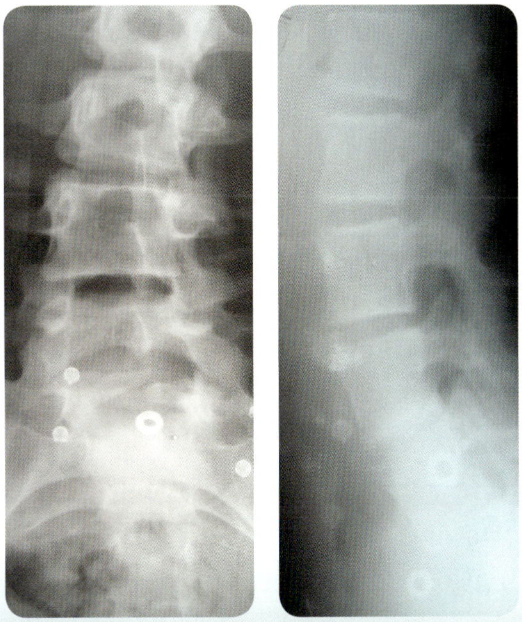

Fig. 5.2.39.

Examination of the patient revealed advanced kyphosis of the thoracic spine, as well as hypotrophy of the gluteal muscles on the left side. We attempted to compensate for the left-sided pelvic tilt with an insole of a height of **15 mm**. The application of pressure on the thoracic and lumbar vertebrae caused the patient severe pain.

The standard treatment, i.e. orthopaedic insole, local paravertebral and transcranial magneto-acoustic therapy, detorsional gymnastics, inflatable rubber collar, was initiated. We advised K. to contact the Kharkov Research Institute of Traumatology and Orthopedics so that they could provide her with a corrective corset and determine whether surgical treatment was necessary. When she was examined 8 months after the start of the treatment, she reported that her appetite had improved. The girl had gained a significant amount of weight. The relative shortening of the left leg had decreased to **3 mm**. The axis of the spine was normalizing. K. could now breathe through her nose, and no longer complained of heart pain and breath-holding. The body temperature was now normal. She wore a corset supplied by the Kharkov Research Institute of Traumatology and Orthopedics. The patient was very satisfied with the results of the treatment.

16. Patient A., a 66-year-old woman who was extremely obese, had been unable to walk for the past 15 years due to intense pain in the shins, feet and lower back. She reported that she had pain and numbness in her hands. She had been treated by internists with phenylbutazone, diclofenac and indomethacin, but there was no positive effect. She complained of severe retrosternal pain and breath-holding. Intense pain in the lower limbs limited her mobility, which together with a good appetite led to weight gain. From time to time, a manual therapist reduced the lumbar spine, whereupon the pain would resolve only for 1–1.5 months, and then all the symptoms recurred.

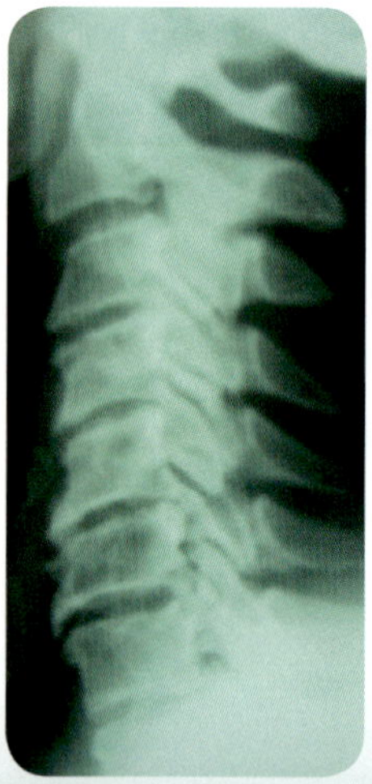

Fig. 5.2.40.

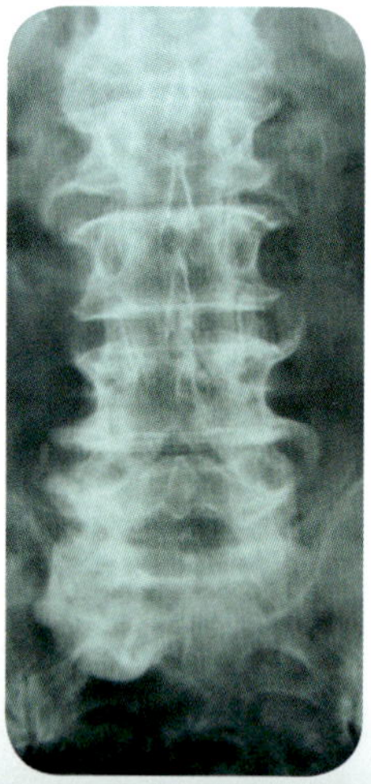

Fig. 5.2.41.

Radiographs of the cervical spine revealed signs of advanced degenerative disc disease and spondylosis (Fig. 5.2.40). In the lumbosacral region, severe osteochondrosis and spondylosis deformans were observed (Fig. 5.2.41).

The examination revealed relative shortening of the right leg (**37 mm**). Palpation of the vertebrae at all levels caused the patient severe pain. There were clinical signs of bilateral plexitis, neuritis of the femoral and obturator nerves, and lumbar ischialgia. Deformation of all joints could be observed.

The standard treatment, i.e. orthopaedic insole, inflatable rubber collar, local magneto-acoustic therapy – paravertebral and in projections of large joints, detorsional gymnastics, was initiated.

When A. was examined 4 months later the relative shortening of the right leg had decreased to **23 mm**. She had become more mobile and the intensity of the pain in the joints of the lower extremities had decreased significantly. The axis of the spine was normalizing. During the 1-year follow-up examination, it was found that the relative shortening of the right leg had decreased to **10 mm**. The patient walked a lot and had obviously lost weight. She was very satisfied with the results of the treatment.

17. Patient N., a 41-year-old man, visited the clinic because of persistent, intense low back pain that worsened after physical activity. He had been treated in Libya (with massages) and had also been to a sanatorium for treatment. However, his condition had not improved.

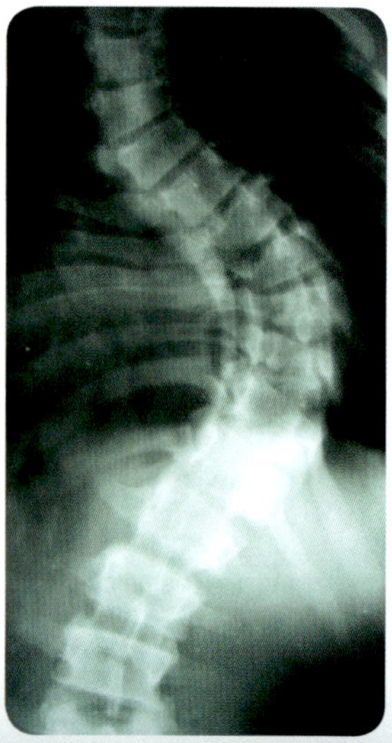

Fig. 5.2.42.

Radiographs of the thoracic and lumbar spine revealed signs of dysplasia, i.e. additional semivertebra at the level of Th_{10}–Th_{11} (Fig. 5.2.42).

Examination of the patient revealed an S-shaped scoliotic spinal deformity of the 2nd–3rd degree and a right-sided rib hump. There was hypotrophy of the gluteal muscles on the left side of the pelvis. We attempted to correct the left-sided tilt of the body with an insole of a height of **23 mm**.

The standard treatment, i.e. orthopaedic insole, local paravertebral magneto-acoustic therapy, detorsional gymnastics, was initiated. When examined after 7 months, N. reported a significant decrease in the intensity of the back pain. The difference in the length of the legs had decreased to **13 mm**.

During a follow-up examination 1 year and 2 months after initiation of treatment, it was seen that the relative shortening of the left leg disappeared, but it was decided to preserve **3 mm** for some months more for maintaining the balance of the spine and pelvis during exercise. The patient had no complaints. Thus, the back pain was not caused by accessory vertebrae, but by the incarceration of spinal roots in the sites of rotational subluxation of the vertebrae along the entire spine. Dysplasia and relative shortening of the left leg were involved in this process due to significant asymmetry of the back muscles.

18. Patient B., a 31-year-old man, had fallen off a ladder one year before visiting our clinic. He complained of dizziness, frequent headaches, weakness and fatigue. He said he could not stand for too long. His vision got blurred when he turned his head suddenly. Further, there was a feeling of pressure in the temples and he had a sensation of flashing lights in both his eyes.

Dopplerography of the cerebral and cervical blood vessels revealed extravasal compression of the vertebral arteries at the level of C_3–C_4 and a right-sided deficit in the blood flow of up to 16%. Radiographs of the cervical spine showed rotational displacement of C_3–C_5, as well as rudimentary cervical ribs at the level of C_7 (Fig. 5.2.43). Radiographs of the thoracic spine revealed kyphotic deformity, osteochondrosis, spondylosis deformans and multiple Schmorl's hernias (Fig. 5.2.44).

The patient was treated by a neurologist after being diagnosed with vegetovascular dystonia (hands sweaty and cold, emotional lability) and vasomotor rhinitis (breathing through the mouth). He was evaluated by a cardiologist because his complaints also included piercing chest pain and breathlessness. According to the cardiologist, there were no pathological changes and the electrocardiograph was normal.

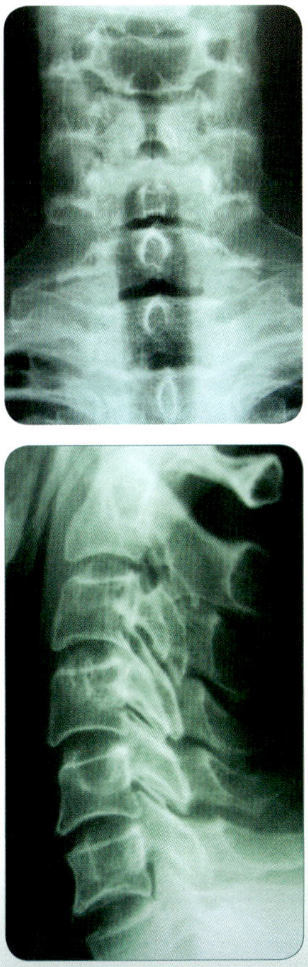

Fig. 5.2.43.

During examination of the patient, we observed rotational displacements of the cervical and thoracic vertebrae. There was an S-shaped spinal deformity of the 2nd degree, mainly in the thoracic region. The patient had bilateral plexitis, neuritis of the femoral nerves and lumbar ischialgia. In addition, there was relative shortening of the left leg (**20 mm**).

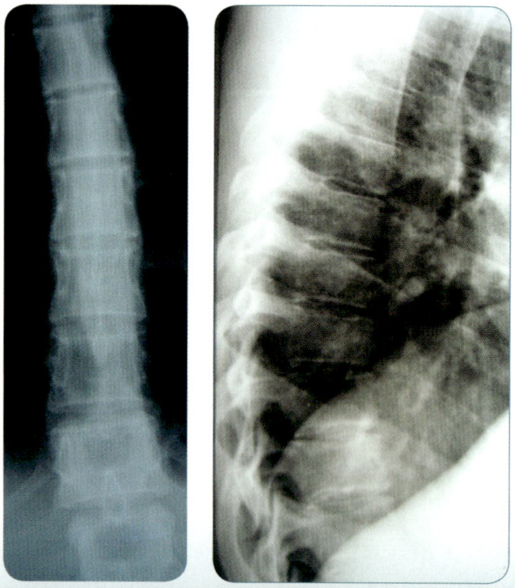
Fig. 5.2.44.

The standard treatment, i.e. orthopaedic insole, detorsional gymnastics, inflatable rubber collar, magneto-acoustic therapy of the local transcranial and paravertebral, including all lumbar and sacral-coccygeal vertebrae, was initiated.

At 6 months' follow-up, it was found that the difference in the length of the legs had decreased to **7 mm**. The headaches and dizziness had resolved, and B. had started to engage in sports activities. There was no pain in the heart. The patient could now breathe through his nose. He was almost healthy and satisfied with the results of treatment.

At 1 year's follow-up, it was found that the axis of the spine had been more or less corrected and the spinal erectors were symmetrical. The left leg remained **3 mm** shorter than the right. The patient had no complaints and was almost healthy. We advised him to continue with the prescribed treatment.

19. Patient C., a 17-year-old young woman, was brought to us by her mother because she had an S-shaped scoliosis (2nd degree) of the thoracolumbar spine. She complained of headaches, constant pain in the heart and breathlessness. Examination by a cardiologist revealed no pathological changes and the ECG was normal. C. also complained of numbness of the fingers and toes, as well as irregular periods.

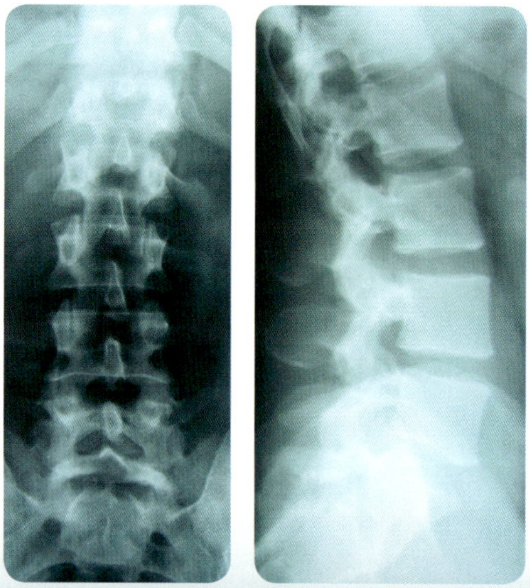
Fig. 5.2.45.

Radiographs of the thoracic and lumbar spine revealed a scoliotic deformity of the 2nd degree and signs of dysplasia, i.e. sacralization of L_5 and lumbarization of S_1 (Fig. 5.2.45).

Examination showed that the girl, who was tall and well built, had rotational displacements in the cervical and thoracic regions, with severe limitation of head movements. Palpation of the spinous processes caused severe pain. There were signs of bilateral plexitis and lumbar ischialgia. Her body was tilted to the right, and we attempted to correct this with an insole of a height of **30 mm**.

The basic treatment (orthopaedic insole, detorsional gymnastics, inflatable rubber collar, local transcranial and paravertebral magneto-acoustic therapy) was initiated.

When C. was examined 5 months after the initiation of treatment, it was found that the difference between the length of the two legs had decreased to **3 mm**. There was no deformation of the spine. She had no complaints. We advised the patient to continue with the prescribed treatment.

At 1 year follow-up, there was no difference in the length of the two legs. The axis of the spine was more or less correct and the spinal extensors were symmetrical. C. was almost healthy and had no complaints.

20. Patient P., a 48-year-old woman, complained of intense headaches, periodic breathlessness and a stabbing pain in the heart. She had suffered from vegetovascular dystonia, coronary artery disease and unstable angina since the age of 24 years. She reported that her head went numb when she turned it and that her scleral blood vessels often ruptured. She also complained of swelling of the legs. Periodically P. had been treated in the department of cardiology.

Doppler ultrasonography of the blood vessels of the head and neck revealed an asymmetrical reduction in the flow of blood in the vertebral arteries in the C_4–C_6 segments. The flow of blood was reduced by 34% on the right side and 40% on the left.

Radiographs of the cervical spine showed signs of degenerative disc disease and deforming spondylosis, with rotational displacement of vertebrae at the level of C_4–C_6, above the physiological curvature (Fig. 5.2.46). Slight deforming changes were noted in the thoracic spine.

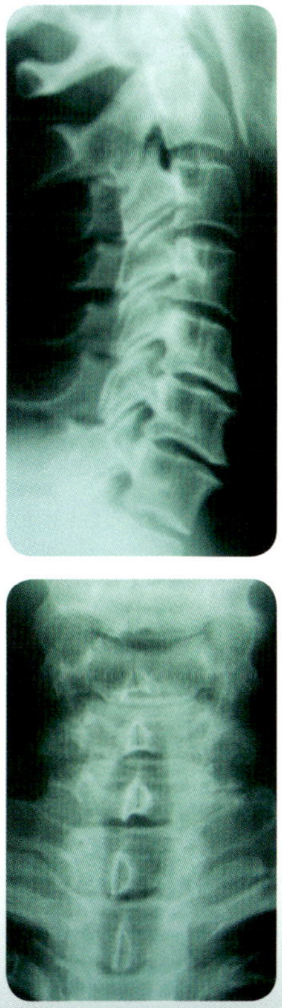

Fig. 5.2.46.

On examination, it was found that the patient had relative shortening of the left leg (**15 mm**). There was rotational displacement of the vertebrae in all regions of the spine, clinically manifested as bilateral plexitis and lumbar ischialgia. Pressure on the spinous processes of the cervical and thoracic vertebrae caused the patient severe pain.

The standard treatment, i.e. orthopaedic insole, detorsional gymnastics, inflatable rubber collar, local magneto-acoustic therapy – transcranial and along the spinal column, was initiated.

At 6 months' follow-up, the difference in length of the two legs was **7 mm**. There was no pain in the heart and the intensity of the headaches had decreased significantly. The patient said that she felt well. At 1-year follow-up, the left leg was **3 mm** shorter than the right. The axis of the spine was normalizing. The patient considered herself healthy because the headaches, breathlessness and heart pain had resolved. However, we advised her to regularly continue with the physical therapy and to wear the insole for another year.

21. Patient K., a 20-year-old man, had been suffering from bronchial asthma for the past few years. He also felt discomfort in the neck. K. had been examined by an ENT specialist, gastroenterologist and endocrinologist, none of whom had found any pathological changes. In recent years, K.'s vision had deteriorated. He also complained of numbness of the fingers. He occasionally felt a stabbing pain in the heart, but the cardiologist had found no pathology. In addition, the patient had convergent strabismus.

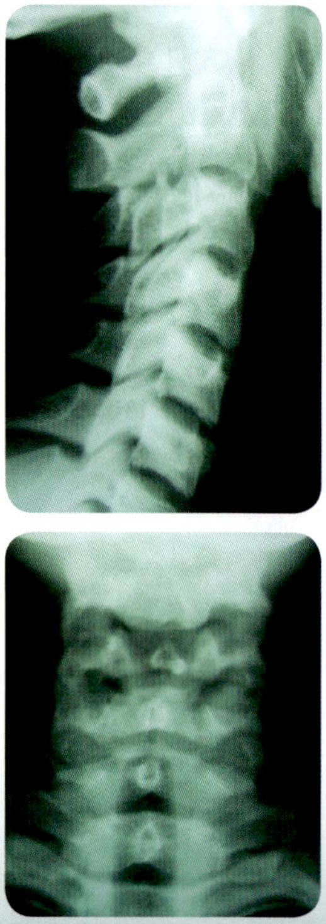

Fig. 5.2.47.

Radiographs of the cervical spine revealed moderate rotational displacements of vertebrae in the typical segments (C_4–C_6), which corresponded to the area above the physiological curvature. There was no bone pathology (Fig. 5.2.47). In the thoracic region, there were moderate signs of degenerative disc disease and spondylosis deformans (Fig. 5.2.48).

Dopplerography of the cerebral and cervical vessels revealed a deficit (of up to 50%) in the flow of blood in the right vertebral artery at the level of the C_3–C_4 segment.

Examination of the patient revealed that he had a scoliotic deformity of the 2nd degree in the thoracic spine, in addition to rotational displacement of the cervical, thoracic and lumbar vertebrae. There was a moderate right-sided rib hump. Hypotrophy of the gluteal muscles in the right half of the pelvis was also evident. We attempted to eliminate the pelvic tilt by prescribing the use of an insole of a height of **18 mm**, to be placed under the right heel. There were signs of bilateral plexitis, neuritis of the femoral and obturator nerves, and lumbar ischialgia.

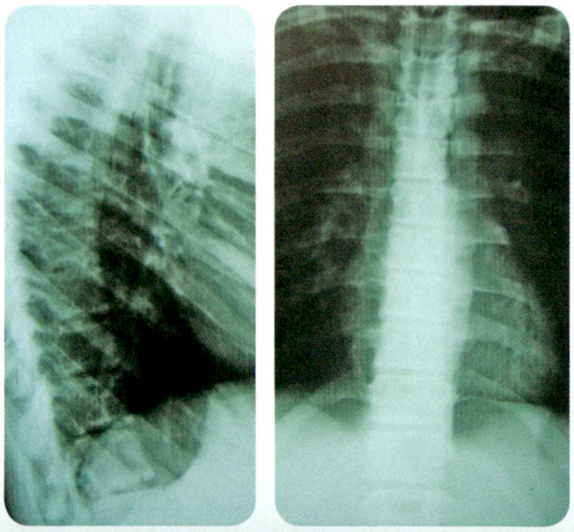

Fig. 5.2.48

The standard treatment, i.e. constant wearing of orthopaedic insole, detorsional gymnastics, inflatable rubber collar, local magneto-acoustic therapy—transcranial and along the spinal column, was initiated. Follow-up examinations were performed every month. During the last examination, which took place 10 months after the initiation of treatment, it was found that there was no more shortening of the right leg and there was no scoliotic deformity (Fig. 5.2.49). The axis of the spine was correct and the spinal erectors had become symmetrical. The patient had no complaints and had a healthy appearance. The attacks of asthma had become rare. K. looks like a healthy person and is very satisfied with the results of treatment.

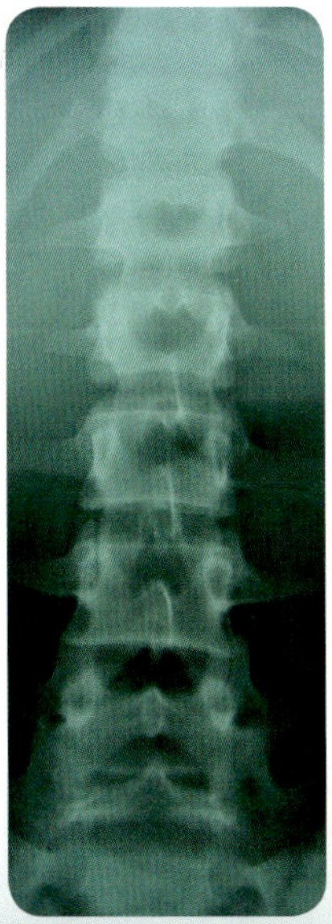

Fig. 5.2.49.

22. Patient T., a 19-year-old young woman, on admission to the clinic, complained of daily headaches, dizziness, nausea, tinnitus and impaired vision. She had very frequent episodes of sudden breathlessness. She had been treated for biliary dyskinesia and vegetovascular dystonia (sweaty hands, emotional lability, touchy, irritable, red dermographism). The patient also had a low blood pressure. Prior treatment had proved ineffective.

Dopplerography of the cerebral and cervical vessels revealed asymmetrical flow of blood in the vertebral arteries at the level of C_3–C_4. The deficit in the blood flow was more marked on the right side and reached up to 55%.

Radiographs of the cervical spine showed rotational displacement of vertebrae at the level of C_3–C_5. In the thoracic region, one could observe a scoliotic deformity, without signs of dysplasia. As for the lumbar region, there was lumbarization of S_1, sacralization of L_5 and asymmetry of the articular processes at the level of L_5–S_1 (Fig. 5.2.50).

Examination of the patient revealed relative shortening of the left leg by **15 mm.** There was a scoliotic deformity of the 2nd–3rd degree in the thoracic region. In addition, there were rotational displacements of the vertebrae at all levels. Clinically, these rotations manifested as bilateral plexitis, neuritis of the obturator and femoral nerves, and bilateral lumbar ischialgia.

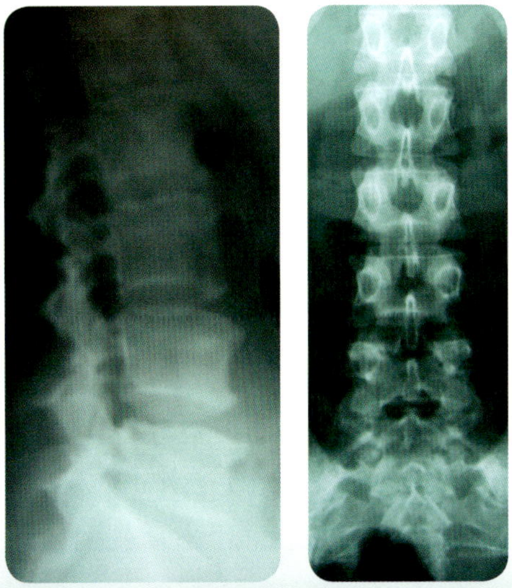

Fig. 5.2.50

The standard treatment, i.e. orthopaedic insole, inflatable rubber collar, local magneto-acoustic therapy—transcranial and along the spinal column, detorsional gymnastics, was initiated. Follow-up examinations were carried out every 1–1.5 months. During the last examination, 8 months after the initiation of treatment, the left leg was found to be **3**

mm shorter than the right. The axis of the spine was normalizing. The patient had no complaints and both she and her parents were very satisfied with the results of treatment because symptoms of various diseases had disappeared. T. continues to be on treatment.

23. Patient D., a 39-year-old woman, on admission to the clinic complained of burning pain in the interscapular region of more than three-an-a-half years' duration. She had a constant pain in the lower back that radiated to both legs. In addition, she suffered from numbness of both hands, headaches and frequent episodes of tachycardia. Many times she was seen in the emergency department. Whatever treatment she had received had been ineffective.

Dopplerography of the cerebral and cervical blood vessels revealed a symmetrical deficit (of up to 50%) in the flow of blood in the vertebral arteries at the level of C_3–C_5.

Radiographs of the cervical spine revealed osteochondrosis and spondylosis deformans, as well as slight rotational displacement at the level of C_3–C_5. As for the thoracic spine, there were signs of advanced degenerative disc disease and spondylosis deformans, together with Schmorl's hernias (Fig. 5.2.51).

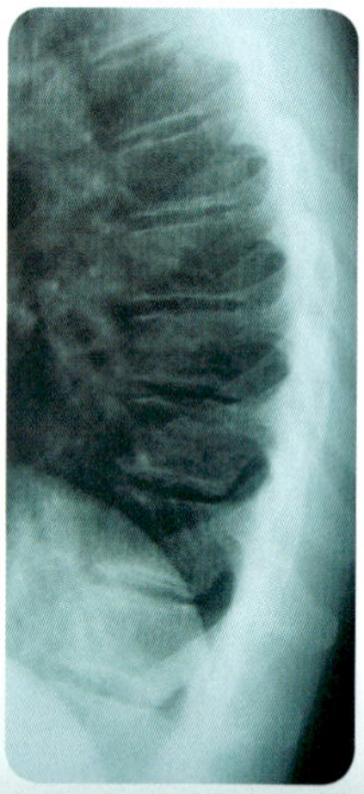
Fig. 5.2.51.

During examination of the patient, kyphoscoliotic deformation of the thorax (2nd–3rd degree) was observed. She had a right-sided rib hump. There was relative shortening of the left leg (**25 mm**), as well as hypotrophy of the left gluteal muscles. D.'s capacity to rotate her head was severely limited. There were rotational displacements of the thoracic vertebrae, with the sites of rotation being painful. The rotations manifested as bilateral plexitis.

The standard treatment, i.e. orthopaedic insole to compensate for the shortening, detorsional gymnastics, local paravertebral magneto-acoustic therapy, inflatable rubber collar, was initiated. After 8 months of treatment, the spinal deformity had been eliminated and the pain had resolved. The axis of the spine was normalizing, while the spinal extensors had become symmetrical. Nonetheless, D. was encouraged to continue with the detorsional gymnastics.

24. Patient Y., a 37-year-old woman, complained of pain 'in the whole body'. She had convergent strabismus and had been suffering from bronchial asthma for several years. She had frequent episodes of breathlessness, extrasystoles and arrhythmias. Y. was being treated for vegetovascular dystonia (red dermographism; sweatiness, coldness and numbness of the hands and feet. In adolescence, she had been actively involved in sports and sustained injuries of the spine several times.

Dopplerography of the cerebral and cervical vessels revealed extravasal compression of the vertebral arteries at the level of C_3–C_5, the deficit in blood flow being up to 25%.

Radiographs of the cervical spine revealed rotational displacement above the curvature (C_3–C_5). Radiographs of the thoracic and lumbar spine revealed scoliotic deformity, signs of advanced deforming spondylosis and degenerative disc disease, Schmorl's hernias and lumbarization of S_1 (Fig. 5.2.52).

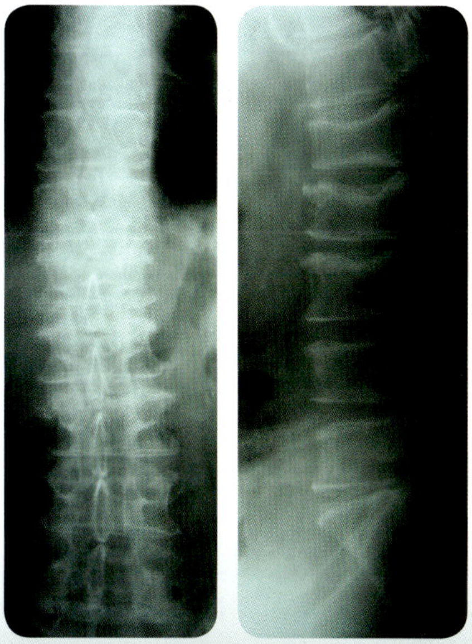
Fig. 5.2.52

On examination of the patient, a scoliotic deformity of the 2nd–3rd degree was noted. In addition, there was a left-sided rib hump. Rotation of vertebrae could be observed in the cervical, thoracic and lumbar regions in the parts where rotation typically occurs. Y.'s capacity to turn her head was severely limited. She had bilateral plexitis and bilateral lumbar ischialgia. The application of pressure on the vertebrae at the sites of rotation was acutely painful for the patient. We attempted to eliminate the right-sided tilt of the pelvis by prescribing the use of an insole of a height of **3 mm**.

The standard treatment, i.e. orthopaedic insole, corrective detorsional exercises, inflatable rubber collar, local magneto-acoustic therapy along the spine, was initiated. When examined after a month, Y. reported a significant improvement in her overall condition. There had been only isolated attacks of asthma and breathlessness. At 5 months' follow-up, the right leg was no longer shorter than the left and the patient had no complaints. The axis of the spine was normalizing and the spinal erectors had become symmetrical. The asthma attacks had resolved.

25. Patient G., a 20-year-old young woman, looked more like a teenager, being very thin as well as short. Her complaints included convergent strabismus, persistent pain in the temples and nape of the neck, frequent pain in the heart, emotional instability and low blood pressure (90/60 mmHg). The neurologist had diagnosed vegetovascular dystonia. G. also complained of heartburn, belching and constant nausea. Though she ate well, she did not gain weight. She said that upon exercising, she felt a pain in the lower thoracic region of the spine. Her periods were not regular. There was a gnawing pain in the abdomen towards the ovaries. The pain was so intense that the patient said it was as if the 'muscles have been separated from the bones'. Her feet and hands were wet and cold.

Control radiography was performed. It revealed rotational displacement of the cervical vertebrae over the physiological curvature (C_4–C_6), as well as congenital anomalies of Th_{10} (wedge-shaped deformation). This had resulted in the development of a lateral curvature in all regions of the spine. Sacralization of L_5 was observed (Fig. 5.2.53).

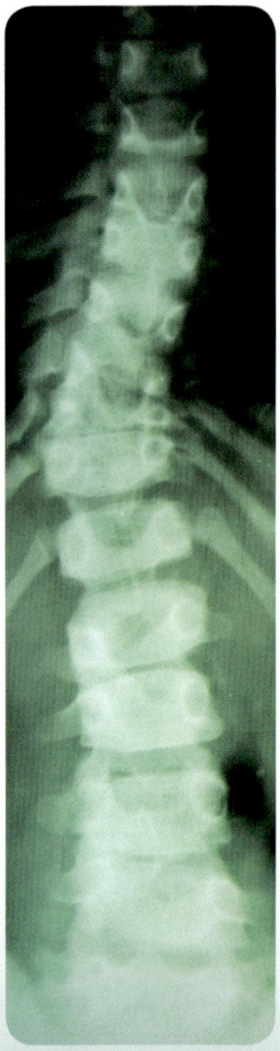
Fig. 5.2.53.

Examination of the patient revealed that she had a scoliotic posture and a chest deformity (left-sided rib hump) which was slightly marked. There was relative shortening of the right leg (**3 mm**). G. was also noted to have a flat-valgus foot on the right side.

The standard treatment, i.e. orthopaedic insole, corrective detorsional gymnastics, inflatable rubber collar, local magneto-acoustic therapy—transcranial and along the spine, was initiated. We advised the patient to use an orthopaedic corset when engaging in physical activities.

When the patient was examined after one-and-a-half months, her general condition was found to have improved. The heartburn, regurgitation and pain in the heart had resolved. Her blood pressure had returned to normal.

At 7 months' follow-up, it was observed that the asymmetry in the length of the legs had been eliminated and the axis of the spine had been corrected to a large extent. The spinal extensors were now symmetrical and the pain in all the regions of the spine had resolved. G. also reported that her menstrual cycle had become regular and said she felt almost healthy. We recommended that she continue with the prescribed treatment, particularly detorsional gymnastics.

26. Patient L., a 43-year-old woman, had been receiving treatment for chronic bronchitis with an asthmatic component for the past 10 years. She told us that she constantly felt a stabbing pain in the heart and also complained of breath-holding and shortness of breath.

She had nodular goitre, which manifested externally as exophthalmos. Among her other complaints were stomachache and belching. She felt spasms in her head when she lay on her back. Her hands went numb when she played the piano (the patient is a musician). She was treated for vegetovascular dystonia (hands cold and sweaty, marked emotional lability).

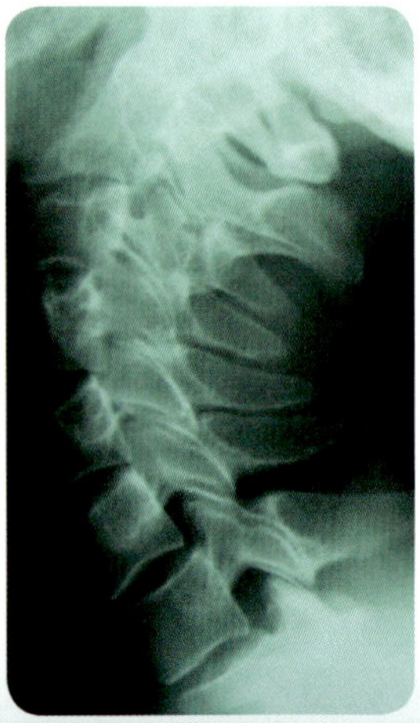
Fig. 5.2.54.

Radiographs of the cervical spine revealed significant rotational displacement of C_4 relative to C_5 (Fig. 5.2.54). Radiographs of the thoracic spine showed signs of osteochondrosis and spondylosis deformans, as well as Schmorl's hernia (Fig. 5.2.55).

Examination of the patient showed that she had a scoliotic

deformity (of the 2nd–3rd degree) of the thoracic and lumbar spine of compensatory muscular origin. We attempted to compensate for the asymmetry of the spinal extensors with an insole of a height of **20 mm**, to be placed under the left heel. L.'s capacity to turn her head was severely limited. Rotational displacement of the vertebrae was observed in the areas where such displacements typically occur. The patient had bilateral plexitis, bilateral neuritis of the femoral and obturator nerves, and left-sided lumbar ischialgia.

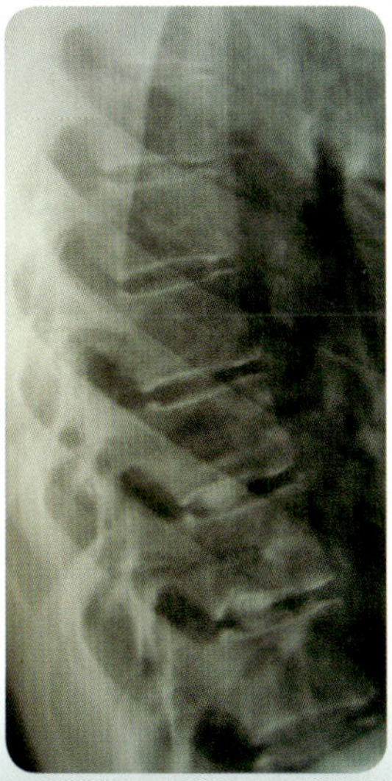

Fig. 5.2.55.

The standard treatment, i.e. orthopaedic insole, physiotherapy, local magneto-acoustic therapy—transcranial and along the spinal column, inflatable rubber collar, was initiated. The patient was trained to perform a set of detorsional exercises. As a result of these, there was a significant reduction in pain in the spine. L. was examined regularly every 1–1.5 months. Her condition improved steadily. During the last examination, 7 months after the initiation of treatment, L. reported that she had had no more attacks of asthma and breathlessness. There were no headaches, and no pain in the extremities, behind the breastbone and in the heart. The exophthalmos had become less pronounced. The patient said there had been significant improvement in her general condition, and she had become active and cheerful. The difference in the length of the legs had decreased to **7 mm** and the axis of the spine was normalizing. L. continued to adhere to the prescribed treatment.

27. Patient V., a 55-year-old woman, complained that she suffered from headaches which were so severe that it was 'terrible to wake up'. She had difficulty standing because of pain in the thoracic spine. She also had severe low back pain, especially when bending forward. Her other complaints included numbness of the hands and feet. She felt a constant pain in the heart. The cardiologist had said that her heart was healthy. Her ECG was normal. V. had been treated for vegetovascular dystonia.

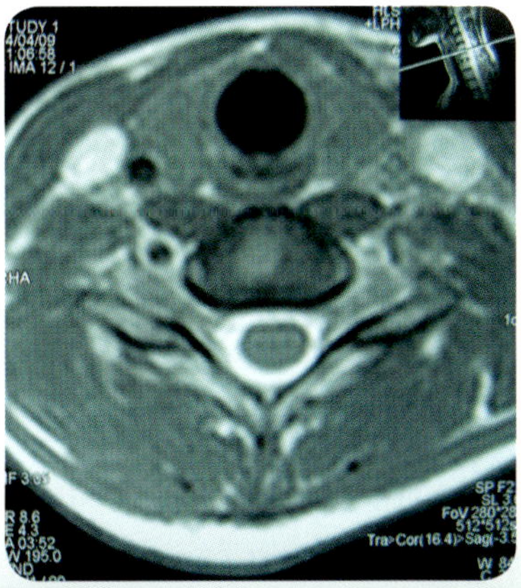

Fig. 5.2.56.

CT scans of the cervical spine revealed marked asymmetry in the diameters of the vertebral foramina at the level of C_4–C_6, above the physiological curvature—a site where mutual rotation of the vertebrae occurs typically (Fig. 5.2.56). Plain radiographs of the same area revealed spondylosis deformans and osteochondrosis (Fig. 5.2.57). Radiograph of the thoracic spine showed widespread osteochondrosis, spondylosis, wedge-shaped deformation of the Th_6–Th_9 vertebral bodies

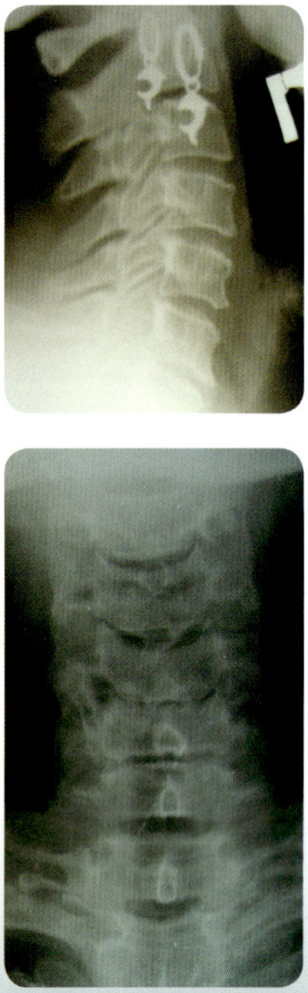

Fig. 5.2.57.

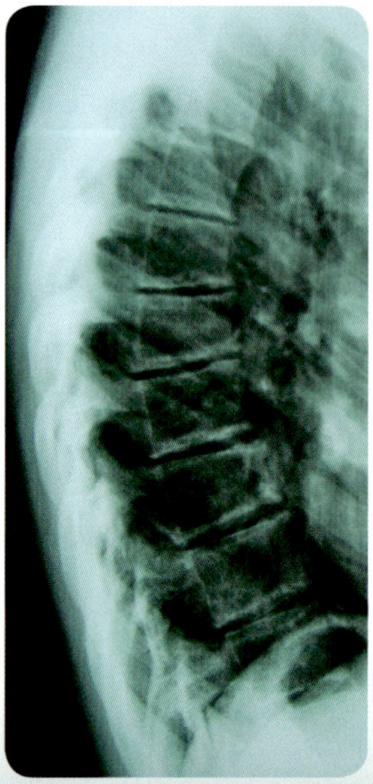

Fig. 5.2.58.

and Schmorl's hernias (Fig. 5.2.58).

On examination, the patient was found to have a scoliotic deformity (of the 2nd–3rd degree) of the thorax, with a slightly marked right-sided rib hump. The body was tilted to the left, and we attempted to eliminate the tilt with the use of an orthopaedic insole of a height of **25 mm**, to be placed under the left heel. Thanks to this insole the horizontal plane of the pelvis was restored and as a result the spinal deformity and muscle asymmetry of the common spinal extensors had almost completely disappeared. For preserving this effect, the patient had to use the orthopaedic insole constantly for quite a long period of time.

V.'s capacity to turn her head was severely limited. She had bilateral plexitis, neuritis of the femoral and obturator nerves, and bilateral lumbar ischialgia.

The standard treatment, i.e. orthopaedic insole, corrective detorsional exercises, inflatable rubber collar, local transcranial and paravertebral magneto-acoustic therapy, was initiated. The patient experienced considerable relief from the pain right from the time she started learning how to perform the detorsional exercises. The patient was examined regularly every 1–1.5 months. Her condition improved progressively. At 6 months' follow-up, she reported that the headaches and pain in the heart had resolved. The pain in the other areas was now negligible. V. could freely bend her trunk in all directions. The axis of the spine was normalizing. The difference in the length of the legs had decreased to **7 mm**. The patient was very pleased with the results of the treatment. She was advised to continue with the prescribed treatment.

The patient was last examined one year after the initiation of treatment. There was no difference in the length of the legs and the axis of the spine was more or less correct. The patient said she felt healthy since the pain had resolved. However, we advised her to regularly continue with the physical therapy and to keep wearing an insole of a height of **3 mm** for another year.

28. Patient M., a 50-year-old man, complained of a dramatic weakening of memory, constant headaches, tinnitus aurium, and severe numbness and coldness of the hands. He could not lie on his back because of pain in the thoracic spine (interscapular region). There was pain all over his body, including the lower back, with the latter radiating to both legs. M. had frequent episodes of breathlessness. A few years before he consulted us, his kidney had been surgically removed as it had been causing him pain. There was constant pain in the left inguinal region, but the surgeon had found no evidence of disease.

CT scan of the brain showed partial atrophy and sclerosis of the cerebral cortex as a consequence of chronically impaired blood supply (Fig. 5.2.59). The radiograph of the cervical spine revealed rotation of the vertebrae at the level of C_5–C_6, with blocking of this segment, probably due to injury. We also observed a reduction in the height of C_6 and ossification of the posterior longitudinal ligament, together with the formation of exostoses (Fig. 5.2.60). In the thoracic region, widespread osteochondrosis and spondylosis deformans, and Schmorl's hernias were observed (Fig. 5.2.61).

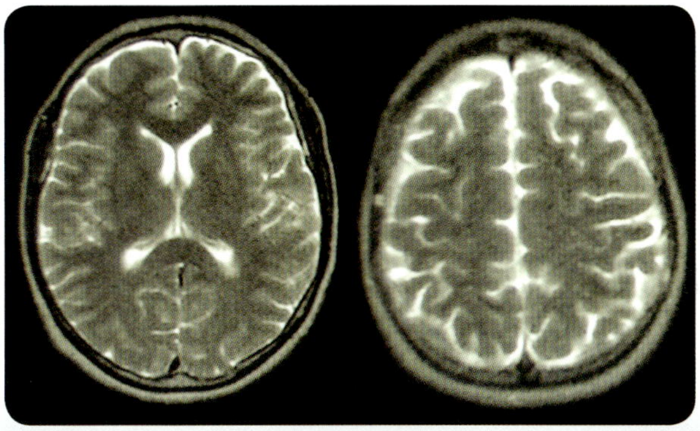

Fig. 5.2.59.

Examination of the patient showed that he had a scoliotic deformity of the 2nd degree and relative shortening of the left leg (**18 mm**). He had bilateral plexitis, neuritis of the obturator and femoral nerves, and bilateral lumbar ischialgia. The range of movements of his head was considerably limited.

The standard treatment, i.e. local magneto-acoustic therapy—transcranial and along the spinal column, inflatable rubber collar, orthopaedic insole, physiotherapy, was initiated. The patient was taught to perform exercises for detorsional correction. The intensity of the back pain decreased significantly after his first few efforts.

The patient was observed over 10 months. During the last examination, it was found that the length of the left leg was **7 mm** less than that of the right. The axis of the spine was normalizing. The spinal muscles (common erector) had

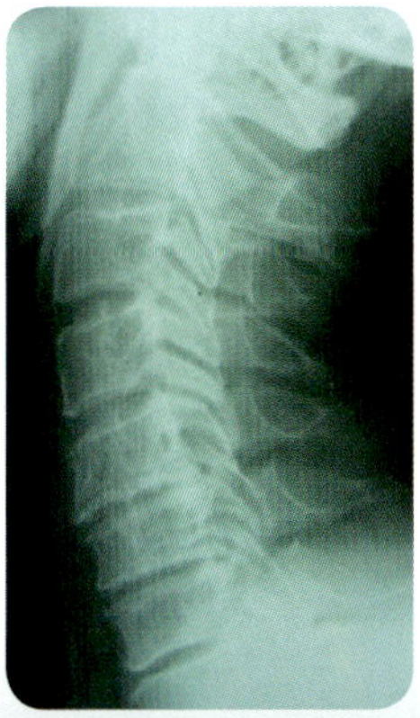

Fig. 5.2.60.

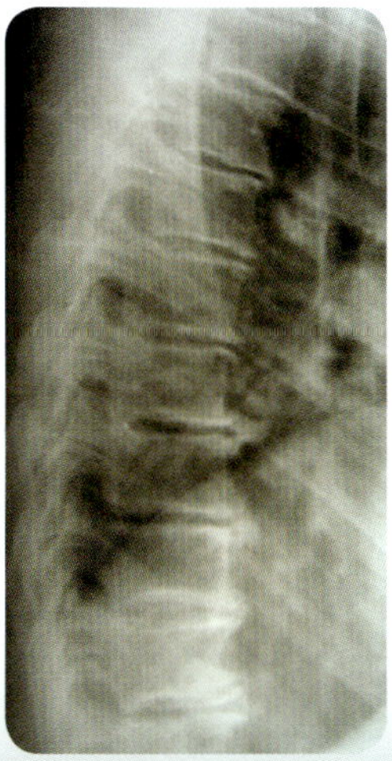

Fig. 5.2.61.

become symmetrical. M. did his detorsional exercises regularly. He reported that he felt almost healthy. We recommended that he continue with the prescribed treatment.

29. Patient D., a 40-year-old woman, complained of dizziness and intense headaches. She had lost consciousness for the first time about 20 years earlier, first in a bathhouse and then in a dormitory. Subsequently, the episodes of loss of consciousness recurred, and she also started suffering from dyspnoea and spells of dizziness. The patient received treatment from neurologists and even neurosurgeons on many occasions. Dyscirculatory encephalopathy, vertebrobasilar insufficiency and vegetovascular dystonia were diagnosed. Treatment in sanatoriums brought temporary relief. D. complained of persistent pain in the interscapular region, saying that it felt like a 'stake being hammered in'.

Radiographs of the cervical spine revealed rotary displacement of vertebrae at the level of C_4–C_6 (Fig. 5.2.62). The CT scan showed no organic changes. Radiograph of the thoracic spine revealed widespread osteochondrosis and spondylosis, as well as Schmorl's hernias (Fig. 5.2.63). Rheoencephalography showed that the flow of blood in the left vertebral artery at the level of C_4 was reduced by 49% and in the right vertebral artery, by 58%. The flow of blood in the internal carotid artery on the right was reduced by 20% and that on the left by 26%.

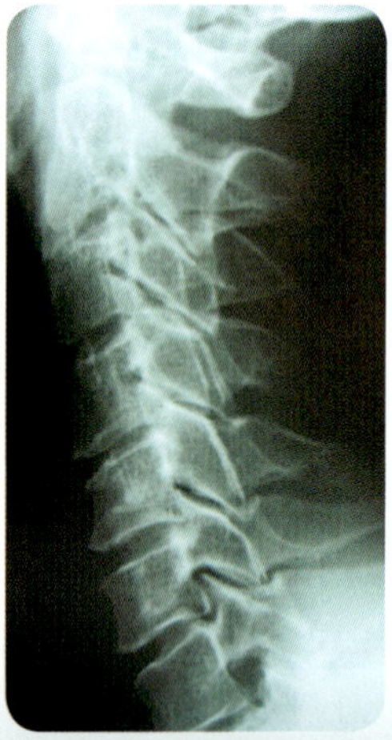

Fig. 5.2.62.

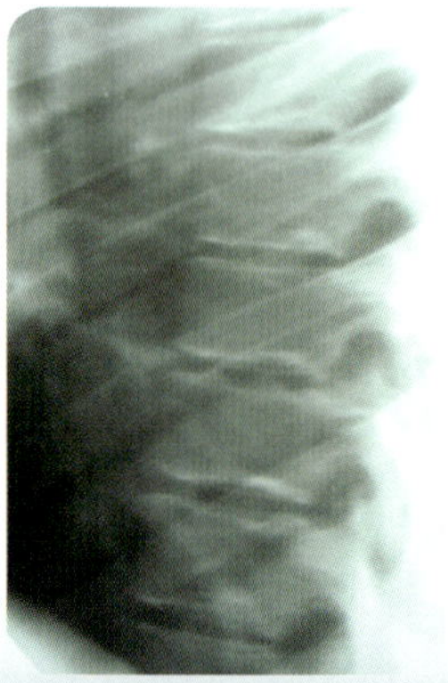

Fig. 5.2.63.

Examination of the patient revealed relative shortening of the right leg by **3 mm**. Her capacity to rotate the head was significantly limited: the range of movement was restricted to less than 40 degrees of the total range of 180 degrees. Bilateral plexitis, neuritis of the obturator and femoral nerves, and lumbar ischialgia were observed. Due to constant dizziness, D. could not walk independently and had to be supported by relatives on both sides.

The standard treatment, i.e. orthopaedic insole, detorsional gymnastics, local magneto-acoustic therapy—transcranial and along the spinal column, rubber inflatable collar, was prescribed. Vitamins were also recommended.

The patient was followed up every month. She gradually began to improve. The dizziness had decreased and there were no more episodes of loss of consciousness. When examined 6 months after the initiation of treatment, D. reported that the dizziness had completely resolved, she had no headaches. There were no more episodes of loss of consciousness. Also, she could walk independently on her own.

She had heeded all the advice and wore the insole regularly. Examination after 1 year of treatment showed that there was no difference in the length of the legs, and the axis of the spine had been corrected to a large extent. D. considered herself healthy and had no complaints. In recent months, she has stopped taking all medication. However, we advised her to continue with the detorsional gymnastics.

30. Patient S., a 50-year-old woman, complained of intense pain in the neck, a marked inability to turn the head fully, severe headaches and dizziness, pain in the interscapular region that radiated to the heart, and periodic breathlessness. She could not raise her right arm because of intense pain in the shoulder joint. Four months before consulting us, she had sustained injuries in a traffic accident. Because of the area in which her residence was located, she could not be provided with specialized medical care, so she was admitted to our clinic for a complete examination and the necessary treatment.

Radiographs revealed a consolidated compression fracture of C_7. There were signs of advanced deforming spondylosis at the same level. One could also observe blocking of the C_6–C_7 vertebrae which were in a state of mutual rotation, as well as ossification of the posterior longitudinal ligament (Fig. 5.2.64).

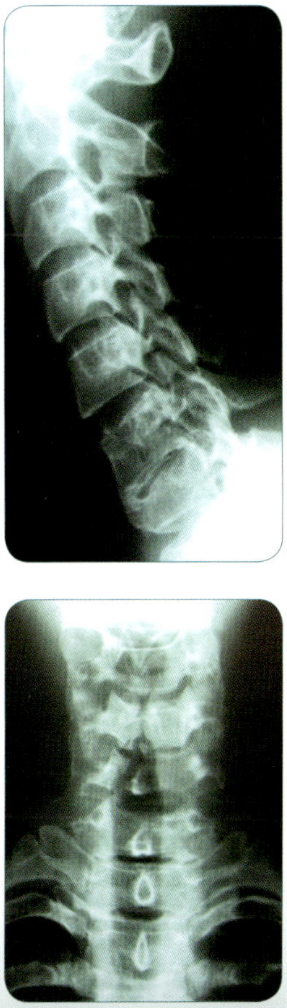

Fig. 5.2.64.

In the thoracic region, there was a consolidated compression fracture of Th_7, which was found to have developed a wedge-shaped deformity (Schemes 5.4 and 5.5). In the lumbar region, sacralization of L_5 and lumbarization of S_1 were observed (Fig. 5.2.65).

On examination of the patient, it was seen that the head was tilted to the right and the total range of its rotational motions did not exceed 40 degrees on either side. She had extremely pronounced signs of bilateral plexitis, more on the right. Paresis of the median nerve of the right wrist was observed (she could not raise the second and the third fingers of this hand). S. had a lateral curvature of the spine, with a right-sided rib hump, as well as hypotrophy of the gluteal muscles on the left side. Relative shortening of the left leg (**20 mm**) was also observed. The patient had bilateral lumbar ischialgia and neuritis of

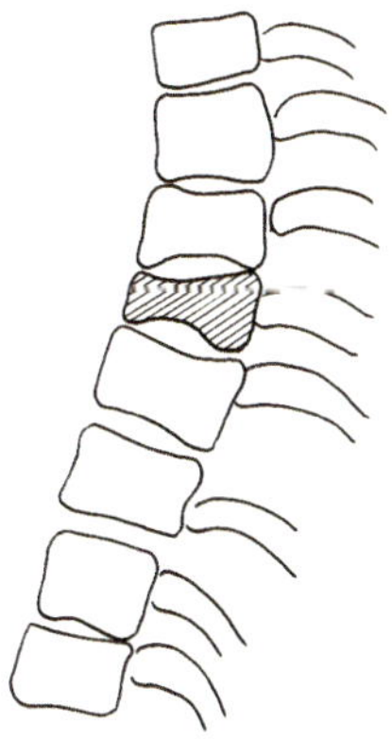

Scheme 5.4

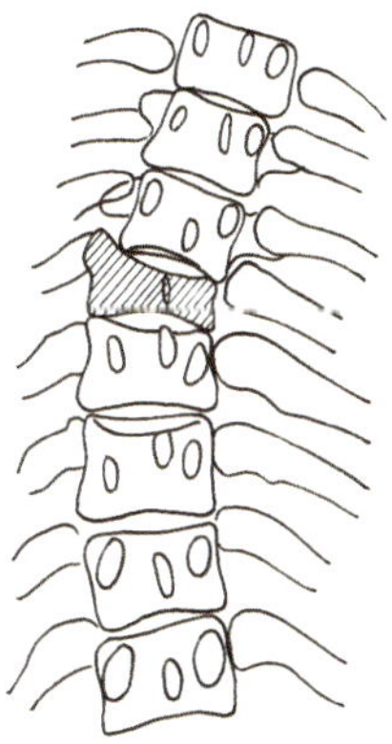

Scheme 5.5

the femoral and obturator nerves.

The standard treatment, i.e. permanent use of an inflatable rubber collar, orthopaedic insole to compensate for the left leg shortening, local magneto-acoustic therapy along the spine, physical therapy aimed to eliminate rotational displacements of the vertebrae, was prescribed. We added vitamin therapy, as well as injections of cocarboxylase and nicotinic acid.

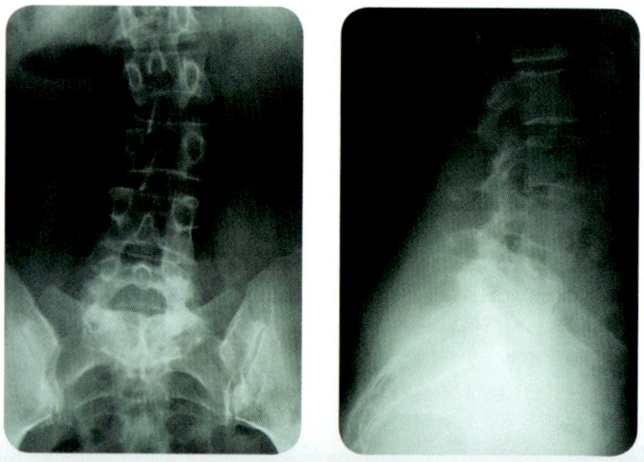

Fig. 5.2.65.

The patient was treated in the hospital for 3 weeks, after which she received treatment on an outpatient basis. She was asked to report for regular weekly examinations. After 2 months, the difference in the length of the legs had decreased to **15 mm**. There were no more headaches and the signs of median nerve neuritis on the right side were now minor. The pain between the shoulder blades had decreased. During the examination carried out 6 months after the initiation of treatment, it was found that the patient was free of all pain syndromes and had only residual symptoms of median nerve neuritis. The difference in the length of the two legs had decreased to **7 mm**. The axis of the spine was on its way to being corrected. We advised the patient to further her recovery in a sanatorium and resort.

31. Patient S., a 41-year-old woman, complained of burning pain in the skin on the back of her head, so much so that she could not place her head on a pillow. She also complained of trichalgia and said that any pressure on her eyeballs caused pain. Her problems had started 13 years ago, when she first began to suffer from dizziness, severe nausea and pain in the right temple.

She said that the spine in the thoracic region 'burns like fire'. The pain had first appeared eight years ago. S. could not straighten her body and could walk only with assistance. She constantly had a feeling of panic and said that nothing helped.

Doppler ultrasound investigation of the cerebral and cervical vessels showed a decrease in the flow of blood in the vertebral arteries at the level of C_3–C_4. The deficit was up to 25% on the right side and up to 54% on the left. Radiographs of the cervical spine revealed rotational displacements of C_4–C_6, with signs of moderate osteoarthritis and spondylosis deformans (Fig. 5.2.66).

Examination of the patient showed that she had a scoliotic deformity of the chest, as well as relative shortening of the left leg (**7 mm**). There was rotational subluxation of the vertebrae in all regions of the spine. Bilateral plexitis, femoral nerve neuritis and lumbar ischialgia were observed.

The standard treatment, i.e. inflatable rubber collar, detorsional exercises for all parts of the spine, magneto-acoustic therapy—local and transcranial as well as along the spine, orthopaedic insole, was prescribed.

When the patient was examined after 1 month, the headaches had become rare, and she no longer suffered from dizziness and a sense of panic. The pain along the spine was now mild.

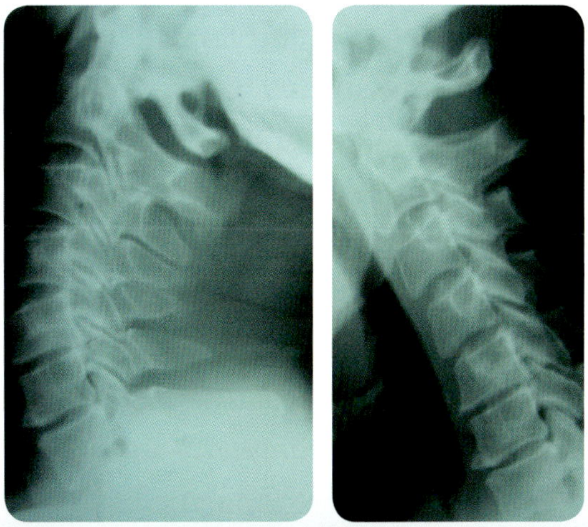

Fig. 5.2.66.

At 5 months' follow-up, the dizziness and headaches had resolved. The patient felt confident enough to walk on her own. Further, the axis of the spine was more or less correct and there was no difference in the length of the two legs. The application of pressure on the spinous processes no longer caused pain. The patient was very satisfied with the results of the treatment and considered herself healthy.

32. Patient S., a 13.5-year-old boy, complained of very intense headaches. One month before consulting us, he had lost consciousness while riding on a tram.

He told us that he could not tolerate physical activity. His other complaints included sweatiness of the hands and feet, emotional lability, tachycardia and shortness of breath. S. was treated by a neurologist and internist for vegetative dystonia, hypertensive–liquorodynamic syndrome and sinus tachycardia. He also suffered from dysbacteriosis. According to his mother, he was a very restless child and cried day and night. When he walked, his legs got tired and he got cramps in the calf muscles.

Dopplerography of the cerebral and cervical vessels revealed extravasal compression of the vertebral arteries at the level of C_3–C_4. There was a bilateral deficiency of blood flow of up to 25%. Radiographs of the cervical spine showed rotational displacement of C_3–C_5 (Fig. 5.2.67). As for the lumbosacral spine, there were rotational displacements of the lumbar vertebrae, lumbarization of S_1 and asymmetry of the articular processes of the L_5–S_1 segment (Fig. 5.2.68).

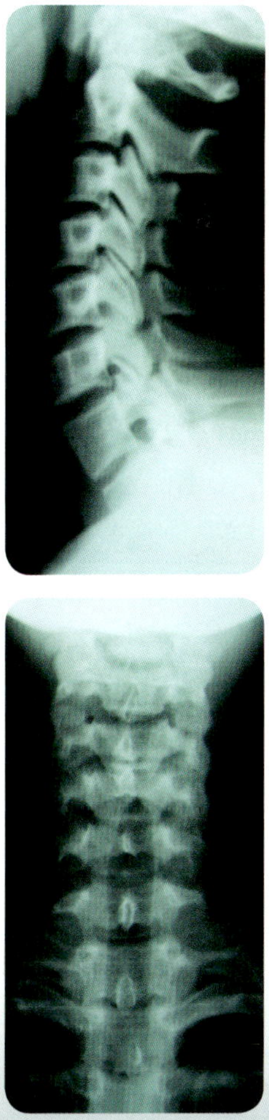

Fig. 5.2.67.

On examination, the patient was found to be very pale, weak and frail. He had a scoliotic posture and an initial manifestation of a rib hump in the form of a right-sided chest deformity, which was of moderate severity. Relative shortening of the left leg (**7 mm**) was observed. S. had bilateral plexitis, bilateral femoral and obturator nerve neuritis, and lumbar ischialgia. The application of pressure on the vertebral spinous processes caused him acute pain.

The standard treatment, i.e. inflatable rubber collar, magneto-acoustic therapy—local and transcranial as well as along the spine, orthopaedic insole, was initiated. The boy's mother was given training in detorsional gymnastics.

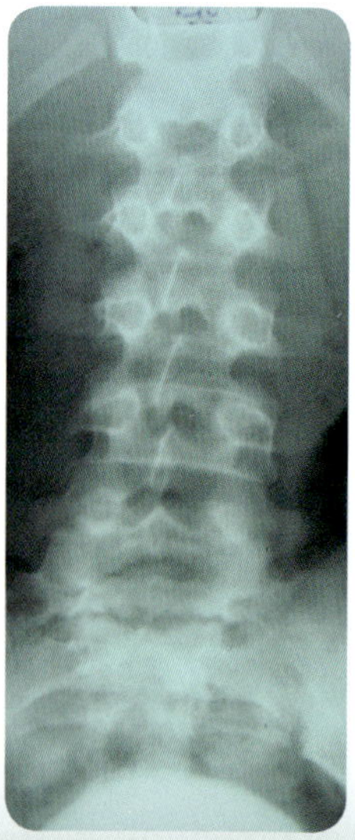

Fig. 5.2.68.

When examined after a month, the patient reported that the headaches had become less severe and there had been no more episodes of loss of consciousness. According to the mother, the boy had become calmer. At 6 months' follow-up, the spine had become straight and the scoliotic posture had been corrected. Relative shortening of the left leg was preserved at **3 mm**. S. did not suffer from headaches any longer and had no neurological symptoms, or episodes of loss of consciousness. We recommended that he adhere to the prescribed treatment for another year, in consideration of the fact that he was still in his growing years.

33. Patient S., a 54-year-old woman, had sustained a head injury (brain concussion) in a road traffic accident 13 years earlier. She had been unconscious for a long time and five of her ribs had been fractured. Her memory had been affected, but it had gradually recovered. However, since the accident, she had been suffering from a constant headache, mostly in the temples and neck.

She said she felt as though 'boiling water is being poured into the head'. S. also said her vision became blurred several times a day, and complained of numbness of the hands and fingers. She could not raise her hands or hold a pen in her right hand. S.'s other complaints included delays of breath and persistent pain in the heart (the ECG was normal). The cardiologist was unable to find any pathology. The patient complained that under the shoulder blades, she felt cold and hot), as if 'a stake is being hammered in'. S. was under treatment for gastritis, pancreatic hypofunction and constipation. Her other symptoms included pain in the feet and cramps in the toes.

Plain radiography revealed pronounced rotational displacement of the cervical vertebrae over the C_3–C_6 curvature (Fig. 5.2.69). As for the thoracic spine, one could observe osteochondrosis and spondylosis deformans, lateral curvature and torsion of the vertebrae at the level of Th_8–Th_9 (Fig. 5.2.70).

CT scans of the lumbar spine showed Schmorl's hernia of a significant size in the L_4–L_5 segment, these vertebrae being mutually rotated (Fig. 5.2.71).

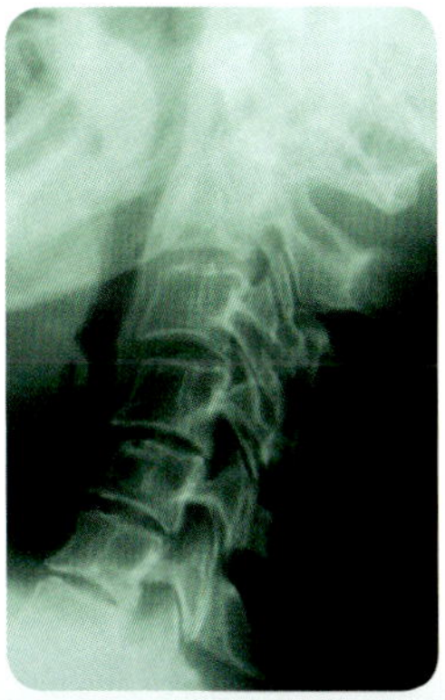

Fig. 5.2.69.

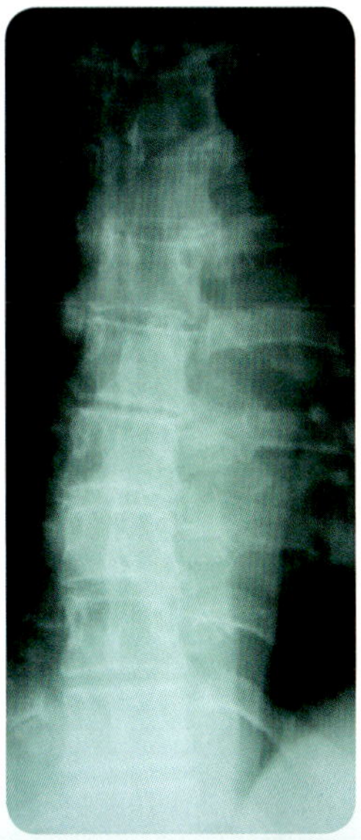

Fig. 5.2.70.

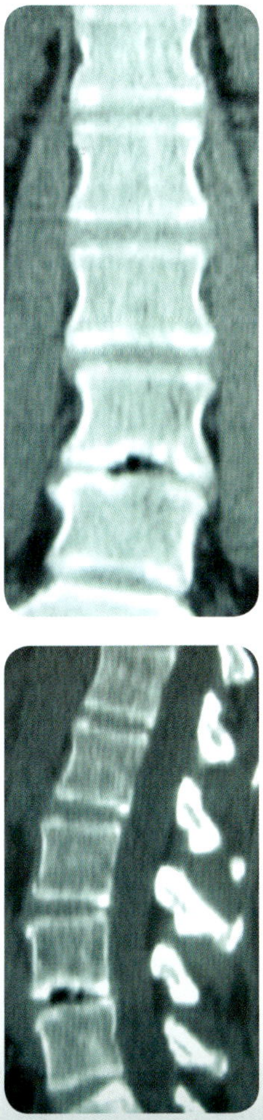

Fig. 5.2.71.

On examination, the patient was found to have a scoliotic deformity of the thoracic and lumbar spine (2nd degree). Hypotrophy of the gluteal muscles on the right side of the pelvis was observed, as was relative shortening of the right leg by **7 mm**. Palpation of the vertebral spinous processes caused the patient acute pain. There were signs of bilateral plexitis, and neuritis of the femoral, obturator and sciatic nerves.

The standard treatment, i.e. inflatable rubber collar, local transcranial and paravertebral magneto-acoustic therapy, detorsional exercises, orthopaedic insole, was initiated.

When examined 8 months later, the patient reported a significant improvement in her general condition. The headaches, numbness of the hands, as well as painful symptoms in other sites had resolved. The difference in the length of the two legs had come down to **3.5 mm**. The axis of the spine was in the process of becoming correct. We advised the patient to continue with the prescribed treatment for another year.

34. Patient B., a 46-year-old woman, complained of persistent headaches, defects in the visual field when making sudden head movements, besides dizziness and presyncopal states. Due to the persistent headaches, she had consulted a neurologist, who had diagnosed her with 'vegetovascular dystonia with increased intracranial pressure'.

Eighteen years ago, B. had sustained injuries in road car accident (RCA). She had received treatment in a district hospital and had taken bed rest for only 2 weeks. Since then till the time she came to consult us, she had been suffering from pain in the neck and lower thoracic region. She could not stand and work for a long time. The pain radiated to the heart. B.'s other symptoms were breath-holding, periodic low back pain, cramps in the calves and freezing feet, whether in winter or summer. Doppler ultrasound investigation of the cerebral and cervical vessels revealed a reduction in the flow of blood in the vertebral arteries at the level of C_3–C_4. The deficit was up to 40% on both sides. An incorrectly fused C_6 fracture, displacement of bone fragments of C_4–C_6 towards the spinal canal and rotational displacement of these were observed on radiographs of the cervical spine. In addition, there was ossification of the posterior longitudinal ligament in the zone of the fracture (Fig. 5.2.72).

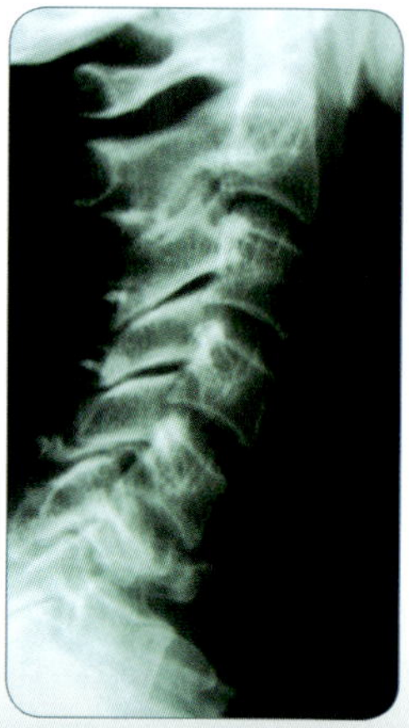
Fig. 5.2.72.

CT scan of the thoracic spine revealed an incorrectly fused compression fracture of the vertebral body of Th_{12} (Fig. 5.2.73).

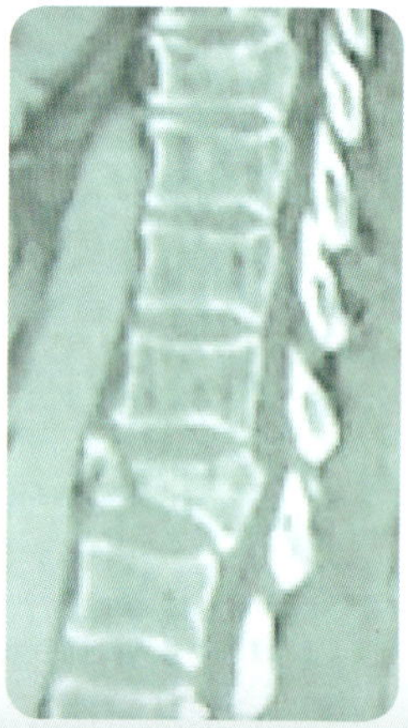
Fig. 5.2.73.

Examination of the patient revealed that she had a scoliotic deformity of the chest with a right-sided rib hump of mild severity. Hypotrophy of the gluteal muscles on the left side of the pelvis was observed. There was relative shortening of the left leg (about **15 mm**). The application of pressure on the thoracic vertebrae caused the patient acute pain. She had bilateral plexitis, and neuritis of the obturator, femoral and sciatic nerves.

The standard treatment, i.e. inflatable rubber collar, local paravertebral magneto-acoustic therapy, physiotherapy, orthopaedic insole, was prescribed. When examined after 2 months, B. reported that there had been a significant improvement in her overall condition. The headaches and dizziness occurred rarely. The pain in the thoracic region (at the site of the trauma) was preserved. At 10 months' follow-up, the difference in the length of the legs had decreased to **3 mm** and the axis of the spine was normalizing. There were no more complaints of heart pain, breath-holding, dizziness and headaches. The patient felt she was almost healthy. She was very conscientious about performing the detorsional exercises. B. continues to use an orthopaedic insole of a height of **3 mm**.

35. Patient K., a 17-year-old young woman, had a significant scoliotic deformity of the chest, of the 3rd–4th degree. It was of a compensatory muscular origin. She also had a moderately pronounced right-sided rib hump. According to the patient's mother, the deformity had progressed over the past few years. The patient complained of headaches, tingling in the heart, breath-holding, persistent pain in the interscapular region, sweatiness of the hands and marked emotional lability. In winter, her hands and feet would freeze. In addition, K. felt heaviness in the stomach, as well as pain in the lower back and knee joints. The neurologist had made a diagnosis of vegetovascular dystonia.

Plain radiography of the thoracic and lumbar regions of the spine revealed a scoliotic deformity, as well as torsion of the thoracic and lumbar vertebrae. As for the lumbosacral region, there was physiological lumbarization of S_1–S_2, sacralization of L_5, spina bifida of S_1 and anomalous tropism of the articular processes in the L_5–S_1 segment (Fig. 5.2.74).

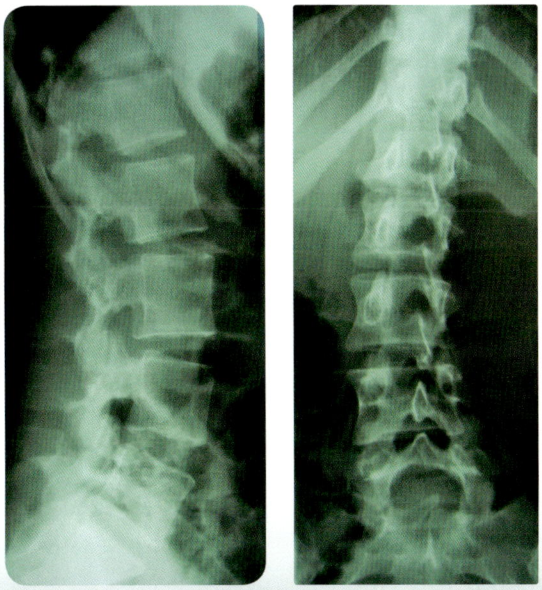

Fig. 5.2.74.

Examination of the patient revealed a considerable tilt of the pelvis to the left and, accordingly, significant curvature of the spine. We attempted to compensate for this with an insole of a height of **40 mm**. She had bilateral plexitis and lumbar ischialgia.

The standard treatment, i.e. orthopaedic insole, inflatable rubber collar, local transcranial and paravertebral magneto-acoustic therapy, scheme of detorsional exercises, was prescribed. The height of the orthopaedic insole was increased gradually, beginning from **15 mm**, to correct the asymmetry of the spinal muscles. Follow-up examinations were carried out every 1–1.5 months on an average. At one year's follow-up, the difference in the length of the two legs had decreased to **18 mm**. K. no longer complained of pain in the back, heart and stomach. The headaches had resolved. The girl and her parents were satisfied with the results of treatment since the deformity of the chest had improved visibly. The axis of the spine was normalizing. K. continued with the recommended treatment focusing on detorsional gymnastics and the use of an orthopaedic insole.

36. Patient E., a 45-year-old woman, had consulted various specialists over the past 6 years, but the intensity of her complaints had gradually increased.

On the day she consulted us, she complained of numbness in the fingers, waking up with a sensation of severe heaviness in the head and neck, tachycardia and frequent extrasystoles. She said that she felt pain along the whole spine in the mornings. Her periods had been painful throughout her life and she had a tendency to constipation. Due to constant pain in the lower abdomen, she had undergone a gynaecological surgery, but the pain persisted. During her school years, E. was actively involved in sports and had sustained a few neck injuries.

Plain radiography of the cervical spine revealed signs of advanced deforming spondylosis and degenerative disc disease, blockade of the C_6–C_7 vertebral bodies and rotational displacement of C_4–C_7 (Fig. 5.2.75). The radiograph of the lumbosacral spine showed lumbarization of S_1, sacralization of L_5, asymmetry of the articular processes in the L_5–S_1 segment and rotational displacement of the lumbar vertebrae (Fig. 5.2.76).

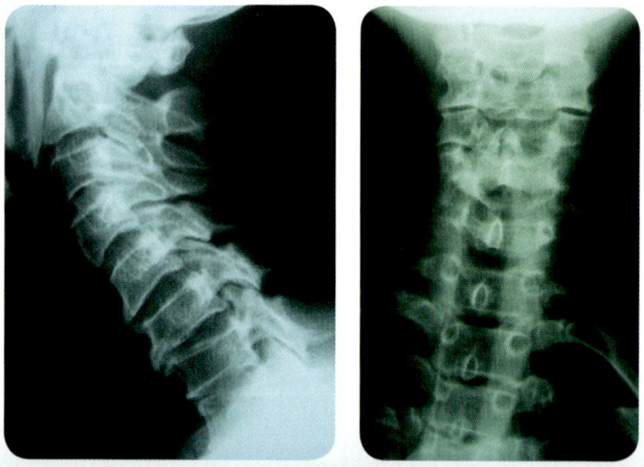

Fig. 5.2.75.

On examination, the patient was found to have a scoliotic posture due to relative shortening of the left leg (up to **20 mm**). She had signs of bilateral plexitis, and neuritis of the femoral, obturator and sciatic nerves.

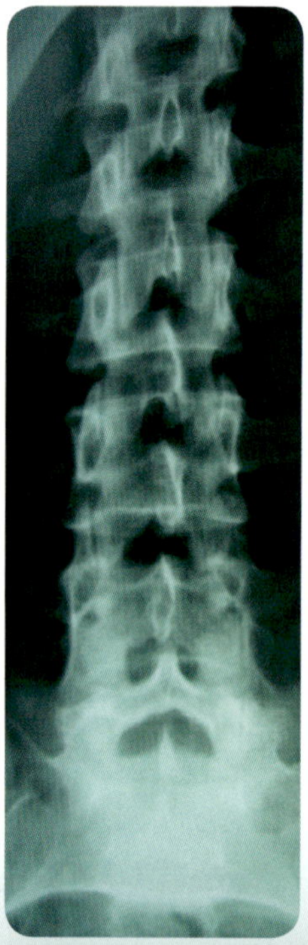

Fig. 5.2.76.

The standard treatment, i.e. inflatable rubber collar, magneto-acoustic therapy—local transcranial as well as along the spine, physiotherapy, orthopaedic insole, was prescribed. The patient was taught to perform detorsional corrective gymnastics during the first consultation itself.

The patient noted that after first derotating movements, the pain in the internal organs and spine had resolved almost completely. Physical therapy and the use of the insole resulted in correction of the vertebral axis.

The long-term results of treatment were assessed 1 year after its initiation. The patient reported a significant improvement in her general condition. There was hardly any pain. Relative shortening of the left leg had decreased to **3 mm**. The axis of the spine was normalizing. We recommended that she continue with the course of treatment.

37. Patient O., a 45-year-old man who came to us for medical assistance, was tall and strong, but nevertheless complained of intense low back pain as well as pain along the spine, and cramps in the leg muscles. He had been diagnosed with convergent strabismus. O. was especially concerned about the extremely painful spasms in the stomach and intestines that occurred periodically and had persisted for several years. They were so intense that during such episodes, he would roll on the floor with his legs crossed, which gave him some relief from the pain. Usually the pain resolved once he was given antispasmodic injections in the emergency department. This positive effect of the medications lasted for a short time and then the pain returned. The surgeon who investigated him found no pathological changes in stomach and intestine.

On examination, the patient was found to have relative shortening of the left leg (**15 mm**). He had a scoliotic posture caused by a pelvic tilt, which we immediately attempted to correct with an orthopaedic insole. O. had acute pain along the spine, as well as bilateral plexitis and lumbar ischialgia.

The standard treatment, i.e. orthopaedic insole, corrective detorsional gymnastics, local magneto-acoustic therapy, was initiated. At 8 months' follow-up, relative shortening of the left leg had reduced to **7 mm**. The axis of the spine was more or less correct. The pain and spasms had resolved completely. The patient performed physiotherapy exercises several times a day. He was encouraged to continue with the prescribed treatment.

38. Patient N., a 25-year-old man, had received treatment from various physicians for spasm of accommodation, polycystosis, calculous cholecystitis and fatty hepatosis. He had constant spinal pain.

On examination, N. was found to have a scoliotic posture associated with a tilt of the body to the left. There was pronounced rotational displacement of the vertebrae in all regions of the spine. The patient was obese. We attempted to eliminate the body tilt and corresponding muscular asymmetry with an orthopaedic insole of a height of **33 mm**, to be placed under the left heel.

The standard treatment, i.e. set of detorsional exercises, inflatable rubber collar, transcranial and paravertebral magneto-acoustic therapy, orthopaedic insole, was prescribed. At the beginning of treatment, the patient was asked to wear an insole of a height of **20 mm**, and after a month, the height was increased by **13 mm**. In addition, local magneto-acoustic therapy was also performed at the base of the skull (projection of the pituitary gland).

When examined 5 months after the initiation of treatment, the patient reported that the pain syndrome, including that in the spine, had resolved. The legs were now of equal length, the pelvic tilt had been eliminated and the spinal erectors were symmetrical. N. had lost weight and it became appropriate for his age. He was last examined one-and-a-half years after the initiation of treatment. He had no complaints; he became a well-set-up young man with no shortening of the left leg. Back muscles were symmetrical. The patient considered himself healthy.

39. Patient D., an 11-year-old girl, had been suffering from bronchial asthma since the age of two. She had pronounced signs of vegetative dystonia (cold and sweaty hands and feet, proptosis, enlarged thyroid gland), as well as divergent concomitant strabismus.

Dopplerography of the cerebral and cervical vessels revealed extravasal compression of the vertebral arteries at the level of C_3–C_5. The blood flow on the right was decreased by up to 30% and on the left, by up to 35%.

On examination, it was found that the patient had a scoliotic posture associated with asymmetry of the back muscles. We asked her to use an insole of a height of **3 mm** to compensate for the relative shortening of the left leg. D. had pain along the spine that severely restricted the movements of her head. In addition, she had signs of bilateral plexitis, and neuritis of the femoral, obturator and sciatic nerves.

The standard treatment, i.e. orthopaedic insole, local magneto-acoustic therapy in all regions of the spine, corrective detorsional gymnastics, inflatable rubber collar, was prescribed.

When examined 6 months after the initiation of treatment, the patient reported that the frequency of asthma attacks had decreased considerably. She did not have any symptoms of neuritis and her posture had become normal. The axis of the spine was more or less correct. We advised the patient to continue with the prescribed treatment.

40. Patient B., a 53-year-old man, complained of headaches and heaviness in the head and said that there was a noise in his head and ears. He also mentioned that his thinking was impaired ('no clarity of thought'). In addition, B. suffered from mixed astigmatism, duodenal ulcer, psoriasis with lesions of the scalp, constricting pain in the heart and neuritis of the right trigeminal nerve (for the past 3 years). His other complaints included burning pain between the shoulder blades (as though 'a stake is being hammered in'), and deep pain in the lower third of the cervical spine, radiating to the right arm.

Dopplerograms of the cerebral and cervical vessels revealed extravasal compression of the vertebral arteries both on the right and left sides at the level of C_3–C_4. The blood flow was decreased by up to 30%. CT scans of the cervical spine showed that physiological lordosis was absent, but abnormal kyphosis was present. There was rotational displacement of vertebrae at the level of C_4–C_6 (Fig. 5.2.77). Asymmetrical contraction of the spinal extensors had given rise to relative shortening of the left leg and a pelvic tilt to the left. We attempted to compensate for this with an insole of a height of **20 mm**.

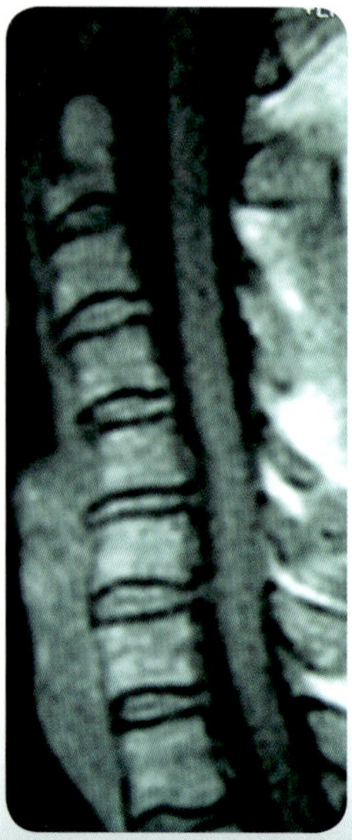

Fig. 5.2.77.

The standard treatment, i.e. detorsional exercises, orthopaedic insole, inflatable rubber collar, local transcranial and paravertebral magneto-acoustic therapy, was prescribed. During an examination 2 months after the initiation of treatment, it was found that there was a significant reduction of pain in the areas that had been painful before treatment. The heart pain and headaches also had resolved. The axis of the spine had become correct. Relative shortening of the left leg had reduced to **10 mm**. At 1.5 years' follow-up, the left leg was **3 mm** shorter than the right. There were no psoriatic plaques. The patient considered himself healthy as the pain had almost totally resolved. He performed detorsional gymnastics regularly, several times a day.

We have given above several examples of our patients who suffered from spinal pain, mostly in the thoracic spine, and the observations we made in these cases. More examples could have been included, were it not for the need to limit the volume of the book. Although the material in this section would be sufficient to facilitate an understanding of the initial condition of the patients and the results of the treatment prescribed, there are other questions that need to be answered. These include how and why patients with chronic conditions were able to get rid of their suffering in a relatively short period of time. What was the secret of their recovery?

We will answer these questions in order.

1. We shall go through the data presented in Figs 5.3 and 5.4, which have been discussed earlier in this chapter. Each organ or group of organs is under the control of certain parts of the central and peripheral nervous systems. Impairment of the control and regulatory functions of these systems inevitably leads to malfunctioning of the cardiovascular, respiratory, digestive, urinary and other systems. It is worth recalling that apart from the nerve plexuses that control a particular system of organs, there are nerves arising from these plexuses that control individual organs, such as the heart, trachea, oesophagus, intestines, liver, gallbladder, pancreas, spleen, kidney, bladder, testis, uterus and vagina. It is quite natural that impairment in the central regulatory system are inevitably reflected in the peripheral part of the nervous system.
2. In all the cases presented in this section, the patients had a lateral curvature of the spine when they sought our help at the beginning of treatment. In the majority of cases, the curvature was caused by unilateral spasm of the long extensors of the spine, excluding cases of accessory or wedge-shaped vertebrae, blockade of vertebrae in a vicious position and other similar conditions. The above-mentioned spasm was associated with structural features of the brain and had been fixed in the vestibular apparatus and cerebellum as a conditioned reflex of 'wrong' vertical body positioning in early childhood. The tilting of the body led to rotation of the vertebrae around their axes in all regions of the spine and to the subsequent development of lateral curvature.

   Thus, blocks (blockades) of spinal motion segments (SMS) were formed, resulting in limited range of motion as well as pain of varying intensity due to traumatization of the nerve endings. The pathological symptoms of the disease depended on the location of these blockades.

3. When analysing the causes of pain in the thoracic spine, one must mention herniation of the intervertebral discs. Herniation occurs relatively rarely because the strong posterior longitudinal ligament prevents displacement of the disc and nucleus. In most cases, pain is associated with deforming arthrosis of the costovertebral joints—a frequent companion of osteoarthritis of the spine. If one considers the fact that the paravertebral sympathetic ganglia forming the sympathetic trunk are located at the level of these joints (on the anterior surface of the costal heads), the cause of girdling intercostal neuralgia with autonomic vasomotor reactions and thoracalgia becomes clear.
4. Correcting the axis of the spine in all its regions, combined with the use of orthopaedic insoles to compensate for the relative shortening of one leg, helped to restore the vertical position of the body and lateral curvature. This led to normalization of functioning of the central and peripheral nervous systems, which ultimately resulted in regression of the pathological symptoms and clinical recovery.
5. Magneto-acoustic therapy, with its anti-oedematous, anti-inflammatory and analgesic effects, also contributed to the process of recovery. This therapy was administered along the entire spine, as well as transcranially (application of the device to the head in the frontal, parietal and occipital zones). The therapy also contributed to normalization of the cerebral and spinal blood flow, resulting in regression of the symptoms associated with ischaemia of the structures mentioned.
6. For patients with pathological symptoms in the cervical and upper thoracic spine, we used an inflatable rubber collar, which provides a soft and dosed relaxation of contracted muscles. It is also used for atraumatic reduction of rotated and displaced vertebrae.
7. Thus, the high level of efficacy of our treatment can be explained by the fact that we were not just treating the symptoms of a disease, but were also correcting the cause or group of causes that had led to its development.

Issues regarding the treatment of patients and the mechanisms of such treatment will be discussed in detail in the concluding chapter.

5.3 Lumbosacral region of the spine

Virtually all our patients, ranging from children to the elderly, had spinal pain predominantly in the lumbosacral region, besides other common complaints. The pain could be localized or radiate to one or both legs, and be associated with cramps and fatigue. We have already provided the reader with information on the nature of spinal pain, drawing on the available literature (*see* Chapter 4 'Spinal pain syndrome and its origin'). Our own observations have confirmed and extended the body of data.

We also found that all patients suffering from spinal pain had lateral curvature of the spine of varying degree. As mentioned earlier, in most cases it was caused by asymmetrical functioning of the common spinal extensors, which results in tilting of the body and pelvis to one side or the other. The development of the spine in a tilted position from early childhood was the cause of asymmetrical development of the vertebral bodies, arches and processes, intervertebral discs, ligaments and other anatomical structures. The result of this asymmetrical development was that zones of instability were formed in all regions of the spine, particularly the lumbosacral region. In accordance with the laws of classical mechanics, the process of rotation was set off in these zones, starting from individual vertebrae, to subsequent torsion of entire segments. This led to the development of a structural scoliotic deformity.

Apart from increasing unilateral spasm of the trunk muscles, there are other factors that weaken the base of the spine (the L_5–S_1 zone) and play a significant role in the mechanism of rotation–torsion. These include shortening of one leg, partial or complete sacralization of L_5, lumbarization of S_1–S_2, posterior defects of the lumbar and sacral vertebrae, anomalous tropism of the articular processes (mainly in the L_5–S_1 spinal mobile segment (SMS) and additional wedge-shaped semivertebrae at different levels of the spine.

We observed that under certain anatomical conditions, rotation of the vertebrae in the lumbosacral region compressed the trunks of the sympathetic and parasympathetic nerves of the lumbosacral plexus (*see* Figs 2.1.34–2.1.42). Impaired functioning of neurological structures led to the development of diseases of the rectum, uterus, ovaries, vagina, etc. Many patients suffered from persistent pelvic pain syndrome, accompanied by signs of urethritis, painful menstruation, chronic constipation, haemorrhoids, anal fistulas, coccyalgia, prostatitis, etc. Impairments in neurotrophic factors and the blood circulation of the lower extremities gave rise to the development of varicose veins and the formation of venous ulcers. In many cases, injury to the lumbosacral plexus could cause various skin diseases and neurological disorders, such as neuritis of the obturator, femoral and sciatic nerves, etc. We observed most of these diseases in our clinical practice and the subject will be discussed further.

All our patients who complained of lumbosacral spinal pain initially underwent radiological evaluation (plain radiography). If necessary, they were referred to a neurosurgeon, neurologist, internist, cardiologist and other specialists. After a final diagnosis was made, the basic therapy was prescribed, except in the case of patients suffering from neurosurgical, oncological and certain specific conditions. The basic therapy included the use of an orthopaedic insole on the side of the shortened leg, detorsional exercises and local paravertebral magneto-acoustic therapy. In some cases, when indicated, we used an inflatable collar for fixation and dosed traction of the cervical and upper thoracic spine.

The results of the treatment were evaluated both in the short term and long term (up to one year). For some cases in which the initial radiographs of the lumbosacral spine were of bad quality, we have presented the relevant schematic images. In order to help the reader understand the material presented here, and in view of the fact that all patients with back pain had dysplastic changes at the level of L_5–S_1, we have divided the patients into three subgroups:

5.3.1. Patients with sacralization of the 5th lumbar vertebra and lumbarization of the sacral vertebrae, as well as abnormalities of the articular processes of the L_5–S_1 SMS

5.3.2. Patients with sacralization of the 5th lumbar vertebra and lumbarization of the sacral vertebrae, posterior clefts of these vertebrae and anomalous tropism of the articular processes of the L_5–S_1 SMS

5.3.3. Patients with low back (lumbar) pain and scoliotic spinal deformity.

Such assignment of patients with scoliosis into the third subgroup should be considered rather conditional (since lateral curvature of the spine was present in all our patients with spinal pain. We once again draw our readers' attention to the fact that initially, our primary aim was to deal with spinal pain, and not to treat scoliosis. This is why we do not have a sufficient number of initial radiographs, especially in the case of children. Often, when parents brought their children to us with the complaints of abnormal vision and vegetative dystonia, our radiological evaluation was not complete and was limited to the cervical spine. This was due to the fact that in the initial stage of our work, we did not have enough knowledge or the confidence to assume that the scheme we had developed for the treatment of vision abnormalities and spinal pain would be just as effective for the elimination of scoliosis.

With the purpose of correcting this situation and evaluating the long-term results of our treatment, we called the patients for follow-up visits at varying intervals and in some cases, with the consent of the parents of children or the adult patients themselves, to perform control radiographic evaluation of the spine. To illustrate this, we shall present a number of clinical cases from our own experience.

5.3.1 Patients with sacralization of L5, lumbarization of sacral vertebrae and anomalous articular processes of L5–S1 spinal motion segment

1. Patient B., a 71-year-old woman, complained of pain, in the thoracic and lumbar spine that had persisted for many years. Earlier in her life, she had been involved in sports activities and sustained a spinal injury.

Radiographs of the thoracic spine revealed osteoporosis, osteochondrosis and spondylosis deformans. In the lumbosacral region, we observed synostosis of the vertebral bodies of L_4–L_5. This was probably of post-traumatic origin. Sacralization of L_5 was also observed. There was blockade of L_4–L_5, which caused compensatory hypermobility at the level of S_1–S_2. This, in turn, led to their separation and compensatory lumbarization of S_1 (Fig. 5.3.1).

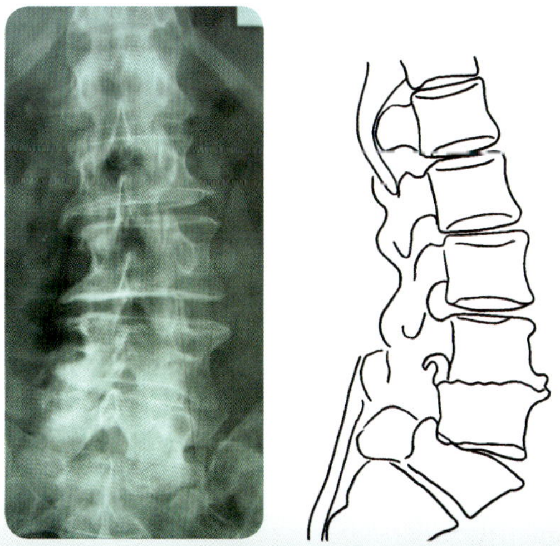

Fig. 5.3.1.

Examination of the patient showed the presence of a severe kyphoscoliotic deformity in the thoracic region. The pelvis was tilted to the left and we attempted to compensate for this with an orthopaedic insole of a height of **10 mm**. B. had clinical signs of bilateral plexitis, and neuritis of the obturator, femoral and sciatic nerves.

The standard treatment, i.e. wearing of orthopaedic insole, detorsional gymnastics, local paravertebral magneto-acoustic therapy, was prescribed. When the patient was examined after a month, the difference in the length of the legs had decreased to **7 mm**. There was also a significant decrease in the pain along the spine. Examined at 3 months' follow-up, the difference in the length of the legs had decreased to **3 mm**. B.

had virtually no complaints. She was encouraged to continue with the recommended treatment during the subsequent year.

On analysing this clinical observation, we arrived at the following conclusions:

a. Compensatory lumbarization at the level of S_1–S_2, associated with tilting of the pelvis to the left, led to the rotation of these vertebrae and injury to the sacral plexus.
b. The treatment prescribed to restore balance in the lumbo-pelvic segment gradually reduced the tilt of the pelvis and helped limit its consequences. This, in turn, contributed to the patient's clinical recovery.

2. Patient Y., a 23-year-old man, presented with the complaints of persistent headaches, neck pain radiating to his arms, and pain in the thoracic and lumbar spine radiating to the legs. The pain was persistent even though he went jogging and played tennis frequently. The patient was obese and tall. Treatment by a neurologist and endocrinologist gave no relief.

Radiography of the cervical spine revealed rotational displacement of the cervical vertebrae at all levels, from C_3 to C_6 (Fig. 5.3.2). As for the lumbosacral region, there was sacralization of L_5, lumbarization of S_1 and impaired tropism (asymmetrical structure) of the articular processes in the L_5–S_1 spinal motion segment (SMS) (Fig. 5.3.3).

Examination of the patient revealed a right-sided scoliotic deformity of the spine. There was a significant pelvic tilt to the left, which we attempted to compensate for with an orthopaedic insole of a height of **30 mm**. Y. had clinical signs of plexitis, lumboischialgia, and neuritis of the obturator and femoral nerves.

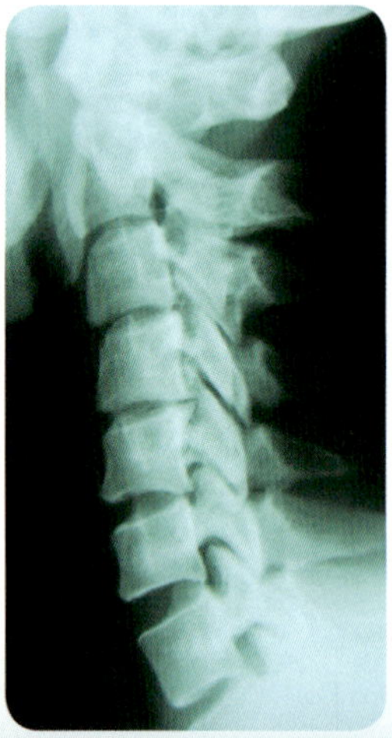

Fig. 5.3.2.

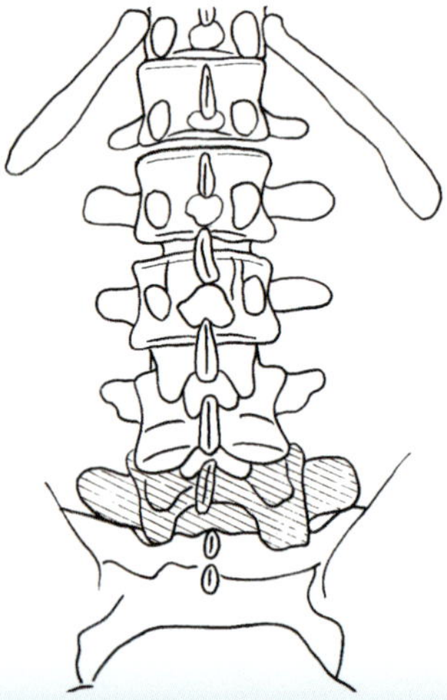

Fig. 5.3.3.

The standard treatment, i.e. wearing of orthopaedic insole, detorsional gymnastics (including exercises involving the cervical spine), local paravertebral magneto-acoustic therapy, was prescribed. We recommended the use of an inflatable rubber collar in order to stabilize the cervical vertebrae. We advised him to start wearing an orthopaedic insole of a height of **15 mm**. During the follow-up examination a month later, the height of the insole was increased by **7 mm**. The patient followed our advice conscientiously. He reported that he had lost weight. At 6 months' follow-up, the relative shortening of the left leg, which was 30 mm at the beginning of treatment, had reduced to **10 mm**. The headaches and pain along the spine had resolved completely.

The patient had become noticeably thinner. He was advised to continue with the prescribed treatment for another 6–7 months.

On analysing this clinical observation, we arrived at the following conclusions:

a. Overweight (moderate obesity) was probably caused by pituitary dysfunction due to significant rotational displacements of the upper cervical vertebrae.
b. Instability and associated rotation of the vertebrae in the thoracic and lumbosacral regions had led to the relative shortening of the left leg by **30 mm**. Dysplastic changes and physiological lumbarization of S_1 relative to S_2 also contributed to this condition.
c. Gradual rebalancing of the lumbo-pelvic segment through the use of an orthopaedic insole and other medical interventions eliminated the causes of spinal pain, and also normalized metabolic processes. As a result, the patient's body weight decreased and the pain resolved.

3. Patient R., a 19-year-old young woman, complained of constant intense pain in the lumbosacral spine of 1-year duration. The pain persisted despite regular measures to keep fit, massages and swimming.

Radiographs of the lumbar spine revealed lumbarization of S_1, sacralization of L_5 and asymmetry of the L_5–S_1 intervertebral articular processes (Fig. 5.3.4).

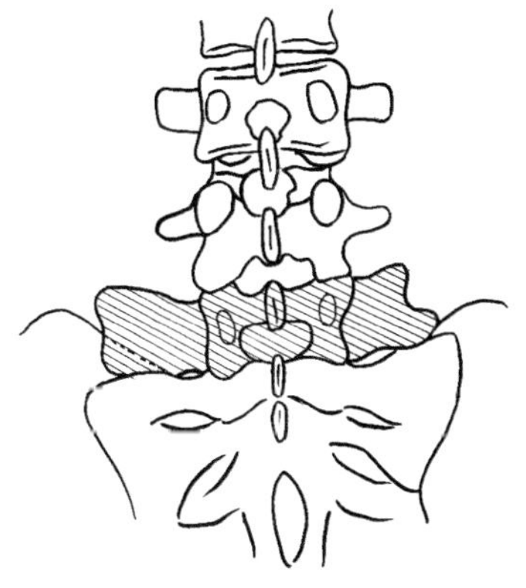

Fig. 5.3.4.

Examination revealed that the girl, who was of a regular build, had a slight scoliotic deformity of the spine. We attempted to correct the tilt of the pelvis to the left with an orthopaedic insole of a height of **18 mm**. She had clinical signs of bilateral lumboischialgia, and neuritis of the femoral and obturator nerves.

The standard treatment, i.e. orthopaedic insole local paravertebral magneto-acoustic therapy and detorsional gymnastics, was prescribed. Initially, an insole of a height of **10 mm** was prescribed and after 2–3 weeks, the height was increased to **18 mm**. The pain resolved immediately after performing the detorsional exercises. At 2 months' follow-up, R. had no complaints. The difference in the length of the legs had decreased to **7 mm**. We scheduled a follow-up examination in 6 months, but the patient did not come.

On analysing this clinical observation, we arrived at the following conclusions:

a. The left-sided pelvic tilt associated with relative shortening of the left leg due to unilateral asymmetry of the spinal muscles had caused rotation of the unfused S_1–S_2 vertebrae.
b. The rotation of these vertebrae caused injury to the sacral plexus and pain in the region.

c. Gradual rebalancing of the lumbo-pelvic segment with the use of an orthopaedic insole, corrective exercises and physiotherapy eliminated the main causes of spinal pain, which helped to cure the patient.

4. Patient K., a 71-year-old woman, complained of back pain which occurred while standing, prolonged sitting or walking, and radiated to the right leg. In adolescence, she had engaged in sports activities and had suffered a spinal injury. She had been under the treatment of a neurologist for many years, but her problems had not subsided completely.

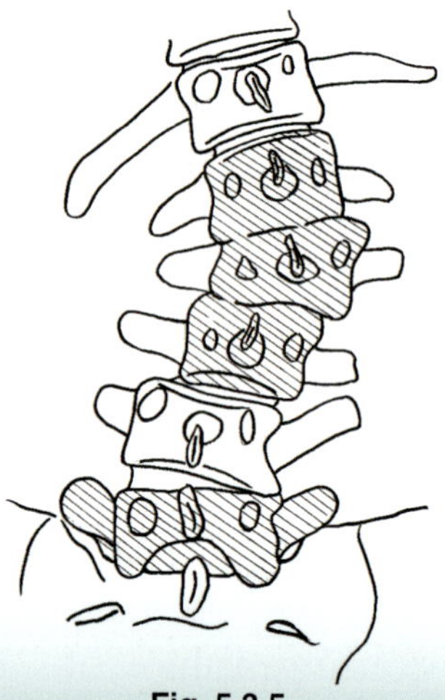

Fig. 5.3.5.

Radiographs of the lumbosacral spine revealed blockade and synostosis of the vertebral bodies of L_1–L_3 in a position of fixed, mutually antithetical rotation with angular deformity. Most likely, this was of traumatic origin. In addition, there was sacralization of L_5, lumbarization of S_1 and maldevelopment of the intervertebral articular processes of the L_5–S_1 SMS (Fig. 5.3.5).

On examination of the patient, left-sided kyphoscoliotic deformity of the thoracic spine was observed. There was a significant tilt of the pelvis to the right, which we attempted to correct with an orthopaedic insole of a height of **30 mm**, to be placed under the right heel. K. had clinical signs of bilateral lumboischialgia, and neuritis of the femoral and obturator nerves.

The standard treatment, i.e. orthopaedic insole, detorsional gymnastics, paravertebral magneto-acoustic therapy, was initiated. When the patient was examined 2 months after the initiation of the treatment, we decreased the height of the orthopaedic insole to **20 mm**. She could now walk a lot and had no difficulty standing up and sitting down. She was very pleased with the results of the treatment. We recommended that she continue with the prescribed treatment for another year without removal of the orthopaedic insole.

On analysing this clinical observation, we arrived at the following conclusions:

a. Blockade of the lumbar vertebrae had created conditions that gave rise to hypermobility of S_1–S_2. This subsequently led to compensatory lumbarization of these vertebrae.

b. The increasing pelvic tilt to the right due to relative shortening of the right leg resulted in rotation of S_1–S_2 and associated injury to the sacral plexus.

c. The gradual restoration of balance in the spinal–pelvic segment helped to fix S_1–S_2 in the correct position and contributed to elimination of the leading causes of pain in the lumbosacral region.

5. Patient B., a 60-year-old woman, had been suffering from low back pain for the past 20 years. She found it difficult to stand up from a seated position, and was unable to stand and walk normally. She had received treatment from neurologists, but it had yielded only short-term relief.

Radiographs of the lumbosacral spine revealed lumbarization of S_1, sacralization of L_5 and marked asymmetry of the intervertebral articular processes in the L_5–S_1 SMS (Fig. 5.3.6).

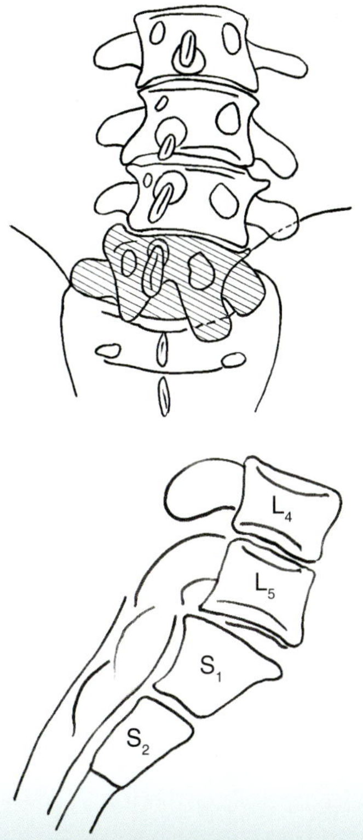

Fig. 5.3.6.

On examination, the patient was found to have clinical signs of bilateral plexitis, femoral nerve neuritis and lumboischialgia. Kyphoscoliotic deformity of the chest was also observed. The pelvis was significantly tilted to the left. We attempted to compensate for this with an orthopaedic insole of a height of **30 mm**, to be placed under the left heel.

The standard treatment was initiated. B. was advised to initially wear an insole of a height of 15 mm, and then in 3 weeks to add another **15 mm**. Detorsional gymnastics and paravertebral magneto-acoustic therapy were also prescribed. At 6 months' follow-up, the difference in the length of the legs was **15 mm**, compared to 30 mm before treatment. B. no longer had difficulty walking and could do so without experiencing any pain. She was very pleased with the results of treatment. We encouraged her to continue wearing the insole and heed all our other recommendations for the next 6–8 months.

On analysing this clinical observation, we arrived at the following conclusions:

a. Compensatory lumbarization of S_1–S_2, associated with significant tilting of the pelvis, caused these vertebrae to rotate and consequently, to injure the sacral plexus.
b. The gradual restoration of balance in the spinal-pelvic segment helped to fix S_1–S_2 in the correct position and contributed to elimination of the leading causes of back pain.

6. Patient P., a 47-year-old man, had been suffering from pain in the lumbosacral spine for the past 10 years. He could not stand for long and could not sleep in a supine position because of the back pain. During the past 2 months, the pain had become constant. In addition, the fingers of his right hand felt numb at night. He had been receiving regular treatment from a neurologist, but there was no appreciable improvement in his condition.

Radiographs of the cervical spine revealed rotational subluxation of C_3–C_6, with signs of degenerative disc disease and spondylosis deformans (Fig. 5.3.7). As for the lumbosacral spine, there was lumbarization of S_1, sacralization of L_5 and anomalous development of the articular processes of the L_5–S_1 SMS (Fig. 5.3.8).

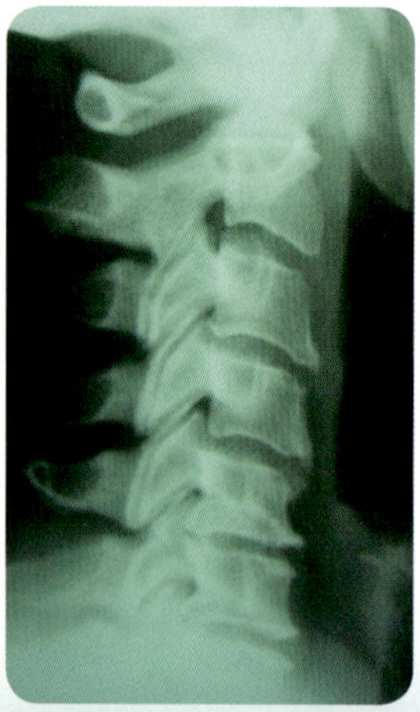

Fig. 5.3.7.

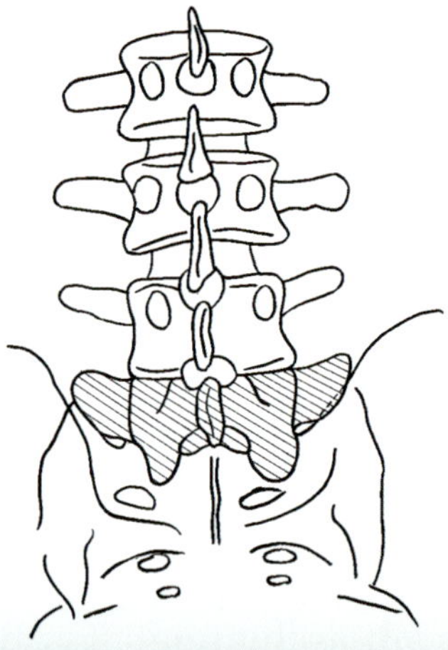

Fig. 5.3.8.

Examination of the patient revealed that he had a right-sided scoliotic deformity of the spine and a pelvic tilt to the left. We attempted to compensate for this with an orthopaedic insole of a height of **7 mm**. He had clinical signs of bilateral plexitis, lumboischialgia, and neuritis of the femoral and obturator nerves.

The standard treatment, i.e. detorsional exercises, local magneto-acoustic therapy – paravertebral and along the spine, orthopaedic insole, was prescribed. During examination after 2 months, it was found that the relative shortening of the left leg had reduced from **7 mm** to **3 mm**. There was slight back pain. B. could stand for long periods of time. At 6 months' follow-up, the left leg was 3 mm shorter than the right. The patient had no complaints.

On analysing this clinical observation, we arrived at the following conclusions:

a. The leading cause of widespread spinal pain was the presence of areas of instability in all regions of the spine.
b. The areas of instability resulted from the pelvic tilt to the left, which was caused by asymmetry of the long spinal extensors, as well as compensatory lumbarization at the level of S_1–S_2.
c. Rebalancing of the spinal–pelvic segment through the use of an orthopaedic insole and detorsional exercises eliminated the major causes of spinal pain.

7. Patient K., a 22-year-old man who was well built and regularly involved in sports activities, complained that he experienced pain in the lumbar spine when he stood or walked for long distances.

Radiographs of the lumbosacral spine revealed lumbarization of S_1–S_2 and anomalous development of the articular processes of the L_5–S_1 SMS (Fig. 5.3.9).

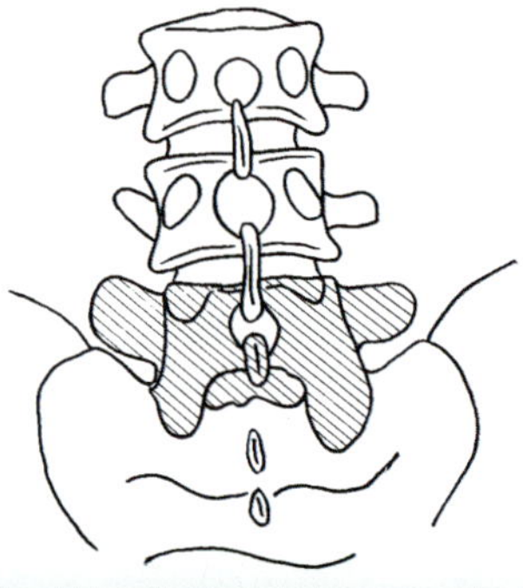

Fig. 5.3.9.

Examination of the patient revealed that his body was tilted to the left. We attempted to compensate for this with an orthopaedic insole of a height of **15 mm**. He had clinical signs of bilateral lumboischialgia and neuritis of the femoral and obturator nerves.

The standard treatment, i.e. orthopaedic insole, detorsional gymnastics, local paravertebral magneto-acoustic therapy, was initiated. During a follow-up examination after 2 months, it was found that the left leg was still 7 mm shorter than the right. The pain had resolved. The patient considered himself healthy.

On analysing this clinical observation, we arrived at the following conclusion:

a. The instability of the L_5–S_1 segment associated with the asymmetrical structure of the articular processes of the vertebrae, in conjunction with lumbarization of the first sacral vertebra and increasing asymmetry of the spinal extensors, created conditions for rotation of L_5–S_1 and the development of facet pain syndrome.

8. Patient N., a 68-year-old woman, complained of dizziness and frequent headaches. Her main complaint was slow intestinal peristalsis. She reported that often, she remained constipated for a week or longer. She had no appetite and suffered from chronic autointoxication. Her other complaints were difficulty in breathing, retrosternal pain, numbness of the legs and cramps in the calf muscles.

Radiographs of the thoracic spine revealed signs of intervertebral osteochondrosis and spondylosis, and Schmorl's hernia at the level of Th_9 (Fig. 5.3.10). The findings with respect to the lumbar spine were sacralization of L_5 the presence of anomalous articular processes, most prominently at the level of L_4–L_5, and lumbarization of S_1–S_2 (Fig. 5.3.11).

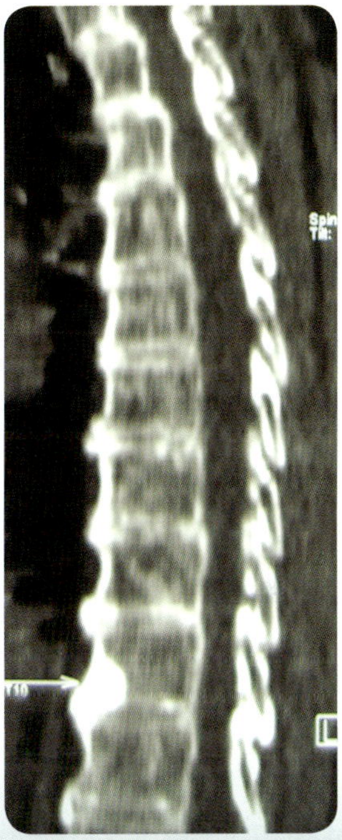

Fig. 5.3.10.

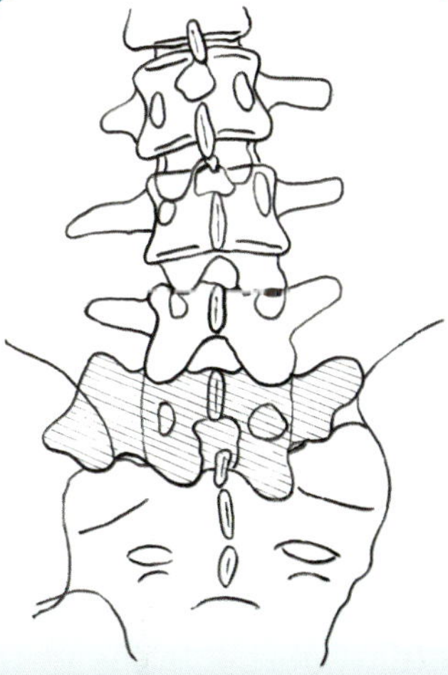

Fig. 5.3.11.

During examination of the patient, it was noted that she a ppeared exhausted. She had kyphoscoliosis of the thoracic spine and her pelvis was tilted to the left. We attempted to compensate for the latter with an orthopaedic insole of a height of **20 mm**, to be placed under the left heel. N. had clinical signs of bilateral plexitis, intercostal neuralgia at the level of Th_7–Th_9, lumboischialgia, and bilateral neuritis of the obturator and femoral nerves.

The standard treatment, i.e. orthopaedic insole, detorsional exercises, paravertebral magneto-acoustic therapy, was initiated. During an examination 3 months later, it was found that the left leg was **10 mm** shorter than the right. Intestinal motility had improved, the patient could breathe more easily and the headaches had resolved. At 6 months' follow-up, the difference in the length of the legs had decreased to **7 mm**. The functioning of the intestines had become regular. The patient reported a significant improvement in her overall condition. At 1 year's follow-up, N. said she now had a good appetite. She had gained some weight and her complexion was normal. There was no chest pain or breath-holding. The patient was very pleased with the results of treatment. We advised her to continue with the prescribed treatment for another year.

On analysing this clinical observation, we arrived at the following conclusions:

a. The numerous complaints of the patient were associated with impaired functioning of the sympathetic and parasympathetic nervous systems, the impairments being caused by deformations in all regions of the spine. The deformations, in turn, were caused mainly by the significant tilt of the pelvis to the left, associated with asymmetry of the long spinal extensors. As a result, zones of instability had formed.
b. Compensatory lumbarization at the level of S_1–S_2 and relative shortening of the left leg by 20 mm had led to the rotation of these vertebrae. This resulted in injury to the sacral plexus and impairment of the functioning of the pelvic organs.
c. Our treatment facilitated rebalancing of the vertebral–pelvic segment and the normalization of S_1–S_2, besides preventing traumatization of the sacral plexus.

9. Patient B., a tall 28-year-old man, complained of constant back pain that occurred after physical exercise, prolonged standing and walking.

Radiographs of the lumbar spine revealed sacralization of L_5 and lumbarization of S_1. Also, there were anomalies of the articular processes of L_1–L_5, most pronounced at the level of L_4–L_5 (Fig. 5.3.12).

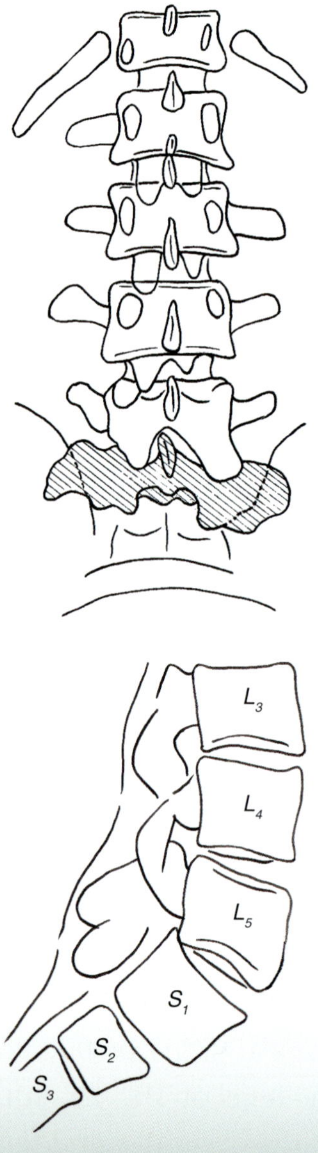

Fig. 5.3.12.

On examination, the patient had a right-sided scoliotic deformity of the chest, and the pelvis was tilted to the left. We attempted to compensate for this with an orthopaedic insole of a height of **15 mm**. B. had signs of bilateral lumboischialgia. Typical rotational displacements of vertebrae were observed in all regions of the spine. There was hypertrichosis in the lumbar region (Fig. 5.3.13). The movement of the cervical spine was limited.

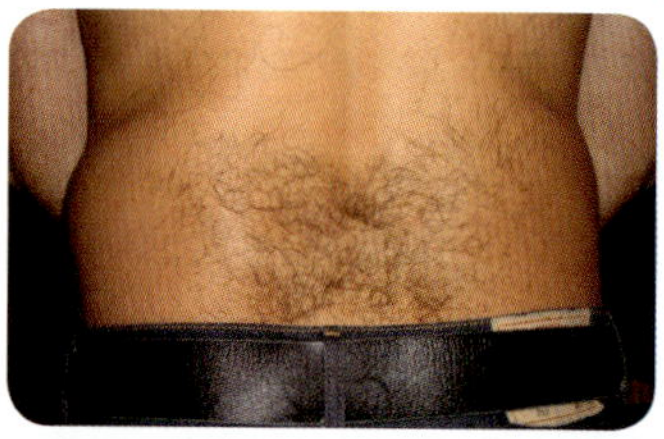

Fig. 5.3.13.

The standard treatment, i.e. orthopaedic insole, detorsional exercises, local magneto-acoustic therapy along the spine, was prescribed. At follow-up examination after 1.5 months, the back pain was found to have resolved. The left leg was **7 mm** shorter than the right. B. continued with all the elements of the therapy. At 3 months' follow-up, the difference in the length of the legs had decreased to **3 mm**. The patient had no complaints and considered himself healthy. However, we advised him to continue with the prescribed treatment for another year. While exercising and taking long walks, he used an insole of a height of 3 mm.

On analysing this clinical observation, we arrived at the following conclusions:

a. Despite the fact that the patient was strong, there was a significant tilt of the pelvis to the left, which had given rise to the development of a zone of instability in the lumbosacral spine. This was facilitated primarily by lumbarization of S_1–S_2, a process which had started in early childhood, as evidenced by hypertrichosis.
b. The gradual restoration of balance in the vertebral–pelvic segment resulted in normalization of functioning of the spine and spinal cord. After 3 months of treatment, the patient recovered completely; he had no complaints.

10. Patient B., a 30-year-old man, informed us that 3 years before consulting us, he had been admitted to the neurosurgical ward of a local hospital because of persistent, severe pain in the lumbosacral spine. The pain radiated to both legs and the legs felt numb. Conservative therapy had no beneficial effect and surgical treatment was proposed. Disc herniation in the L_4–L_5 segment was removed. Six months after the surgery, the pain recurred. One year before consulting us, the patient had undergone a second operation in the neurosurgical department for transpedicular fixation of L_2–L_4. The postoperative period was uneventful. The second operation, too, brought no relief to the patient.

During the initial examination in our clinic, the patient complained of lumbar pain radiating to both legs. He walked with the help of crutches because he felt shaky. He said, 'the legs do not hold'.

Radiographs of the lumbosacral spine revealed sacralization of L_5 and lumbarization of S_1. Asymmetry of the intervertebral articular processes of the transitional L_5–S_1 SMS was clearly visible. Figure 5.3.14 shows what L_5–S_1 SMS looked like after stabilizing surgery with two metal plates and four screws.

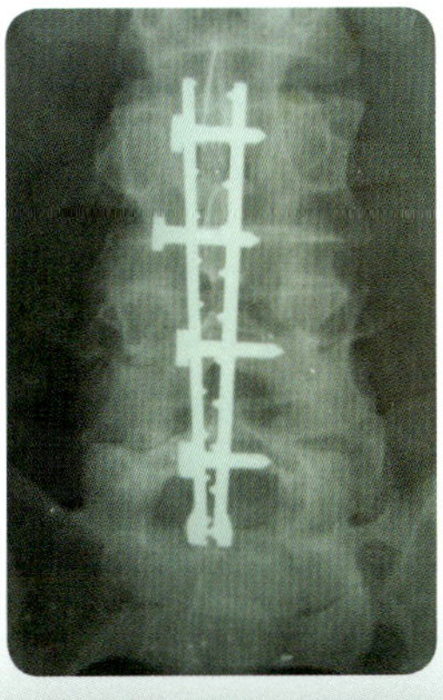

Fig. 5.3.14.

Examination of the patient showed that he had a kyphoscoliotic deformity of the spine and the pelvis was tilted to the left. We attempted to compensate for this with orthopaedic insole of a height of **17 mm**. B. had bilateral lumboischialgia, and neuritis of the femoral and obturator nerves.

The standard treatment, i.e. orthopaedic insole, local magneto-acoustic therapy along the spine, detorsional exercises, was prescribed. During examination a month later, the patient reported that there had been a significant decrease in the intensity of the back pain. At 2 months' follow-up, the difference in the length of the legs was **10 mm**. The patient said he felt more confident about walking and had started using a cane instead of crutches. At 6 months' follow-up, the difference in the length of the legs had decreased to **7 mm**. The spinal pain was negligible. The patient was very satisfied with the results of the treatment. He could now walk even without a cane. We advised him to continue with the treatment for another year.

On analysing this clinical observation, we arrived at the following conclusions:

a. The tilt of the pelvis to the left, resulting from asymmetry of the spinal muscles, caused rotational displacement of the dysplastically changed L_5–S_1–S_2 vertebrae. Rotation of S_1–S_2 was possible because they were not fused and also due to compensatory lumbarization.

b. Facet pain persisted because of a relative shortening of the left leg by 17 mm.

c. The neurosurgical operations did not eliminate shortening of the left leg and, consequently, the cause of facet pain syndrome. This is why there were no positive changes in patient's health condition.

d. Gradual rebalancing of the vertebral–pelvic segment with the help of an insole, corrective exercises and magneto-acoustic therapy eliminated the most important causes of spinal pain and promoted recovery of the patient.

11. Patient S., an 11-year-old boy, told us that 6 months before consulting us, he had felt pain in his left knee after a physical education class, and a month later, his right knee had also become painful. He had no fever and the rheumatological tests were negative. Paediatric orthopaedists had not found any pathological changes in the musculoskeletal system. The results of the blood tests were normal. However, due to the increasing pain in the knees and the suspicion of brucellosis, the boy was hospitalized in a clinic for infectious diseases. The treatment proved ineffective. S. found it difficult to climb stairs and could not walk long distances because of the pain.

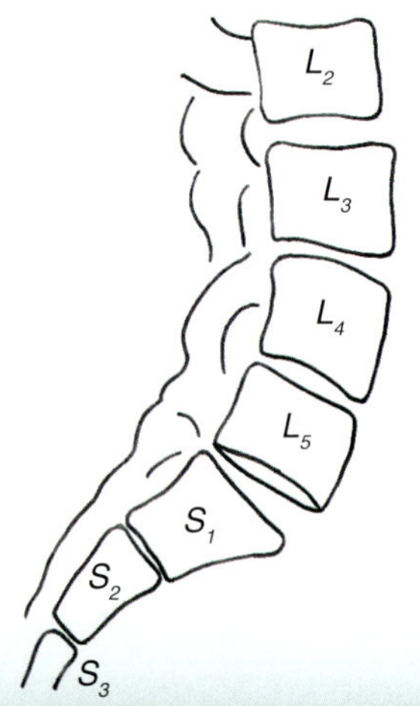

Fig. 5.3.15.

Radiographs of the knee joints did not reveal any pathological changes in the bones. In the lumbosacral region, physiological lumbarization of S_1–S_2 was observed (Fig. 5.3.15).

Examination of the patient revealed that the pelvis was tilted to the left, which had given rise to a right-sided lateral curvature of the spine. There was a relative shortening of the left leg. We attempted to compensate for this with an insole of a height of **3 mm**. The boy had severe radicular pain syndrome, and suffered from bilateral neuritis of the obturator, femoral and sciatic nerves.

The patient went through with the first session of detorsional exercises during the examination. This did away with the rotational displacement of the sacral vertebrae. The neurological symptoms disappeared immediately, to the extent that the patient was able to easily climb the stairs to the fifth floor of the clinic and run down easily.

The standard treatment, i.e. orthopaedic insole under the left heel, detorsional exercises, local magneto-acoustic therapy along the spine, was prescribed. On 1 month's follow-up, the pain in the knee joints had resolved. The patient considered himself completely healthy. We recommended that he complete the full course of physiotherapy and wear the insole for another year.

On analysing this clinical observation, we arrived at the following conclusions:

a. In our view, the pain in the knee joints and lumbosacral region was caused by compression of the nerve roots passing through the intervertebral foramina at the level of L_5–S_1–S_2. Rotation of the sacral vertebrae had led to compression of the nerve roots.
b. The restoration of balance in the spinal–pelvic segment led to correction of the rotation of these vertebrae, which eased the pressure on the nerve roots forming the sacral plexus. This resulted in resolution of the pain and restoration of the range of movements of the lower limbs.

12. Patient P., a 55-year-old man, complained of headaches, mostly on the left side, which had been bothering him for the past year and a half. He said here was a constant pain in his left eye, 'as if it is being taken out'. His other complaints were pressing retrosternal pain, shortness of breath, persistent back pain ('burns like fire'), occasional numbness of the right leg, and very frequent cramps in the calf muscles and toes. He could not walk long distances or stand for long because of pain in the knee joints. In adolescence, P. had sustained a spinal injury and had received non-surgical treatment.

Radiographs of the lumbar spine revealed blocking synostosis of L_5–S_1 (probably of post-traumatic origin), lumbarization of S_1, sacralization of L_5 and asymmetry of the intervertebral articular processes of the transitional L_5–S_1 SMS (Figs 5.3.16, 5.3.17). Radiographs of the knee joints did not reveal any pathological changes in the bones.

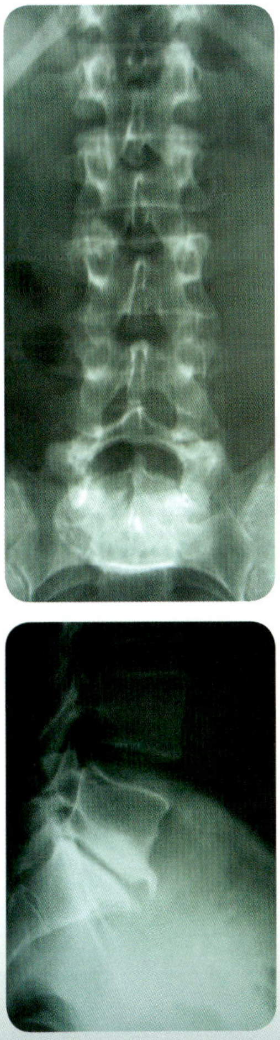

Fig. 5.3.16.

Examination of the patient revealed the presence of a spinal deformity, together with a right-sided rib hump and left-sided pelvic tilt. We attempted to compensate for the tilt with an orthopaedic insole of a height of **10 mm**, to be placed under the left heel. P. had clinical signs of left-sided plexitis, bilateral neuritis of the femoral and obturator nerves, and right-sided lumboischialgia.

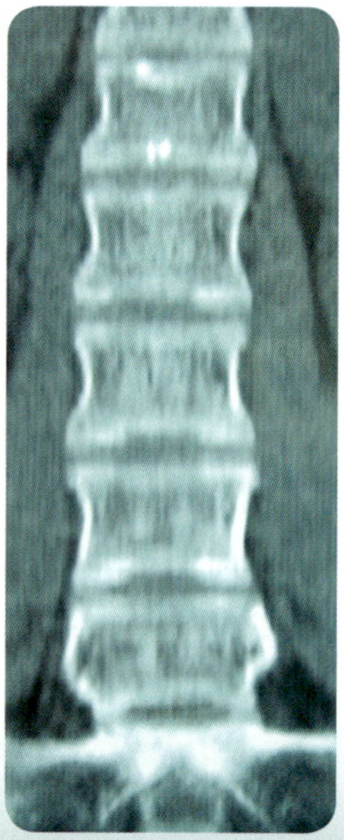

Fig. 5.3.17.

The standard treatment, i.e. wearing of orthopaedic insole, detorsional exercises, local magneto-acoustic therapy along the spine, was prescribed. At 2 months' follow-up, shortening of the left leg had reduced from 10 mm to 7 mm. The headaches, heart pain and shortness of breath had resolved. The patient still felt some pain in the lumbar region and in the knees. At 7 months' follow-up, the length of the legs had become equal. The axis of the spine was now correct and the spinal extensors had become symmetrical. The patient had no complaints and considered himself healthy. We recommended that he continue with the course of treatment, including the use of an insole of a height of **7 mm**, for another year.

On analysing this clinical observation, we arrived at the following conclusions:

a. Compensatory lumbarization of S_1–S_2 was probably due to long-standing post-traumatic synostosis of L_5–S_1.
b. The tilt of the pelvis to the left, a product of asymmetry of the trunk muscles, induced rotational displacement of vertebrae along the entire spine, in the sites where rotation typically occurs. The result was widespread spinal pain syndrome.
c. Rebalancing of the vertebral–pelvic segment corrected the rotation of the vertebrae and, consequently, reduced spinal pain.

13. Patient H., a 16-year-old girl, had injured her neck and back while exercising in school one-and-a-half years before consulting us. She was unable to bend or straighten her body, and had been admitted to the neurological ward of a local hospital. She was treated conservatively, the methods including manual therapy. However, the treatment did not prove to be beneficial. After the first session of manual therapy, H. developed enuresis, which had persisted since then. Moreover, she reported that her menstrual cycle had become irregular. Endocrinological impairments, such as increased facial pilosity, had also emerged.

Radiographs of the lumbosacral spine revealed no pathological changes. The only thing that could be observed was physiological lumbarization of S_1–S_2 (Fig. 5.3.18).

Examination of the patient showed a scoliotic deformity of the chest and a significant tilt of the pelvis to the right. We attempted to eliminate this with an orthopaedic insole

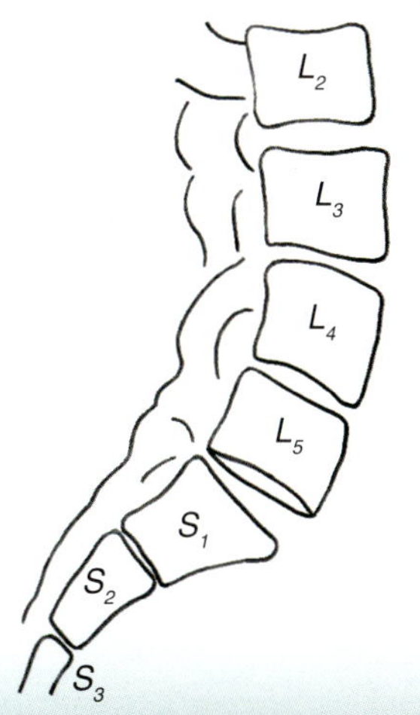

Fig. 5.3.18.

of a height of **10 mm**, to be placed under the right heel. H. had neurological signs of pronounced bilateral neuritis of the femoral, obturator and sciatic nerves.

The standard treatment, i.e. detorsional gymnastics, use of orthopaedic insoles in all types of shoes, transcranial and local paravertebral magneto-acoustic therapy, inflatable rubber collar, was prescribed. The patient was admitted to our hospital. Within 3 days of treatment, the pain and enuresis had resolved. She was discharged and asked to report as an outpatient. At 2 months' follow-up, there was no difference in the length of the legs. There had been no recurrence of the pain or urinary incontinence. At 8 months' follow-up, the patient said she had no complaints. Besides the other improvements mentioned earlier, her menstrual cycle had become normal and the facial pilosity had decreased. However, we recommended that she continue with the prescribed treatment for another year. When we examined H. one-and-a-half years later, we found that her face was clean and smooth, and the excessive pilosity had subsided. She had no complaints and considered herself healthy.

On analysing this clinical observation, we arrived at the following conclusions:

a. The neurological symptoms (facet syndrome) were caused by abrupt compression of the lumbar and sacral roots in the L_5–S_1 intervertebral foramina, as well as at the level of the S_1–S_2 sacral foramina, due to the rotation of the vertebrae.
b. The main cause of rotation of the vertebrae was trauma to the lumbar spine, associated with an impairment in the lumbar–pelvic balance on account of the gradually increasing spasm of the spinal extensors on the right side.
c. The disappearance of excessive facial pilosity can probably be explained by normalization of pituitary function as a result of elimination of subluxations of the cervical vertebrae.

14. Patient S., a 65-year-old woman, complained that for 10 years, she had been suffering from faecal incontinence, which had been preceded by constipation and vaginismus. She had been treated by a neurosurgeon, but to no avail. She would get cramps in her legs when she straightened them at night.

Radiographs of the lumbosacral spine revealed sacralization of L_5, lumbarization of S_1 and asymmetry of the intervertebral articular processes of the transitional L_5–S_1 SMS (Fig. 5.3.19).

On examination of the patient, we observed a significant tilt of the pelvis to the left and the development of a lateral curvature of the spine. We attempted to compensate for this with an orthopaedic insole of a height of **25 mm**, to be placed under the left heel. S. had clinical signs of bilateral neuritis of the femoral, obturator and sciatic nerves. At the time of examination, she was asked to perform a few detorsional exercises, after which the intensity of the neurological symptoms decreased significantly.

The standard treatment, i.e. orthopaedic insole, detorsional exercises, local magneto-acoustic therapy along the spine, was initiated. When the patient was examined 2 months later, the difference in the length of the legs had decreased to **20 mm**. The faecal incontinence had become almost completely controlled by the patient.

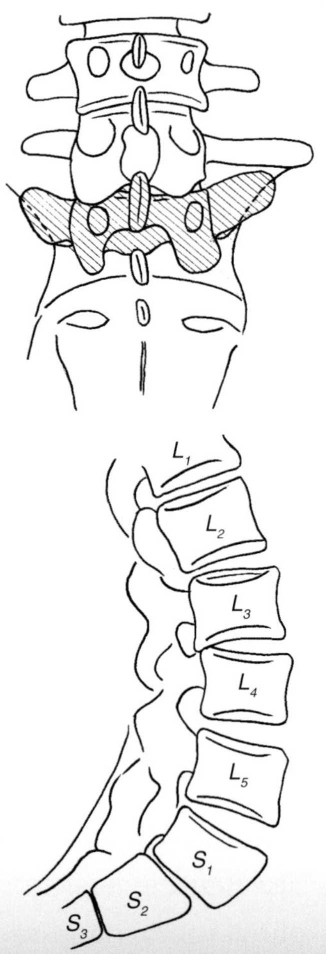

Fig. 5.3.19.

Frequency of the leg cramps had decreased considerably. At 8 months' follow-up, the difference in the length of the legs had decreased to **7 mm**. The leg cramps had resolved. The patient had regained more or less full control over intestinal functioning, but the problem of involuntary defecation still occurred on several occasions (during sleep). During examination one year after the initiation of treatment, it was found that the difference in the length of the legs had decreased to **3 mm**. S. had now gained full control over intestinal functions. She considered herself healthy and was very pleased with the results of the treatment. We recommended that she continue with the prescribed treatment for another year and a half.

On analysing this clinical observation, we arrived at the following conclusions:

a. The patient's pelvic disorders arose from impairment of functioning of the sacral nerve plexus. The nerves had got compressed due to rotation of the vertebrae at the level of L_5–S_1 and S_1–S_2.
b. Elimination of the pelvic tilt led to normalization of the position of the vertebrae and thus, to elimination of the causes and consequences of impaired functioning of the sacral plexus.

15. Patient A., a 63-year-old woman, had earlier been admitted to one of the city's hospitals due to her complaint of intense pain in the lower back and right hip. The pain was so intense and persisted for such long periods that only large doses of the strongest analgesic drugs brought relief. The pain intensified with any movement of the right leg. She was diagnosed with coxarthrosis and hip replacement surgery was recommended.

Radiographs of the pelvis revealed deforming changes of the head of the right femur (Fig. 5.3.20). To provide relief from pain in the right hip, the attending physician applied skeletal traction to the right tibial tuberosity. However, the pain persisted.

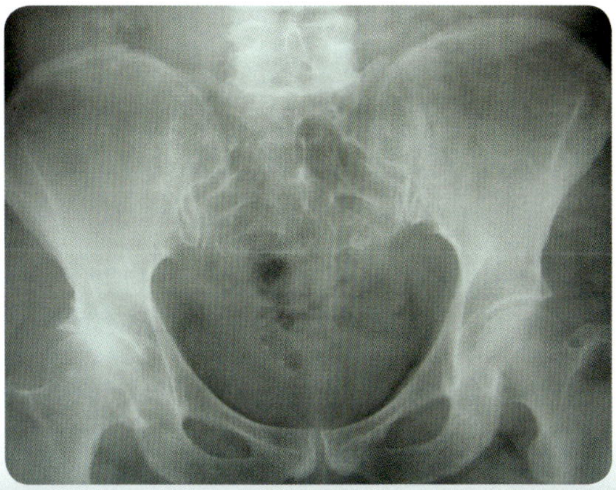

Fig. 5.3.20.

During examination of the patient, we observed that she was in severe pain, typical of neuritis of the obturator, femoral and sciatic nerves. In an attempt to address the source of the intense pain which, in our view, was not consistent with the degree of destruction of the femoral head, we decided to perform a simple twist of the pelvis to the right and left after removing the load on a Beller's frame. This manipulation was enough to bring immediate relief from the acute signs of neural compression. After this, the devices for skeletal traction were withdrawn and the patient began to sit up in bed. By evening, she was on her feet. Examination of the patient in the upright position revealed that there was a significant pelvic tilt to the right and relative shortening of the right leg by **30 mm**.

The standard treatment, i.e. detorsional gymnastics, local magneto-acoustic therapy in the lumbosacral region and area of the right hip joint, was prescribed. For the first four days, the patient wore an insole of a height of **10 mm** to compensate for the shortening of the right leg, after which the height was increased to **20 mm**. The more she walked, the better she felt. After 10 days, she had no complaints and was discharged from the hospital. We recommended that the height of the insole be increased to **30 mm** in 2 weeks and that she should continue with all the measures that had been prescribed for another year.

At 3 months' follow-up, the patient reported that she had no complaints and could walk properly and with confidence. The right hip joint was no longer a source of trouble. Regular monitoring by an orthopaedic surgeon was recommended.

On analysing this clinical observation, we arrived at the following conclusions:

a. The significant tilt of the pelvis, caused by relative shortening of the left leg by 30 mm, had given rise to an imbalance in the vertebral–pelvic segment and rotation of the lumbar and sacral vertebrae around their axes.
b. Abrupt narrowing of the spaces between the transverse and articular processes of the 5th lumbar and 1st sacral vertebrae, as well as rotation of S_1 relative to S_2, had led to compression of the lumbar and sacral nerves, mainly on the right side.
c. The long-standing pelvic tilt to the right had put excessive pressure on the head of the right femur and led to pathological reorganization of the latter.

d. The pain in the right hip was caused by the destructive process affecting the femoral head and neuritis of the sciatic nerve.
e. Twisting of the pelvis to the right and left facilitated the repositioning (reduction) of the lumbar and sacral vertebrae and freed the nerves from compression, thus bringing relief from pain. The use of an orthopaedic insole under the right heel facilitated the restoration of balance in the vertebral–pelvic segment. Local magneto-acoustic therapy helped to reduce oedema of the nerve trunks.

16. Patient F., a 70-year-old woman, complained of constant pain in the lumbar region of 10 years' duration. During the past few years, she had been suffering from severe pain in and numbness of the legs, and could not stand or walk. At the age of 23, she had sustained a spinal injury while engaging in a sports activity. F. had been treated by traumatologists and neurologists. By the time she came to consult us, she had developed an additional problem, i.e. a tendency to constipation.

Radiography of the lumbar spine revealed spondylolisthesis at the level of L_4–L_5, with blocking of L_5–S_1; lumbarization of S_1–S_2, which was most likely of a compensatory nature (Fig. 5.3.21); and sacralization of L_5 (the transverse processes were significantly enlarged) (Fig. 5.3.22).

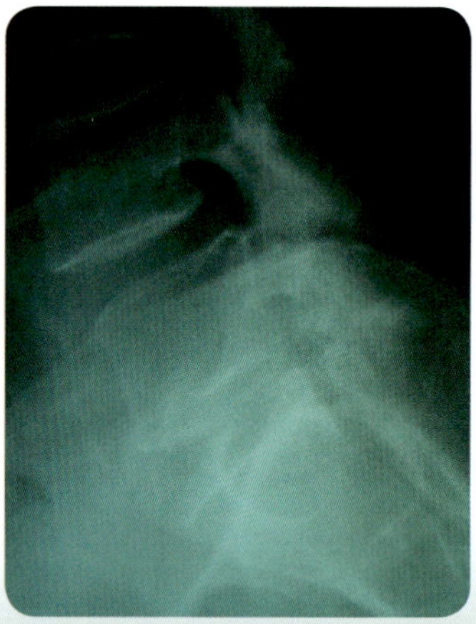
Fig. 5.3.21.

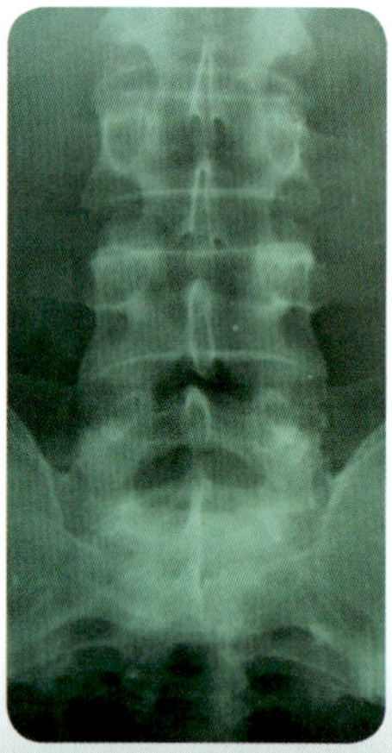
Fig. 5.3.22.

On examination of the patient, we observed a significant left-sided pelvic tilt, kyphoscoliotic spinal deformity and relative shortening of the left leg. We attempted to compensate for the latter with an orthopaedic insole of a height of **20 mm**. F. had clinical signs of bilateral neuritis of the obturator, femoral and sciatic nerves.

The standard treatment, i.e. orthopaedic insole under the left heel, detorsional exercises, local magneto-acoustic therapy along the lumbosacral spine, was prescribed. At 2 months' follow-up, the left leg was still 15 mm shorter than the right. The intensity of the pain had decreased significantly. F. could easily walk for long distances and the numbness of the legs had subsided. At 6 months' follow-up, the difference in the length of the two legs had decreased to **10 mm**. There was no pain in the legs and the patient's intestinal function had been restored. She had no complaints and was satisfied with the results of the treatment.

On analysing this clinical observation, we arrived at the following conclusions:

a. Hypermobility of L_4–L_5 had led to blockade at the level of L_5–S_1 which, in turn, had resulted in compensatory lumbarization of S_1–S_2.
b. The lumbar–pelvic balance was impaired because of a gradual increase in the tilt of the pelvis to the left, resulting from spasm of the spinal extensors on the right. This led to rotational displacement of L_4 relative to L_5, and S_1 relative to S_2, and thus compression of the nerves of the lumbosacral plexus. Sacralization of L_5 also contributed to this process.
c. Restoration of the vertebral–pelvic balance through the use of an insole corrected the rotational displacement of L_4–S_1–S_2. This led to a gradual cessation of the spinal pain. Local magneto-acoustic therapy and detorsional exercises also had a significantly positive effect.

17. Patient K., a 29-year-old woman, told us that 9 months before consulting us, she had started to feel a severe pain in the sacrum every time she rose from the bed abruptly. The pain had not resolved despite the treatment she had received in different neurological clinics. Manual therapy had also proved ineffective. On the day of consultation, K. also complained of constant pain in all regions of the spine, tinnitus, dizziness, blurred vision, a pricking sensation in the heart and breath-holding. She had a congestive liver. Her periods were irregular and her bowel function was impaired—constipation alternated with diarrhoea. Her other complaints were urinary urgency, cramps in the calf muscles and freezing cold feet, whether in the winter or summer. She wore warm socks even in summer.

Radiographic evaluation revealed flattening of cervical spine lordosis, rotational displacement of the vertebrae above the curvature (C_3–C_5), and moderate signs of degenerative disc disease and spondylosis deformans (Fig. 5.3.23). As for the lumbosacral spine, lumbarization of S_1–S_2 and asymmetry of the intervertebral articular processes between L_5 and S_1 were observed (Fig. 5.3.24). CT scans of the lumbosacral spine (Fig. 5.3.25) revealed advanced deforming spondylosis at the level of L_5–S_1–S_2–S_3, as well as of both sacroiliac joints. The changes were indicative of chronic traumatization of the endplates of these vertebrae.

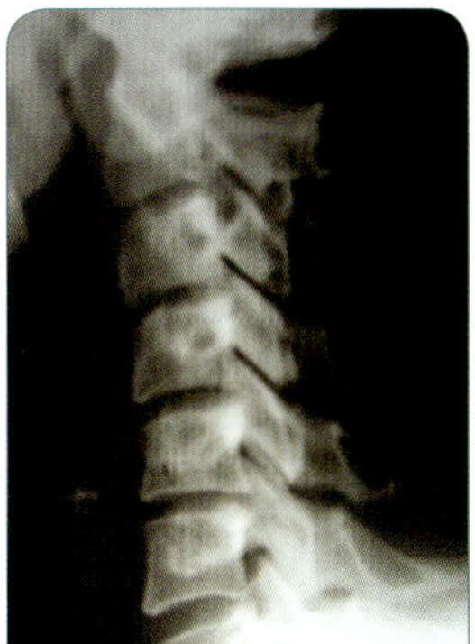

Fig. 5.3.23.

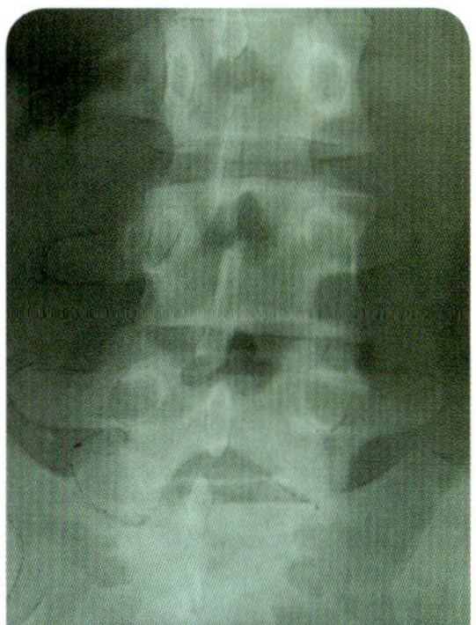

Fig. 5.3.24.

On examination of the patient, we observed that she had a pronounced lateral curvature of the spine and a significant tilt of the pelvis to the left. We attempted to compensate for this with an insole of

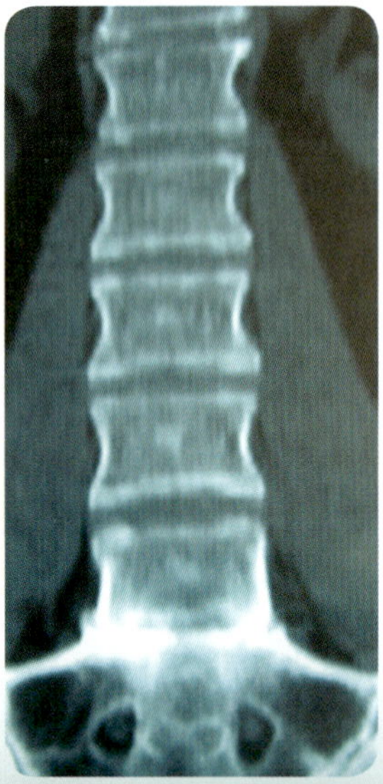
Fig. 5.3.25.

a height of **55 mm**, to be placed under the heel. K.'s ability to rotate her head was significantly limited. The application of pressure on the spinous processes of the cervical and thoracic vertebrae caused her acute pain. She had clinical signs of bilateral plexitis, and neuritis of the femoral, obturator and sciatic nerves.

The standard treatment, i.e. orthopaedic insole, corrective detorsional exercises, local transcranial and paravertebral magneto-acoustic therapy, inflatable rubber collar to stabilize the cervical spine, was prescribed. The insole prescribed was initially of a height of **15 mm** for the purpose of adaptation. Regular use of the insole for 2 months helped reduce the relative shortening of the left leg to **25 mm**.

At 3 months' follow-up, the left leg was 10 mm shorter than the right. The axis of the spine was correct and the spinal muscles were no longer asymmetrical. The pain had resolved and the functioning of the intestines was normal. The dizziness and tinnitus had also resolved. At 6 months' follow-up, the left leg was **3 mm** shorter than the right. The bowel and bladder were functioning normally. The pain that the patient had been suffering from in different parts of the body had virtually resolved. She now considered herself healthy. However, we recommended that she continue with the treatment for at least another 6 months.

On analysing this clinical observation, we arrived at the following conclusions:

a. One of the leading factors responsible for the development of disease was the significant tilt of the trunk and pelvis to the left, which had been caused by spasm of the spinal extensors on the right side. We compensated for this tilt with an orthopaedic insole of a height of 55 mm.
b. In accordance with the laws of biomechanics, such a significant tilt of the trunk resulted in rotational displacement of vertebrae in all regions of the spine (cervical, thoracic, lumbar and sacral), ultimately leading to compression of the spinal nerves and other neural structures.
c. Long-standing, repeated rotation of the lumbar and sacral vertebrae, caused by dysplastic changes in L_5–S_1–S_2, led to the development of deforming spondylosis and narrowing of the intervertebral foramina at all levels. This, along with instability of L_5–S_1–S_2, ultimately caused continuous traumatization of the lumbosacral plexus. This, in essence, was the cause of the widespread spinal pain syndrome.
d. Gradual restoration of the vertebral–pelvic balance through the use of an orthopaedic insole, combined with detorsional gymnastics and magneto-acoustic therapy, led to the gradual elimination of pain and clinical recovery of the patient.

5.3.2 Patients with sacralization of vertebra L5 and lumbarization of sacral vertebrae, posterior clefts and anomalous tropism of articular processes of L5–S1 SMS

1. Patient Z., a well-built 64-year-old man, told us that almost 20 years ago, he had fallen off the bars while practising gymnastics and had injured his back. There were no fractures, and the pain had gradually resolved completely. During his entire life, he had been engaged in recreational athletic gymnastics. A year before he consulted us, the back pain recurred. Physical activity aggravated the pain. Z. was treated by various physicians, but all methods of treatment proved ineffective.

Radiography of the lumbosacral spine revealed a wedge deformity of L_4 (probably a sign of long-standing consolidated fracture), synososis of L_4 with L_5, spondylosis deformans, sacralization of L_5 and lumbarization of S_1. There was pronounced anomalous tropism of the articular processes at the level of the L_5–S_1 SMS, and a cleft of the posterior arch of S_1 (Fig. 5.3.26).

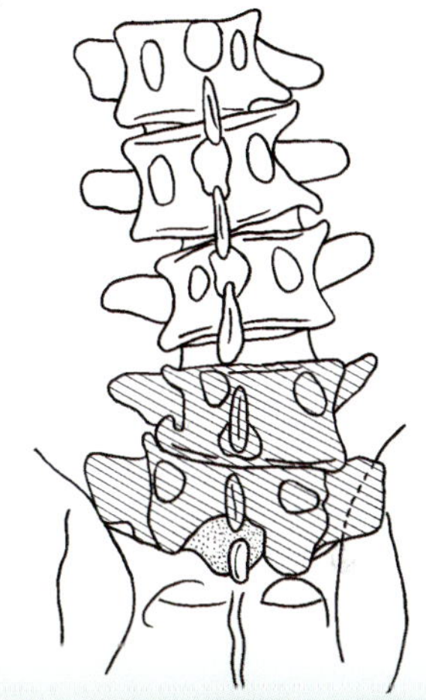
Fig. 5.3.26.

Examination of the patient showed that he had a mild scoliotic deformity of the thoracic and lumbar spine, and the pelvis was severely tilted to the left. We attempted to counterbalance the tilt with an orthopaedic insole of a height of **20 mm**, to be placed under the left heel. Z. had clinical signs of bilateral lumboischialgia, and neuritis of the femoral and obturator nerves.

The standard treatment, i.e. insole, local paravertebral magneto-acoustic therapy and detorsional exercises, was prescribed. The height of the insole prescribed was initially 10 mm. This was increased to **20 mm** after 1–1.5 months. When the patient was examined 2 months later, the left leg was **10 mm** shorter than the right. He reported that the intensity of the back pain had decreased. At 4 months' follow-up, the pain had decreased further and Z. had no complaints. We advised him to use the orthopaedic insole for anothcr 6–8 months.

On analysing this clinical observation, we arrived at the following conclusions:

a. Shortening of the left leg by 20 mm had caused a pelvic tilt, which led to an imbalance in the vertebral–pelvic segment, as well as rotation of the lumbar and sacral vertebrae around their axes.
b. Severe narrowing of the space between the transverse and articular processes of L_5–S_1, as well as rotation at the level of S_1–S_2, resulted in compression of the

corresponding lumbar and sacral nerves and caused bilateral lumboischialgia, together with neuritis of the femoral and obturator nerves.

c. By reducing the pelvic tilt through the use of an orthopaedic insole, we normalized the positioning of the vertebrae concerned, thus eliminating the causes and consequences of impaired function of the lumbar and sacral plexuses.

2. Patient K, a 72-year-old man, complained of persistent back pain of more than 10 years' duration. The pain radiated to the left buttock. K. also suffered from cramps in both legs. He had been an athlete in the past and had once suffered a trauma to the spine by falling off the horizontal bar. Five years before consulting us, he had started training (active gymnastics, jogging) to improve his level of fitness. This led to an increase in the mild back pain and pain in the left leg. During examination, K. complained of headaches, dizziness and diplopia following abrupt turning of the head. His upper and lower extremities were always cold.

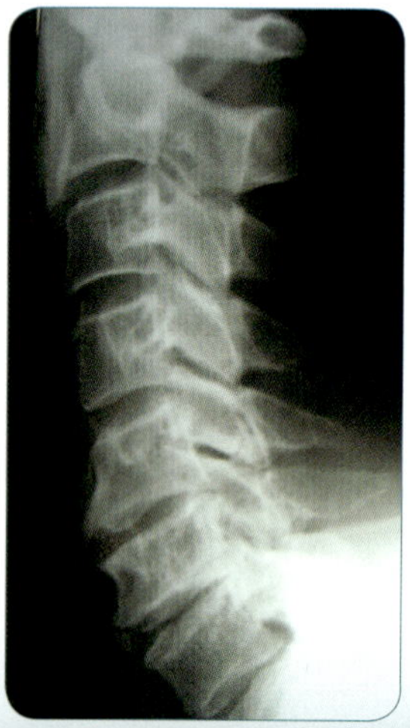
Fig. 5.3.27.

Radiographs of the cervical and thoracic spine demonstrated severe osteochondrosis and deformitive spondylosis (Figs 5.3.27, 5.3.28). Signs of lateral deformity, osteochondrosis and deformative spondylosis were also observed in the lumbar spine. Synososis of L_4–L_5–S_1, a cleft of the posterior arch of S1 and lumbarization of S1 were in evidence as well (Fig. 5.3.29).

On examination of the patient, a severe kyphoscoliotic deformity of the thoracic spine was observed. There were signs of bilateral plexitis, and neuritis of the femoral and obturator nerves. The symptoms of lumboischialgia were more pronounced on the left side. We attempted to compensate for the severe tilt of the pelvis with an orthopaedic insole of a height of **30 mm**.

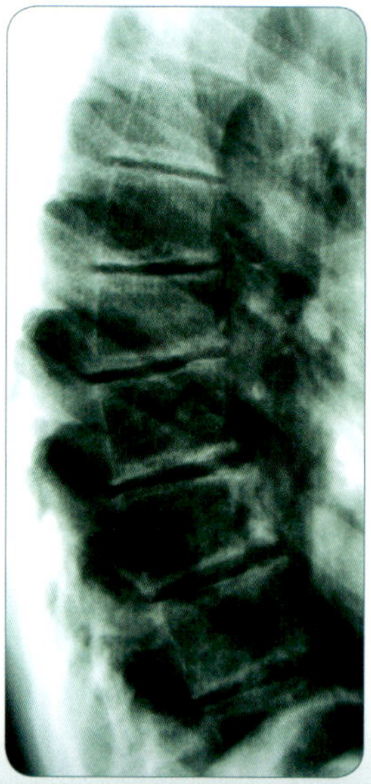
Fig. 5.3.28.

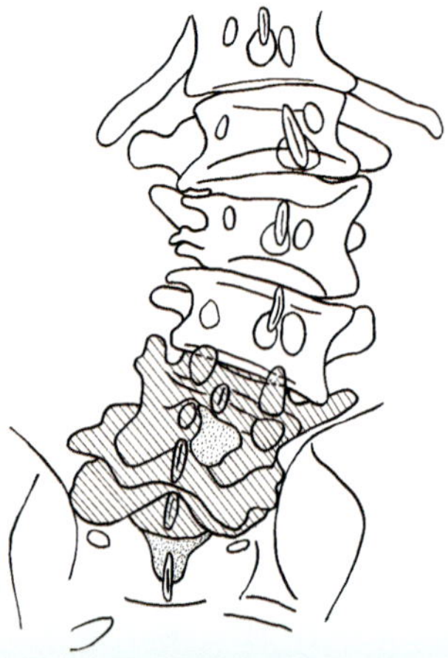
Fig. 5.3.29.

The standard treatment, i.e. local magneto-acoustic therapy in all regions of the spine, inflated rubber collar for the cervical spine, detorsional exercises, an insole initially of a height of 10 mm, was prescribed. When examined 2 months later, the patient reported a decrease in the intensity of the back pain. The height of the insole was increased to **20 mm**. At 6 months' follow-up, K. was able to walk confidently, the cramps and pain in the left leg had resolved, and the headaches and dizziness had decreased significantly. A year after the initiation of treatment, the left leg was still **15 mm** shorter than the right. The headaches and dizziness had resolved, while the back pain and pain in the left leg had decreased.

On analysing this clinical observation, we arrived at the following conclusions:

a. The widespread spinal pain syndrome was associated with the long-standing tilt of the pelvis to the left and relative shortening of the left leg by **30 mm**. Physical strain, trauma and increasing asymmetry of the spinal muscles had led to instability at all levels of the spine. The sites at which the back pain was more pronounced corresponded to the dysplastic changes at the level of L_4–L_5–S_1–S_2.
b. The widespread osteochondrosis and deformative spondylosis were compensatory in nature, being aimed at stabilizing the vertebrae. The restoration of the spinal–pelvic balance through the use of an orthopaedic insole led to a gradual reduction of the pelvic tilt and abolition of its consequences.
c. The use of the orthopaedic insole, detorsional exercises and magneto-acoustic therapy allowed us to significantly improve the general condition of the patient.

3. Patient K., a 65-year-old woman, complained that she could not sit, rise, lie down or walk. She suffered from intense pain along the spine, predominantly in the interscapular region which radiated to the heart. She also suffered from pain in the lumbosacral spine that radiated to the right hip and knee joints. Her symptoms had started more than 10 years ago, immediately after a road accident (pelvic trauma with injury to the roof of the right acetabulum). She had received conservative treatment. Later on, she was treated in neurological hospitals and sanatoriums for a constant dragging pain in the projection of the right sciatic nerve and right knee. However, these treatments gave her only short-term relief.

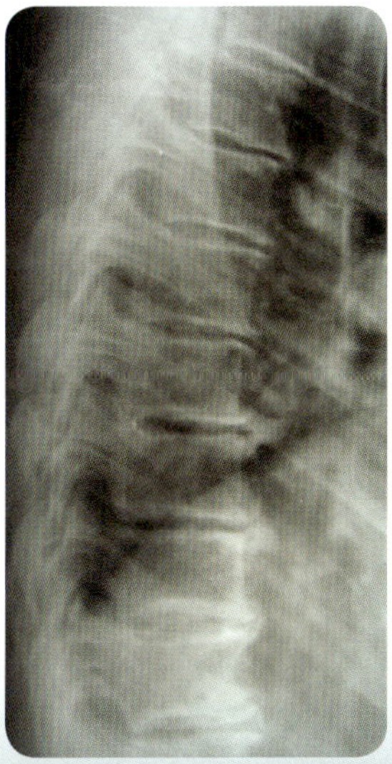
Fig. 5.3.30.

Radiographs of the spine revealed signs of osteochondrosis and deforming spondylosis of the thoracic spine (Fig. 5.3.30), deforming changes of the right hip joint, spina bifida of S_1 (Fig. 5.3.31), and osteoarthrosis of the right knee joint as a consequence of an undiagnosed fracture of the external condyle of the tibia (Fig. 5.3.32).

Examination of the patient revealed a severe pelvic tilt to the right, which we attempted to compensate for with an orthopaedic insole of a height of **10 mm**. External deformation of the right crus (genu valgum) was observed (Fig. 5.3.33).

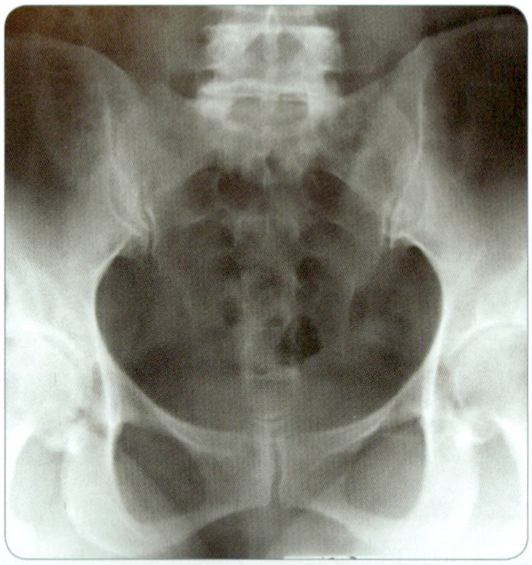

Fig. 5.3.31.

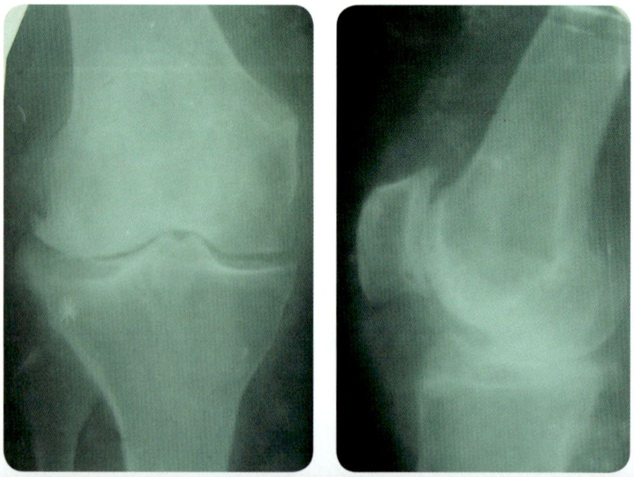

Fig. 5.3.32.

Palpation along the vertebral column caused the patient significant pain. She had clinical signs of bilateral neuritis of the obturator, femoral and sciatic nerves, as well as acute pain in the region of S_1–S_2. Movements of the right hip and knee joints were restricted and painful.

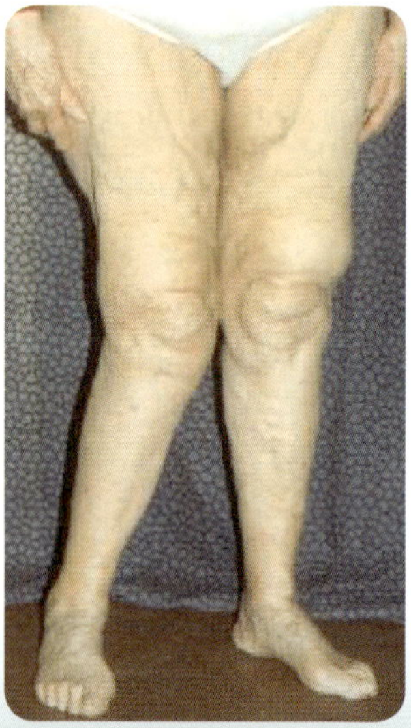

Fig. 5.3.33.

The standard treatment, i.e. application of **10 mm** orthopaedic insole under the right heel, detorsional exercises, local magneto-acoustic therapy along the vertebral column, right hip and knee joints, was prescribed. The patient was trained to perform detorsional exercises. During examination 2 months later, it was found that the pain along the vertebral column had decreased significantly, allowing the patient to 'walk freely, lie down, sit and rise'. The difference in the length of the legs had decreased to **7 mm**. K. did all the exercises regularly. The pain in the large joints persisted.

At 4 months' follow-up, the constant pain in the right hip and knee joints had decreased significantly but continued to persist. For this reason, we recommended a knee-joint replacement surgery, which was neglected by the patient. She continued to wear an insole of a height of **7 mm** under the right heel and followed the other treatment we had given her.

When we examined K. 8 months after the initiation of treatment, we found that the pain in the right knee had not abated and advised her to undergo a corrective osteotomy of the right tibia instead of a knee replacement surgery (post-surgery radiograph Fig. 5.3.34).

At follow-up one-and-a-half years after the operation, the right leg was found to be **3 mm** shorter than the left. There were no signs of a pelvic tilt. The axis of the lower extremities was correct (Fig. 5.3.35). The pain in the right knee joint had decreased and the joint space was almost normal (Fig. 5.3.36). Since the pain in the right hip joint had become negligible, K. rejected our suggestion to undergo a joint replacement surgery. She was very pleased with the results of the treatment.

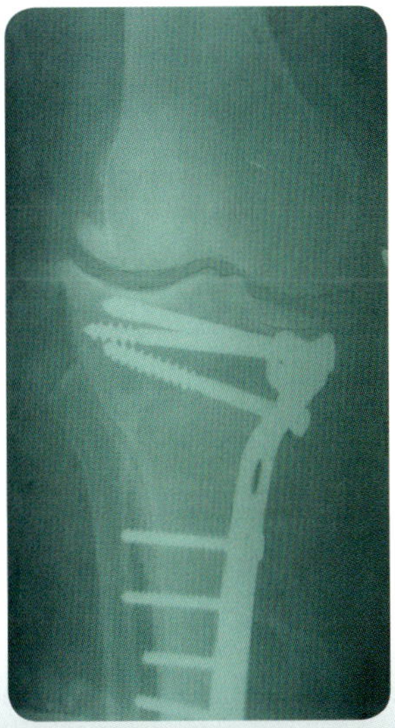

Fig. 5.3.34.

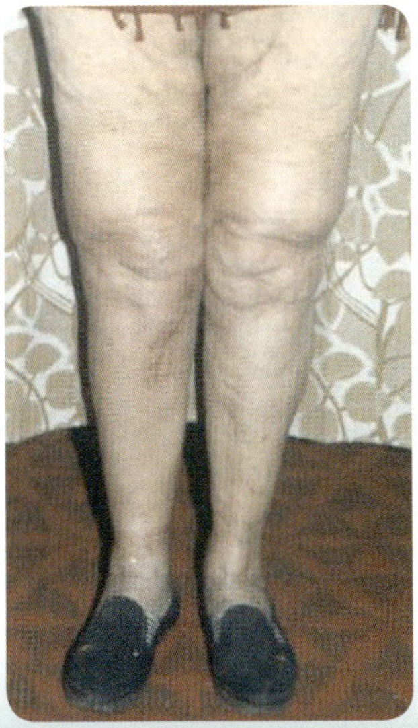

Fig. 5.3.35.

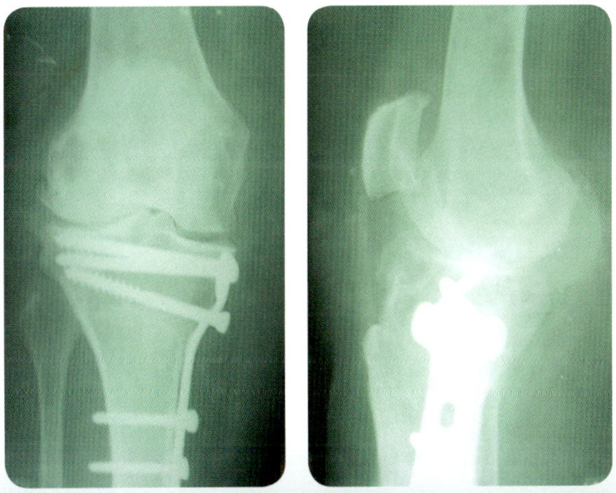

Fig. 5.3.36.

On analysing this clinical observation, we arrived at the following conclusions:

a. A combination of spinal–pelvic instability, relative shortening of the right leg and a tilt of the trunk to the right led to a change in position of the trunk and extremities. At the root of these processes was trauma to the right hip and knee joints.
b. Due to the processes mentioned above, an uneven load was placed on the articular surfaces of the hip, knee and talocrural joints. The long-standing incorrect load on these joints gave rise to deformative arthrosis. Osteochondrosis and deforming spondylosis developed for the same reason.
c. The patient was able to make a gradual recovery due to the reduction in the pelvic tilt, restoration of balance and correct biomechanics in the spinal–pelvic segment, detorsional exercises and local magneto-acoustic therapy. Surgical correction of the axis of the right crus contributed significantly to the positive results of our treatment.

4. Patient T., a well-built 20-year-old man, had consulted us for the first time 3 years earlier because of severe pain in the lumbar region. We discovered that he had relative shortening of the left leg by **3 mm**. After performing detorsional correction, the pain had resolved. The patient was given certain recommendations for further treatment. However, T. failed to heed our advice and there was a recurrence of pain, which was very intense, especially after physical activity. When the patient was prone or at rest, the pain did not occur.

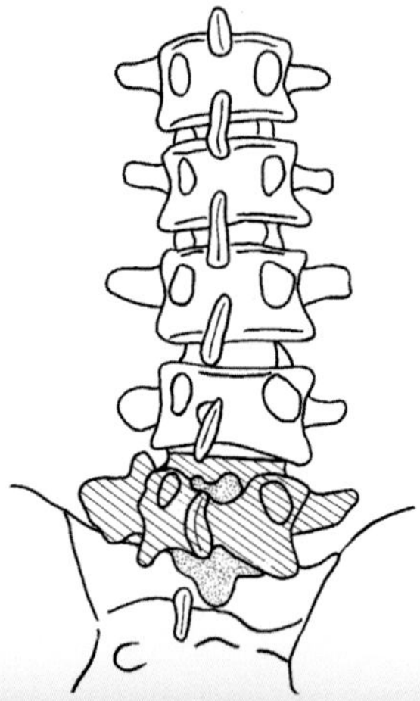
Fig. 5.3.37.

Radiographs of the lumbar spine revealed signs of dysplasia—lumbarization of S_1, sacralization of L_5, spina bifida of S_1, asymmetrical development of the interarticular processes of L_5 in the L_5–S_1 SMS (Fig. 5.3.37).

During examination of the patient, it was found that he had a scoliotic deformity of the thoracic and lumbar spine. We attempted to correct this with an orthopaedic insole of a height of **18 mm**, to be placed under the left heel. He had a severe pain syndrome, as seen by bilateral plexitis, and neuritis of the obturator, femoral and sciatic nerves. Palpation of the spinous processes of the cervical, thoracic and lumbar vertebrae caused the patient considerable pain.

The standard treatment, i.e. orthopaedic insole, detorsional exercises and local magneto-acoustic therapy along the spine, was prescribed.

At 2 months' follow-up, the difference in the length of the legs had decreased from 18 mm to 7 mm. The axis of the spine was correct and the spinal extensors had become symmetrical. Palpation of the spinous processes of the cervical, thoracic and lumbar vertebrae was not painful any more. The pain in the lumbar spine had resolved. The patient did not report to us after this.

On analysing this clinical observation, we arrived at the following conclusions:

a. The patient's unwillingness to wear an orthopaedic insole of 3 mm height under the left heel led to increasing asymmetry of relative shortening of legs. As a result, by the time the patient came for a re-examination 3 years later, an insole of a height of 18 mm was required.
b. The pain in the lumbar spine could be explained by compression of the nerves of the lumbar plexus upon rotation of L_5 relative to S_1, as well as rotation of S_1 relative to S_2.
c. Lifting heavy loads proved to be harmful since the defects of the posterior part of S_1 contributed to prolapse of the meninges, as well as compression of the spinal cord and probably, of some of the cauda equina nerves. By reducing the pelvic tilt with the help of an orthopaedic insole, we eliminated the causes of the rotation of dysplastically changed vertebrae, thus creating conditions conducive to recovery.

5. Patient E., a 43-year-old man, complained that he suffered from intense pain in the lumbar and sacral regions on physical exertion. He also had pain in the legs. He tired very easily and did not feel any pain when he was at rest. He had been suffering from these problems for more than a year.

Radiographs of the lumbosacral spine revealed lateral deformity of the spine, together with rotation of the vertebrae around their axes. In addition, we observed osteochondrosis and deforming spondylosis, spina bifida of S_1, anomalous tropism of the articular processes of L_5 of the L_5–S_1 SMS and lumbarization of S_1. There were marginal osteophytes which had developed on the bodies of L_2–L_4 vertebrae (Fig. 5.3.38).

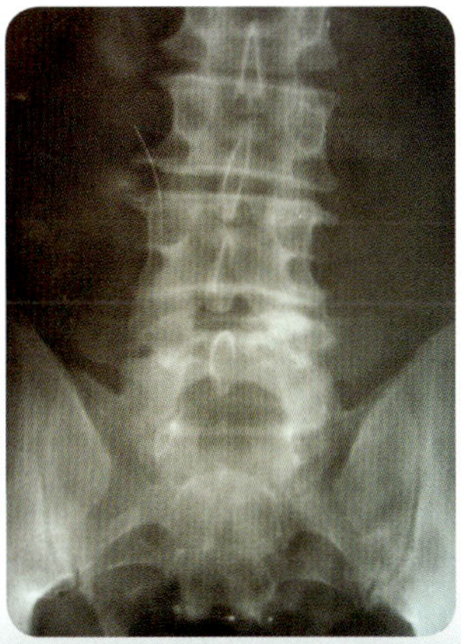

Fig. 5.3.38.

On examining the patient, we noted that his muscles were very strong. He had hypertrichosis in the lumbar region (Fig. 3.5.39), a lateral deformity of the thoracic and lumbar spine, and a pelvic tilt which resulted in shortening of the left leg by **7 mm**. We attempted to correct this through the use of an orthopaedic insole. There were clinical signs of bilateral neuritis of the femoral, obturator and sciatic nerves.

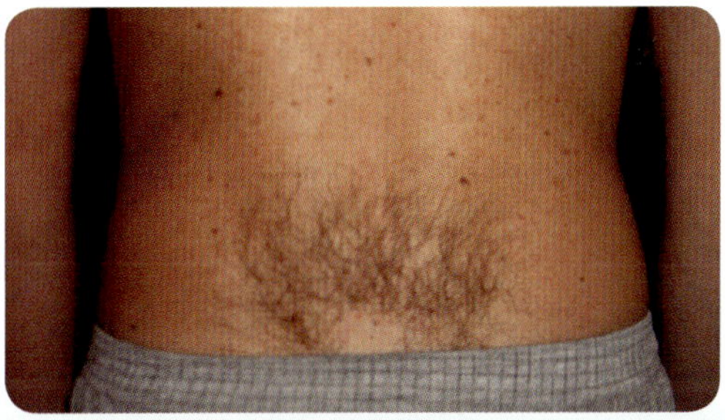

Fig. 5.3.39.

The standard treatment, i.e. orthopaedic insole, detorsional exercises and magneto-acoustic therapy in the paravertabral region, was prescribed. When the patient was being taught exercises during the first consultation, he experienced relief from the pain in all areas, especially in the region of the sacral bone.

At 2 months' follow-up, the patient was free from pain in the lumbosacral region even during periods of physical activity. He regularly wore an orthopaedic insole of **7 mm** height under his left heel and performed detorsional exercises. We advised him to continue with the prescribed treatment for another year.

On analysing this clinical observation, we arrived at the following conclusions:

a. The dysplastic changes of the vertebral bodies of L_5–S_1 were inherited, as evidenced by the presence of hypertrichosis. Asymmetry of the spinal extensors played the key role in the pathological process in this case, gradually creating an imbalance in the spinal–pelvic segment. The body tried to correct the imbalance by blocking the motion of the lumbar vertebrae, but as it turned out, this was not sufficient. The pelvic tilt increased progressively with physical strain and this led to the rotation of L_5, S_1 and S_2 around their axes. Compression of the nerves of the lumbar and sacral plexuses resulted in the neurological symptoms mentioned above.

b. One of the major factors which caused the pain syndrome was the cleft of the posterior arch of S_1 (spina bifida of S_1). The rotated vertebrae of L_5–S_1 extruded the meninges of the spinal cord and probably some of the cauda equina nerves as well. Compression of the cord and meningeal hernia caused intense pain and fatigue in the legs. The negative factors did not come so much into play when the patient was in the prone position; thus, the pain disappeared. The aim of prescribing an insole was to restore the spinal–pelvic balance and minimize the possibility of rotation of the vertebrae.

6. Patient D., a 39-year-old woman, when she consulted us, complained of low blood pressure and tachycardia, saying that she felt as if 'my heart is popping out of my chest'. She often lost consciousness, even if she had not been through any strain. It could happen during a conversation, before a meal or during a meal. The loss of consciousness could last for minutes or even hours. She felt sick (nervous breakdown) during conversations. D. could not stand, walk or even sit for a long period of time due to intense pain in the lumbar spine. She had been treated by neurologists, neurosurgeons and psychiatrists. The Evminov board and several other methods had been tried, but all the treatments had proved ineffective.

CT scans revealed severe asymmetry of the foramina of the transverse processes of the cervical vertebrae at the level of C_5–C_7 (Fig. 5.3.40). Doppler ultrasound scanning of the cervical and cerebral vessels showed a symmetrical deficiency of blood flow of up to 45% in the vertebral arteries (on both sides) at the level of C_2–C_5. Radiographs showed evidence of spina bifida of L_5 and S_1, sacralization of L_5 and severe asymmetry of the interarticular processes of L_5 (Fig. 5.3.41).

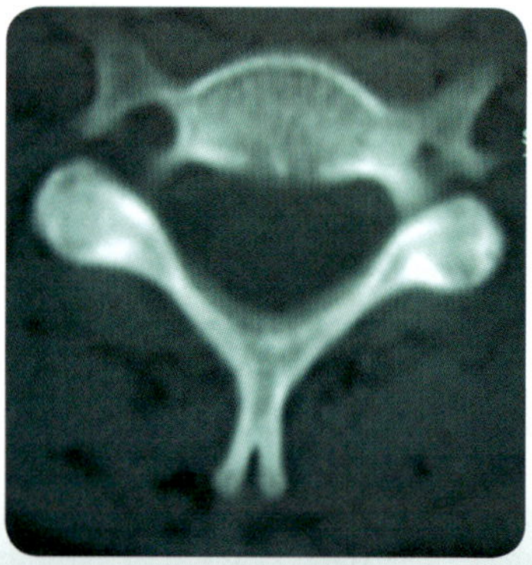

Fig. 5.3.40.

During examination of the patient, we observed signs of bilateral plexitis, a severe pelvic tilt, right-sided scoliotic deformity and relative shortening of the left leg by **30 mm**. D. had clinical signs of bilateral neuritis of the femoral, obturator and sciatic nerves.

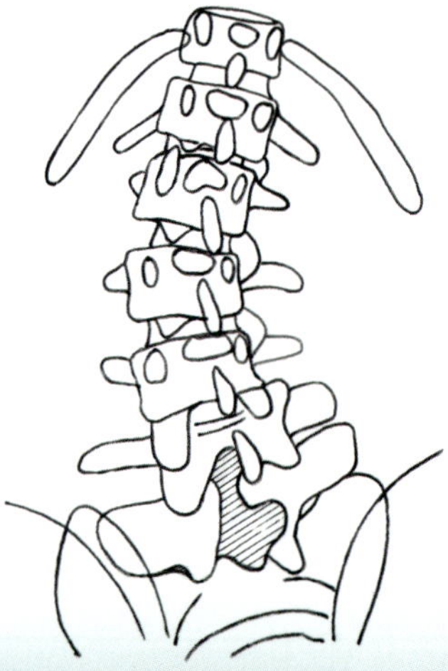

Fig. 5.3.41.

The standard treatment, i.e. orthopaedic insole, detorsional exercises, local magneto-acoustic therapy at all levels of the spine, daily use of an air-inflated rubber cervical collar, was prescribed. From the beginning, she started to apply an orthopaedic insole of a height of **10 mm**. A month later, this was increased to **20 mm** and another month later, to **30 mm**. At 5 months' follow-up, D. reported that there had been only a few episodes of tachycardia since she had started the treatment, while the episodes of loss of consciousness had ceased altogether. The pain in the lumbar spine and legs had also resolved. She had been following our advice conscientiously, actively performing all the recommended scheme of therapeutic measures. Relative shortening of the left leg was **20 mm**.

At 8 months' follow-up, the difference in the length of the legs had decreased to **7 mm**. The axis of the spine had normalized to a great extent. D. said she felt well and considered herself healthy since all her previous complaints had regressed. She had no episodes of loss of consciousness. The patient could now lead an active and independent life. Nonetheless, we advised her to continue with the prescribed treatment, including the use of an orthopaedic insole, for another year.

On analysing this clinical observation, we arrived at the following conclusions:

a. The leading factor responsible for the patient's condition was the pelvic tilt, which developed due to spasm of the spinal extensors on the right. (We attempted to compensate for this tilt through the use of an orthopaedic insole of a height of **30 mm**.)
b. The pelvic tilt caused deformation of the cervical, thoracic and lumbar spine. In keeping with the laws of biomechanics, this resulted in rotation of the vertebrae at different levels of the spine, in the sites where rotation typically occurs. The rotation of vertebrae in the cervical spine, along with signs of congenital stenosis of the transverse foramina and stenosis of the intervertebral foramina (due to osteochondrosis and deformative spondylosis), led to impairment of the cerebral blood flow, as well as of the functioning of the upper and lower cervical sympathetic ganglia, with the associated consequences.
c. The rotation of the vertebral bodies of L_4–L_5–S_1, which had clefts in their posterior arches, gave rise to the formation of a spinal meningeal hernia. This caused pain in the lower extremities.
d. By restoring the spinal–pelvic balance with the help of an orthopaedic insole, we eliminated the causes of rotational displacement of the vertebrae and thus the syndrome of widespread pain.

7. Patient B., an 18-year-old young man, complained of long-standing constant pain in the lower thoracic and lumbosacral regions that radiated to both legs. He could not walk or stand for a long period of time. He also had a tendency to constipation.

Radiographs of the spine revealed a scoliotic deformity of the thoracic and lumbar spine (caused by dysplasia of the thoracic and lumbar vertebrae), and wedge-shaped vertebrae at the level of Th_{10}–Th_{11} and L_1–L_4. In addition, the patient had spina bifida of L_5–S_1. Physiological lumbarization of S_1, as well as rotation and dislocation of the vertebrae were also observed. There were signs of left-sided sacralization of L_5 (Fig. 5.3.42).

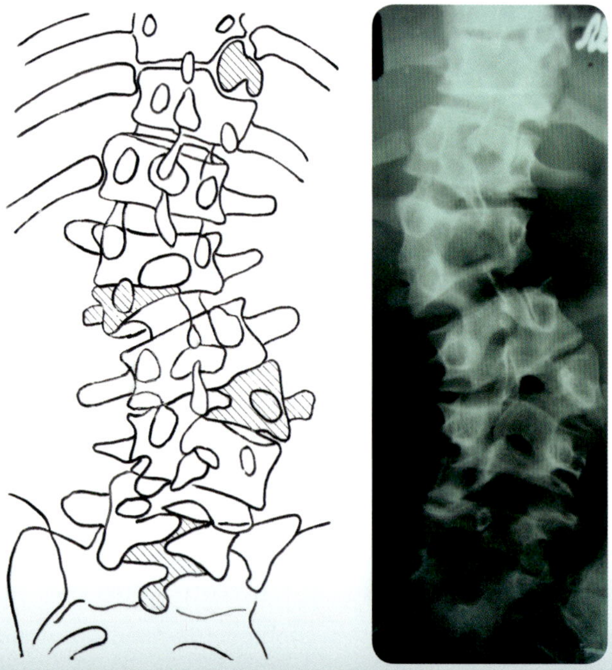
Fig. 5.3.42.

Examination showed that the body was tilted to the left. We attempted to reduce this tilt with the help of an orthopaedic insole of a height of **15 mm**. An S-shaped deformity of the thoracic and lumbar spine was observed. There were distinct signs of bilateral neuritis of the femoral, obturator and sciatic nerves.

The standard treatment, i.e. orthopaedic insole, detorsional exercises, local magneto-acoustic therapy along the lumbosacral region, was prescribed. During examination 6 months later, it was found that though the lumbar spine still had a scoliotic deformity, the pain in all regions of the spine had resolved. The difference in the length of the legs had decreased to **10 mm**. At 10 months' follow-up, the left leg was **7 mm** shorter than the right. The intestines had started functioning normally. The patient was able to walk a great deal without experiencing any pain in the legs. Though he had no complaints, the deformity of the lumbar spine had still not been eliminated. We advised him to continue with the prescribed treatment for another year.

On analysing this clinical observation, we arrived at the following conclusions:

a. In this case, we came across the relatively rare combination of wedge-shaped vertebrae and defects of the posterior arches of L_5–S_1.
b. The pelvic tilt, which developed due to the presence of wedge-shaped vertebrae and spasm of the spinal extensors, led to the rotation and dislocation of the vertebrae mentioned above. The defects of the posterior arches of L_5–S_1 set the stage for spinal meningeal hernia and subsequent compression of the nerves and spinal cord, which caused spinal pain syndrome and dysfunction of the pelvic organs (constipation).
c. The use of an orthopaedic insole to compensate for the relative shortening of the left leg by **15 mm** resulted in partial restoration of the spinal–pelvic balance, but did not change the position of the wedge-shaped vertebrae. However, even this was sufficient to reduce the symptoms reported by the patient during the first examination.

8. Patient M., a strong-built 37-year-old woman, complained of emotional lability, sensation of 'pricking' in the heart and episodes of breath-holding. Her wrists were cold and sweaty. She had been treated by a neurologist, who had diagnosed her with vegetovascular dystonia. Her major complaint was constant back pain, predominantly on the right side, which appeared even with slight flexion–rotation of the body. M. also suffered from frequent cramps in the calf muscles, as well as acute pain in the right groin. She had been suffering from these problems for a couple of years, but during the preceding year, the symptoms had worsened. M. also had a tendency to constipation.

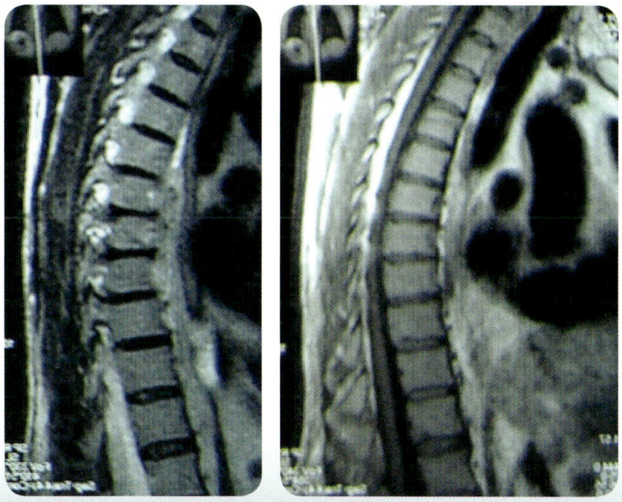

Fig. 5.3.43.

CT scans of the thoracic spine revealed signs of spondylosis deformans and multiple Schmorl's hernias (Fig. 5.3.43). Radiographs of the lumbar spine showed that there was a cleft in the posterior arch of S_1 and lumbarization of this vertebra, as well as significant asymmetry of the intervertebral joints between the L_5 and S_1 vertebrae (Fig. 5.3.44).

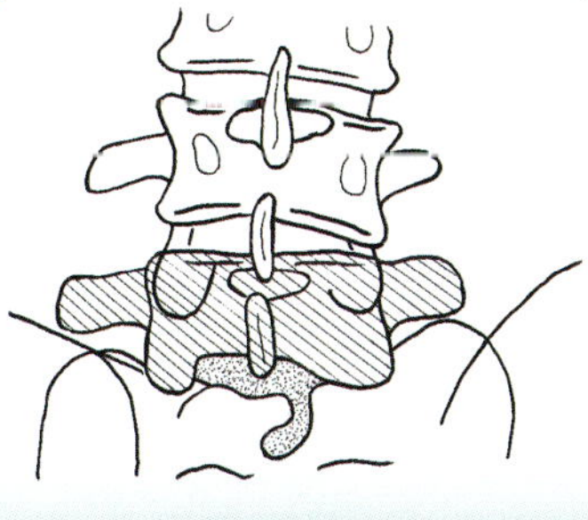

Fig. 5.3.44.

On examination, the patient was found to have a left-sided scoliotic deformity of the thoracic spine and a pelvic tilt, which we attempted to correct with an orthopaedic insole of a height of **10 mm** under the right heel. There were clinical signs of bilateral plexitis and lumboischialgia. M. also had enlarged subcutaneous veins on both legs, predominantly on the right calf, which is a sign of long-standing impairment of venous blood flow (Fig. 5.3.45).

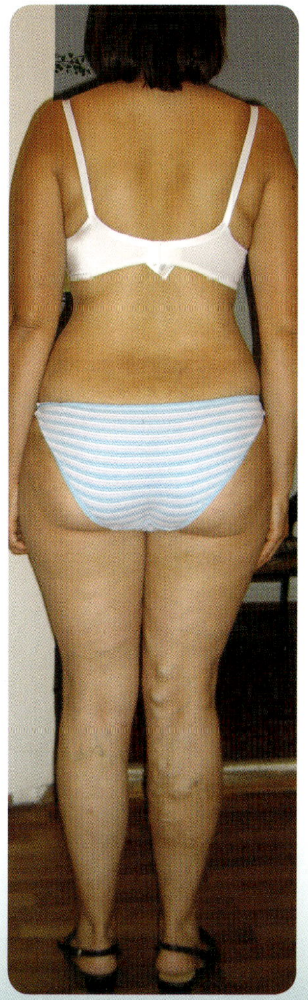

Fig. 5.3.45.

The standard treatment, i.e. orthopaedic insole, detorsional exercises, local magneto-acoustic therapy along the spine, was prescribed. At 3 months' follow-up, the right leg was 3 mm shorter than the left. The patient reported a significant improvement in her general condition. The pain in the lumbar spine had resolved, and there were no more leg cramps or episodes of 'pricking' of the heart and breath-holding. Intestinal functioning was normal. We advised her to continue with the prescribed treatment for the next 6 months.

On analysing this clinical observation, we arrived at the following conclusions:

a. The relative shortening of the right leg, which gradually became shorter over the years, was caused by unilateral spasm of the spinal muscles and led to tilting of the pelvis. This, in turn, resulted in the development of zones of instability at all levels of the spine.
b. Hard physical work resulted in the formation of Schmorl's hernias and corresponding pain syndrome in the thoracic part of spine.
c. Rotation of the dysplastically changed L_5–S_1 vertebrae caused herniation of the spinal meninges, which led to pain and spasm of the muscles in the lower extremites, a deficiency of blood flow in both legs and impairment of functioning of the pelvic organs.
d. Restoration of the spinal–pelvic balance through the use of an orthopaedic insole and detorsional exercises excluded the reasons for the rotation and displacement of the vertebrae, thus improving the patient's overall condition and reducing the burden of existing complaints.

9. Patient K., a 32-year-old man, had developed a pain in the lumbar spine, radiating to the right hip joint after he had lifted a heavy load almost 6 months before consulting us. The local neurologist had treated him for 'lumboischialgia' but to no avail. One month earlier, K. had felt a similar pain in the left hip joint that radiated to the groin.

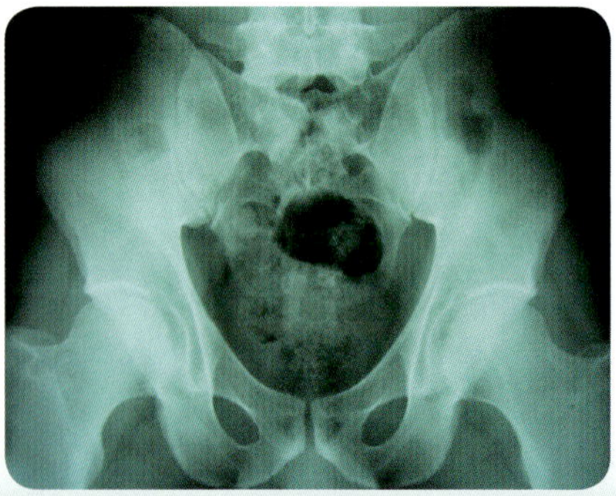

Fig. 5.3.46.

Plain radiographs revealed no pathological changes in either hip joint (Fig. 5.3.46). However, they showed the presence of a cleft in the posterior arch of S_1, sacralization of L_5, anomalous tropism of the articular processes of the L_5–S_1 SMS and lumbarization of S_1 (Fig. 5.3.47).

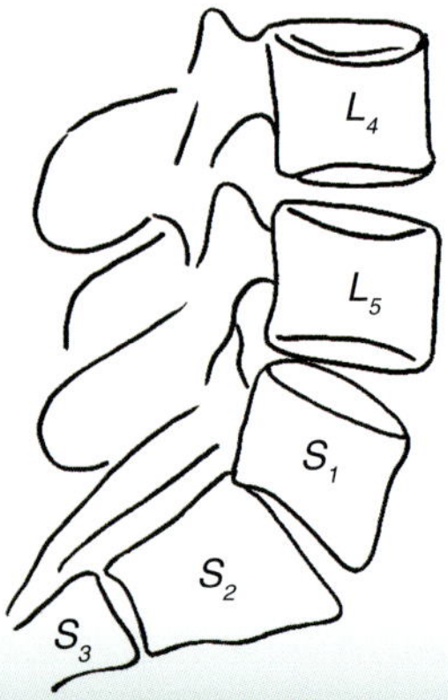

Fig. 5.3.47.

On examination, the patient was found to have a right-sided scoliotic deformity of the thoracic spine and a pelvic tilt, which we attempted to correct with an orthopaedic insole of a height of **3 mm**. Clinical signs of bilateral plexitis, and bilateral neuritis of the femoral, obturator and sciatic nerves were present.

The standard treatment, i.e. orthopaedic insole under the left heel, detorsional exercises, magneto-acoustic therapy along the lumbosacral spine, was prescribed. When examined 2 months later, the patient reported that the pain in the hip joints and lumbar region had resolved. We advised him to continue with the prescribed treatment for another 6 months.

On analysing this clinical observation, we arrived at the following conclusions:

a. The major factor responsible for the patient's condition was the tilt of the body to the left, caused by spasm of the spinal extensors on the right side.
b. This tilt of the body led to the rotation and dislocation of vertebrae, predominantly in the lumbosacral spine. This was facilitated by the dysplastic changes in L_5–S_1. The resultant compression of the nerves of the lumbar and sacral plexuses gave rise to neurological symptoms.
c. The use of an orthopaedic insole contributed to the restoration of the spinal–pelvic balance, which eliminated the causes of rotation and dislocation of L_5–S_1 and thus brought about clinical recovery.

10. Patient M., a 70-year-old woman, complained of severe pain in the lower extremities and cramps in the calf muscles. In her youth, she had suffered multiple injuries of the spine while engaging in sports activities. She used the most powerful analgesics to get relief from the pain. She was given a course of radiotherapy and administered intra-articular injections of steroids, which had no positive effect. Following this, a joint replacement surgery (the right knee) was planned.

Radiographs of the knee joints revealed signs of deforming osteoarthrosis. Radiographs of the lumbar spine showed distinct signs of deforming spondylosis of all lumbar vertebrae, wedge-shaped deformity of L_4, synostosis between L_3–L_4 (probably of post-traumatic origin), sacralization of L_5, lumbarization of S_1, anomalous tropism of the articular processes of L_5 and spina bifida of S_1 (Fig. 5.3.48).

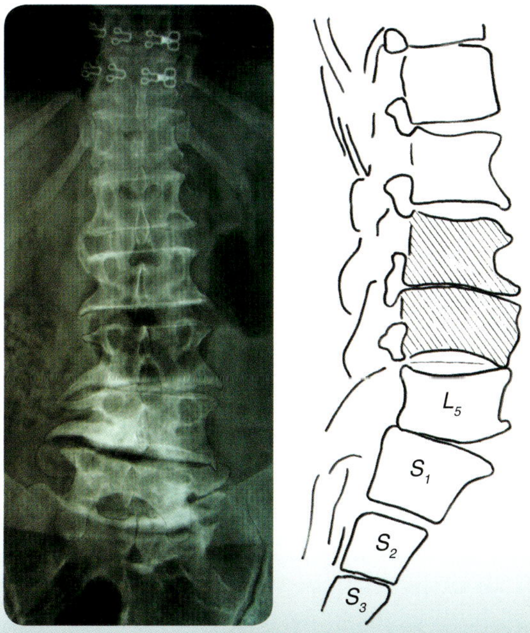

Fig. 5.3.48.

During examination of the patient, it was observed that there were signs of hypotrophy of the left buttock. The calves and toes of both legs were externally rotated. The valgus deformity was more pronounced on the left side (Fig. 5.3.49). We attempted to reduce the pelvic tilt with an orthopaedic insole of a height of **20 mm**. M. had clinical signs of bilateral plexitis, and bilateral neuritis of the femoral, obturator and sciatic nerves.

The standard treatment, i.e. orthopaedic insole, detorsional exercises, magneto-acoustic therapy along the vertebral column, was prescribed. We initially recommended the use of an insole of a height of **10 mm**, and this was increased to **20 mm** a month later.

When examined 2 months later, the patient reported that the intensity of the pain in the lumbar region and knee joints had decreased. At 6 months' follow-up, the spasm and cramps in the legs had resolved, while the pain in the knee joints had decreased significantly. The difference in the length of the legs had decreased to **15 mm**. At 1 year's follow-up, the difference in the length of the legs had come down to **10 mm**. The pain had become negligible and she could walk for long stretches. M. was very pleased with the results of the treatment. Nevertheless, we recommended that she continue with the prescribed treatment for the next 1–1.5 years using the insole of **10 mm** height under the left heel.

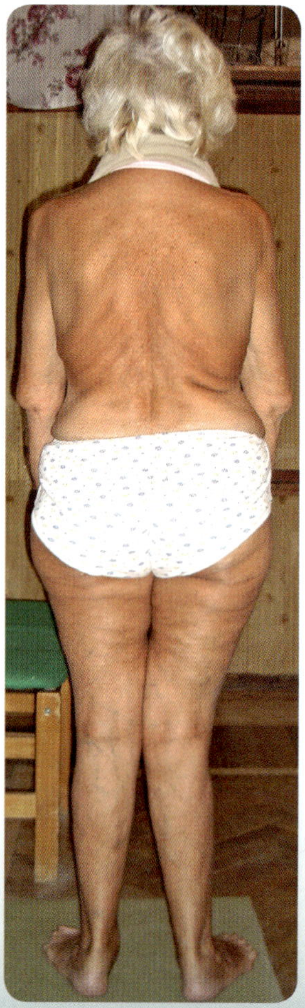

Fig. 5.3.49.

On analysing this clinical observation, we arrived at the following conclusions:

a. Relative shortening of the left leg by 20 mm and the associated pelvic tilt had given rise to instability of the spinal–pelvic segment.
b. Severe injuries to the spine as well as dysplastic changes of the L_3–L_4–L_5–S_1 vertebrae contributed to the progression of this pathological condition. The long-standing asymmetrical load on the spine and large joints caused deformative arthrosis, osteochondrosis and deforming spondylosis.
c. Elimination of the pelvic tilt, which is the major factor responsible for all skeletal changes, due to the use of an orthopaedic insole gradually restored the impaired biomechanics of the musculoskeletal system and helped to obtain positive results of the prescribed treatment.

11. Patient K., a 61-year-old woman who was overweight, complained of pain in the lumbar region which radiated to the left leg. She attributed her excessive weight to the use of prednisolone and diprospan. For the past 10 years, she had been receiving treatment for rheumatoid arthritis, which had manifested as pain in the wrists, shoulders and knee joints. Later, she had developed pain in the lumbar region.

CT scans of the lumbar spine (Fig. 5.3.50) revealed distinct signs of osteochondrosis, deforming spondylosis and Schmorl's hernias. Radiographs of the lumbosacral spine showed signs of osteochondrosis and deforming spondylosis, marginal osteophytes and spina bifida of S_1 (Fig. 5.3.51).

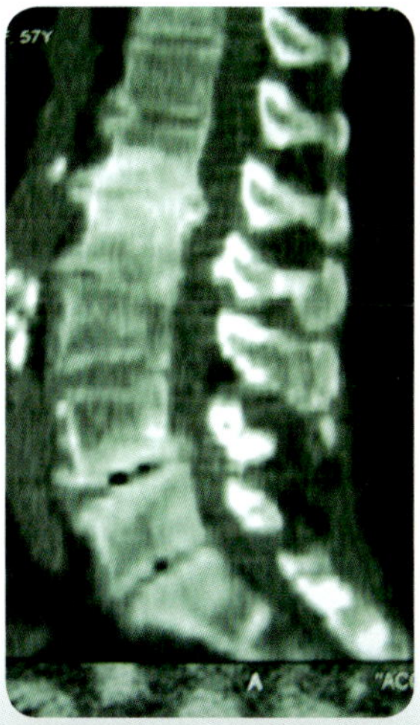

Fig. 5.3.50.

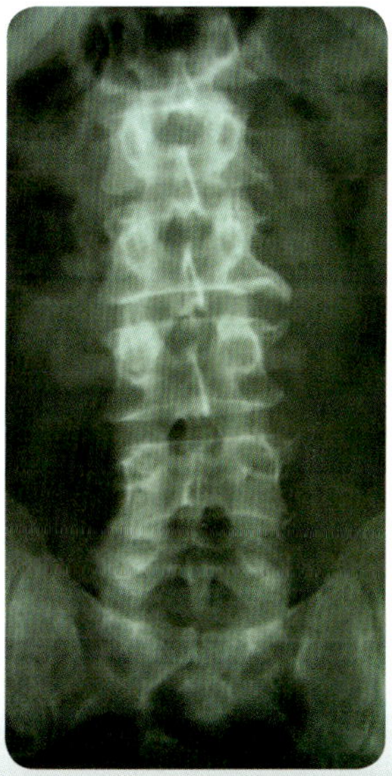

Fig. 5.3.51.

Examination of the patient showed that she had severe kyphoscoliotic deformation of the thoracic spine, as well as a severe pelvic tilt, which we attempted to compensate for with an orthopaedic insole of a height of **30 mm** placed under the right heel. Her face was hyperaemic. There were clinical signs of bilateral plexitis, lumboischialgia, and bilateral neuritis of the femoral, obturator and sciatic nerves. Varus deformation of the right knee joint was observed.

The standard treatment, i.e. orthopaedic insole, detorsional exercises, local magneto-acoustic therapy along the spine, was prescribed. We initially recommended the use of an insole of a height of **15 mm**, to be increased to **30 mm** in 1–1.5 months. At 6 months' follow-up, the difference in the length of the legs had decreased to **20 mm**. The intensity of the pain had decreased significantly and K. had become slightly thinner. We advised her to continue with the prescribed treatment for a year and then to come for an obligatory check-up.

On analysing this clinical observation, we arrived at the following conclusions:

a. In our opinion, the pain in the upper and lower extremities was initially a manifestation of a widespread syndrome of fibromyalgia. Signs of dysplasia of the 5th lumbar and 1st sacral vertebrae, associated with progressive asymmetry of the trunk muscles, also contributed significantly to the development of the above-mentioned pain syndrome.
b. Long-term hormonal therapy adversely affected the patient's metabolism and led to obesity. Excessive body weight caused the trunk to tilt further to the right, which resulted in deformation of the right knee joint and a distinct facet pain syndrome in the lumbar spine.
c. The defect of the posterior arch of S_1 played a major role in the development of the spinal pain syndrome, as it was a zone of herniation of the spinal meninges.

d. Physicians should be careful not to be misled by the variety of clinical signs of such a pathological condition when trying to determine its origin. Progressive tilting of the pelvis and consequent violation of the biomechanics of the spine lead to increasing relative shortening of one of the legs, which in its turn provokes further tilting of the pelvis and so on. This is why we believe that such relative shortening is the root of the problem which must be addressed as soon as possible.

12. Patient S., a 28-year-old man, had had a fall and injured his right knee a year before consulting us. He was diagnosed by an orthopaedic surgeon as having a contusion of the knee joint without bone pathology. S. was treated for one month, but to no avail and in fact his left knee joint started hurting as well. During his first visit to us, he complained of pain in both knees and said he could not walk because of the pain. Moreover, he suffered from a constant intense headache and his hands turned numb if he raised them above his head.

Radiographs of the knee joints did not reveal any signs of bone pathology. In the lumbosacral spine, lumbarization of S_1 (Fig. 5.3.52), a cleft in the posterior arch of S_1 and anomalous tropism of the articular processes of the L_5-S_1 SMS could be observed (Fig. 5.3.53).

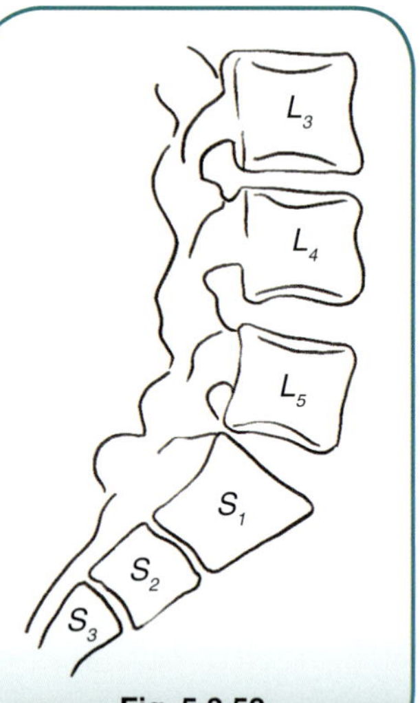

Fig. 5.3.52.

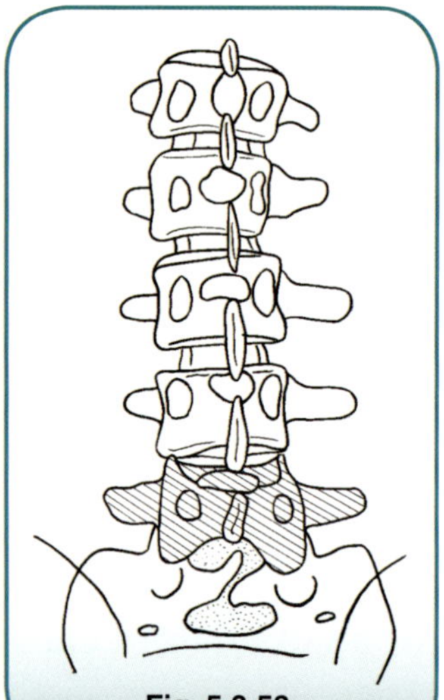
Fig. 5.3.53.

On examination, the patient was found to have clinical signs of bilateral plexitis, and bilateral neuritis of the femoral, obturator and sciatic nerves. He had a pelvic tilt, which we attempted to correct with an orthopaedic insole of a height of **3 mm** under the right leg.

The standard treatment, i.e. orthopaedic insole, detorsional exercises and local magneto-acoustic therapy along the paravertebral region, was prescribed. At 3 months' follow-up, neither of the knee joints was painful. The headaches and numbness of the hands had resolved. S. considered himself healthy. Nonetheless, we advised him to continue with the prescribed treatment for another 6 months.

On analysing this clinical observation, we arrived at the following conclusions:

a. Relative shortening of the right leg by 3 mm led to imbalance of the spinal–pelvic segment. Dysplasia of the 1st sacral vertebra, i.e. the defect of its posterior arch and asymmetry of the articular processes of L_5 contributed to the development of the spinal pain syndrome.
b. When the patient fell and injured his right knee, the dysplastically changed L_5-S_1-S_2

vertebrae became displaced and the facet pain syndrome emerged.

c. The protrusion of the spinal meninges through the defect in the posterior arch of S_1 led to the development of meningeal hernia and severe pain in the lower extremities.
d. The gradual restoration of balance in the spinal–pelvic segment through the use of an orthopaedic insole, detorsional exercises and magneto-acoustic therapy took care of the major factors responsible for the spinal pain, thus promoting recovery of the patient.

13. Patient T., a well-built 46-year-old man, suffered from intense pain in the lumbar region that radiated to both legs. The pain would occur after he lifted relatively small weights, when his trunk was rotated. He had had such episodes of pain earlier in his life too, during training.

CT scans and radiographs of the lumbosacral spine revealed signs of dysplasia and deformative spondylosis of L_5–S_1, lumbarization of S_1 (Fig. 5.3.54), sacralization of L_5, spina bifida of L_5–S_1, and asymmetry of the articular processes of L_5–S_1 (Fig. 5.3.55). Distinct deforming changes in the sacroiliac joints and of the L_5–S_1–S_2 SMS provided evidence of multiple dislocations in the past of the upper sacral vertebrae relative to L_5.

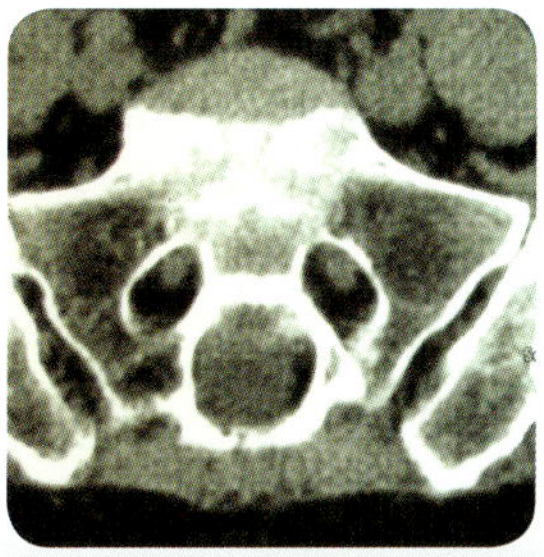

Fig. 5.3.54.

On examination, the patient was found to have hypertrichosis of the skin in the lumbar region as an external sign of dysplastic changes in L_5–S_1 SMS (Fig. 5.3.56). He also had signs of bilateral plexitis and lumboischialgia. The pelvis was tilted to the left resulting in the development of a right-sided scoliotic deformation of the spine. There was relative shortening of the left leg by **20 mm**. The patient was taught detorsional exercises during the first examination and after he performed them, the pain in the lumbar region disappeared.

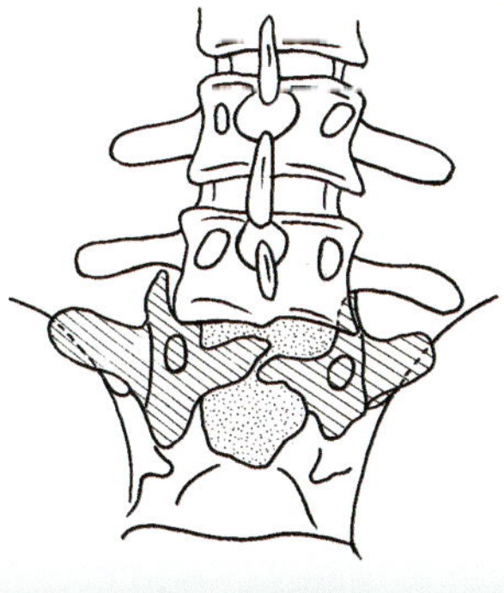

Fig. 5.3.55.

The standard treatment, i.e. orthopaedic insole of 20 mm height under the left leg, detorsional exercises and local magneto-acoustic therapy, was prescribed. During examination 2 months later, it was found that the difference in the length of the legs had decreased to **10 mm**. There was no pain in the lumbar region. T. regularly performed the detorsional exercises. At 4 months' follow-up, the patient had no complaints at all. The difference in the

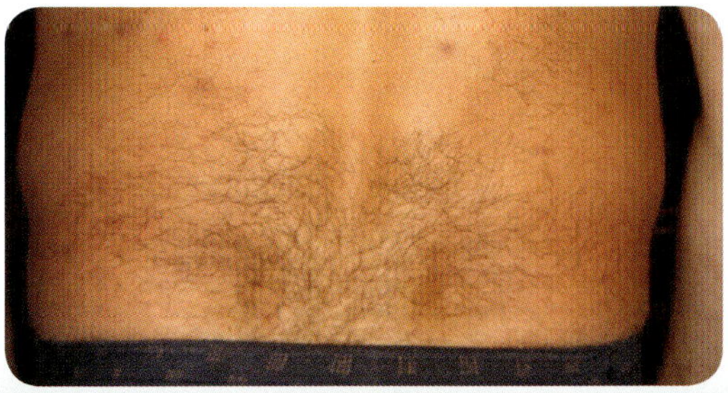

Fig. 5.3.56.

length of the legs had decreased to 3 mm. We advised him to use the insole regularly during physical activity and to continue with the prescribed treatment for another year.

On analysing this clinical observation, we arrived at the following conclusions:

a. The progressive relative shortening of the left leg, associated with several types of dysplasia of the 5th lumbar and 1st sacral vertebrae, caused instability of the spinal–pelvic segment at the level of L_5–S_1.
b. Dysplastic changes of the L_5–S_1 vertebrae were inherited, as was evident from the presence of hypertrichosis.
c. Progressive tilting of the pelvis due to physical exertion led to rotation of the 5th lumbar and 1st sacral vertebrae around their axes. The patient's neurological symptoms were caused by compression of the nerves of the lumbar and sacral plexuses.
d. The main factor that caused pain were the clefts in the posterior arches of L_5–S_1. Rotation of the vertebrae at this level led to compression of the spinal meninges in the area of the defect. This caused the acute pain in the lumbar region, radiating to both legs.
e. The use of an orthopaedic insole, continuation of detorsional exercises and magneto-acoustic therapy helped to restore the stability of the spinal–pelvic segment and eliminate all the factors that had been causing spinal pain, thus promoting clinical recovery of the patient.

14. Patient L., a 35-year-old man, complained of pain in the lumbar region of 7–8 months' duration. The pain appeared when he had bent low to dig potatoes. Chiropractics, massage, grinding and sagging on the horizontal bar did not improve his condition.

CT scans of the lumbar spine showed sacralization of L_5 and lumbarization of S_1 (Fig. 5.3.57). The scans also revealed the presence of a cleft in the posterior arch of the 1st sacral vertebra and asymmetry of the articular processes of the L_5–S_1 SMS (Fig. 5.3.58).

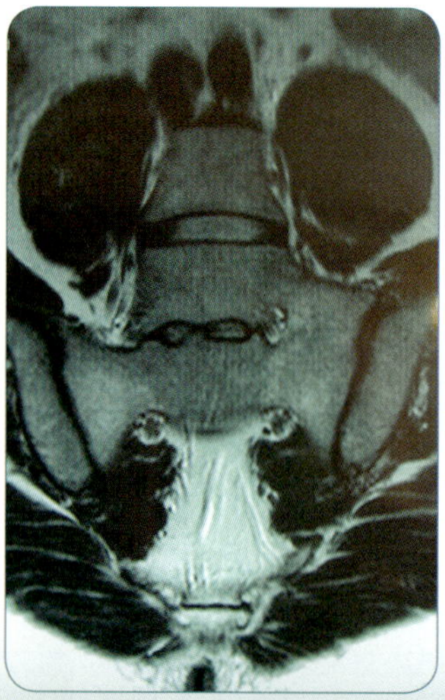

Fig. 5.3.57.

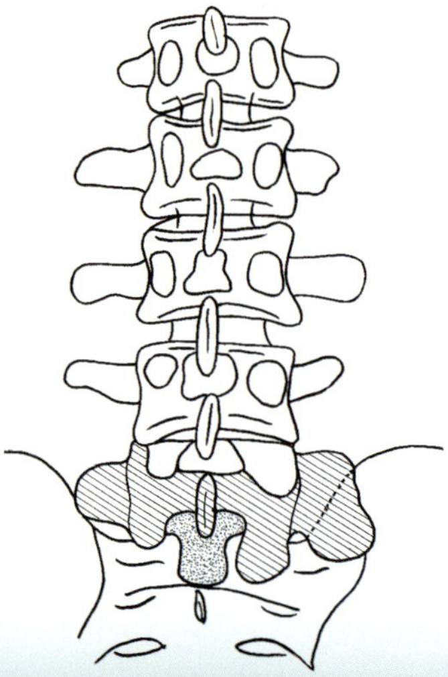

Fig. 5.3.58.

On examination, the patient was found to have a left-sided scoliotic posture. We proposed to reduce the tilt of the body through the use of an orthopaedic insole of a height of **3 mm**. The application of pressure on the lower lumbar and upper sacral vertebrae gave rise to pain. L. also had bilateral lumboischialgia.

The standard treatment, i.e. magneto-acoustic therapy along the paravertebral region, orthopaedic insole under the right heel and detorsional exercises, was prescribed. When learning the detorsional exercises in our clinic, L. reported that the very first movement had resulted in the disappearance of the pain in the sacrum. At 3 months' follow-up, although the relative shortening of the right leg had been corrected, we advised the patient to use an orthopaedic insole for another year. He had no complaints and considered himself healthy.

On analysing this clinical observation, we arrived at the following conclusions:

a. Relative shortening of the right leg created conditions that led to the impairment of balance in the spinal–pelvic segment at the level of L_5–S_1 SMS.
b. Rotation and dislocation of the dysplastically changed vertebrae (L_5–S_1) occurred when the patient engaged in physical activity in which the body was bent forward (such as digging potatoes). This caused facet pain syndrome.
c. The defect in the posterior arch of S_1 eventually led to prolapse of the spinal meninges and development of meningeal hernia, accompanied by a severe pain syndrome.
d. We reduced the pain by eliminating the factors that had caused the rotation of L_5–S_1 and restored the pelvis to its correct position. This was achieved with the help of an orthopaedic insole, detorsional exercises and local magneto-acoustic therapy.

15. Patient Sh., a 16-year-old young man, mentioned urinary incontinence (enuresis) as his major complaint. He urinated twice or thrice at night. Moreover, he complained of frequent headaches and said his hands went numb when he raised them above his head.

Radiographs of the lumbosacral spine (Fig. 5.3.59) showed sacralization of L_5, lumbarization of S_1 and a cleft in the posterior arch of the 1st sacral veretebra (spina bifida of S_1).

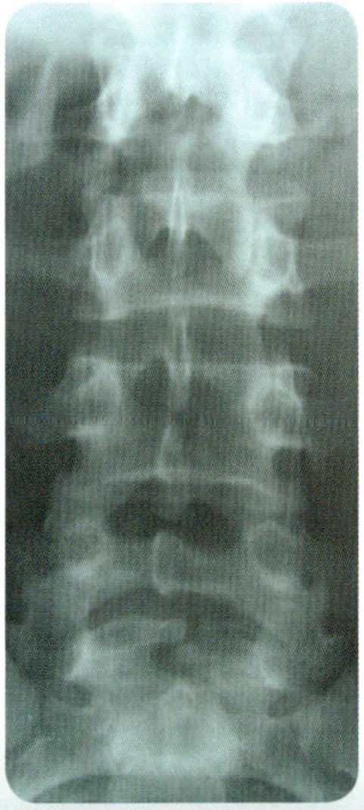

Fig. 5.3.59.

On examination, it was observed that the patient had clinical signs of bilateral plexitis, and bilateral neuritis of the femoral, obturator and sciatic nerves. We also observed relative shortening of the left leg by **7 mm**, which had caused a left-sided pelvic tilt and the development of a scoliotic posture.

The standard treatment, i.e. orthopaedic insole of 7 mm under the left heel, detorsional exercises, local magneto-acoustic therapy along the lumbosacral area, was prescribed. When examined 4 months after the initiation of treatment, Sh. reported that the episodes of nocturnal urinary incontinence had become rare—they occurred a few times a week. He had been wearing the orthopaedic insole regularly. At 7 months' follow-up, the episodes of urinary incontinence had ceased altogether. Relative shortening of the left leg had decreased to **3 mm**. Sh. had no complaints. We advised him to continue with the prescribed treatment for another 6 months.

On analysing this clinical observation, we arrived at the following conclusions:

a. The patient's neurological disorders were caused by rotation of the cervical, thoracic and lumbar vertebrae and compression of the neural structures corresponding to them. The rotation of the vertebrae was the result of the pelvic tilt to the left and development of areas of instability.
b. Dysplastic changes of L_5–S_1 and the cleft in the posterior arch of the 1st sacral vertebra promoted the above-mentioned disorders.
c. Presence of this defect, spina bifida of S_1, led to prolapse of the spinal meninges and development of hernia. We consider this to be a cause of urinary incontinence.
d. By removal of the pelvic tilt and eliminating the factors that caused rotation of the vertebrae at all levels of the spine, we were able to cure the neurological disorders and restore urinary bladder control.

16. Patient G., a 21-year-old young man, who was well built and actively engaged in sports, informed us that at the age of 14–15 years, he had fallen from the upper berth of a train and lost consciousness. He had not received any treatment and had recovered gradually without medical assistance. One year before consulting us, he had collided with another player while playing football and had received a strong blow on his head, as a result of which he had lost consciousness. Since then, he had been suffering from headaches, and pain in the upper cervical region, which increased during abrupt rotation of the head. There was also pain in the lumbosacral spine. In addition, the patient got cramps in the gastrocnemius muscles at night, suffered from blurred vision and had occasional episodes of breath-holding. He was treated in the sports centre, but there was no improvement in his condition.

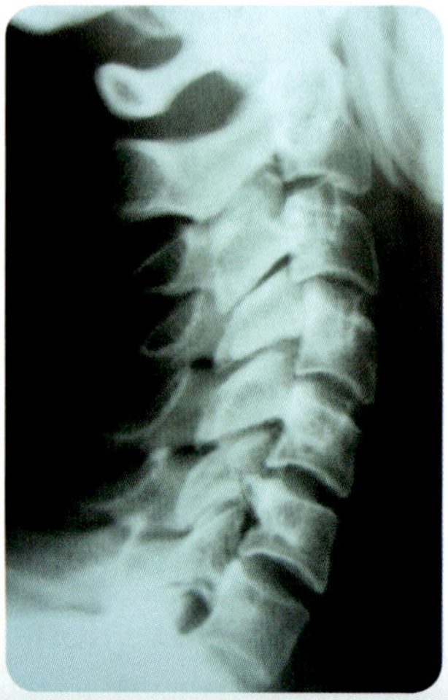

Fig. 5.3.60.

Radiographs revealed rotation and dislocation of the C_3–C_4 vertebrae, a huge exostosis on the posterior surface of C_6 (probably corresponding to the area of injury) (Fig. 5.3.60), anomalous tropism of the articular processes of the L_3–L_5–S_1 SMS, and lumbarization and spina bifida of S_1 (Fig. 5.3.61).

During examination of the patient, a right-sided scoliotic deformity of the thoracic spine was observed. The body was tilted to the left. We proposed to compensate for this with an orthopaedic insole of a height of **15 mm**.

The standard treatment, i.e. detorsional exercises, local magneto-acoustic therapy, orthopaedic insole, was prescribed. Initially, the height of the insole prescribed was **10 mm**, but this was increased to **15 mm** after 2 weeks. At 6 months' follow-up, relative shortening of the left leg had decreased to **3 mm**. G. reported a significant improvement in his overall condition. There was no more dizziness, the episodes of apnoea had ceased and the pain in the legs had resolved. We advised him to continue with the prescribed treatment for another year.

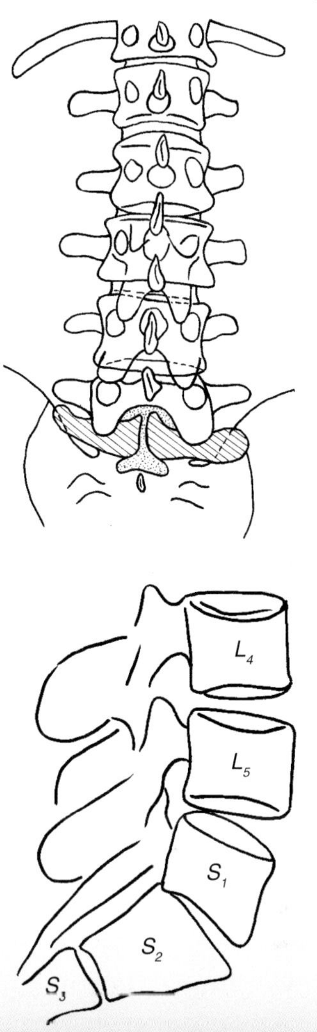

Fig. 5.3.61.

On analysing this clinical observation, we arrived at the following conclusions:

a. Despite the fact that the patient systematically pursued sports activities, the spinal extensors were asymmetrical. This led to a pelvic tilt and the development of areas of instability at all levels of the spine.
b. Rotation and dislocation of vertebrae occurred in the areas of instability, causing traumatization of the cervical, thoracic, lumbar and lumbosacral plexuses and giving rise to the corresponding neurological symptoms. The patient's symptoms were provoked by repeated trauma of the spine and dysplastic changes in the L_3–L_5–S_1 vertebrae.
c. Restoration of the spinal–pelvic balance through the use of an orthopaedic insole under the left heel reduced the underlying factors causing the rotation and displacement of vertebrae, and the complaints associated with them.

17. Patient K., a 33-year-old man, had first suffered from pain in the spine 15 years earlier, after a session of physical training. Sports was his mainstay, and he played football, trained with dumbbells and enjoyed fencing. Gradually, this pain started occurring regularly whenever he would stand or lift loads, mostly during winter. When he was 19–20 years old, he had suffered from pain in his groin and the caecum following urination. The urologist and surgeon had excluded any pathology. He was treated by a neurologist, but there was no improvement in his condition.

Radiographs of the lumbar spine showed lumbarization of S_1, sacralization of L_5, spina bifida of S_1 and distinct asymmetry of the interarticular processes of the L_4–L_5–S_1 SMS (Fig. 5.3.62).

On examining the patient, we found that he had bilateral lumboischialgia, which was more pronounced on the right side. He had a scoliotic posture and a pelvic tilt to the left, which we attempted to correct with an orthopaedic insole of a height of **10 mm**.

The standard treatment, i.e. detorsional exercises, local magneto-acoustic therapy and application of orthopaedic insole, was prescribed. At 1 month's follow-up, the difference in the length of the two legs had decreased to **3 mm**. The patient had no complaints. At 3 months' follow-up, the left leg was not shorter than the right one any more. The patient considered himself healthy. We advised him to wear an orthopaedic insole of a height of 3 mm during physical exertion of any kind.

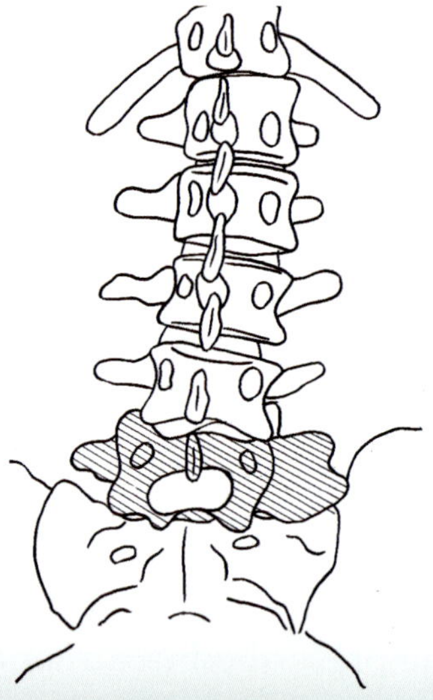

Fig. 5.3.62.

On analysing this clinical observation, we arrived at the following conclusions:

a. Among the various factors that can cause this pathological condition, we believe that the most important is the instability of the lumbosacral spine, resulting from the stable tilting of the pelvis due to asymmetry of the muscles of the trunk.

b. Physical exertion promoted not only the development of the body's muscles, but also instability at all levels of the spine, as well as rotational displacement of the vertebrae. The dysplastic changes in L_5–S_1 facilitated this process.

c. Meningeal hernia in the area of the defect of the posterior arch of S_1 caused neurological disorders. Spinal pain was also caused due to traumatization of the nerve roots due to enlarged interarticular processes, the so-called 'facet' pain syndrome.

d. Reduction in the pelvic tilt corrected the rotation of all the vertebrae and promoted gradual recovery of the patient. Apart from the orthopaedic insole, magneto-acoustic therapy, with its anti-oedematous and analgesic effects, and detorsional exercises played a significant role.

5.3.3 PATIENTS WITH LUMBAR PAIN SYNDROME AND SCOLIOTIC DEFORMATION OF THE SPINE

1. Patient Sh., a 24-year-old woman, who had had scoliosis since childhood, complained of frequent headaches, a tendency to get easily fatigued and emotional lability. Her wrists were constantly sweaty and cold, and her hands went numb when she raised them above her head. She had also suffered from pain in the heart

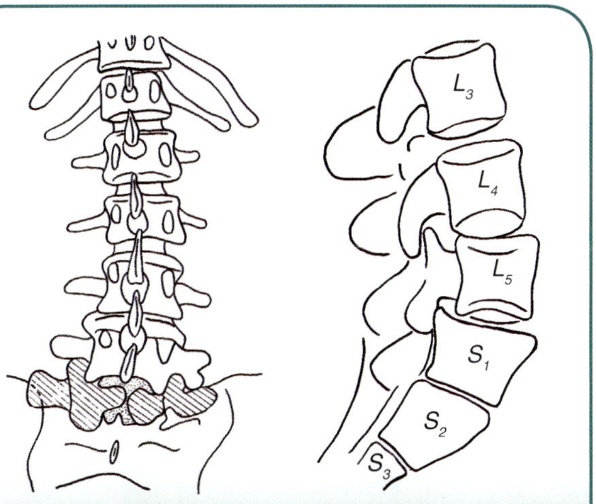

Fig. 5.3.63.

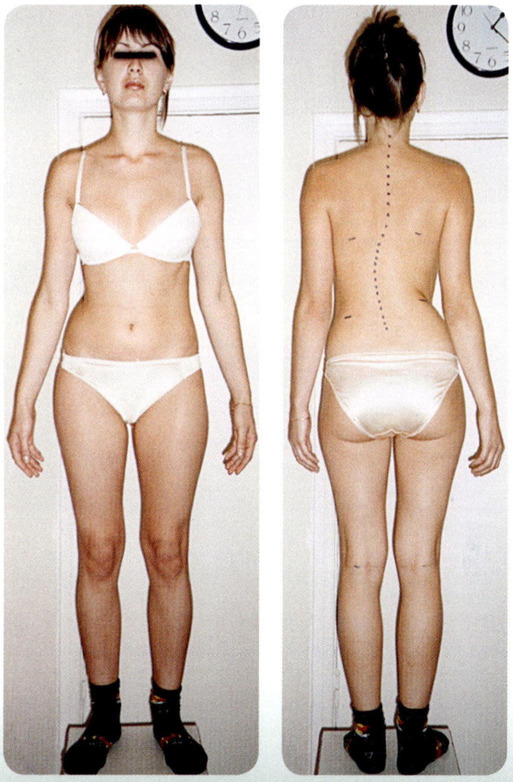

Fig. 5.3.64.

and tachycardia since the age of 16–17 years, lumbar pain and cramps in the gastrocnemius muscles. Sh. had been treated by neurologists and traditional healers.

Radiographs of the lumbar spine revealed spina bifida of L_5, sacralization of L_5 and physiological lumbarization of S_1 (Fig. 5.3.63).

During examination of the patient, scoliotic deformation (grade 3) of the thoracic and lumbar spine was observed (Fig. 5.3.64). We planned to compensate for the lateral deformity of the spine with an orthopaedic insole of a height of **30 mm**, to be placed under the left heel. Sh. had clinical signs of bilateral lumboischialgia, neuritis of the femoral and obturator nerves, and neuritis of the left trigeminal nerve.

The standard treatment, i.e. detorsional exercises, an orthopaedic insole initially of a height of **20 mm**, magneto-acoustic therapy along the paravertebral region, was prescribed. During the follow-up visit 3 months later, the height of the insole was increased by 10 mm. A deformation of the thorax (costal hump) was visible. The pain syndrome had become negligible. Due to her work abroad, the next follow-up examination was performed only 1 year and 7 months after the initiation of treatment. Sh. reported that she no longer suffered from pain in the heart or cramps in the calf muscles. Her posture had become correct and the asymmetry of the gluteal muscles had decreased significantly (Fig. 5.3.65). The left leg was still **10 mm** shorter than the right. She had no complaints and considered herself 'almost' healthy. Sh. continued to adhere to the prescribed treatment. At 2.5 years' follow-up, the patient reported that she had no complaints. The length of both legs was equal, the posture was correct, and the volume of the right and left gluteal muscles was equal (Fig. 5.3.66).

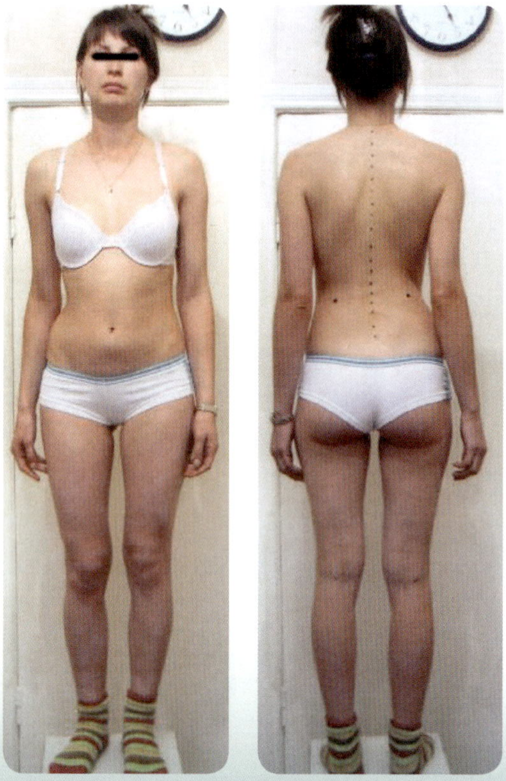

Fig. 5.3.65.

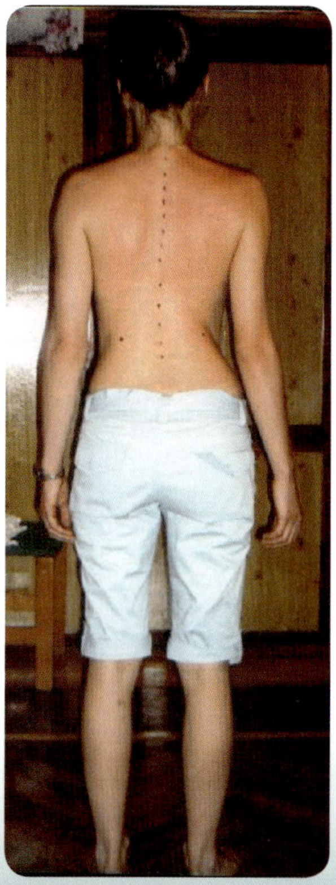

Fig. 5.3.66.

2. Patient P., an 11-year-old girl, had been receiving treatment for scoliosis of the thoracic and lumbar spine since the age of 6. She complained of recurrent headaches, as well as retrosternal and interscapular pain. She also suffered from vegetovascular dystonia.

Radiographs of the spine showed sacralization of L_5, lumbarization of S_1 and S_2, clefts in the posterior arches of the 5th lumbar and 1st sacral vertebrae, and asymmetry of the articular processes of the L_3, L_4 and L_5 vertebrae (Fig. 5.3.67).

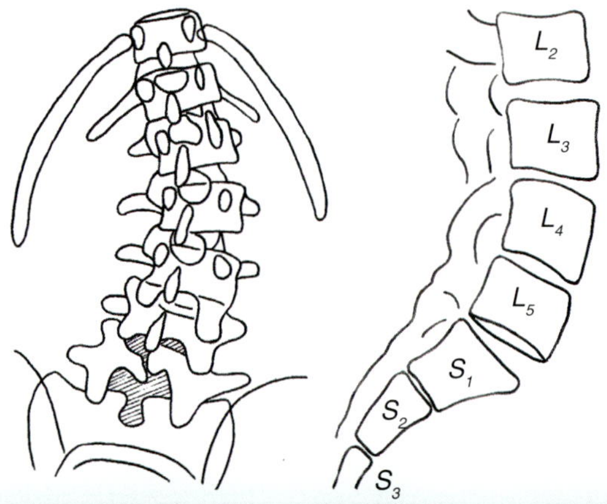

Fig. 5.3.67.

On examination of the patient, scoliotic deformation (grade 3) of the thoracic and lumbar spine was observed (Fig. 5.3.68; start of treatment). We planned to compensate for the tilt of the pelvis to the left with an orthopaedic insole of a height of **45 mm**, to be placed under the left heel. P. had signs of bilateral lumboischialgia, and neuritis of the femoral and obturator nerves.

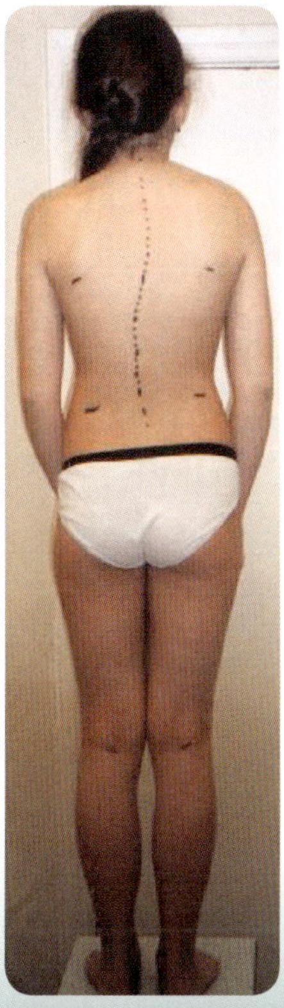

Fig. 5.3.68.

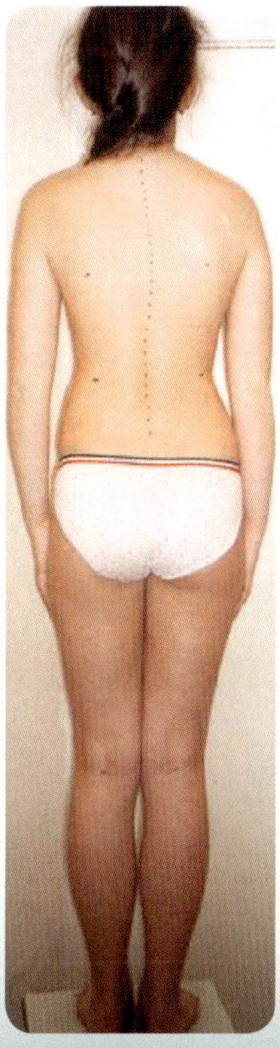

Fig. 5.3.69.

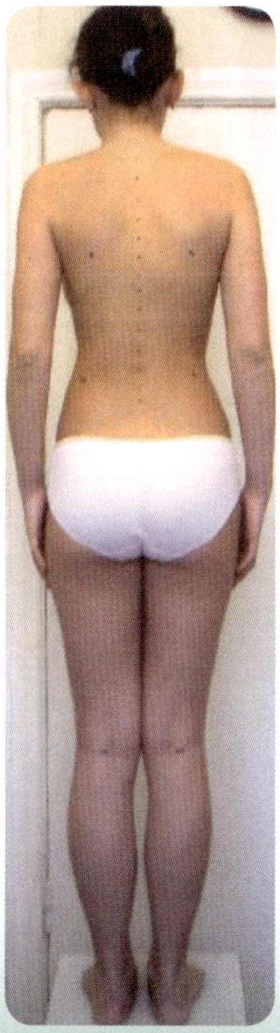

Fig. 5.3.70.

The standard treatment, i.e. magneto-acoustic therapy along the paravertebral region, detorsional exercises, orthopaedic insole, was prescribed. During the first examination, we prescribed the use of an insole of a height of **15 mm**. Two weeks later, we increased the height to 20 mm and a month later, to 35 mm. At 4 months' follow-up, the axis of the spine had straightened considerably and there was also a significant decrease in the asymmetry of the gluteal muscles (Fig. 5.3.69; 4 months later). The spinal pain had become negligible. The difference in the length of the legs had decreased to **20 mm**. At one year's follow-up, it was **7 mm** (Fig. 5.3.70; 1.5 years later). The deformity of the thorax had been corrected to a large extent. The patient had no complaints. Nonetheless, we advised her to continue with the prescribed treatment for another year as she was still in her growing years.

3. Patient T., a 14-year-old girl, had a severe scoliotic deformation of the thoracic and lumbar spine and suffered from a severe spinal pain syndrome, which, as her mother mentioned, was associated with inherited spinal hernia. During the first week after her birth, she had undergone surgery in which a haemostatic sponge was used to effect closure of the bone defect of the sacral vertebrae. T.'s other complaints were constipation, enuresis and accommodation spasm.

Radiographs revealed signs of sacralization of L_5, an extremely enlarged transverse process on the right side of L_5, physiological lumbarization of S_1, asymmetry of the articular processes of the L_5–S_1 SMS and defects of the posterior arches of the 1st–3rd sacral vertebrae (Fig. 5.3.71).

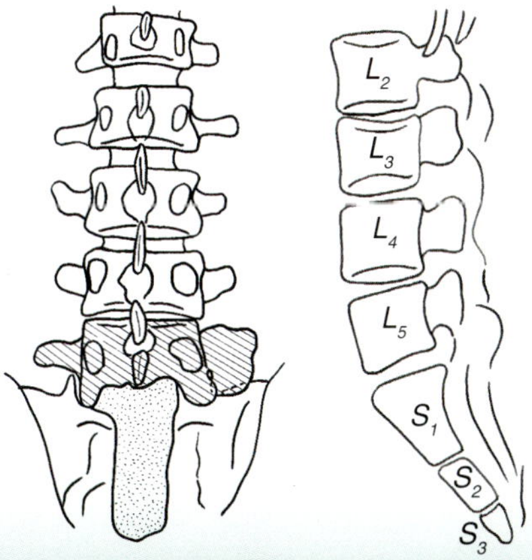

Fig. 5.3.71.

On examination of the patient, scoliotic deformation (2nd–3rd grade) of the thoracic and

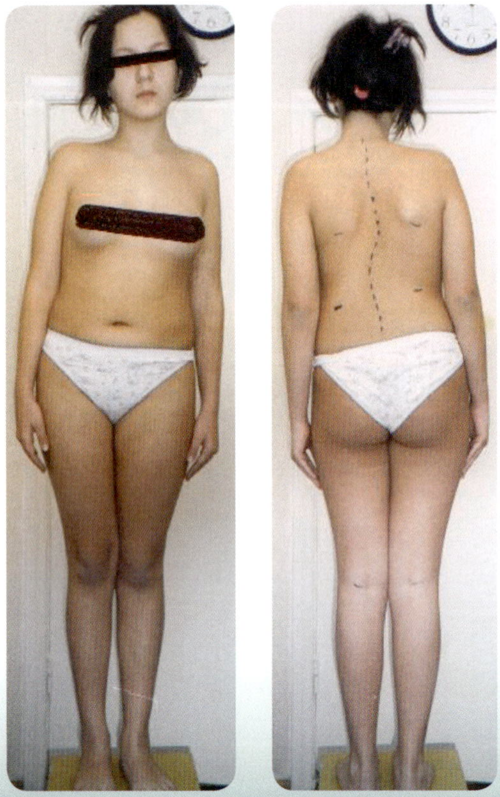

Fig. 5.3.72.

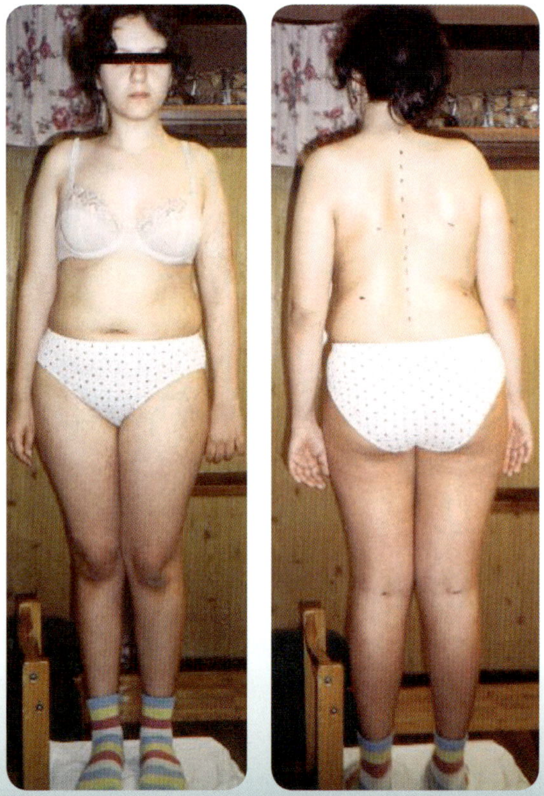

Fig. 5.3.73.

lumbar spine was observed (Fig. 5.3.72). She had a pelvic tilt, which we planned to compensate for with an orthopaedic insole of a height of **40 mm**. Clinical signs of bilateral lumboischialgia and neuritis of the femoral and obturator nerves were present.

The standard treatment, i.e. orthopaedic insole, detorsional exercises, magneto-acoustic therapy along the vertebral column, was prescribed. Initially, we recommended an insole of a height of **15 mm**. The girl and her mother were trained to perform the exercises. Three weeks later, we increased the height of the insole to **30 mm** and after another 3 weeks to 40 mm.

Thus, we totally compensated for the relative shortening of the left leg. At 1 year's follow-up, the difference in the length of the legs was **7 mm** (Fig. 5.3.73). Palpation of the vertebrae was no longer painful and the axis of the spine had been corrected. She performed the entire scheme of treatment procedures. Enuresis and constipation were rare. T. had been following all our advice. She and her mother were satisfied with the results of the treatment. We advised T. to continue with the prescribed treatment for another year.

4. Patient L., a 14-year-old girl, visited us with her mother, who informed us that 2 years earlier, she had noticed a progressively growing deformity in her daughter's thorax. Whatever treatment she had received for her problem (massage, swimming, electroprocedures, treatment in sanatoriums) had proved ineffective. The girl suffered from constant headaches and severe spinal pain. She had recurrent retrosternal pain and emotional lability. She also had episodes of apnoea.

Radiographs revealed right-sided scoliotic deformation of the thoracic spine and left-sided deformation of the lumbar spine (grade 3), physiological lumbarization of the sacral vertebrae, spina bifida of S_1, and severe asymmetry of the intervertebral joints of the L_4–L_5–S_1 vertebrae (Fig. 5.3.74).

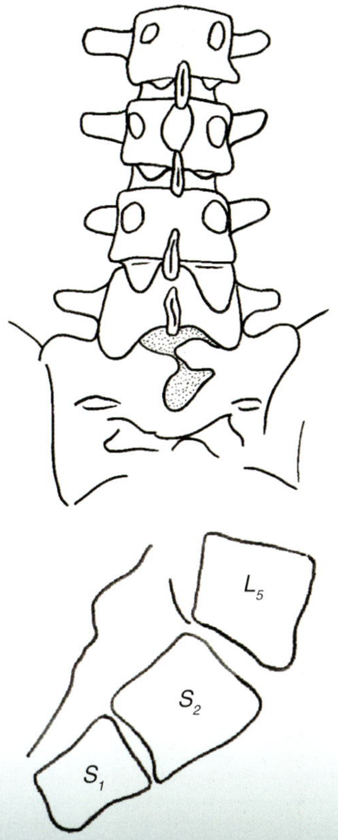

Fig. 5.3.74.

On examining the patient, we found that rotation of the head to the left was limited and there was lateral deformity of the thoracic and lumbar spine. The gluteal muscles as well as pelvic bones on the left side were severely underdeveloped and there was a pelvic tilt. We planned to correct this through the use of an orthopaedic insole of a height of **47 mm** (Fig. 5.3.75). L. had clinical signs of bilateral lumboischialgia, as well as neuritis of the femoral and obturator nerves.

The standard treatment, i.e. magneto-acoustic therapy along the paravertebral region, detorsional exercises, orthopaedic insole of a height of **15 mm,** was prescribed. The height of the insole was increased gradually and 4 months after the initiation of treatment, the patient started to wear an insole of a height of **47 mm**. At 6 months' follow-up, the difference in the length of the legs had decreased to **40 mm** and the axis of the spine was normalizing. The volume of the gluteal muscles was slowly being restored. L. had no pain in the spine any more. Magneto-acoustic therapy was stopped. At 8 months' follow-up, the axis of the spine was correct, while the asymmetry of the pelvis and gluteal muscles had become negligible. The left leg was still **20 mm** shorter than the right. L.

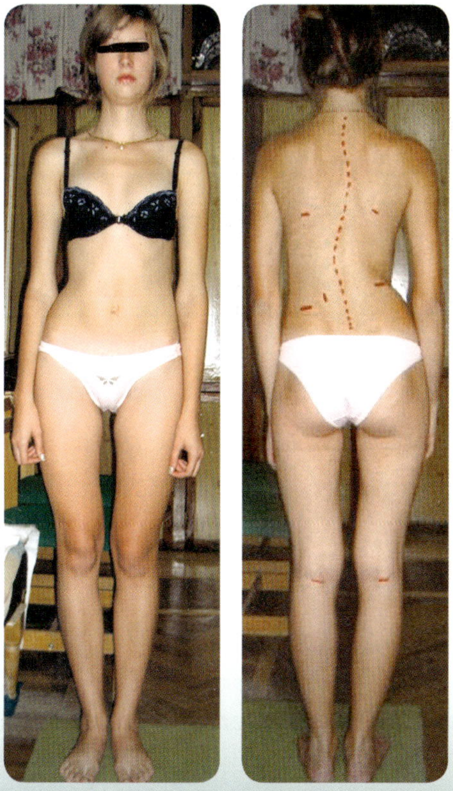
Fig. 5.3.75.

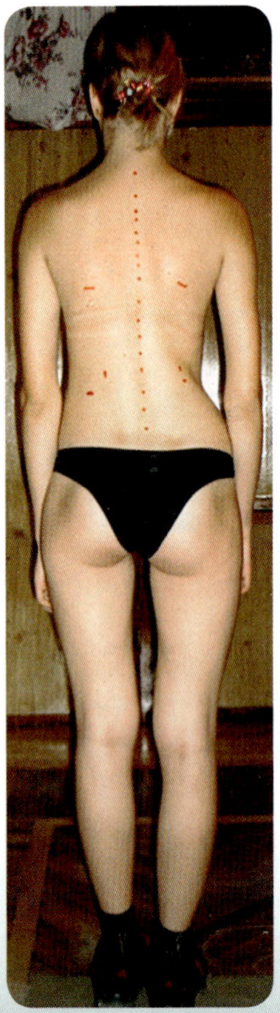
Fig. 5.3.76.

followed our advice conscientiously. At 2 years' follow-up, the axis of the spine was correct, the volume of the gluteal muscles and pelvic bones on the left side had been more or less restored (Fig. 5.3.76). L. had no complaints, but the left leg was still **7 mm** shorter than the right, because she had not used the orthopaedic insole regularly. We advised her to continue using the insole and to perform detorsional exercises.

5. Patient V., a 14-year-old boy, visited us together with his parents, who were worried about the progressive scoliotic deformity of the child's spine. The boy had a severe pelvic tilt to the left. At the age of 10, he had had Perthe disease on the left side. His orthopaedic surgeon had suggested that it was due to this that there was a progressive deformation of the spine, associated with destruction of the head of the left femoral bone. V. complained of persistent pain in the lumbar region that radiated to both legs, which often became fatigued and turn numb. Plain radiographs of the pelvis showed that the structure of the left head of the femoral bone was solid and the pathological process had resolved completely. There were signs of sacralization of L_5, predominantly on the left side, and clefts in the posterior arches of the 5th lumbar and 1st sacral vertebrae (Fig. 5.3.77).

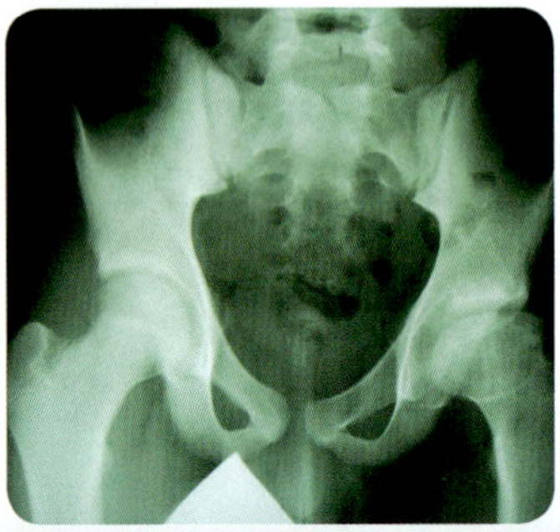
Fig. 5.3.77.

Examination of the patient, right-sided scoliotic deformation of the thoracic spine and left-sided scoliotic deformation of the lumbar spine (grade 2–3) were observed. There was a severe pelvic tilt, which we planned to compensate for with an orthopaedic insole of a height of **35 mm** (Fig. 5.3.78). Clinical signs of bilateral lumboischialgia, as well as neuritis of the femoral and obturator nerves, were present.

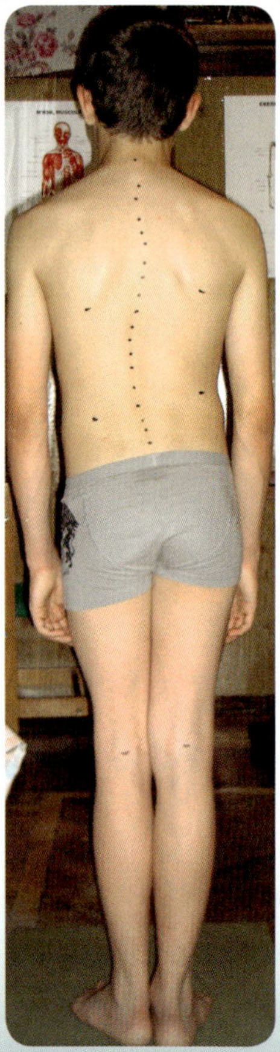
Fig. 5.3.78.

The standard treatment, i.e. orthopaedic insole, local magneto-acoustic therapy, detorsional exercises, was prescribed. We initially recommended the use of an orthopaedic insole of a height of **10 mm**. Every third week, we increased the height by **10 mm** until it reached the height required for total compensation. At 3 months' follow-up, there was a significant decrease in the pain in the spine and extremities, as also in the deformation of the spine. The relative shortening of the left leg had decreased to **25 mm**. Application of magneto-acoustic therapy was stopped. At 9 months' follow-up, the axis of the spine was correct, the spinal extensors were symmetrical and the spinal–pelvic balance had been restored (Fig. 5.3.79). The patient had no complaints. Since the left leg was still 10 mm shorter than the right, we recommended the use of an orthopaedic insole and continuation of detorsional exercises for another 6 months.

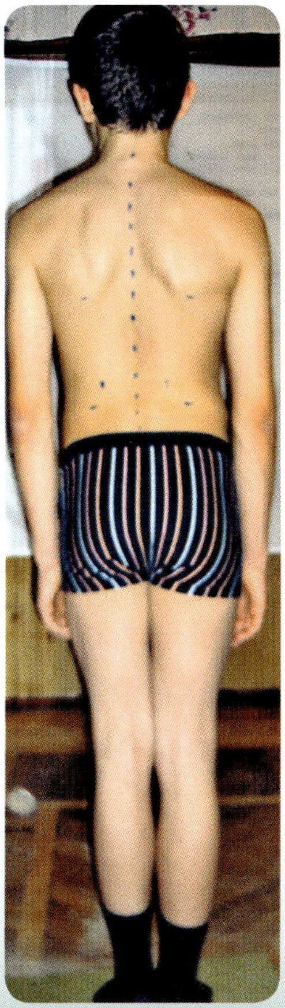

Fig. 5.3.79.

6. Patient K., a 26-year-old woman, complained that she had been suffering from headaches for more than 5 years. She also mentioned episodes of apnoea, pain in the heart, 'terrible' pain in the left shoulder, emotional lability, the feeling that all her bones were 'crunching', heartburn, stomach cramps and a tendency to constipation. Further, K. said she could not sit because of pain in the back. When in the prone position, she felt a severe pain in the left lumbosacral joint.

Radiographs revealed signs of sacralization of L_5, lumbarization of S_1–S_2 and lateral deformity of the spine (Fig. 5.3.80).

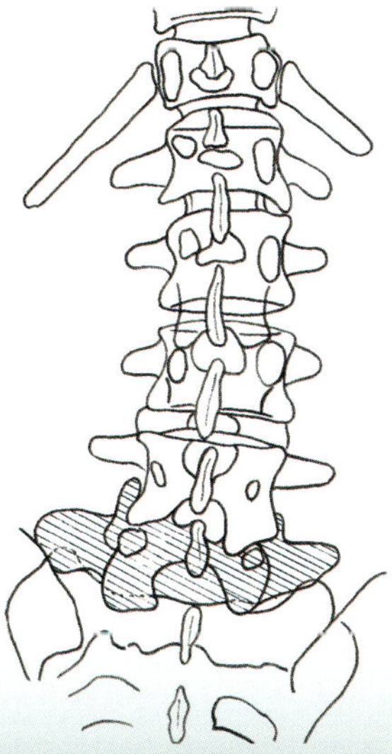

Fig. 5.3.80.

On examination of the patient, right-sided scoliosis of the thoracic and left-sided scoliosis of the lumbar spine were observed. There was a pelvic tilt, which we planned to compensate for with an orthopaedic insole of a height of **7 mm**. There was also minimal hypotrophy of the muscles of the left buttock compared to the right one (Fig. 5.3.81). K. had distinct clinical signs of bilateral plexitis, as well as neuritis of the femoral and obturator nerves. Palpation of all the vertebrae caused the patient pain.

The standard treatment, i.e. magneto-acoustic therapy along the paravertebral region, orthopaedic insole of a height of **7 mm** under the left heel, was prescribed. Control examination 3 months after initiation of treatment showed that the difference in the length of the legs had decreased to **3 mm**. At 1 year's follow-up, the legs were of equal length and the axis of the spine was correct. The functioning of the stomach and intestines had normalized. The size of the costal hump had decreased (Fig. 5.3.82). K. had no complaints. To correct the remaining deformity of the thorax, we advised her to use an orthopaedic insole of a height of **3 mm** and perform detorsional exercises. We asked her to come for a follow-up visit a year later.

7. Patient C., a 16-year-old girl, was brought to us by her mother, who had noticed a progressive deformity of the child's spine and the presence of right-sided torticollis. C. complained of pain in her eyeballs and weakening of vision. She felt very irritable, and her palms were always sweaty and cold. In addition, the girl suffered from pain in the arms and legs, as well as along the vertebral column. She could not sit for long and her legs became fatigued very easily.

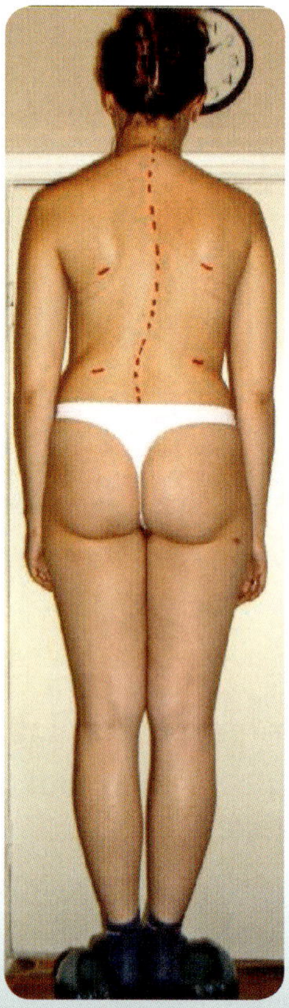

Fig. 5.3.81.

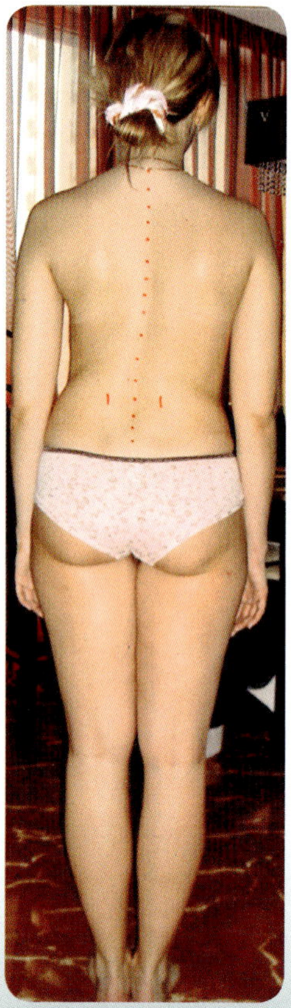

Fig. 5.3.82.

Radiographs of the spine revealed lateral deformity of the spine (grade 1–2), sacralization of L_5 and lumbarization of S_1 (Fig. 5.3.83).

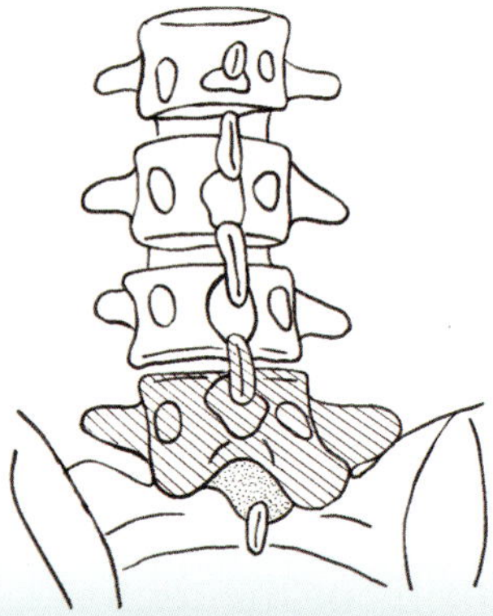

Fig. 5.3.83.

On examination of the patient, right-sided scoliotic deformation of the thoracic and left-sided scoliotic deformation of the lumbar spine were observed (Fig. 5.3.84). We planned to compensate for the pelvic tilt with an orthopaedic insole of a height of **10 mm**. Clinical signs of bilateral plexitis, as well as neuritis of the femoral and obturator nerves were present.

The standard treatment, i.e. orthopaedic insole, detorsional exercises and magneto-acoustic therapy along the paravertebral region, was prescribed. Control examination 7 months after initiation of treatment (Fig. 5.3.85) showed that the difference in the length of the legs had decreased, there were no signs of torticollis and the axis of the spine was correct. The gluteal muscles had become symmetrical and her palms were dry and warm. The patient had no complaints and she and her mother were very satisfied with the results of the treatment.

8. Patient M., a 44-year-old man, complained of pain in the lumbar region and lower extremities. The intensity of the pain, which appeared after physical activity

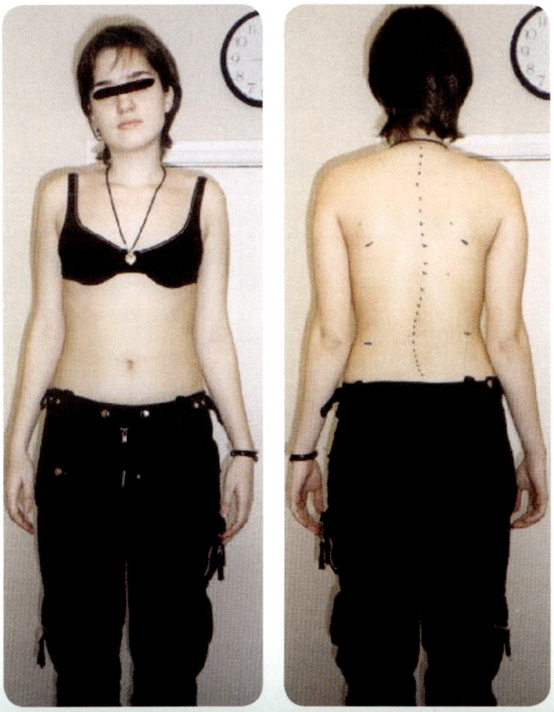

Fig. 5.3.84.

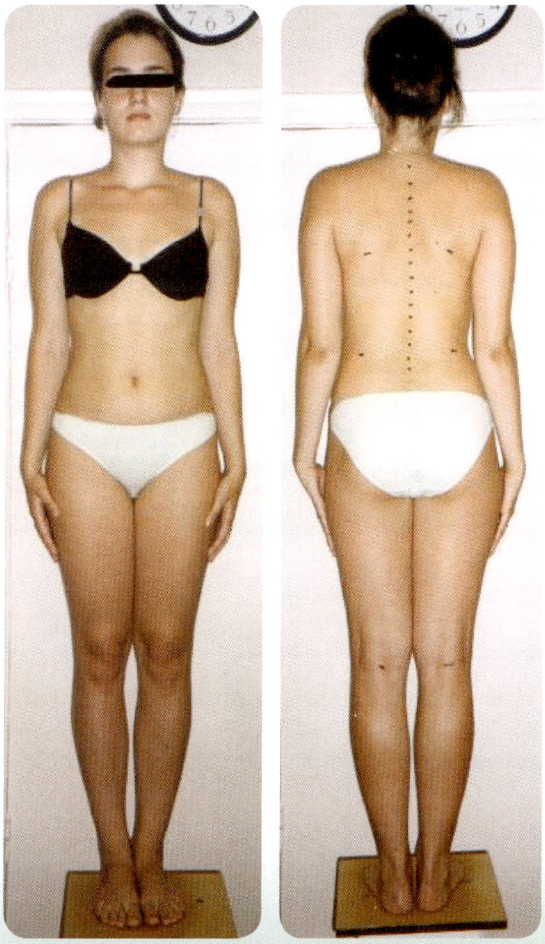

Fig. 5.3.85.

and was associated particularly with weight-lifting training, had increased in recent years.

CT scans revealed advanced deformative changes in the lumbar spine, predominantly at the level of L_5–S_1, and lumbarization of S_1 (Fig. 5.3.86).

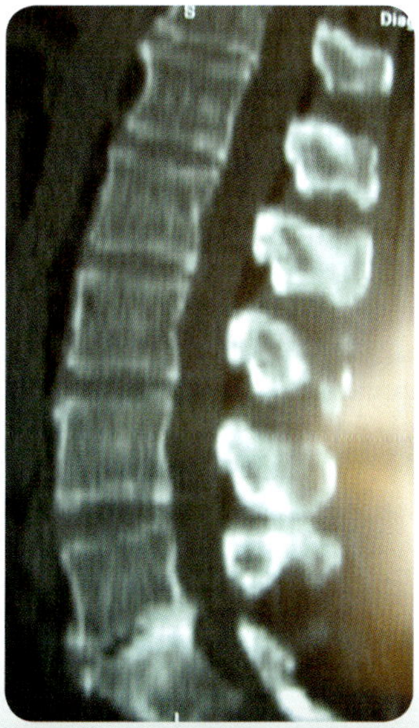

Fig. 5.3.86.

Examination showed that the man, who was well built, had a lateral deformity (grade 2) of the spine (right-sided scoliosis of the thoracic and left-sided scoliosis of the lumbar spine). We planned to counterbalance this with an orthopaedic insole of a height of **18 mm**. Slight hypotrophy of the left glutei was observed (Fig. 5.3.87).

The standard treatment, i.e. orthopaedic insole, detorsional exercises, magneto-acoustic therapy along the paravertebral region, was prescribed. Control examination 7 months after initiation of treatment showed that the axis of the spine had become correct and the length of the two legs was identical. His body had become symmetrical (Fig. 5.3.88). M. had no complaints.

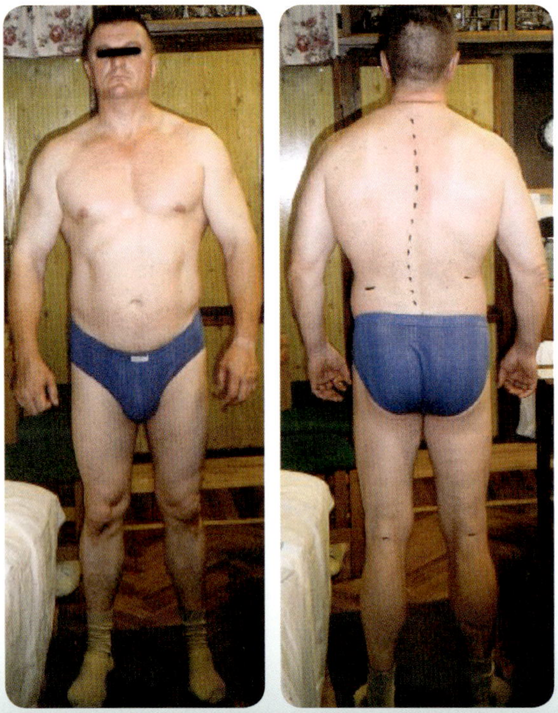

Fig. 5.3.87.

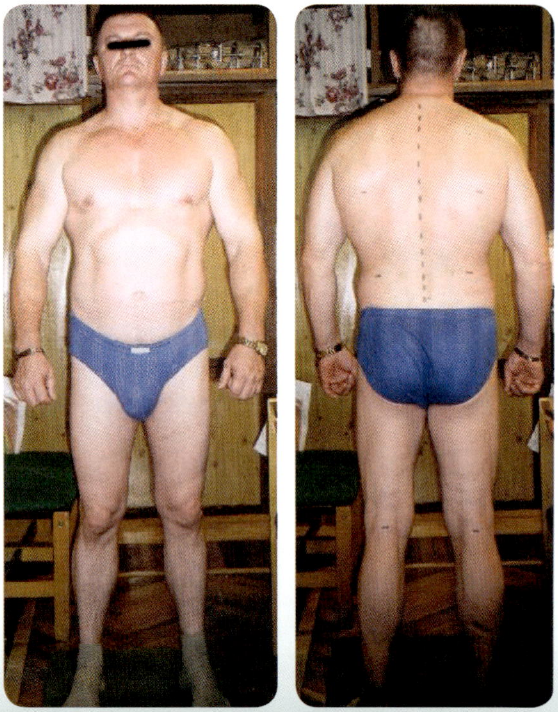

Fig. 5.3.88.

Application of magneto-acoustic therapy was stopped. In our view, the pain in the sacral region resolved because of restoration of the symmetry of the spinal extensors, as well as stability of the spinal segment concerned. We also eliminated the causes of rotation of the S_1–S_2 vertebrae. From our point of view, the main cause of the pain was the rotation of the 1st sacral vertebra relative to the 2nd and not the deformative changes in the area of L_5–S_1. The rotation led to traumatization of the nerves.

9. Patient C., a 15-year-old girl, complained of headaches, signs of vegetovascular dystonia (tachycardia, aggression), irregular and painful periods, pain in the lower extremities and cramps in the calf muscles at night.

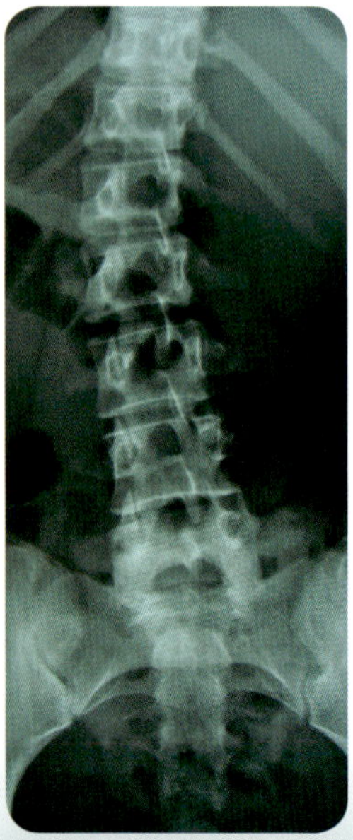

Fig. 5.3.89.

Radiographs (Fig. 5.3.89) revealed a scoliotic deformity of the spine and physiological lumbarization of S_1.

On examination of the patient, a lateral deformity of the spine (grade 2), predominantly in the lumbar region, was observed. This was associated with a right-sided costal hump. There was also evidence of hypotrophy of the muscles in the left gluteal region (Fig. 5.3.90). The trunk was tilted to the left. We planned to compensate for this with an orthopaedic insole of a height of **37 mm** under the left heel.

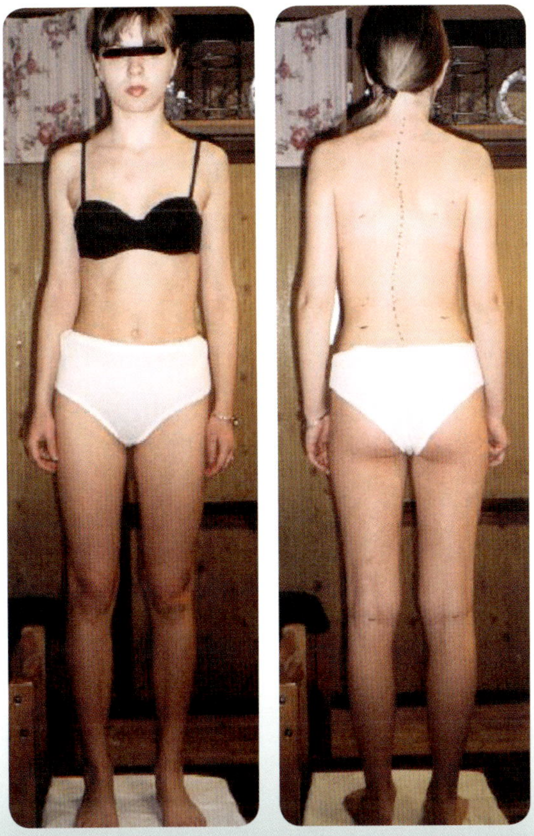

Fig. 5.3.90.

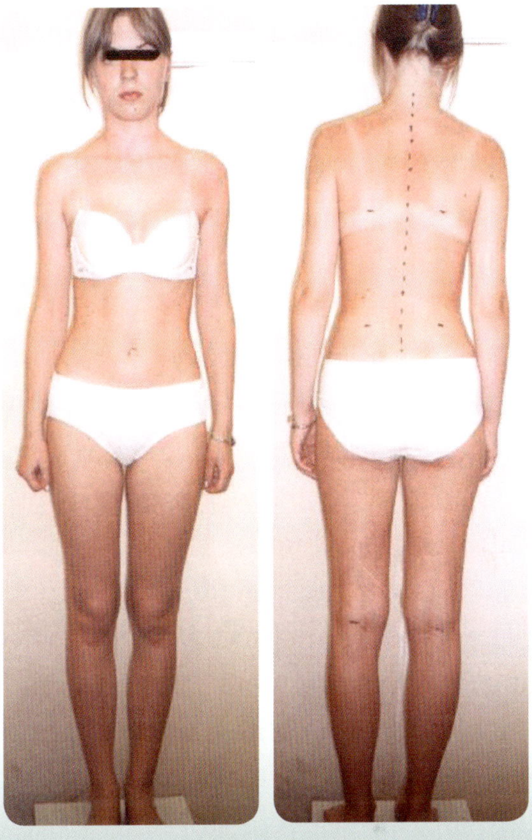

Fig. 5.3.91.

The standard treatment was prescribed. It included usage of an orthopaedic insole, detorsional exercises and magneto-acoustic therapy along the paravertebral region.

Initially, we prescribed an orthopaedic insole of a height of 15 mm. The height was increased every third week until it reached **37 mm**. At one year's follow-up, the difference in the length of the legs had decreased to **10 mm**. C. had no complaints. Her periods had become regular and painless. At 2 years' follow-up, the legs were of equal length, the patient's trunk had become symmetrical and the axis of the spine was correct (Fig. 5.3.91). She considered herself healthy. Radiographs of the lumbar spine revealed a reduction in the lateral deformity, although lumbarizaton of S_1 persisted (Fig. 5.3.92).

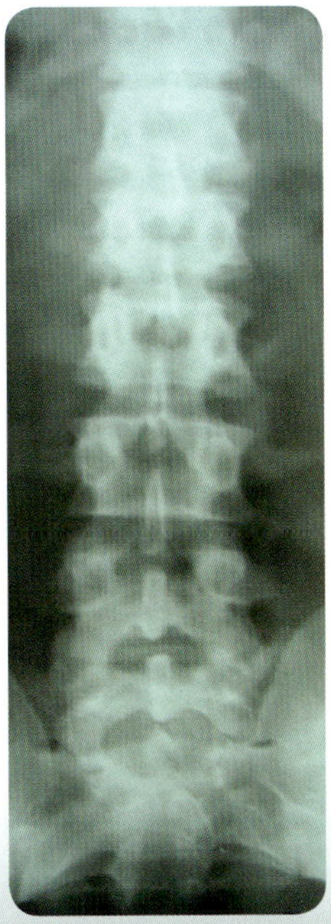

Fig. 5.3.92.

It might be interest for the reader that the patient's mother was treated simultaneously for scoliosis associated with relative shortening of the left leg by a similar 37 mm. The duration of correction of the lateral deformity and the speed of reduction of the relative shortening of the left leg was similar for mother and daughter in spite of the difference in their age.

10. Patient K., a 10-year-old boy, complained of pain in the umbilical region and the lower abdomen. He was examined by a paediatric surgeon, who suspected acute appendicitis and umbilical hernia, but no pathological changes were found.

When we examined him, we found that he had right-sided scoliosis and left-sided torticollis. He complained of pain in the lower extremities. He said he could not stand for long, and found it difficult to walk and run. He also had frequent headaches and said his vision was growing weaker.

Radiographs revealed physiological lumbarization of S_1–S_2 (Fig. 5.3.93).

On examining the patient, we found that he had convergent strabismus and left-sided tortocollis. His trunk was tilted to the left and there was a right-sided scoliotic deformation in the thoracic region (Fig. 5.3.94). We planned to compensate for the tilt of the body with an orthopaedic insole of a height of **10 mm**, to be placed under the left heel. Asymmetry of the spinal extensors was evident on palpation.

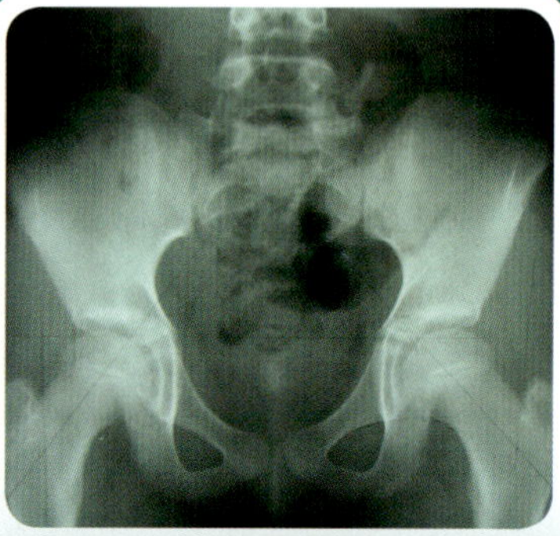

Fig. 5.3.93.

The standard treatment, i.e. magneto-acoustic therapy along the paravertebral region, detorsional exercises (which the mother was trained to perform), orthopaedic insole of a height of 10 mm, was prescribed. At 8 months' follow-up, there were no signs of lateral deformation of the spine. The length of the legs was equal and the

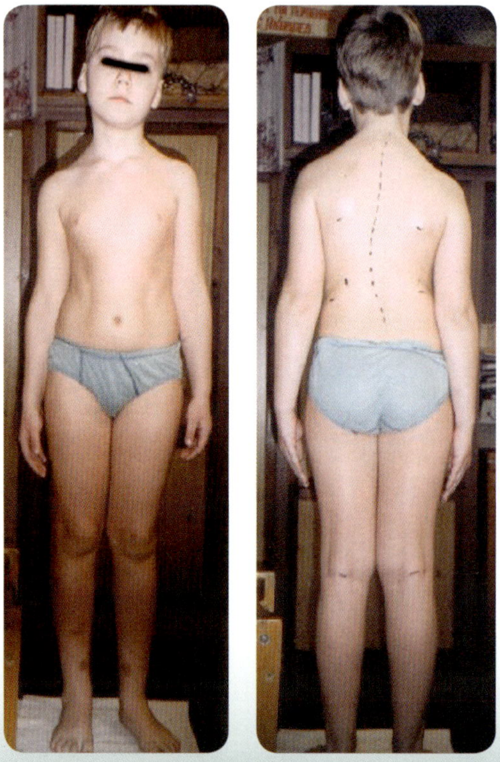

Fig. 5.3.94.

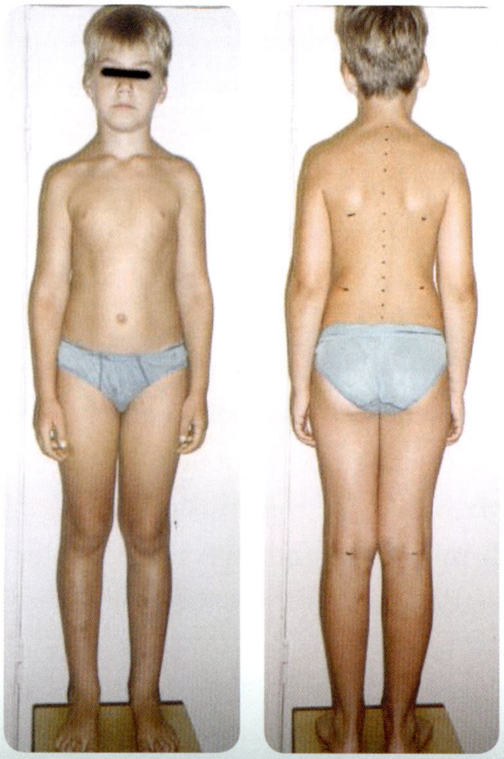

Fig. 5.3.95.

positioning of the eyeballs had normalized (Fig. 5.3.95). The pain had resolved. K.'s mother was very pleased with the results of the treatment. However, since the boy was still in his growing years, we recommended the use of an orthopaedic insole of a height of **3 mm** under the left heel when he went to school or engaged in physical activity (running, jumping). We advised him to visit a paediatric orthopaedic surgeon for annual check-ups.

11. Patient Ch., a 14-year-old girl, complained of a constant headache and said that when she suddenly turned her head, everything grew dim and she felt faint. Her other complaints were emotional lability and coldness and sweatiness of the hands. She received treatment for vegetovascular dystonia, but with no relief.

On examination of the patient, lateral deformity of the spine—right-sided in the thoracic spine and left-sided in the lumbar spine—was observed. There was distinct hypotrophy of the gluteal muscles, as well as underdevelopment of the pelvic bones (Fig. 5.3.96). The body was tilted to the left. We planned to compensate for this with an orthopaedic insole of a height of **38 mm** under the left heel. Clinical signs of bilateral plexitis, as well as neuritis of the femoral and obturator nerves were, present.

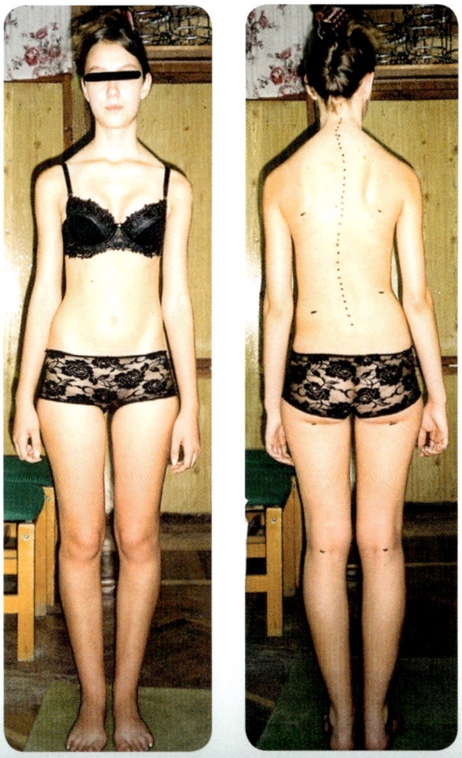

Fig. 5.3.96.

The standard treatment, i.e. orthopaedic insole, magneto-acoustic therapy along the paravertebral region, detorsional exercises, was prescribed. We initially recommended an insole of a height of **10 mm**. We increased the height by another **10 mm** a month later. The height was gradually increased further and within 3 months, it was brought up to **38 mm**.

On 8 months' follow-up, we found that the difference in the length of the legs had decreased to **20 mm**. The axis of the spine was in the process of being corrected. The volume of the gluteal muscles was in the process of being restored. There was no pain in the spine. The magneto-acoustic therapy was stopped. At 1.5 years' follow-up, the left leg was **15 mm** shorter than the right. At 3 months' follow-up, the difference in the length of the legs was **7 mm**.

When Ch. was examined 2 years after the initiation of treatment, she had no complaints. The length of the legs was equal, the posture was correct. Asymmetry of pelvic bones had decreased significantly (Fig. 5.3.97). Nonetheless, due to the fact that the patient was in her growing years, we advised her to use an orthopaedic insole of a height of 7 mm under the left heel and to be regular with the detorsional exercises.

12. Patient P., a 6-year-old boy, was brought to us by his grandmother from a suburban region of Odessa due to a progressive deformity of his spine.

He complained of a constant headache, as well as pain in his arms, legs, the interscapular region and along the vertebral column.

Examination showed that the child had an S-shaped lateral deformity of the spine (grade 2)—right-sided in the thoracic spine and left-sided in the lumbar spine. Asymmetry of the spinal extensors was also observed. He had a pelvic tilt to the left side, which we planned to compensate for with an orthopaedic insole of a height of **3.5 mm.** Clinical signs of bilateral plexitis and lumboischialgia were present. Rotation of the head to either side was distinctly limited. Also, the right scapula protruded posteriorly (Fig. 5.3.98).

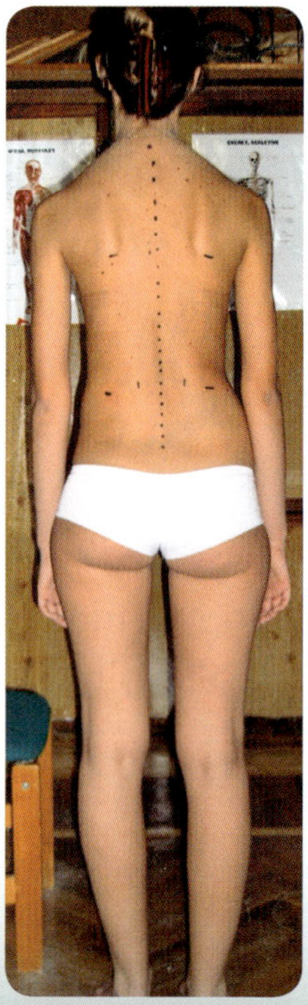

Fig. 5.3.97.

The standard treatment was prescribed. P.'s grandmother was taught to perform magneto-acoustic therapy, using her own apparatus, and to help the boy perform detorsional exercises. We advised the patient to use an orthopaedic insole of a height of **3.5 mm** under the left heel, regardless of the footwear he wore.

Control examination 2 months after the initiation of treatment showed that there was no shortening of the legs and the axis of the spine was correct. The posterior protrusion of the right scapula had become less pronounced (Fig. 5.3.99). P. had no complaints. The magneto-acoustic therapy was stopped. However, since the boy was still growing, we advised him to continue with the prescribed treatment (orthopaedic insole and detorsional exercises) for another 4 months. At 1 year's follow-up, the symmetry of the body, including that of the trunk muscles, had

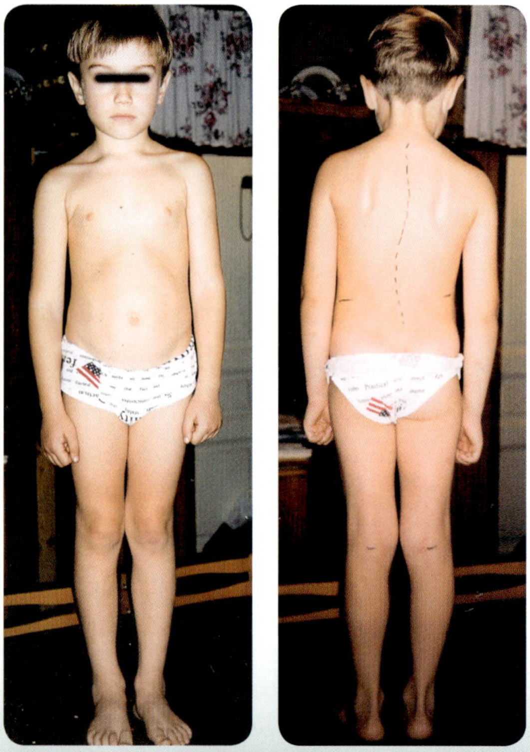

Fig. 5.3.98.

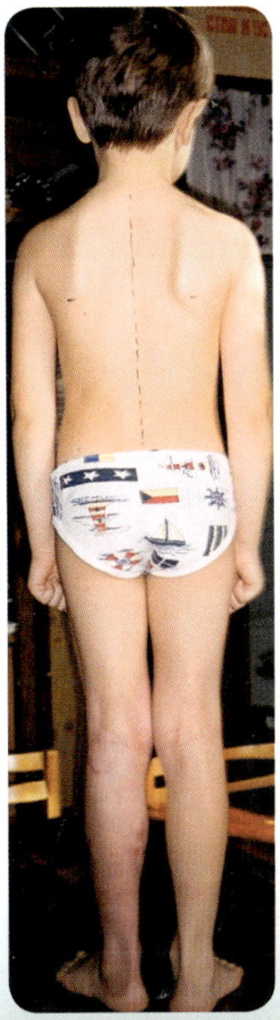

Fig. 5.3.99.

been restored (Fig. 5.3.100). The patient had no complaints and his relatives were very satisfied with the results of the treatment.

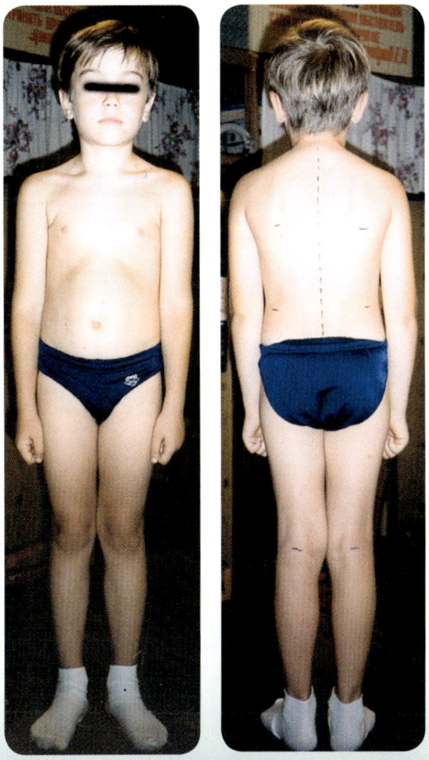

Fig. 5.3.100.

13. Patient C., a 2-year-old girl, was brought to us by her mother because she had a constant headache, as well as pain in the arms and legs. The child could not run and mostly remained seated. The paediatric ophthalmologist diagnosed her with congenital myopia and esotropia. Ultrasound dopplerography of the cervical and cerebral vessels revealed a deficit in blood flow (of up to 40%) in the vertebral arteries of both sides at the level of C_3 and C_4.

During examination of the patient, distinct signs of deformity of the thorax were evident. She had a scoliotic posture and we also noticed protrusion of the right scapula, which heralds the formation of a right-sided costal hump. C. had relative shortening of the left leg, which we planned to compensate for with an orthopaedic insole of a height of **3.5 mm**. Signs of hypotrophy of the muscles of the left gluteal region were present. The child was also diagnosed with planovalgus deformity of the feet (Fig. 5.3.101).

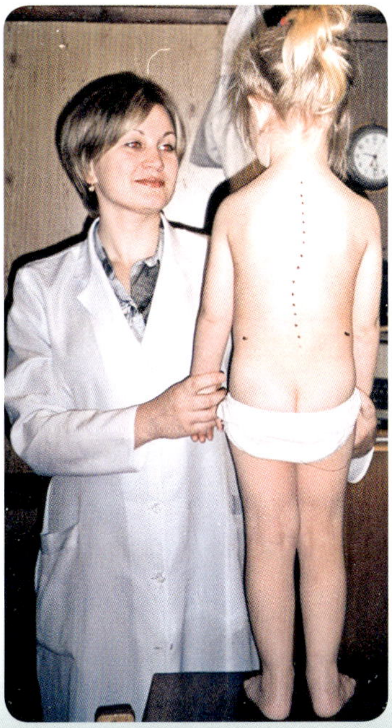

Fig. 5.3.101.

The standard treatment was prescribed. Her mother was trained to perform magneto-acoustic therapy using a portable apparatus, and to help the child perform detorsional exercises. We advised her to continue with the magneto-acoustic therapy for the next 2 months and to ensure that the insole was used in all kinds of footwear over the following year.

At 1 year's follow-up after initiation of treatment, we found a positive effect. C.'s vision had improved.

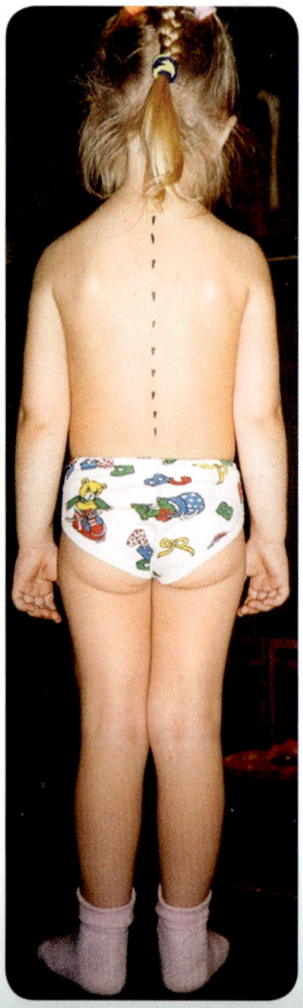

Fig. 5.3.102.

She no longer experienced pain on palpation of the spine and the axis of the spine was correct. She had no complaints. The planovalgus deformity of the feet was now insignificant (Fig. 5.3.102). However, since C. would continue to grow for a number of years, we advised her mother to ensure that the orthopaedic insole was used in the shoes that the girl wore outdoors.

Control examination was done 10 years after the initiation of treatment. We invited the patient to come for evaluation of the long-term results of treatment. She considered herself healthy. Her vision had normalized, there was no strabismus, and the headaches had resolved as well. She led a normal and active life, like any other teenager. Her body had become symmetrical, there was no lateral deformity of the body, and the volume of the spinal extensors was now equal on both sides (Fig. 5.3.103). The girl and her parents were satisfied with the results of the treatment.

An analysis of this case allows us to conclude that long-term restoration of the correct posture can be achieved by promoting the 'physiologically correct' conditioned reflex of the vertical position of the body when the patient is still a child, through the use of our therapeutic scheme. We did not observe any recurrence of the lateral deformity. This was confirmed by long-term follow-up examinations of other patients of the age of 8–10 years. We concluded that improving children's health should be performed at the earliest possible age to eliminate the initial signs of scoliosis. This could prevent different diseases not only in teenagers but adults as well, protecting them against diseases later in life.

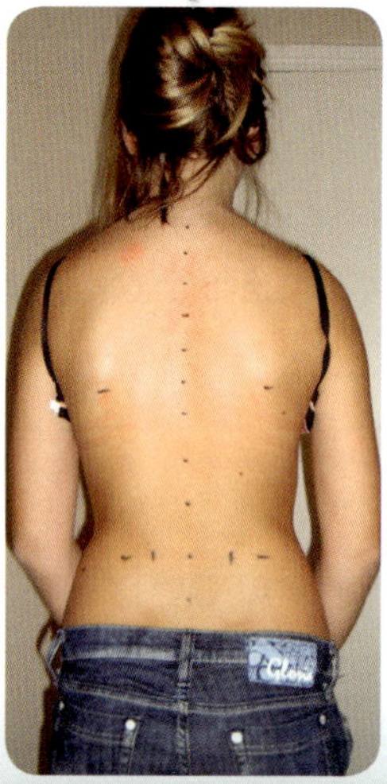

Fig. 5.3.103.

We have now finished presenting some of our clinical cases pertaining mostly to pain in the lumbosacral region of the spine, as well as pain in this region combined with lateral deformity of the spine. In the majority of cases, the prescribed treatment proved to be effective and yielded good results, which was evident with correction of scoliotic deformity of the spine and elimination of spinal pain in its different clinical forms.

We consider it necessary to explain the results obtained by us. We grouped all cases of spinal pain in accordance with the factors that caused them and compared our data with those from other studies. *Our analysis led us to the following conclusions.*

a. In the majority of patients, lumbosacral pain was associated with different types of dysplasia. The type that stands out most is asymmetry (the form, size and location) of the intervertebral joints between L_5 and S_1 vertebrae. According to S.A. Reinberg (1964), this anomaly comprises more than 30% of all cases of hypoplasia of the skeleton. The asymmetry of the intervertebral joints is of great functional importance and can lead to the rotation of vertebrae at the level of L_5–S_1 SMS and the subsequent development of a zone of instability. The dislocation of elements of the articular joints results in compression of the spinal nerve as it is. This is how unilateral spinal pain syndrome develops.

b. According to the data of the same author, rarely, i.e. in 20% of all cases of dysplasia, one can observe clefts in the posterior part of the vertebral bodies and arches of the lumbar and sacral vertebrae (posterior clefts). This is known as 'spina bifida posterior'. More frequently, i.e. in almost 30%–50% of patients who undergo radiography, incomplete clefts of S_1 may be observed. Incomplete clefts of L_5 are rare, while in 3%–5% cases, the posterior part of the whole sacral canal remains open ('spina bifida sacralis totalis'). When the patient jumps, exerts physically, or turns sharply, his body tilts to left or right side and, as a result, the spinal meninges may protrude into these clefts and form spinal hernias (meningocele).

While examining such patients (adults and even children), we observed 'hypertrichosis' (increased pilosity of the skin) in the area of the sacrum. Previously, in Chapter 2, we have given already the explanation of its origin. Hypertrichosis develops due to irritation of the skin nerves.

Compression of the spinal meninges, and sometimes even of the elements of the cauda equina, causes a syndrome of extremely intense pain. This is clinically manifested as lumbosacral pain, often without radiation to the lower extremities. The clinical picture of chronic meningeal hernia is characterized by the persistence of symptoms and low efficacy of therapeutic measures.

c. One of the most important causes of the development of spinal pain syndrome is partial or total (true) sacralization of L_5. This anomaly of the transverse processes of the L_5 vertebra occurs among 5%–7% of all patients with spinal pain. When the distance between the transverse processes of L_5 and S_1 decreases due to their rotation, unilateral or bilateral compression of the nerves occurs and a syndrome of extremely intense pain develops. Figures 5.3.104 and 5.3.105 illustrate some of the types of dysplasias mentioned above.

d. Ten to fifteen per cent of patients with spinal pain syndrome in the lumbosacral region have hernias of the intervertebral discs. The hernias are associated with osteochondrosis and deforming spondylosis, which alter the structure of a disc and lead to the development of cracks in the disc if the patient suffers an injury or lifts heavy weights. These cracks provide a route for the nucleus pulposus to shift

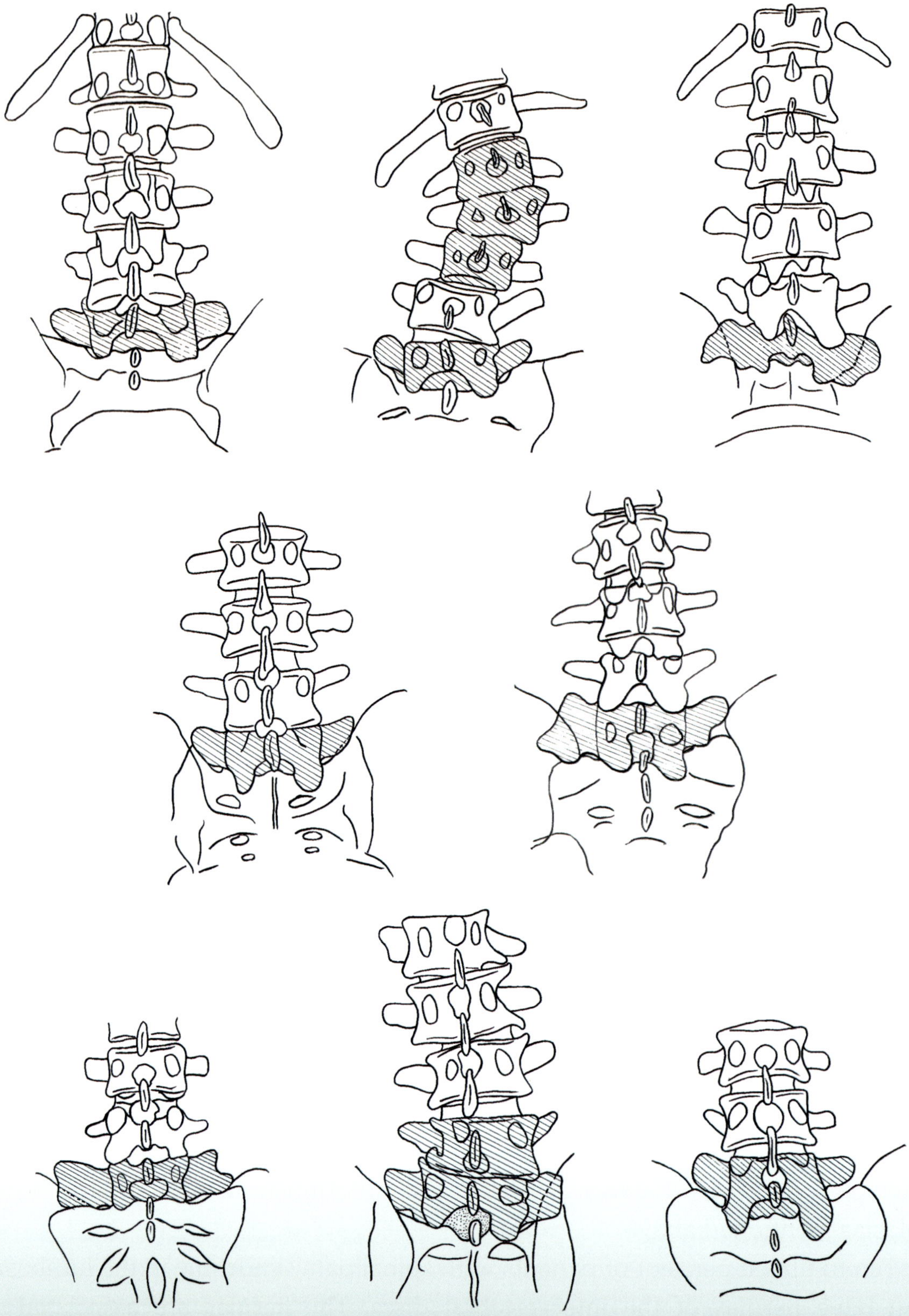

Fig. 5.3.104.
Types of sacralization of L_5 and lumbarization of S_1 and asymmetry of the intervertebral articular processes of transitional L_5–S_1 SMS

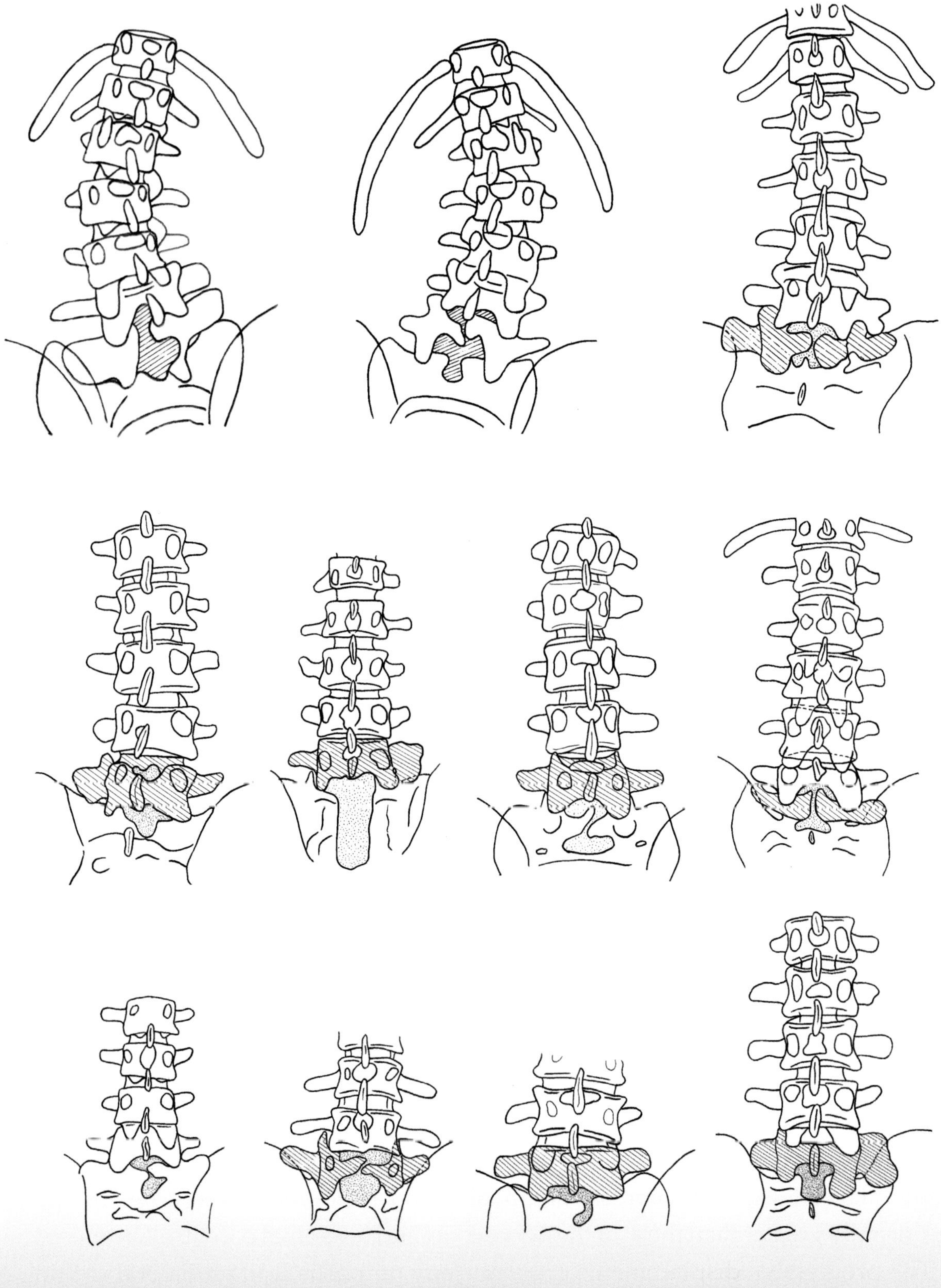

Fig. 5.3.105.
Types of sacralization of L_5 and lumbarization of S_1; anomalous tropism of articular processes of transitional L_5–S_1; SMS associated with posterior cleft of the lumbar and sacral vertebrae

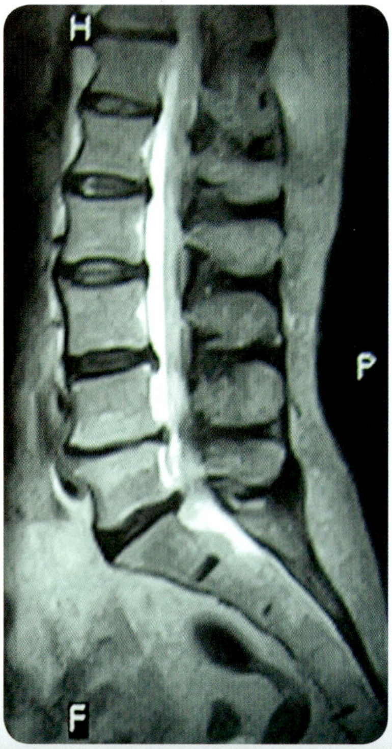

Fig. 5.3.106.
Herniated discs at the level of L_3–L_4–L_5, lumbarization of S_1

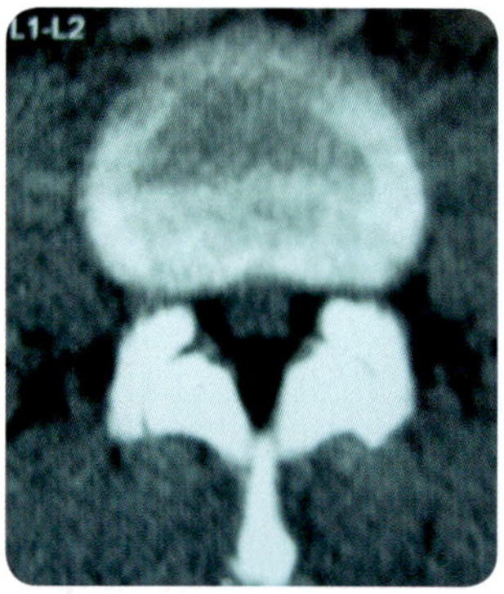

Lumbar spine; transverse section at the level of L_1–L_2; diameter of the spinal canal is larger than the diameter of the spinal cord

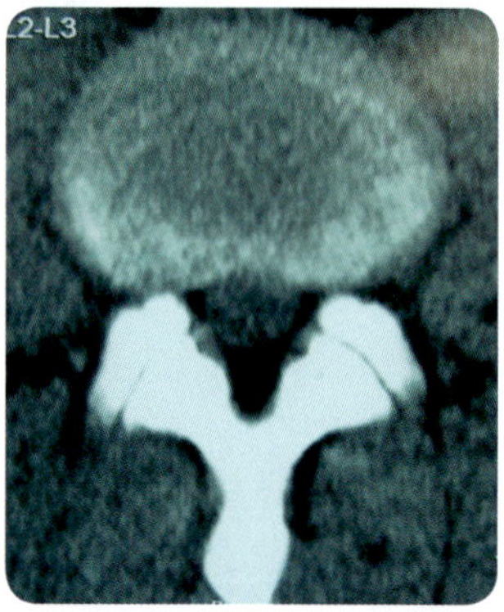

Lumbar spine; transverse section at the level of L_2–L_3; the diameter of the spinal canal is larger than the diameter of the spinal cord

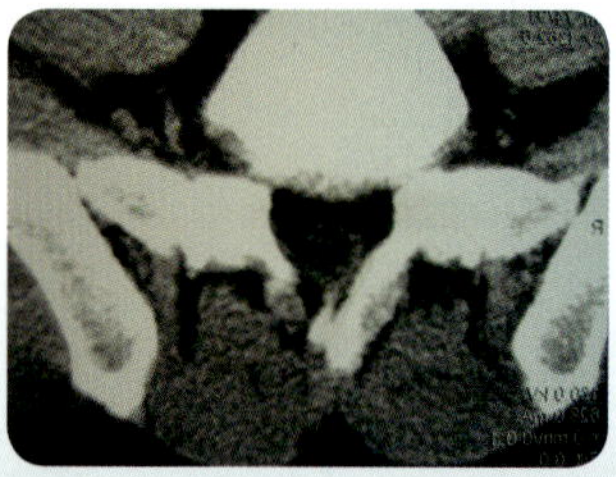

Lumbosacral spine; transverse section at the level of L_4–L_5; diameter of the spinal cord is much smaller than the diameter of the spinal canal

Fig. 5.3.107.
Ratio of diameters of the spinal cord and the spinal canal at different levels of the lumbosacral spine

towards the spinal cord and its rootlets. The conditions for such hernial protrusion are the most favourable at the level of L_5–S_1, where the thickness of the posterior longitudinal ligament is the least (about 1 mm). In these situations, patients are referred for computer scanning of the lumbar spine. CT scanning can detect one or more protrusions of the nucleus pulposus and can also determine the degree of displacement into the spinal canal (Fig. 5.3.106).

However, radiological findings do not provide enough evidence to conclude whether the disc hernia is the cause of pain. According to the findings of Professor I.A. Movshovich (1964), which were confirmed by our observations, the diameters of the intervertebral foramen (*see* Fig. 3.2.12) and the spinal canal (Fig. 5.3.107) are significantly greater than those of the nerve roots and the spinal cord itself, respectively.

The progressive displacement of the nucleus pulposus leads to lateral shifting of these structures, which gradually adapt to their new position, thus minimizing the possibility of acute injury to the spinal cord.

In our opinion, these days there is a tendency to overestimate the role of disc herniation in the development of lumbar pain. We have repeatedly observed cases in which surgery (removal of herniated discs) has had only a short-term beneficial effect. In the majority of cases, the clinical course of hernias is asymptomatic and they are detected incidentally.

But if true disc herniation is behind of only 10%–15% of cases of back pain, what is the aetiology in the remaining 85%–90% of cases?

e. The more patients we examined, the more we came across cases in which low back pain developed even in the absence of hernias and dysplasias. This held good for children, adolescents, well-built young people and even professional athletes, including world champions. We eventually came to the conclusion that the leading cause of pain was traumatization of the lumbosacral plexus, with non-consolidated and thus mobile sacral vertebrae.

Textbooks of radiology describe lumbarization of the sacral vertebrae, in which the S_1–S_2 vertebrae, and rarely S_3, are unfused. However, these books do not contain any information on the role of this type of dysplasia in the development of pain syndrome. Comparing the clinical signs of pain in our patients with the data obtained from their radiographs, we found that lumbarization of S_1 was present in 100% of cases with back pain syndrome (Fig. 5.3.108). This sign of dysplasia, the opposite of sacralization, was sometimes combined with other signs of dysplasia or occurred independently.

We have divided all cases of lumbarization into two types.

The first type: is typical for young adults. The fusion of the sacral vertebrae usually begins from the lower vertebrae upwards at the age of 13–14 years. The fusion of the upper vertebrae ends by the age of 23–25 years. This type of lumbarization is 'physiological'.

The second type: in which the 1st, 2nd and even 3rd sacral vertebrae are separated from each other throughout the person's life. Functionally, these additional 6th, 7th and 8th lumbar vertebrae even have discs between them (Fig. 5.3.109). Similar data have been presented by S.A. Reinberg (1964).

In our clinical experience, lumbarization of S_1, which was found in all individuals who had spinal pain and were 25 years of age or older, was associated with factors such as lifting heavy loads, intensive training and repeated injuries, which may have dated back to the youth of older patients. We term this type of lumbarization 'compensatory-adaptive', since it is essentially a mechanism to adapt to significant loads. It should be considered 'pathological' due to the fact that 'one or a few of the transitional vertebrae create a zone of instability in the lumbosacral spine'. This is the weak spot (locus minoris resistentiae) of the spine where, under certain anatomical conditions, the sacral vertebrae turn around their axes during rotation or bending of the body. This leads to rotation of the vertebrae lying above, which results in the development

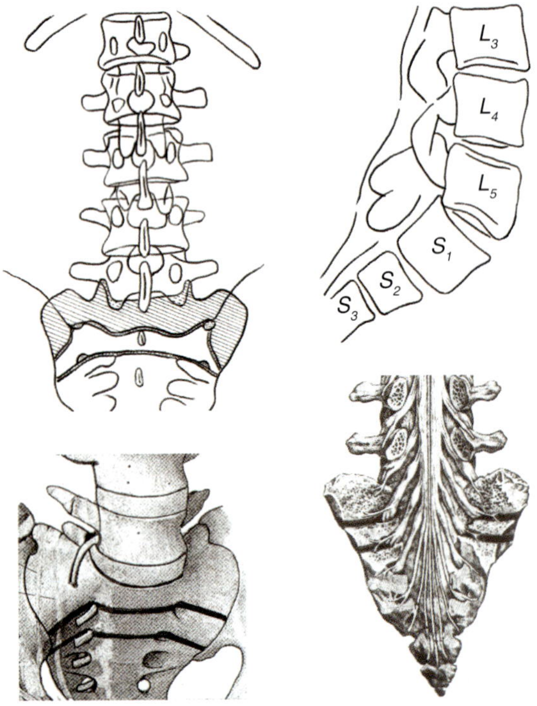

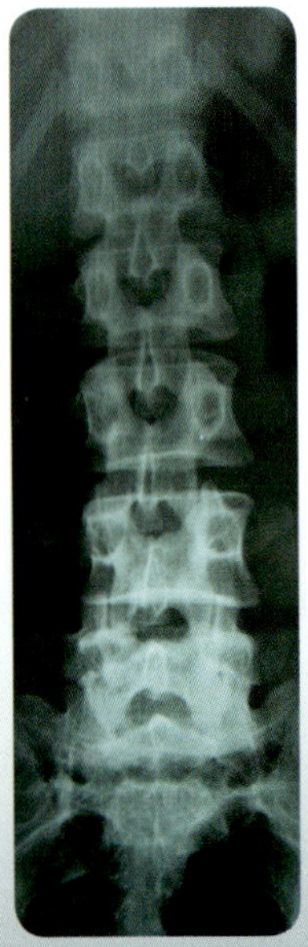

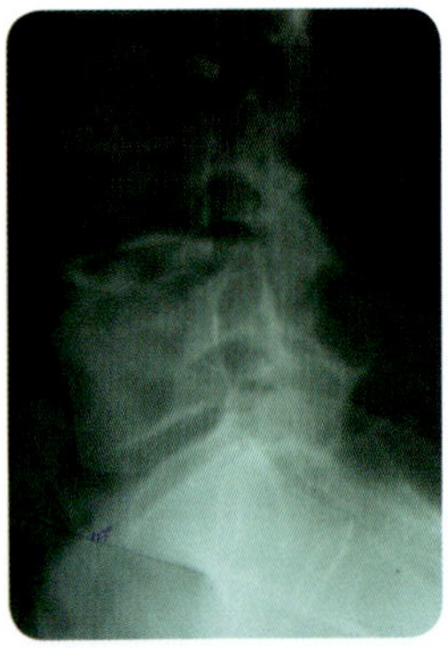

Fig. 5.3.108.
Dysplastic changes in the sacral vertebrae—lumbarization of S_1–S_2

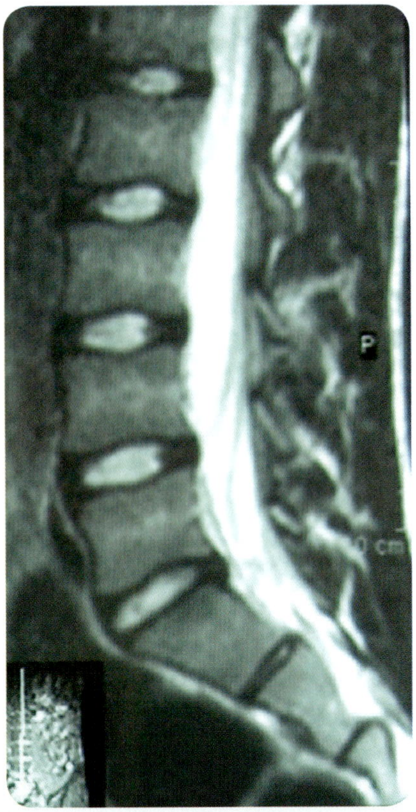

Fig. 5.3.109.
Computed tomography of lumbosacral spine; multiple hernial protrusions (L_2–L_5); lumbarization of S_1–S_2, intervertebral disc is seen between them

of a lateral curvature of the spine. The rotation of the sacral vertebrae traumatizes the nerves of the sacral plexus, giving rise to syndrome of pain of high intensity.

We observed that the rotation of L_5 relative to S_1 and of S_1 relative to S_2 was initiated by a unilateral increase in tonus of the spinal extensors, which led to tilting of the pelvis to the side where the weaker muscles were located, and consequently, to development of relative shortening of the leg on this side.

In the course of our experience, we observed that this chain of events occurred regularly in thousands of our patients with spinal pain.

Thus, when relative shortening of the leg occurred on the left side and the pelvis was tilted to the left, the injury to the sacral nerves, and the pain in the sacrum, hip and lumbosacral joints, calf and often foot, were also localized predominantly on the left side. When relative shortening of the leg occurred on the right, these symptoms occurred on the right side.

We have seen clear evidence that in the majority of cases, there is a complete regression of pain, or a substantial decrease in its intensity, following atraumatic (conducted by the patient) reduction of the displaced sacral vertebrae even in presence of other types of dysplasia. This confirms the important role of the reciprocal displacement of the 5th lumbar and 1st sacral vertebrae in the development of spinal pain.

Signs of lumbarization can be determined by regular radiographs and by CT scanning (Fig. 5.3.110). Unfortunately, when evaluating the CT scans, radiologists did not indicate the presence of diastasis between S_1 and S_2, even in cases in which the diastasis was of a high degree, and the intervertebral disc between these vertebrae was clearly visible (Fig. 5.3.109). Instead, they described the herniated discs in detail. Signs of deforming changes at the level of L_5–S_1–S_2 and deforming changes of the sacroiliac joints were usually not described properly. We believe that the radiographic signs indicated long-standing, repeated rotation of the vertebrae in this region which had occurred due to instability of the L_5–S_1 SMS (Figs 5.3.111–5.3.113).

As mentioned earlier, our search of the available national and foreign literature did not yield a single study that analysed cases of spinal pain due to lumbarization of S_1–S_2. It seems that this issue did not draw the attention either of radiologists or clinicians. Our explanation of this situation is that radiologists, vertebrologists, neurologists, other practitioners and patients as well firmly believe that lumbar pain

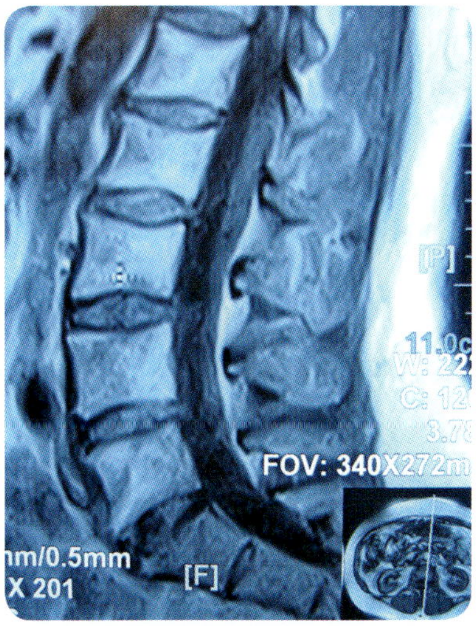

Fig. 5.3.110.
Herniated disc (L_3–L_4), blockade of L_5–S_1 segment; lumbarization of S_1–S_2 with intervertebral disc between these vertebrae

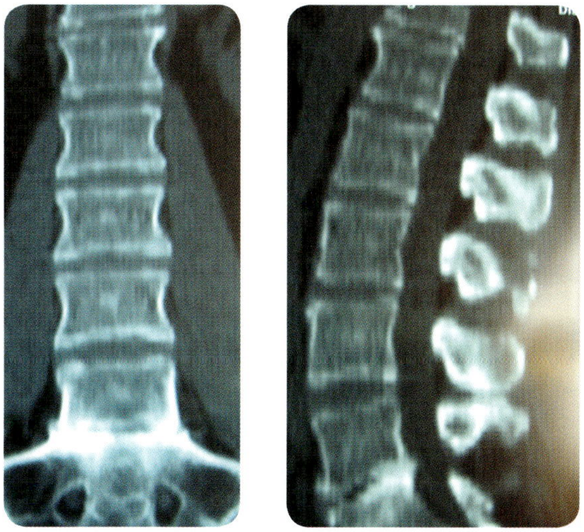

Fig. 5.3.111.
Spondylosis deformans of L_5–S_1 segment, deforming changes in the sacro-vertebral joints; compensatory lumbarization of S_1

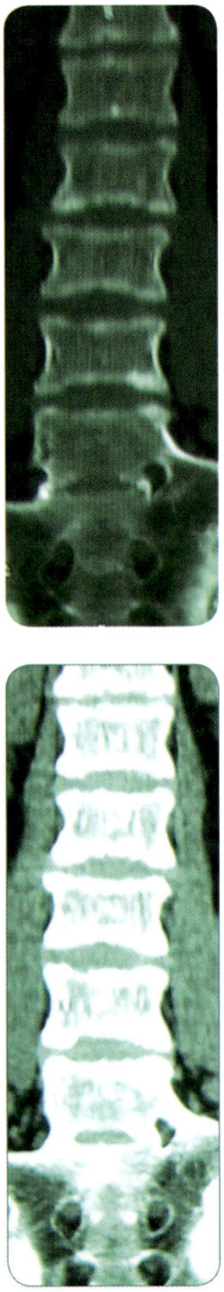

Fig. 5.3.112.
Left-sided sacralization of L_5; compensatory lumbarization of S_1–S_2; deforming changes in the right and left sacroiliac joints

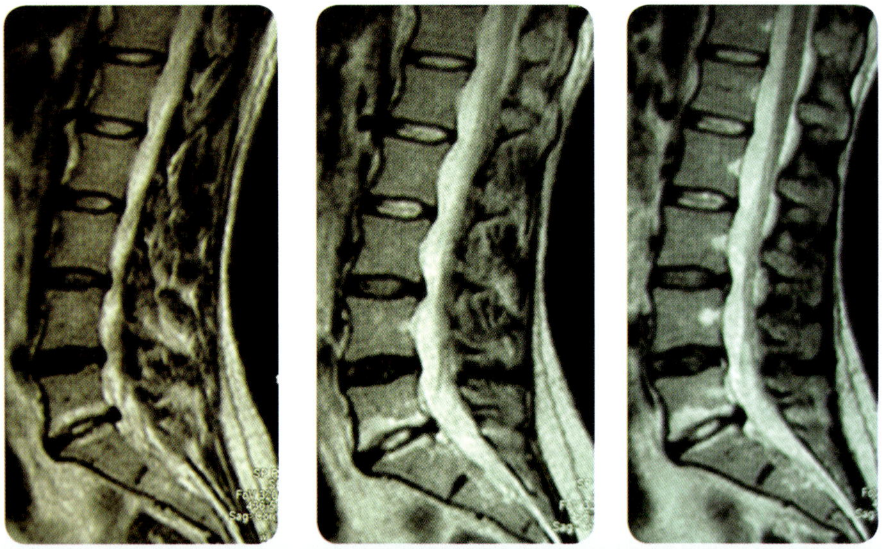

Fig. 5.3.113.
Herniated L_5–S_1 disc associated with blockade of the segment of post-traumatic origin and asymptomatic for 25 years; osteochondrosis; protrusion of L_3–L_4 disc

can be associated only with hernias of the disc. Moreover, they think these are clearly visible on CT scans. The complexity of the role of the radiologist lies in the fact that usually he is not involved in the clinical examination of the patient and does not know his complaints. Therefore, the radiologist is not in a position to correlate radiological findings with the patient's complaints.

Among adults, lumbar pain may also be caused by spondylolisthesis ('S'), which is an anterior dislocation or slippage of L_5 relative to S_1 (Fig. 5.3.114). When true sacralization of the transitional vertebrae occur, i.e. when the sacrum consists of six vertebrae, the development of 'S' of L_4 is possible. We have found that the most common causes of 'S' of L_4–L_5 were traumas and heavy physical exertion which resulted in spondylolysis, i.e. formation of a defect in the vertebral arches. Spondylolysis usually leads to the development of 'S' (Fig. 5.3.115).

Very often, spondylolisthesis is not accompanied by pain and, therefore, radiological evaluation is of crucial importance. Physicians are very apprehensive about handling such patients as they fear that their manoeuvres on the patient's spine might cause displacement of the vertebrae and trauma to the spinal cord. We did not come across cases among our patients in whom the pain was in the area of spondylolisthesis. Usually, the site of pain was below the level of dislocation.

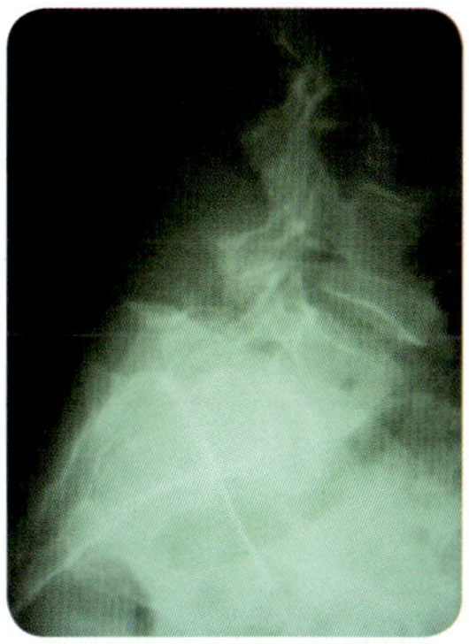

Spondylolysis of L_5, spondylolisthesis of L_5; blockade of L_5–S_1 segment; compensatory lumbarization of S_1

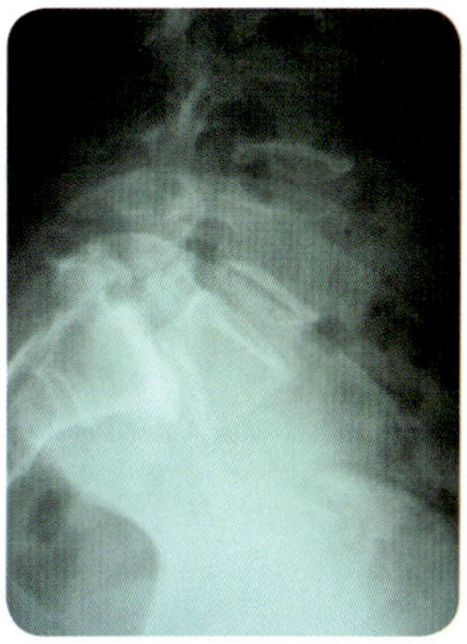

Spondylolysis of L_5, spondylolisthesis of L_5; spondylosis deformans of L_5–S_1 segment with its blockade; compensatory lumbarization of S_1

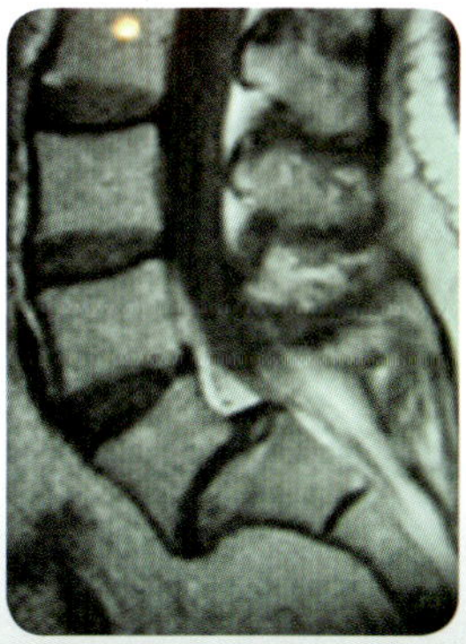

Spondylolysis of L_5, spondylolisthesis of L_5; blockade of L_5–S_1 segment; compensatory lumbarization of S_1

Fig. 5.3.114.
Types of spondylolisthesis of L_5

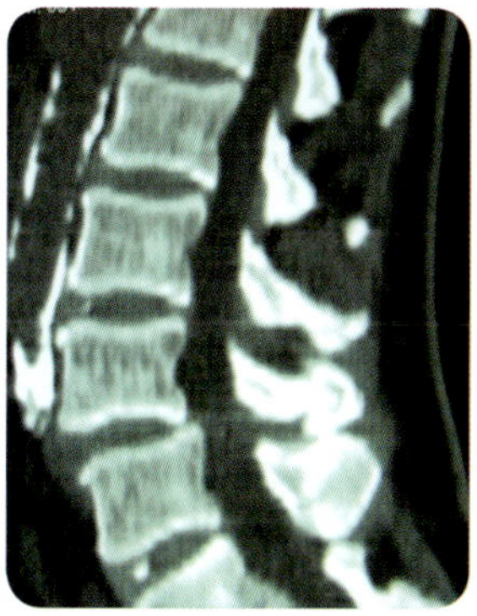

Spondylolisthesis of L_4; blockade of L_4–L_5–S_1 segments; compensatory lumbarization of S_1

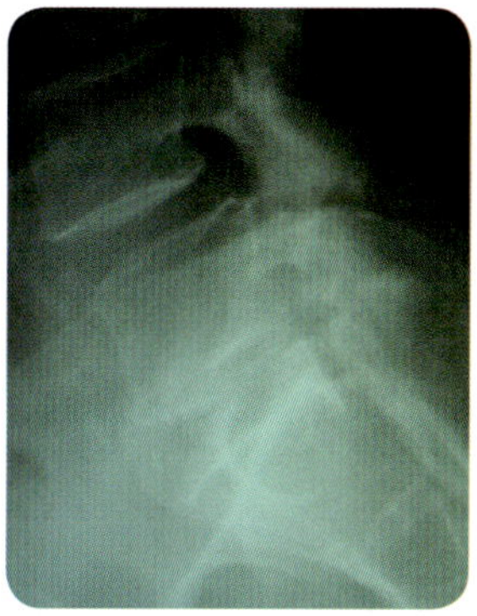

Spondylolisthesis of L_4; blockade of L_5–S_1 segment; compensatory lumbarization of S_1

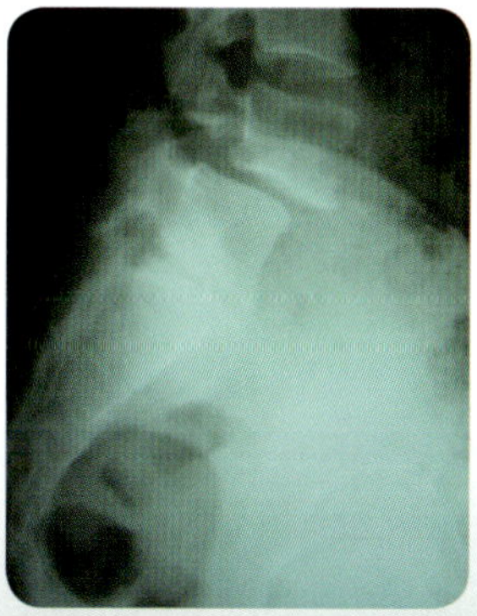

Spondylolysis of L_4 led to spondylolisthesis of this vertebra; lumbarization of S_1 of compensatory–adaptive origin

Fig. 5.3.115.
Variants of L_4 spondylolisthesis

Professor M.I. Sitenko discusses this subject in his report, 'Low back pain from orthopaedic perspective' (4th Ukrainian Congress of Surgeons, 1936). The vertebrae in the area of 'S' are blocked by bony and cartilaginous outgrowths. This causes hypermobility of S_1-S_2 which, in turn, results in lumbarization of the compensatory-adaptive type. Such hypermobility can result in an increased range of motion in the area of S_1-S_2 if physiological lumbarization happens to be present already. In both cases, the lumbosacral plexus is traumatized.

f. Pain in the lumbar region can be caused by other, more rare causes, such as benign or malignant tumours, specific and non-specific inflammatory processes, fractures, spinal stenosis, degenerative disc disease in a background of deforming spondylosis and deforming arthrosis of the costo-vertebral joints. *It is important to remember that back pain could be of non-vertebrogenic origin.* Of particular importance are reflected pain, psychogenic pain and myofascial pain syndrome (MFPS), also known as fibromyalgia or chronic fatigue syndrome. A patient with the latter suffers, among other things, from widespread musculoskeletal pain, which lasts for more than 1–3 months and affects the neck, shoulders, back and lower extremities. Myofascial pain syndrome might affect the patient's sleep and cause a constant headache, depression, dysmenorrhoea, female urethral syndrome, etc.

Though the aetiopathogenesis of lumbosacral spinal pain syndrome seems to be infinitely complex, the doctor has to understand the nature of the syndrome by making a thorough study of the patient's medical history (anamnesis vitae et morbi), as well as examining the patient, his plain radiographs (at least of two projections) and CT scans, which are of great informative value as well.

g. Let us take the example of a patient who played football till a few days ago and suddenly starts suffering from an extremely intense spinal pain. It is with great fear that he reads the conclusion of the radiologist, who has diagnosed him with disc hernia. However, we know now that disc hernia is not necessarily the cause of the pain and it is not true that only surgery can relieve it. Well-educated neurosurgeons, vertebrologists and neurologists must find the real cause of pain. In cases of true, irreducible disc hernia, the problem should be solved radically. However (excuse us for repeating ourselves), such a situation occurs only in 10%–15% of all cases. The others could, and probably should, be treated non-surgically.

We fully agree with the conclusions that S.A. Reinberg (1964) has made while studying the causes of spinal (lumbar) pain syndrome and its association with different types of dysplasia of the spine. In his opinion, it is not the anomaly of the vertebrae that play the major role in causing spinal pain, but the complications arising from these anomalies, caused by some unknown factor. Our years of experience with patients enabled us to understand that this reason was the rotation of vertebrae (around their axes) at all levels, first and foremost of S_1 which, in turn, was caused by asymmetry of the trunk muscles.

Thus, in our view, traumatization of the nerves of the sacral plexus, caused by the displacement of S_1–S_2 in the area of their physiological or pathological non-fusion, is the main cause of lumbosacral pain.

h. The original purpose of our outpatient and clinical work was to help people suffering from pain in the cervical, thoracic and lumbosacral regions of the spine. It appeared that such pain was always associated with the presence of a lateral deformity of the spine, of varying degrees. As our clinical experience grew, we came to understand the role of asymmetry both of the body and spinal extensors in the development of these deformities. When dysplastic changes in the lumbosacral spine were present (lumbarization of S_1–S_2 is the most important) the above-mentioned asymmetry caused a misbalance in the lumbosacral region as well as the rotation of vertebrae at the level of L_5–S_1 and progressive development of scoliosis.

The presence of lumbarization of S_1–S_2 was so important that only this particular sign and even minimal (3 mm) relative shortening of one leg (more often the left one) was enough to give rise to the development of a lateral deformity. The manifestation of the deformity, which was always associated with spinal pain, depended on the extent of shortening of the leg. In turn, reducing the difference between the length of the legs led to correction of the spinal axis and the consequent amelioration of spinal pain.

Thus, the basic cause of scoliosis is asymmetry of the trunk and, in particular, of the spinal extensors, as mentioned several times earlier. Orthopaedic insoles play a very important role in the reduction of lateral deformities of the spine. They not only restore the balance of the lumbosacral spine, but also promote the development of the 'physiologically correct' reflex of the vertical body position. Systematic detorsional exercises strengthen this reflex. Our evaluation of the long-term results of the treatment of patients with scoliosis supports this conclusion. We found that the deformity did not recur even 11–13 years after the completion of treatment.

Our data also confirmed the conclusions of Professor A.B. Sitel, the main chiropractor of the Ministry of Health of the Russian Federation, the head of the Russian Centre for Chiropractics. According to the newspaper *Paradigm* (Moscow, 2001, 'Physical activities cause irreparable harm to one's health'), excessive physical activity at school damages a child's health. We found that it was true that the more a teenager trained physically, the more expressed was his spinal deformity. Our explanation for this is that when the shortening of a leg is not compensated for, unilateral spasm of the spinal extensors increases during physical activity. Thus, every child, teenager and even an adult should use an orthopaedic insole before beginning training and should train under the guidance of a sports physician or orthopaedic surgeon. These issues are discussed in the next chapter.

We now conclude Chapter 5, in which the association between various human diseases and spinal deformities has been discussed. The chapter is based on the results of our clinical experience with more than 8000 patients who were of different ages and suffering from pain in all regions of the spine, combined with dysfunction of various organs and tissues. Patients with a scoliotic deformity of the spine have also been included. On the basis of our daily practice, we were able to conclude that there is a definite relationship between the pathogenesis of many human diseases and pathological changes in various regions of the spine. Our theoretical proposition that 'diseases in adulthood are associated with spinal deformities in childhood' was recognized as a scientific discovery and awarded a diploma by the Ukrainian Academy of Original Ideas in 1995. Our study of the mechanisms of lateral deformity of the spine allowed us to establish that 'scoliotic deformity is to be expected when there are zones of instability in all regions of the spine, resulting from asymmetry of the spinal extensors, which is caused, in turn, by functional asymmetry of the brain's hemispheres'. This finding was also recognized as a scientific discovery and awarded a diploma by the Ukrainian Academy of Original Ideas in 2008.

We observed that impaired functioning of any part of the central or peripheral nervous system, caused by trauma due to the displacement of vertebrae at all levels, had a negative effect on the functioning of all internal organs. Although such impairments were not directly responsible for the specific, non-specific, inflammatory and non-inflammatory diseases, or for tumours, the development of the diseases was a consequence of impairment of the complex system of innervations. This is because the latter lowered the activity of the immune system and consequently, decreased the body's resistance to infectious agents and other negative factors.

The standard treatment prescribed for all patients included, apart from the use of an orthopaedic insole and detorsional exercises, local magneto-acoustic therapy, the analgesic, anti-inflammatory and anti-oedematous effects of which helped to strengthen the immune system.

The next chapter gives a detailed description of the treatment methods used for our patients.

6 Treatment of patients with spinal deformities and spinal pain

THE PATIENTS VISITING OUR CLINIC had certain similar complaints. These ranged from headache, dizziness and loss of consciousness to numbness of the digits of the upper and lower extremities, cardialgias, episodes of apnoea, retrosternal pain, and local or radiating pain in the lumbosacral region. The severity of the symptoms depended on the patient's age and the duration of the disease. Usually, patients came to us after treatment failures, being dissatisfied with the previous results.

Regardless of age, all the patients had lateral deformity of the spine and asymmetry of the spinal muscles, and felt pain when the spinous processes of the cervical, thoracic and lumbar vertebrae were pressed. Elderly patients also complained of constant pain in the joints of the upper and lower extremities. The corresponding neurological signs—plexitis, intercostal neuralgia, lumboischialgia, neuritis of the femoral and obturator nerves—were also observed.

The primary aim of our treatment was not only to eliminate spinal pain and lateral deformity of the spine, but also to eliminate the underlying causes which induced them. As we have mentioned earlier, our main concern was to treat patients who were not suffering from neurosurgical, specific or oncological conditions. The majority of our patients with scoliosis were children or young people who were suffering from idiopathic scoliosis of the 1st–3rd degree, and who came to us with complaints such as dysopia, vegetovascular dystonia, nocturnal urinary incontinence, persistent headaches, bronchial asthma, endocrinological disorders, pain in the lower extremities and chronic fatigue.

Before presenting our data, we would like to share the information that we obtained from the literature on this subject. Thousands of studies on spinal pain had established the important role played by the intervertebral disc (nucleus pulposus) and its herniation; intervertebral joints and the consequences of compression of their capsules and meniscoids; stenosis of the spinal canal and intervertebral foramina, as well as osteochondrosis and spondylosis deformans. The role of instability and the functional blockade of spinal motion segments at different levels was also recognized.

Surgical and non-surgical (conservative) methods were used to relieve the spinal pain caused by osteochondrosis and other factors mentioned above.

In recent decades, surgical intervention seems less necessary for the treatment of diseases of the spine. Thus, according to the data provided by Nordemar (Sweden, 1991), out of thousands of people with serious diseases of the spine, no more than 1% were treated surgically. B.M. Rachkov (1995) held that only 2%–5% of cases of spinal diseases should be treated surgically. In contrast with the 1960s–1980s when intervertebral disc herniations were often treated surgically, these days, more and more physicians tend to recommend 'complete rest' which allows us to achieve the same results as with surgical intervention.

Surgery could be the preferred line of treatment when it is necessary to stabilize certain segments of the spine in order to prevent prolapse of the nucleus pulposus directly towards the spinal canal or to remove a fragment of an already prolapsed nucleus.

As far as the conservative treatment of the spinal pain syndrome is concerned, one can recommend manual therapy (MT) or therapeutic physical training (TPT), combined with physiotherapy, reflexotherapy, blockades (injections), general and spot massage, etc. These methods have gained widespread recognition due to their low degree of invasiveness and high efficacy. Both MT and TPT consist of performing movements that have a therapeutic purpose. In TPT, these movements are performed by the patient, while in MT, they are performed by the practitioner.

Manual therapy has evolved from the 'miraculous' remedies prescribed centuries ago to medically approved effective methods of treatment practised by well-educated professionals and approved by the Ministry of Health of the USSR, Russian Federation and Ukraine. The first reference to MT can be traced to the works of Klaudius Galen and Hippocrates, but its birth as a scientific method is associated with the name of A. Still, who established the School of Osteopathy in the town of Kirksville (England) in 1874. The general course of studies lasted for 2 years. Among the physicians associated with the development of MT are K. Levit, J. Sachse and W. Janda (1993). The work of the famous MT therapist from the US, Michael Kale, which was aimed at correction of the spine in the C_1–C_2 region (stem location), came to be known worldwide.

Great contribution to the theory and practice of MT have been made by Russian and Ukrainian specialists such as G.H. Gruntovsky, V.A. Kislitsa (1982), N.A. Kasian (1985), V.Y. Fischenko (1989), I.Z. Samosyuk (1992), A.A. Buryanov (1997), I.N. Krapivka (1997), G.A. Ivanichev (1998), D.D. Cherkes-Zade (2000) and Y.Y. Popelyansky (2003).

Therapeutic physical training developed parallel to MT. It was practised for the treatment of spinal pain from ancient times in India, China, Korea, Vietnam, Japan and other countries, where exercises were developed hundreds of years ago. The various therapeutic methods were quite similar and differed from each other only in the number of exercises (from hundreds to thousands) and their duration.

In fact, all TPT methods are united by one primary goal, which is to restore physiologically correct functioning of the spine by means of aligning, reducing functional blockades, and restoring flexibility and mobility. This is clear from the statement of the 18th century French practitioner, Tissot: 'All remedies across the world will not replace the therapeutic value of motions. Treatment of spinal pain should be effective if it includes not only medications, but patient's active physical exercises, done under supervision of the doctor.'

There is another interesting fact: rites performed by people of different religions include motions of the body (flexion, extension, tilting, bobbing and so on). While watching a congregation of Christians, Muslims, Jews or others, one is tempted to believe that these motions have been incorporated into religious rites not only for a spiritual purpose but to strengthen the body as well.

Among the active supporters of TPT are: V.I. Dikul, V.A. Ivanchenko—founders of the Moscow centre for rehabilitation of spinal patients (1988), G.A. Goryanoy (1991), R. Nordemar (1991), K.V. Bobrischeva (1994), P.G. Bragg (1997), A.A. Unanov (2001), J. Sutcliffe (2002), V.V. Evminov (2002), A.I. Dyadyk (2005) and A.B. Sitel (2006).

It would be appropriate to introduce the reader to the seminal work of H. Gelb and P. Siegel (1990), who analysed their experience, spanning decades, in the treatment of patients suffering predominantly from headaches and recognized the role of the temporo-mandibular joint in the genesis of headaches. They found that misalignment of the upper and lower jaws increases the tension of the facial muscles, which can cause headache, as well as pain in the neck, shoulder and even spine. According to Gelb and Siegel, phenomena such as ringing and whistling noises in the ear, dizziness, disorientation, short-term loss of consciousness, and pulsating, dumb or continuous headaches are associated with malocclusion as well as a difference in the length of the lower extremities. Shortening of one leg leads to predominantly unilateral tension in the spinal and cervical muscles, which they felt was the cause of widespread pain syndrome. They prescribed an orthopaedic footwear to eliminate the difference in the length of the legs, restore the correct posture and help the muscles to relax. Moreover, an oral acrylic insole was recommended to fix the correct occlusion. They also proposed a scheme of detorsional TPT, which included nearly 120 exercises that were characterized by slow, rhythmic motions and were aimed at stretching and normalizing the tonus of the body's muscles. In the course of our clinical work, we have tested various schemes of TPT and would like to discuss some of these (Fig. 6.1).

The schemes developed by Pol S. Bregg and R. Nordemar (1991) and J. Sutcliffe (2002) include exercises for pregnant women, as well as postpartum exercises. They also include special exercises for correcting the posture and easing acute and chronic back pain. In the case of patients with scoliosis, the authors emphasize the need to

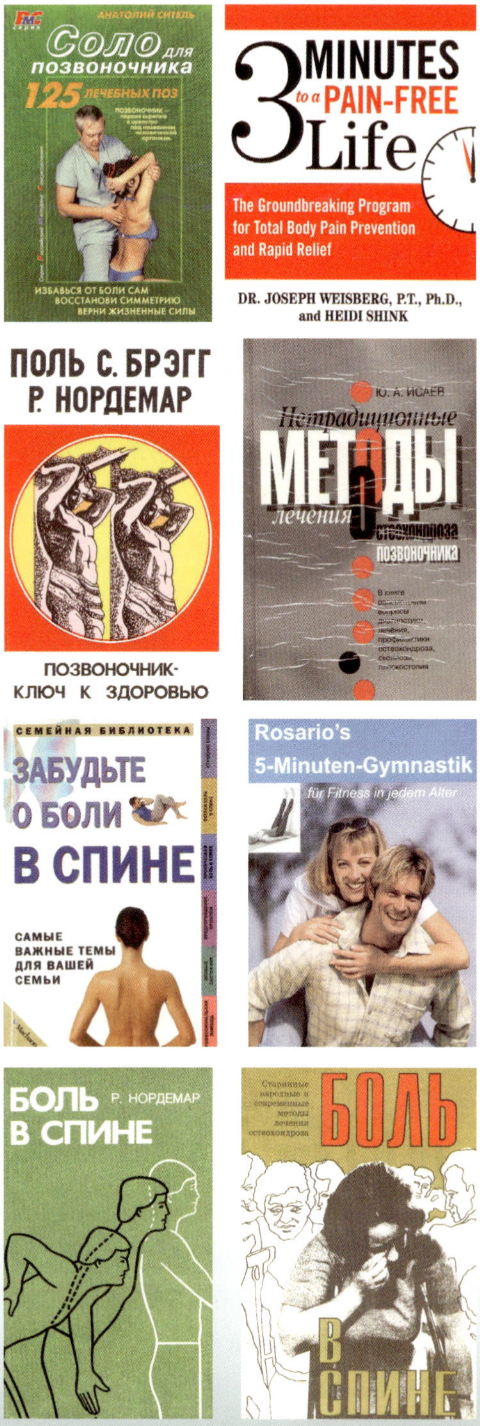

Fig. 6.1.

measure the length of the legs and prescribe the use of an orthopaedic insole to eliminate any difference between their length (Fig. 6.2).

In his book, Professor A.B. Sitel (2006) describes 125 postures aimed to correct the axis of the spine along with treatment for different types of spinal pain and headaches, cardialgias, lung diseases, etc.

Rosario Schiano's (2005) scheme is of great practical interest. It includes exercises for the trunk, and upper and lower extremities which should be performed for 5 minutes every day to reduce different forms of spinal pain syndrome. Much like Rosario Schiano, we came to the conclusion that there is no need to perform hundreds of time-consuming exercises to benefit from therapeutic movements.

These conclusions find an echo in the seminal work of the US authors J. Weisberg and H. Shink (2005). On the basis of 30 years of experience in treating patients with widespread spinal pain syndrome, they recommended a scheme consisting of six basic exercises, on each of which the patient has to spend just 30 seconds. According to the authors, the recommended duration of tension of different muscles performed in maximal static effort is therapeutically the most optimal. This method of treatment has been used in over 10,000 patients between 9 and 98 years of age and has proved to be of great therapeutic efficacy. The exercises that are performed daily include bending of the body in the lumbar, thoracic and cervical regions; touching the floor with the palms, when legs are spread wider than the shoulders; fixation of the body in an upright position with the arms extended upward while sitting on the floor with the legs crossed.

J. Weisberg and H. Shink argued that acute or chronic muscular pain is a manifestation of biomechanical dysfunction. Thus, only recommended therapeutic

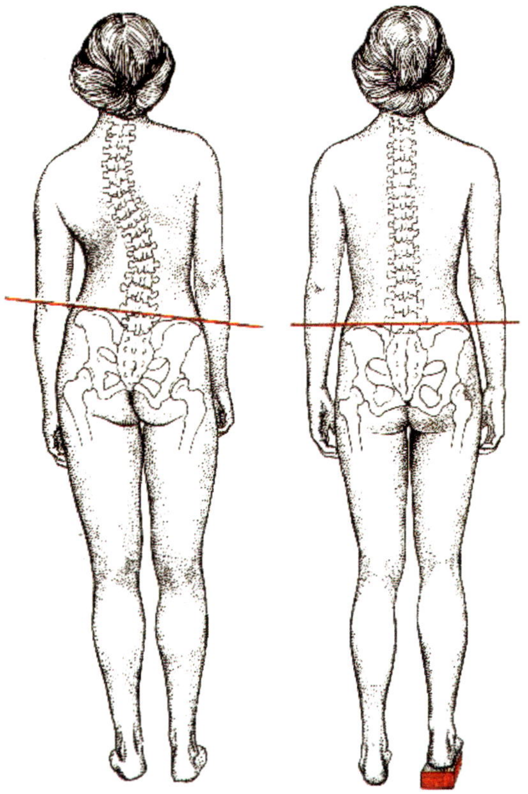

Relative shortening of the right leg; S-shaped scoliotic deformation of the spine

Shortening of the right leg is compensated for with a shoe insole; the pelvic tilt is removed; the axis of the spine is correct

Fig. 6.2.
Curvature of the spine in shortening of the right leg

movements can reduce pain. These movements aim to stretch the muscles that are in spasm, strengthen them and stabilize the correct posture. Adhering regularly to this scheme of treatment ensures that the pain does not recur.

Thus, the treatment of widespread spinal pain with MT and TPT was aimed at reducing and correcting the abnormal tension of muscles, caused by disharmony in the body.

While comparing the efficacy of various treatment methods, we found that all the authors had underestimated the role of anomalies of the lumbar and sacral vertebrae associated with relative shortening of one leg. Though they were aware of these anomalies, they had not fully appreciated the correlation between spinal pain and lumbarization of the 1st or even the 2nd sacral vertebra. In our opinion, lumbarization gives rise to the sudden rotation of S_1 relative to L_5 and S_2, which causes compression of the rootlets of the sacral plexus and thus acute pain.

There was no clear understanding of the principles governing the use of orthopaedic insoles to reduce asymmetry of the spinal muscles and thus correct the position of the spine relative to the pelvis. Though it was accepted that an insole should be used, uncertainty remained as to how to estimate the proper size of the insole or how to determine the duration for which the patient should wear it. The mechanism by which the use of an insole helped cure pain was not clearly understood either.

The answers to these and other questions will be found in the following discussion of our method of treating spinal deformities and spinal pain. The reader is already familiar with the aetiopathogenesis of lateral (scoliotic) deformity of the spine, which has been discussed in Chapter 3.

6.1 Our system of treatment of spinal deformities and spinal pain

Between February 1996 and February 2013, we treated more than 8100 patients of less than 1 year to 90 years of age for spinal pain syndrome and various neurological disorders associated with spinal deformities. The largest group (32.88%) consisted of patients who were 28–50 years of age. Sixty per cent of treated patients were women.

The general examination, conducted in the standing and lying positions, was preceded by thorough history-taking. The patients also went through preliminary examinations by a neurologist, paediatrician, neurosurgeon, oncologist and other specialists, depending on the nature of their complaints. In addition, they underwent X-ray examination, computed tomography, Doppler ultrasound scanning of the cerebral and cervical blood vessels, and other necessary studies.

Young patients usually complained of weakening of the vision (myopia, astigmatism, amblyopia, strabismus, nystagmus, etc.), sometimes accompanied by headaches, dizziness, vertebral artery syndrome, memory loss, irritability and manifestations of vascular dystonia, as well as vertebrobasilar syndrome.

Elderly patients had similar complaints, but due to deformities of the thoracic and lumbosacral spine resulting from osteochondrosis, spondylosis deformans and intervertebral disc herniations, they also complained of retrosternal pain, episodes of apnoea, extrasystoles and other signs of thoracalgia, as well as lumbalgia, as described in the previous chapters.

6.1.1 Evaluation of the general status of the patient

In 89.3% of the patients we examined, the left half of the body was underdeveloped. This was clinically manifested by asymmetry of the face, trunk and extremities (*see* Chapters 1 and 3). As for the face, we found that the features of the left half (including the ear, eyelid, eyebrow and nasolabial fold) were much lower than those of the opposite half. The left eyelid was thinner. The head was flexed and fixed to the right. In the same 89.3% of patients, an examination of the trunk revealed a deformation of the thorax—the right clavicle and left costal arc protruded anteriorly, and from the dorsal view, a costal hump could be observed on the right side. There was right-sided deformity (curvature) of the thoracic spine and left-sided deformity in the lumbar region. Among the other things we observed were unilateral underdevelopment of the pelvis, i.e. the bones of the left side were smaller than those on the right and the volume of the gluteal muscles also differed. Tilting of the pelvis to the left side and its flexion causes pathological changes in the axis of the lower extremities, leading to the development of varus (inwards) or valgus (outwards) deformation of the calf and toes. This clinical picture was observed in all patients who had shortening of the left lower extremity.

Underdevelopment of the right half of the body was seen in only 10.7% of all patients. All deformities of face, trunk and extremities described earlier were on the opposite side of the body.

The severity of the clinical symptoms varied and depended on the degree of shortening of one of the lower extremities, gender, age and the duration of the disease.

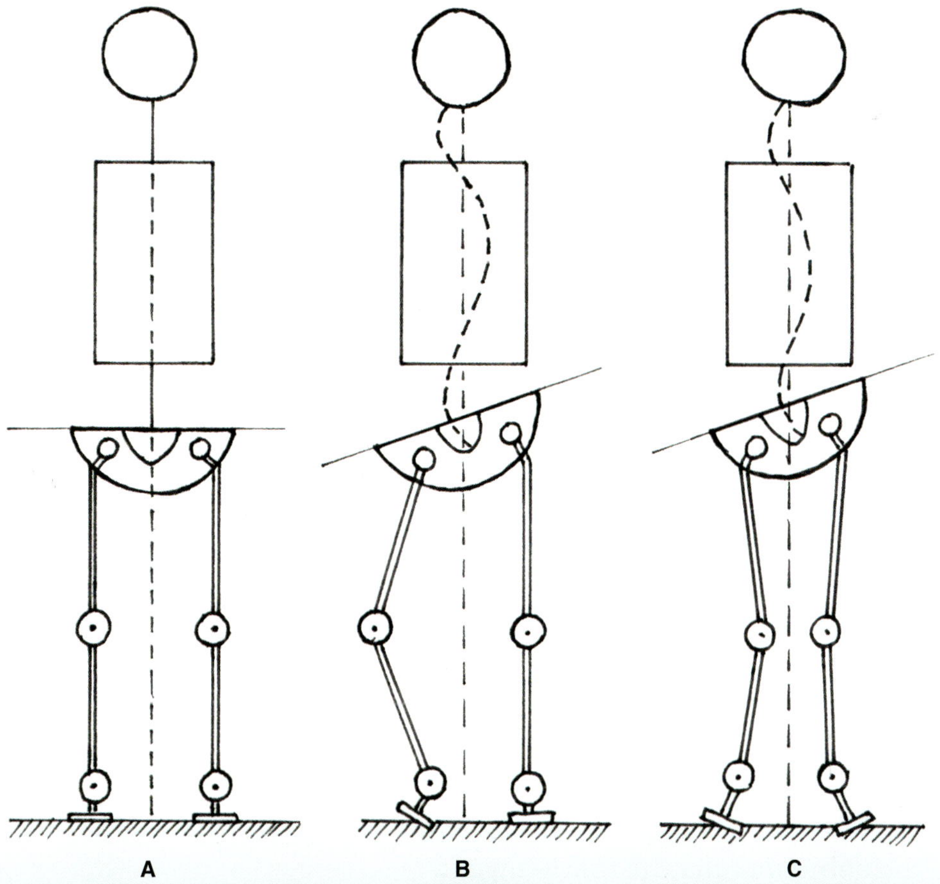

Fig. 6.3.
Deformations of the lower limbs depending on the position of the torso and pelvis
A - symmetrical length of the lower extremities **B** - relative shortening of the left leg, pelvic tilt towards the left side; formation of varus **(B)** or valgus **(C)** deformity

While examining elderly patients, we observed that long-standing body flexion to the right or left led not only to deformation of the trunk, but also of the extremities (*see* Figs 1.7 and 6.3). This unequal load gave rise to osteoarthrosis of the large joints, which later required surgical replacement. *The most important element of the general examination is an assessment of the length of the lower extremities*. The necessity of this practice becomes clear when one considers the fact that every single patient who was examined had a right-sided or left-sided pelvic tilt and shortening of one of the lower extremities on the same side. As we gained an understanding of the nature and various causes of such shortening, we were able to define our methods of treatment further.

As mentioned in Chapter 3, functional asymmetry of the anterior central gyrus of the human brain results in unilateral spasm of the spinal extensors. The spasm causes the pelvis to tilt towards the side of the weaker muscles, which leads to lateral deformation of the spine. The shortening of one leg during this process is known as relative, because the absolute length of both lower extremities is equal.

Mild asymmetry of the trunk muscles is typical of all human beings and is a physiological norm. The deterioration towards pathological changes (decompensation) begins if the body's resources to regulate its vertical posture becoming insufficient. This leads to biomechanical failure of the musculoskeletal apparatus. The causes of decompensation include the following:

- Intensive training of sportspersons
- Regular and excessive physical exertion, including weightlifting
- Long hours of sitting at a table, e.g. before a PC, or of playing a musical instrument
- Trauma to the backbone
- Suddenly lifting a heavy weight, etc.

Once the process of decompensation has begun, it progresses if its causes remain unaddressed. This gradually leads to a further increase in muscular asymmetry, the degree of the pelvic tilt and the extent of the relative shortening of one of the lower extremities (more often the left one). The extent of the relative shortening and whether it is on the right or left side are genetically determined. Thus, when a daughter has shortening of one leg, generally her mother, and even her grandmother, have the same problem on the same side. The same holds good for a son, his father and grandfather.

As mentioned earlier in this book, shortening of the leg can also be absolute, which means that there is shortening of one or two segments of the extremity. The causes of absolute shortening include the following:

- Consolidation of a fracture of a hip or knee with angular deformity
- Consequences of poliomyelitis, which causes shortening of one leg due to one-sided

underdevelopment of an affected segment

- Unilateral osteochondropathy of the femoral head
- Unilateral congenital hip luxation
- Valgus or varus deformation of a hip and/or knee and/or foot due to rachitis
- Hyperparathyroid bone disease
- After resection of a tumour affecting a segment of a bone
- After resection of a bone segment due to osteomyelitis
- Inherited underdevelopment of a hip and/or knee
- Unilateral varus or valgus deformity of the feet of varying aetiology.

In our experience, absolute shortening of a leg happened very rarely (no more than 1% of all cases). In such cases surgical treatment is required.

As for relative shortening, we first determined the extent of shortening and then used an orthopaedic insole to correct it. An insole of the required height was inserted under the patient's heel from behind.

These measurements were performed in an upright position from behind, while

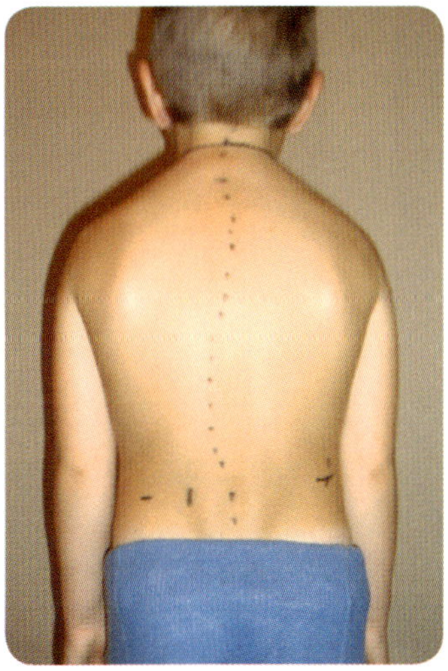

Boy of 4 years. Kyphoscoliotic posture. In the thoracic region the axis of the spine is shifted to the right. Volume of the spinal extensors on the right is much more than that on the left. Relative shortening of the left leg is 3 mm.

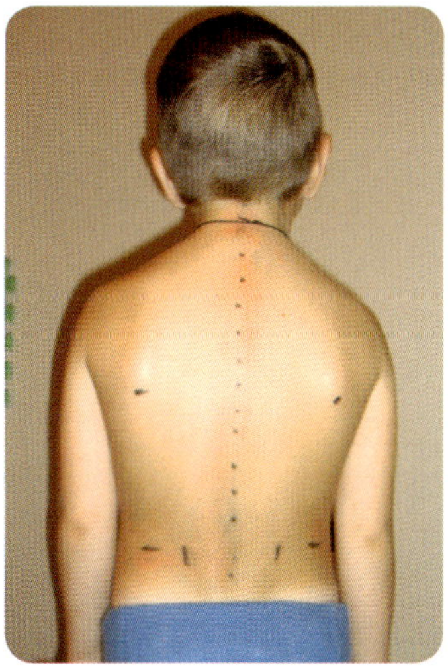

Application of 3 mm orthopaedic insole under the left heel led to restoration of symmetry of the spinal extensors. Axis of the spine is correct.

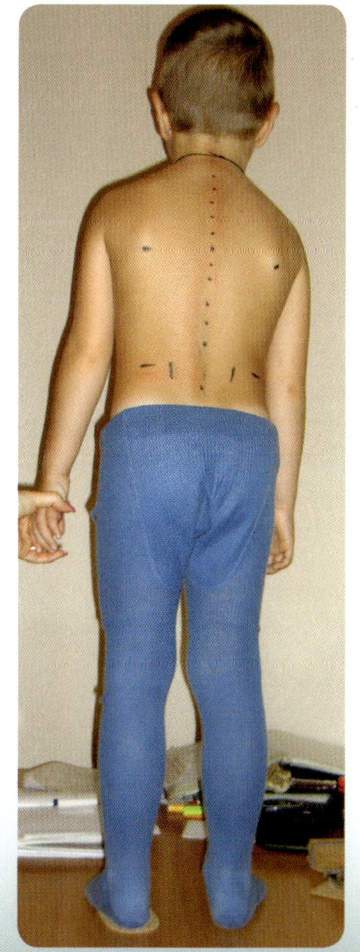

Fig. 6.4.A

putting insoles of different thicknesses under the heel. The criterion we used for determining whether we had chosen an insole of the correct thickness (or height) was the volume of the spinal extensors. We were putting insoles under the heel of the shortened leg until the volume of these muscles became equal on both sides of the body (Fig. 6.4. A–B). According to our observations, the extent of relative shortening of the leg among patients of different genders and ages could vary from 3 mm to 55 mm.

It is worth mentioning that the use of an orthopaedic insole allowed us to significantly reduce relative shortening of the leg and correct a lateral pelvic tilt even in adult patients. This leads us to the essential question as to what exactly happens to the leg, body and brain to facilitate correction? What kinds of changes occur to make rebalancing and correction of the pelvic tilt and lateral deformity possible? This issue will be discussed later.

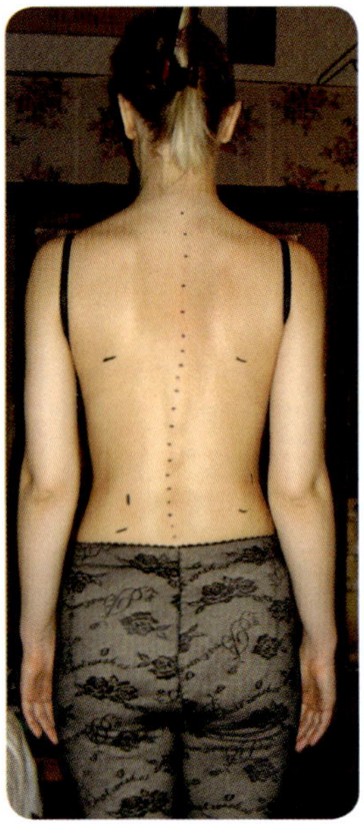

Woman of 23 years. Volume of the spinal extensors on the right is much more than that on the left side. Relative shortening of the left leg is 38 mm. Axis of the spine in the thoracic region is shifted to the right.

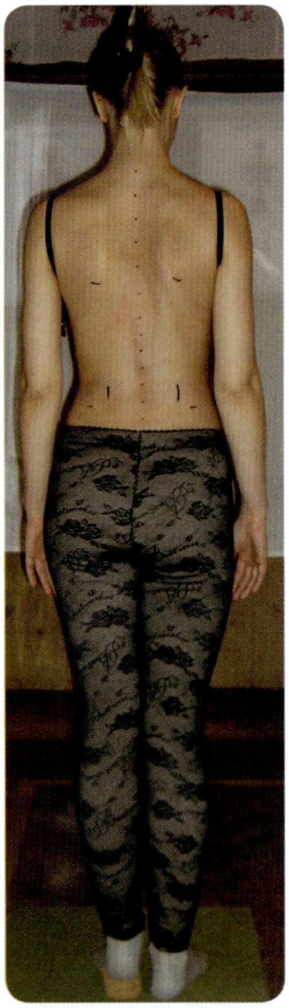

Application of 38 mm orthopaedic insole under the left heel led to the restoration of symmetry of the spinal extensors. Axis of the spine is correct.

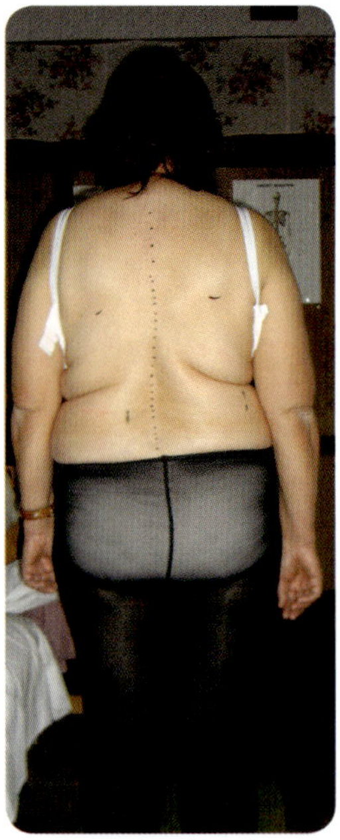

Woman of 57 years. Volume of the spinal extensors on the right is much more than that on the left side. Relative shortening of the left leg is 30 mm. Volume of the left half of the pelvis is lesser than that of the right. Axis of the spine is shifted to the right.

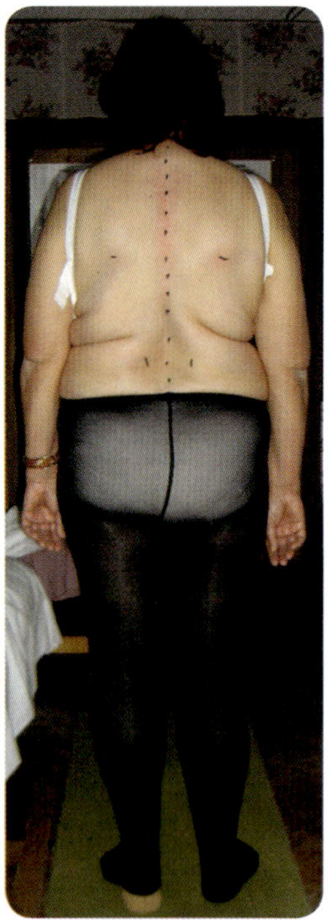

Application of 30 mm orthopaedic insole under the left heel led to the restoration of symmetry of the spinal extensors. Axis of the spine is correct.

Fig. 6.4.B

6.1.2 Therapeutic mechanisms of orthopaedic shoe insole

The vertical position of a human body is controlled by the cerebellum, which is responsible for the coordinated muscle contractions necessary for motion, and the vestibular apparatus, which is the organ of static balance. The latter is located in the pyramid of the temporal bones. The cerebellum and two vestibular organs function in coordination with each other. While the latter contributes to the body's sense of balance, the cerebellum receives impulses from the loaded bones, muscles and other anatomical structures of the lower extremities through the pathways of the spinal cord. This 'muscle sense' together with our tactile and visual sensations allow us to coordinate our movements and control the position of the body in space (F. Ivanov. *Fundamentals of Normal Anatomy* in 2 volumes, 1949). This is the essence of the teachings of Professor I.M. Sechenov (1866) on proprioception (I.M. Sechenov, *Physiology of the Nervous System*, Moscow, 1866).

The functional asymmetry of the cerebral hemispheres, which develops *in utero* itself and persists after birth, gives rise to unilateral spasm of the spinal extensors and leads to lateral deformation of the spine, initially in the form of physiological scoliosis. As the newborn grows older, the asymmetry of the trunk muscles gets fixed in the cerebellum, which is the repository of conditioned reflexes. During the period of 6–8 months when the baby first learns to stand and then walk confidently, the 'conditioned reflex of vertical body position' forms. Unfortunately, what this reflex fixes in the cerebellum is an incorrect, unilaterally flexed position of the body. Thus, it should be called 'vicious'. The scoliotic deformation gradually becomes structural and is combined with torsion of wedge-shaped vertebrae, including the cervical.

The result is the setting up of a 'vicious circle': progressive, generally unilateral impairment of the cerebellar blood flow, caused by compression of the vessels and nerves in the cervical spine, which leads to unilateral underdevelopment of the cerebellum and consequently, unilateral impairment of its function, i.e. keeping the body in the vertical position. This process results in even greater flexion of the spine, and the greater the flexion, the greater the impairment of blood flow to the cerebellum and so on.

However, this 'vicious circle' can be broken. Based on Professor I.I. Pavlov's theory of conditioned reflexes, we understand that lateral habitual deformation of the spine can be modified by developing the conditioned reflex of the correct vertical body position. To achieve this, one should use an orthopaedic insole under the heel of the shortened lower extremity. By restoring the correct vertical position of the body, the insole forms a feedback system between the position of the body in space and the vestibular organs of the human being. As a result, this position becomes fixed in the cerebellum as a new correct reflex.

The development of such a reflex takes a lot of time. If primarily an incorrect reflex has been forming for 6–8 months, the formation of a new correct reflex (in adults) would probably take the same period of time.

When the new correct reflex of the vertical body position has been fixed in the cerebellum and unilateral spasm of the spinal muscles has decreased, the conditions are ideal for restoration of the vertical position of the body and for the reduction of a lateral deformity of the spine. It was for this reason that at the end of our treatment, the axis of the spine normalized and the scoliotic deformation disappeared.

The period of time for which one should wear an orthopaedic insole depends on the extent of relative shortening of the lower extremity and the age of the patient. It should be mentioned that in the case of a child, who will continue to grow, the insole should be worn for a longer time, at least for the same period as an adult.

We would like to draw the reader's attention to the other important facts. First, when a patient is to regularly use an insole in all kinds of shoes and when the initial shortening of one leg was significant, the size of the insole should be increased gradually so that the spine and joints of the extremities can adapt to the new position of the body. This allows one to minimize the discomfort in the spine and the shortened extremity. Secondly, during restoration of balance in the spinal–pelvic segment and reduction in shortening of the leg, the height of the insole should also be decreased gradually.

Relative shortening of the leg decreases by 3–5 mm when an insole is used constantly for a mean period of 10–14 days, independent of the extent of the initial shortening. It is to be noted that premature withdrawal of the insole could interrupt the formation of the new reflex, and preserve the asymmetrical traction of the spinal muscles. The use of an insole for a period that is longer than necessary can cause asymmetry of the spinal muscles on the opposite side. Thus, the use of an insole should be supervised by the practitioner. Children should be examined at least once in 3–4 weeks and adults, once in 1.5–2 months.

Even after the symmetry of the spinal muscles has been completely restored in adult patients, especially in those involved in physical work, they should constantly wear an insole of a height of 3 mm while working.

Thus, development of the correct posture, correction of deformities of the spine, and development of the conditioned reflex of the body's correct position are based on the laws of neurophysiology and biomechanics.

6.1.3 DETORSIONAL THERAPEUTIC PHYSICAL TRAINING (TPT)

Apart from the orthopaedic insole, correction of the spinal axis at different levels through the use of TPT is one of the main elements of the treatment scheme.

In 1960, for the first time in the history of orthopaedics in the Soviet Union, two doctors of the Moscow Orthopedic Hospital, A.M. Reisman and F.I. Bagrov (*Detorsional Exercises in Physiotherapy for Scoliosis* [of the 2nd and 3rd degrees], Medgiz, Moscow, 1960, 42 pp.) embarked on a study of the role of torsional and detorsional exercises for the treatment of scoliosis of the 2nd and 3rd degrees. Physical exercises which bring about reverse torsion of the vertebrae were termed 'detorsional' by the authors, meaning that the exercises oppose torsion.

The authors confirmed that biomechanical disorders of the musculoskeletal system of a human are the main factors responsible for the development of scoliosis. They also outlined the leading role of the m. erector trunci in torsion of the vertebrae and alignment of the spine.

Detorsional exercises (DE) should be used to achieve the following goals:

1. Rotation of vertebrae to the side opposite the torsion in the area of the scoliotic deformation
2. Correction of scoliosis through alignment of the tilted pelvis and restoration of the spinal–pelvic balance
3. Stretching of contracted muscles and strengthening of stretched muscles in the thoracic and lumbar spine.

The indications for DE are S-shaped scoliosis of the thoracic and lumbar spine, isolated (partial) scoliosis of the thoracic and lumbar spine, and C-shaped scoliosis. The major indication for DE is idiopathic scoliosis.

Depending on the aetiology and grade of scoliosis, the clinical and radiological findings should be considered while using DE.

Scoliosis of the 1st degree: There is no torsion and thus DE is not indicated.

Scoliosis of the 2nd degree: When there is progressive deformity of the spine and thorax (muscular ridge, rib hump, tilting of the trunk, etc.), one should prescribe DE for the purposes of treatment and prevention. DE is of maximal efficacy at this stage.

Scoliosis of the 3rd degree: This stage is characterized by structural changes in the vertebral bodies and severe deformation of the ribs, along with progressive changes in the musculo-ligamentous apparatus of the trunk. DE should be prescribed to prevent further torsion and to decrease pain.

The scheme of DE that we developed was similar for all patients of different ages, and consisted of rotation in the lumbar, thoracic and cervical spine. Adult patients were taught to perform these exercises under the practitioner's guidance; afterwards they performed them at home. The exercises consisted of 10 turns to the right and left for each segment of the spine (Fig. 6.5. A-B-C). Children performed these exercises under their parents' guidance.

The scheme of detorsional movements, usually performed once a day, took only

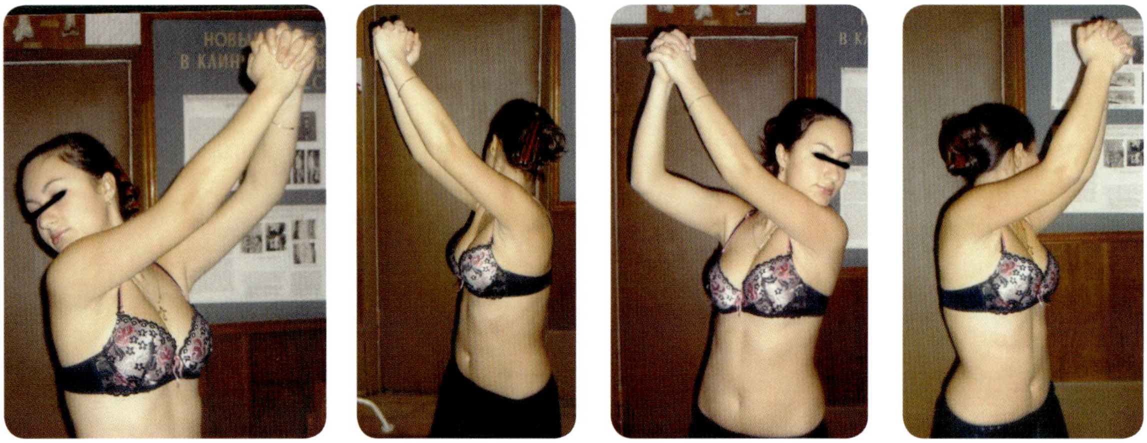

1 2 3 4

A. Rotational movements in the cervical spine (to the right and to the left)

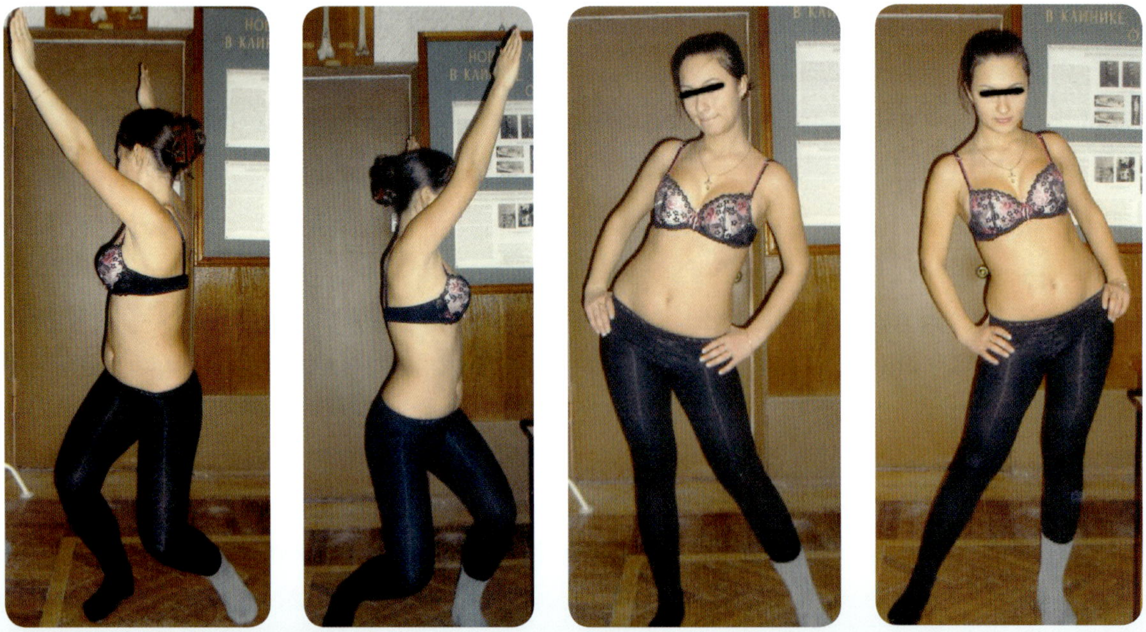

B. Rotational movements in the thoracic spine (to the right and to the left)

C. Rotational movements in the lumbar spine (to the right and to the left)

Fig. 6.5.
A set of detorsional exercises for different regions of the spine

60 seconds of the patient's time. However, a patient with extra time could perform DE two or three times a day without running the risk of damaging his health.

On the basis of the follow-up data on patients who performed DE, we were able to establish that in cases in which lateral deformation of the spine was associated with spasm of the muscles of the trunk, even several rotational movements of the pelvis were sufficient to reduce muscular spasm and lateral deformity of the spine (Fig. 6.6. A-B-C).

For a long time, we had been searching for an answer to the question as to what exactly happens to a patient on performing these exercises. How does just a simple rotation of the body allowed us to achieve such results? At last, we found the answer in the work of Professor I.M. Sechenov (1866). One of his major discoveries was the phenomenon of so-called central inhibition—the mechanism of partial or total disruption of the reflex. The morphological basis for this process is located in the brain's thalamus. A human being acquires the ability to group motions through the fixation of associated reflexes. However, these reflexes may be inhibited due to the influence of other motions.

Thus, one can assume that a few rotations of the body in the direction opposite to the

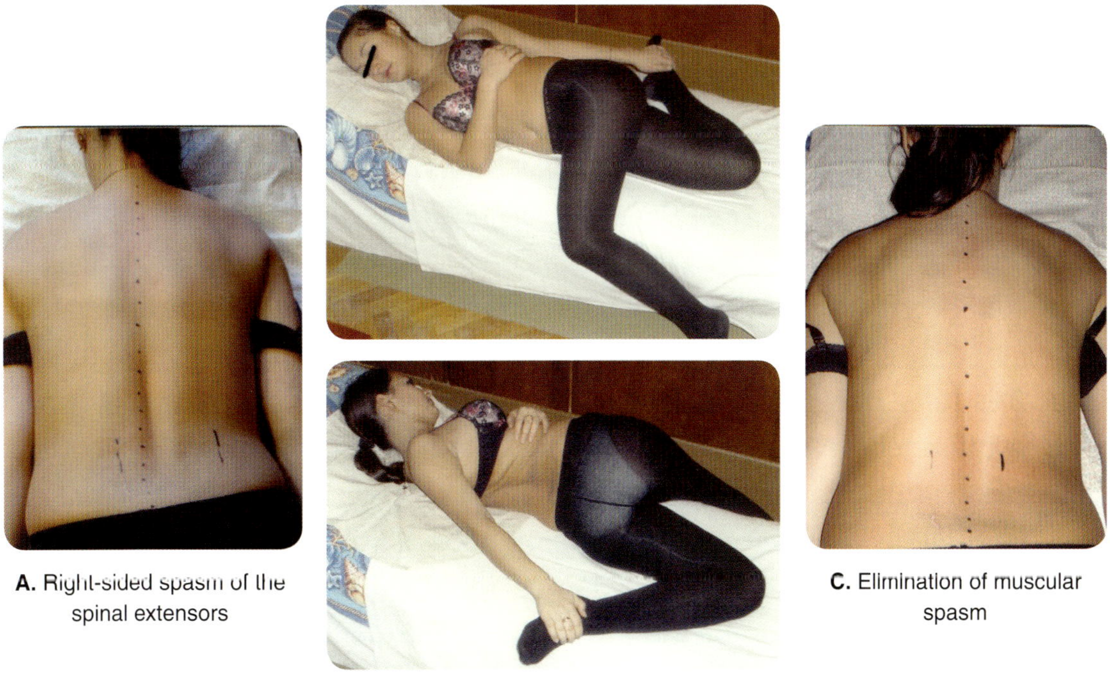

A. Right-sided spasm of the spinal extensors

B. Rotational movements of the pelvis to the right and to the left in lying position

C. Elimination of muscular spasm

Fig. 6.6.
Elimination of spinal extensor spasm with rotational movements of the pelvis while lying on a couch

torsion lead to a disruption of the reflex arc (anterior frontal gyrus–spinal extensors) and, consequently, to the disruption of the conditioned reflex of the incorrect body position. We have witnessed this phenomenon during the treatment of thousands of our patients.

In our view, 'central inhibition' can explain many things we experience, for example, when a strong desire to urinate disappears immediately because of a sudden danger or some other extraordinary circumstance. Most probably the efficacy of TPT, massage, MT and reflex therapy in reducing spinal pain could be explained by the mechanism of 'central inhibition'.

As we already know, chiropractors, masseurs and TPT specialists achieve good results in the reduction of spinal pain and lateral deformity of the spine. The scheme of TPT can align the axis of the spine in 10–15 sessions. However, the situation can turn around in several weeks or months; the lateral spinal curve can appear again, indicating that the reflex of incorrect body position has relapsed.

Our guess is that it happens because these treatments are not intended to replace the incorrect reflex of the vertical position of the body with the development of the correct one. The transformation of the incorrect reflex requires considerable time and the use of an orthopaedic insole, in accordance with the principles described earlier.

To summarize the above, we concluded that correction of the axis of the spine at different levels, using detorsional TPT in combination with an orthopaedic insole, which compensates for relative shortening of a lower extremity and promotes the correct vertical position of the body, led to the restoration of the spinal–pelvic balance and stable correction of lateral deformity of the spine. Under these conditions, the functional status of the central and peripheral nervous systems normalized, leading to resolution of the pathological symptoms and clinical recovery of the patient.

Detorsional correction of vertebrae in children created optimal conditions for their development and, what is most important, served as active prophylaxis for internal diseases. In adults, detorsional correction helped to reduce signs of brachial plexitis, thoracalgia of vertebral origin, particularly cardialgia, and lumbosacral plexitis.

As mentioned in Chapter 5, in all cases of spinal pain in the lumbosacral region, application of DE led to a reduction in torsion of S_1 relative to L_5 and S_2 in the area of lumbarization. As a result, patients obtained relief from acute lumboischialgia due to the easing of compression of the lumbosacral plexus. In addition, DE brought a gradual improvement in the condition of those suffering from chronic lumbar pain.

To maximize the positive results of our treatment, we combined the methods described above with physiotherapy (magnetic therapeutic devices of our construction), which we shall now discuss.

6.1.4 LOCAL MAGNETO-ACOUSTIC THERAPY

This method of the treatment of deformities of the spine and spinal pain consists of physiotherapy, or more specifically, local magneto-acoustic therapy. For this treatment, we use a multipurpose source of magnetic fields, the 'PDMT' apparatus, which we designed in collaboration with Professor I.G. Herzen, Professor K.S. Ternovoy, and the engineers E.L. Apotovsky, D.S. Faerman and A.A. Artemenko (Fig. 6.7). (We were awarded an invention certificate [No. 784060] for the apparatus by the USSR from 1 August 1980, and another invention certificate [1140297] from 22 November 1982.)

In recent years, a portable apparatus for magneto-acoustic therapy (the 'MAVR' series) has come into wide use. It was designed by us in collaboration with the engineers E.L. Apotovsky and V.L. Roisin (USSR patent No. 32881 from 26 September 1990 and Ukraine patent No 4119 from 27 December 1994) (Fig. 6.8). In contrast to other sources of magnetic field, the MAVR apparatus generates an electromagnetic field in combination with sound waves. There are two levels of frequency: 50 Hz and 100 Hz. The level of induction varies from 11 to 17 mTl. Treatment with this apparatus has a high therapeutic efficacy because the vibrating magnetic plate provides the tissues with a micro-massage. Moreover, the electromagnetic and acoustic impacts potentiate each other and provide anti-oedematous, anti-inflammatory and analgesic effects. This therapeutic influence is achieved due to stimulation of self-synchronization of the biorhythms of pathologically changed

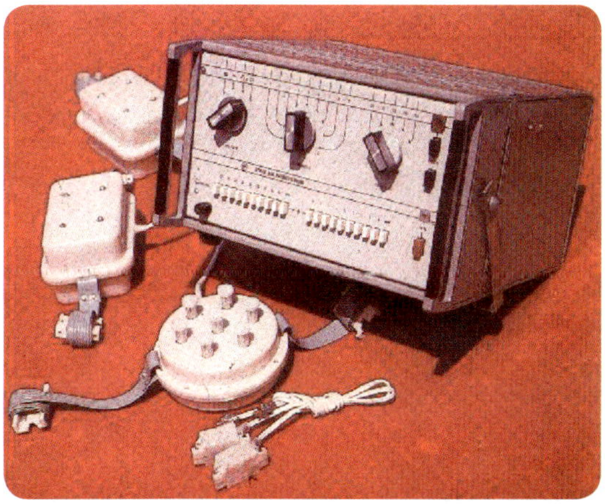

Fig. 6.7.
General view of 'PDMT' device for magneto-acoustic therapy

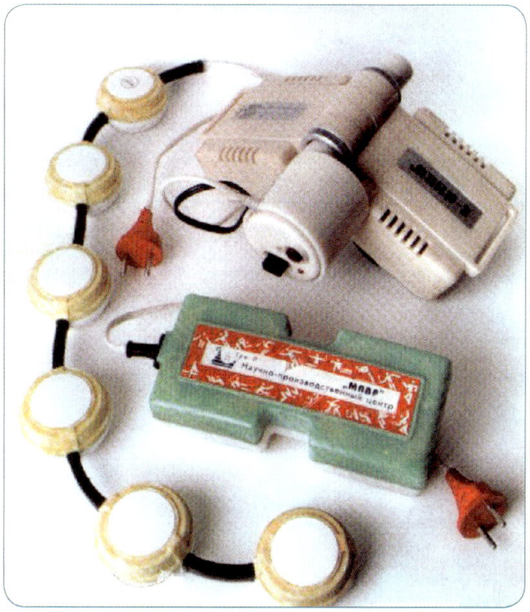

Fig. 6.8.
General view of MAVR-series device for magneto-acoustic therapy

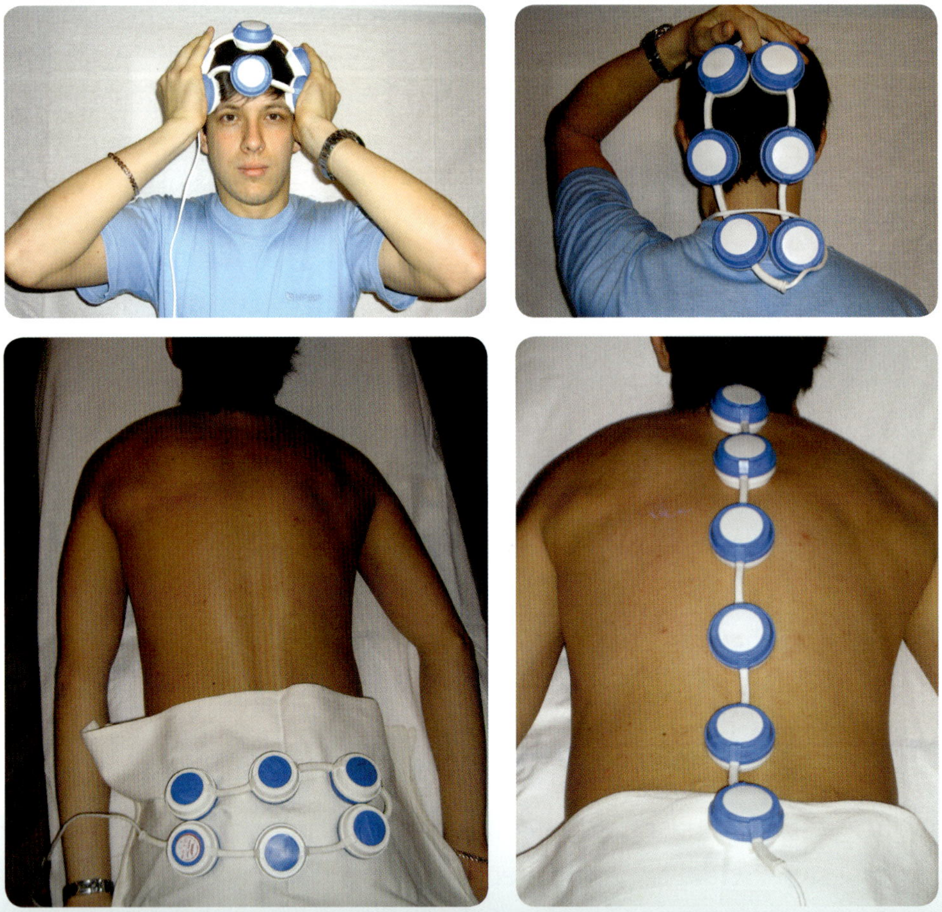

Fig. 6.9.
Zones of application of MAVR device to different parts of the body

tissues, accelerating the process of their recovery.

The PDMT and the MAVR series of devices are in use since 1990 in almost all physiotherapy departments of polyclinics (outpatient hospitals) and hospitals of the former Soviet Union.

As far as vertebrology is concerned, the apparatus for magneto-acoustic therapy is used on the whole body. It is applied along the spine, including the cervical, thoracic and lumbosacral regions, and can also be used for trans-cranial stimulation (for this purpose, the apparatus is applied directly to the head) (Fig. 6.9).

The therapy facilitates the restoration of the blood flow in the brain and spinal cord, which leads

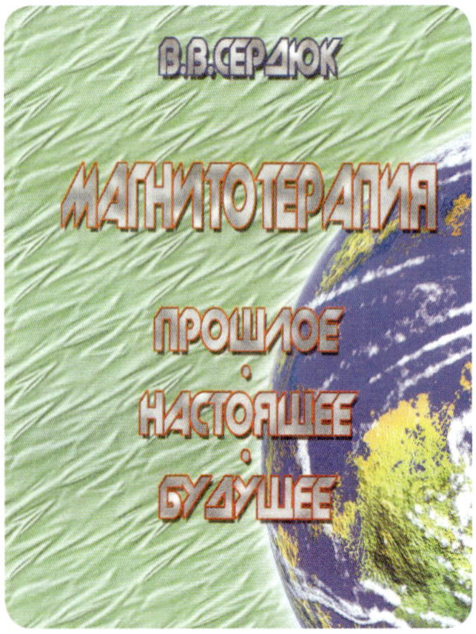

Fig. 6.10.
The monograph *'Magnetotherapy: Past, Present and Future': A Reference Guide*

to a reduction in the pathological symptoms that have arisen in the brain and spinal cord due to ischaemia. If the reader wishes to, he can refer to our monograph on magneto-acoustic therapy (V.V. Serdyuk, *Magnetotherapy: Past, Present and Future: A Reference Guide*, Azimuth-Ukraine K, 2004, 536 pp.)—(Fig. 6.10). In this monograph, the mechanisms of influence of the magnetic field on living organisms are discussed in detail. An extensive review of the national and foreign literature on the clinical application of this method is also presented.

6.1.5 AIR-INFLATABLE COLLAR-CORRECTOR OF CERVICAL AND UPPER THORACIC SPINE

The addition of the rubber air-inflatable collar-corrector in our arsenal of therapeutic measures allowed us to improve the efficacy of our treatment significantly. The major advantage of the collar is its ability to provide gentle relaxation of muscles that are in spasm, as well as atraumatic reduction of rotated and displaced cervical and upper thoracic vertebrae. This is very important while treating children, in whom manipulations of the vertebrae are very dangerous due to the risk of trauma. The collar-corrector is also used in adults (Fig. 6.11), especially those with signs of advanced osteochondrosis and deformative spondylosis of the cervical spine. Reduction of deformed vertebrae by the usual manual methods can cause avulsion of osteophytes.

Finally, atraumatic, dosed traction of the cervical vertebrae is indicated for the large group of patients with signs of fibromyalgia, vertebrobasilar insufficiency, vertebral artery syndrome, and long-standing traumas of the cervical vertebrae, in which rotational displacement is made permanent by ossified ligaments. Atraumatic, dosed traction should be performed for 10 minutes twice a day. The duration of the treatment is four weeks. In the case of children, the duration of the treatment should be reduced.

On the basis of our many years of experience with the use of the air-inflatable collar, we recommend that it should be used not only in traumatology and orthopaedics, but also in neurology, ophthalmology and even psychiatry.

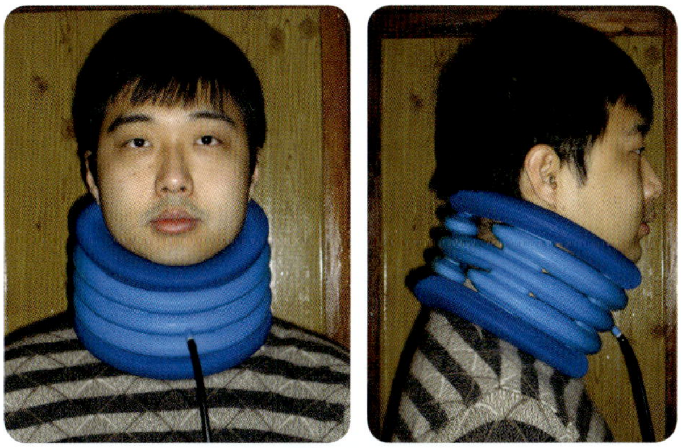

Fig. 6.11.
Photo of a patient with inflatable collar

6.1.6 New treatment methods for strabismus, trigeminitis and lateral deformation of the spine

Establishment of the regularity of genesis of human diseases because of spinal deformities due to asymmetrical functioning of the cerebral hemispheres was validated by the diplomas on discoveries (*see* author's website: www.orthopedics.com.ua). This information became the theoretical basis for the development of the new methods of treatment (*see* Epilogue).

Let us first describe the 'Treatment method for strabismus' (Ukraine patent No. 48900, 15 August 2002), which we developed in collaboration with the paediatric ophthalmologist A.N. Komashko. We have already described the practical use of this method for the treatment of children with impaired vision. This method excludes the necessity of undergoing surgery. Now we will focus on the essence of the method.

The problem of how to treat strabismus continues to preoccupy ophthalmologists all around the globe. This can be explained by the fact that the existing methods of conservative and surgical treatment have a low efficacy and carry a high risk of recurrence. This is because of a number of reasons.

First, the correction of strabismus in children does not have a lasting positive effect because the patient is growing continuously. During the period of growth, the biomechanics of the body muscles, including the eyeball muscles (EB), change and this inevitably leads to the recurrence of strabismus.

Another cause for recurrence is no less important. Ophthalmologists treat the eye without paying attention to the patient's skeleton. As we know from anatomy, the reflective associated movements of the striated muscles are controlled by *n. oculomotorius*, *n. trochlearis* and *n. abducens*. The motor nucleus of the latter is located in the pons Varolii, while the nuclei of the former two are located in the pedicles of the brain (pedunculi cerebri). Compression of these structures by rotated and dislocated C_1–C_2–C_3 vertebrae impairs the functioning of these nerves and consequently, of the muscles.

We have also established the role played by another negative factor, which is inadequate blood supply. This adversely affects the functioning of the muscles and all other anatomical structures of the EB. Our practice of systematically asking patients to undergo Doppler scanning of the cerebral and cervical vessels brought to light the fact that all patients with strabismus and other disorders of vision had symmetrical or asymmetrical compression of the vertebral arteries and veins at the level of C_3–C_4, with the deficiency in the blood flow in these vessels being 30%–50% or even more. The extent of compression of the vertebral arteries, veins and sympathetic trunks depended on the degree of vertebral torsion and on the structural features of the transverse processes and intervertebral foramina. Long-standing unilateral compression of the vertebral artery led to a deficiency in the blood supply and unilateral underdevelopment of the cerebellum. This, in turn, resulted in a tilt of the body and fixing of the tilted position as a reflex of incorrect vertical body position.

While treating our patients, we saw that the restoration of the correct position of the EB was possible only after the upper, middle and lower cervical ganglia, as well as the ganglia of the four upper thoracic vertebrae had been released, i.e. decompressed. *Thus, the treatment of strabismus should begin with the restoration of blood supply and innervation of the EB muscles, instead of surgery.* As Chapter 5 contains a detailed description of these processes, we would like to present the essence of our invention. In addition to the traditional treatment of strabismus, which consists of the use of corrective lenses and special exercises, we decided to perform detorsional correction of the cervical spine to reduce compression of the upper cervical sympathetic ganglia. When a patient has an S-shaped scoliosis on the left side, detorsional correction of the cervical spine should be performed at the level of C_1–C_2 to the right (Fig. 6.5 [1–2]), and when a patient has an S-shaped scoliosis on the right side, detorsional correction should be performed toward the left at the same level (Fig. 6.5 [3-4]). The course consists of 35–40 sessions, which should be performed once a day. In the case of children, we taught the parents to perform the detorsional exercises for the child. We believe that when financially possible, it is advisable to use an air-inflatable rubber collar to reduce rotary subluxation of the cervical and upper thoracic vertebrae instead of performing detorsional correction. Magneto-acoustic therapy (along the neck and collar area, 30 procedures for 10 minutes a day), using the MABP-series device, was prescribed for all patients. This treatment scheme also included use of the orthopaedic insole on the side of the shortened leg, which helped to reduce the pelvic tilt.

Almost every single patient with strabismus suffered from pain in the EB and also had acute pain at the exit of the branches of the trigeminal nerve (*n. trigeminus*) at the upper edge of the orbit, the maxilla and mandible. Patients with osteochondrosis and deformative spondylosis, who additonally had persistent headaches, dizziness, episodes of short-term loss of consciousness and burning pain in the occipital region, had similar complaints. All these patients were diagnosed with trigeminitis. Usually, in such situations, the pain is intense and persistent, and can be relieved only with very strong analgesic drugs. The problem of how to treat this condition is urgent as there is no clear understanding of its origin.

We made a thorough analysis of various textbooks of anatomy, atlases and anatomical macro-preparations under the guidance of Professor V.N. Romanenko (Department of Normal Human Anatomy of Odessa National Medical University). This helped us to conclude that the development of trigeminitis could be combined with trauma to the trigeminal nerve in the area of the trigeminal ganglion (ganglion trigeminale) (Fig. 5.1.9) and its nuclei in the area of the pons Varolii (Fig. 5.1.10) at the level of the C_1–C_2 vertebrae. We believe that compression of the pyramidal part of the medulla oblongata occurs due to the rotation of these vertebrae in scoliotic deformation of the cervical spine.

Thus, in order to ease the compression of the trigeminal ganglion and its nuclei in the area of the pons Varolii (Pons) and the medulla oblongata, we need to deal with the rotation of the cervical vertebrae and its cause, i.e. scoliotic deformation of the spine. We invented our own method to accomplish this. Called the 'Treatment method for inflammation of trigeminal nerve (trigeminitis)' (awarded a knowhow certificate [No. 024] by the Ukranian Academy of Original Ideas on 28 March 2005), it was developed in collaboration with the paediatric ophthalmologist A.N. Komashko. The essence of the method is detorsional correction of the 1st–2nd cervical vertebrae, in combination with a long course of TPT and the use of an orthopaedic insole under the heel of the shortened leg. The scheme of procedures also includes magneto-acoustic therapy, using the PDMT or MAVR series of devices on the cervical collar area and the sites of nerve endings. Our clinical studies have proved the high clinical efficacy of this method of treatment. An understanding of the importance of the use of an insole in the formation of the correct conditioned reflex of vertical body position served as the basis for the development of another invention, the 'Method of correction of different lengths of lower extremities' (awarded a knowhow certificate [No. 025] by the Ukrainian Academy of Original Ideas on 28 March 2005). The invention pertains to the development of a new reflex through the use of an orthopaedic insole placed under the shorter leg. The insole compensates for the relative shortening of the leg. The size of an insole ranges from a few millimetres to a few centimetres, and the duration of its use depends on the extent of shortening.

We have estimated that when there is a shortening of one leg by 3 mm, the patient has to use a corrective insole constantly for 10–14 days. This period is enough for development of the correct reflex of vertical body position.

When the shortening of one leg is 7 mm or more, the patient should wear an insole for a longer period of time. The time taken to develop the new reflex is shorter in the case of children than adults, which can be explained by certain features of the central nervous system in young people (it is more receptive to new skills). That is why adult patients were asked to wear an insole for a much longer period of time (up to one year and even longer) than children. Sometimes it is necessary for the patient to wear the insole for another period later to consolidate the reflex that has been formed.

We also favour the mass production of specially designed perambulators for newborns (meant for the child in prone position) and older children (meant for the sitting position). This, together with regular adherence to the therapeutic measures, is one of the most important ways of treating and preventing scoliotic and kyphoscoliotic deformations of the spine. We also recommend the production of a specially designed bicycle for children of pre-school and school age. Both of these inventions received a knowhow certificate by the Ukrainian Academy of Original Ideas (No. 023) on 28 March 2005, 'Method of correction of lateral deformation of the spine', as well as the author's certificate of Ukraine for 'Device for the correction of lateral deformation of the spine' (No. 035, 28 March 2005).

The use of a special perambulator during the first months of a child's life helps in the formation of the correct posture and the prevention of deformation of the spine. In the case of older children, whose parents consult a physician much later than they ideally should have, the use of a special bicycle helps to restore the correct body position as fast as possible. Regular use of the bicycle promotes consolidation of the new reflex of correct vertical body position.

On the basis of a study of the short- and long-term results of the clinical application of the scheme of methods used by us for the treatment of deformities of the spine, we were able to establish the following.

1. No matter how complex the clinical picture of widespread pain syndrome was in the majority of cases, *the main cause of the disease was shortening of one of the lower extremities*. This caused an imbalance of the spinal–pelvic segment, the development of zones of instability and subsequent development of deformities of the spine, as well as different diseases, which have been described above.

2. In the majority of patients with idiopathic scoliosis of the 2nd or 3rd degree and a costal hump, *wearing an orthopaedic insole over a long period of time (1.5–2 years) reduced lateral deformation of the spine and led to a total reduction or significant partial reduction of the costal hump*. In these cases, surgery should not be performed and in many cases, the patient should be advised to stop wearing a brace. It is advisable to regularly follow the set of treatment methods suggested by us at the earliest age possible. For example, we are of the view that a person should start with these treatment methods at the age of 1–1.5 years, as this would prevent the progression of spinal deformities, and effectively promote prophylaxis of Perthes disease and diseases of the large joints. The reduction in the pelvic tilt enabled us to enhance the efficacy of the treatment of patients with planovarus and planovalgus deformities of the feet.

3. *The instability of vertebrae in the lumbosacral spine, which led to traumatization of the corresponding neural plexuses, was the main cause of acute pain in the L_5–S_1 SMS, persistent pain syndrome, fibromyalgia, etc.* Impairment of innervation, which was predominantly unilateral, and hence improper functioning of the leg muscles, was the major cause of varicose vein disease and even the formation of trophic ulcers on the foot on the same side. The use of an orthopaedic insole placed under the heel of the shortened leg allowed us to restore the spinal–pelvic balance and thus eliminate the cause of vertebral instability.

4. *The reduction in pelvic tilt with the help of an orthopaedic insole restored equal distribution of body weight on the large joints of the lower extremities.* This slowed down the progression of valgus and varus deformity of the extremities and led to a significant decrease in the pain syndrome even in elderly patients. The importance of equal distribution of load on the large joints of the lower extremities was evident also in patients who had already undergone joint (knee and/or hip) replacement surgeries before consulting us. Many such patients suffered from persistent pain syndrome even after surgery. This could be due to the persistence of the pelvic tilt, which did not allow the replaced joint to function properly. Only an orthopaedic insole could solve this problem and consequently do away with the pain in the replaced joint.

5. *An understanding of the aetiology and pathogenesis of myopia, strabismus and other eye diseases* allowed us to come up with new, highly effective methods of treatment. They opened huge opportunities to provide qualified help to citizens of various groups. It became clear that there was a need for close cooperation between ophthalmologists and orthopaedic surgeons. The earlier one starts to treat spinal problems in children with impaired vision, the better the results. The adoption of this approach should ultimately result in a decrease in the number of adult patients.

6. It should be recognized that our scheme of treatment methods should be used *for children with bronchial asthma, endocrine disorders (obesity and diabetes), skin diseases (psoriasis), vegetative dystonia, nocturnal enuresis, etc.,* which have been discussed in Chapter 5. The clinical experience accumulated by us in the treatment of children suffering from the above-mentioned conditions clearly indicates that there is ample scope for further studies in this area, with close collaboration among vertebrologists and paediatricians, endocrinologists, dermatologists, neurologists and other specialists.

7. The long-term results of our treatment were investigated over follow-up periods of 10–12 years. We could see that the spinal extensors remained symmetrical in all patients, irrespective of age, who regularly performed the scheme of detorsional TPT. However, under certain circumstances, e.g. after trauma or falling down, sudden lifting of a heavy weight and giving up on TPT, the symmetry of the muscles was disturbed, leading to a recurrence of spinal pain and lateral deformity of the spine. In such cases, we advised the patient to wear an orthopaedic insole again to restore the spinal–pelvic balance and thus align the axis of the spine and decrease the spinal pain.

8. The high efficacy of our treatment methods has been confirmed by our long-standing experience with patients suffering from spinal deformities and spinal pain syndrome and, on the basis of this, we would like to recommend these methods to orthopaedic surgeons, endocrinologists, neurologists and other specialists.

Conclusions

WE HAVE GIVEN A VAST AMOUNT OF INFORMATION in this book and have attempted to present our analysis from the first steps in understanding the importance of the problem of body asymmetry, the variety of spinal deformities and spinal pain to the nature of these processes. I want to recall the opinion of the prominent orthopaedic surgeon A. Schantz (1908) who said that spinal diseases are among the darkest areas of pathology. And this is true!

However, in the march of science, there are times when the quantitative accumulation of knowledge inevitably leads to a process of rethinking and the development of new ideas, new ways of understanding things and new discoveries, which will raise the problem to a new stage in the evolution of our thinking.

1. We are aware that this book does not completely solve the problem of scoliosis and spinal pain. However, we hope that it will open the door to that area of knowledge which will help physicians and researchers to look at these problems differently and unconventionally, and will raise the quality of treatment, thus making their work maximally professional. But as knowledge is unlimited, it is possible that future researchers will be able to write new pages in the book of knowledge about scoliosis and spinal pain. We heartily wish them success!
2. When we started on this work, we had several objectives in mind: to clarify the nature of body asymmetry, associated scoliosis and other spinal deformities; to establish whether these deformities have a possible influence on development of a variety of human diseases; and finally, to understand the nature of spinal pain. The ultimate goal was to come up with curative and preventive measures aimed at eliminating them.
3. It is essential for a living organism (human beings, animals, plants, even single cells) to have an asymmetrical structure. There is no life without asymmetry. In human beings, asymmetry manifests itself in various clinical signs, including unequal contraction of the spinal extensors. The latter is caused by the asymmetrical functioning of the cerebral hemispheres, particularly the anterior central gyrus, which controls the movements of the body. This results in a pelvic tilt towards the weaker muscles and relative shortening of the lower extremity, as well as the

development of lateral deformity of the spine. Since this deformity is typical for all people, it may be called physiological.

4. The process of development of the vertebral bodies, arches and processes, as well as intervertebral discs, ligaments and other anatomical structures, takes place on the base of the lateral deformity of the spine. The result is unilateral underdevelopment of these structures which, in turn, gives rise to zones of instability in every segment of the spine. In accordance with the laws of biomechanics, even a small pelvic tilt is enough to induce rotation of vertebrae around their axis in the cervical, thoracic, lumbar and, most importantly, sacral spine, the area where the vertebrae are not fused.
5. Thus, the process of torsion of wedge-shaped vertebrae begins and true or structural scoliosis starts to develop. The degree of curvature depends on the extent of shortening of the leg, the condition of the muscles; the patient's living conditions, nutrition and level of physical activity, and other factors. Genetic factors are also of great importance. The mechanism of development of lateral deformity of the spine is consistent across the human race, regardless of gender, age and nationality.
6. So far, we have discovered the essence of the pathogenesis of what is termed idiopathic scoliosis, which comprises more than 90% of all lateral deformities of the spine. In our view, the term 'idiopathic scoliosis', or spinal deformation of unknown aetiology, should be replaced with another term 'Scoliosis: spinal muscles asymmetrical deformation of a reflex origin'.
7. Examination of a multitude of patients who belonged to all age groups and had scoliotic deformity of the spine enabled us to answer another question which our predecessors had pondered over. This was the question on the origin of human diseases.
8. On the basis of our studies, we established that rotational displacement of vertebrae, which begins in early childhood and increases gradually as a person matures, has an adverse effect on the development of all organs and systems. This invariably becomes a basis for the development of different pathological conditions. This is how children are forming a reserve army of future adult patients.
9. Our clinical observations helped us to uncover the mechanisms of acute local pain in the area of the L_5–S_1 SMS, as well as of persistent pelvic pain syndrome and fibromyalgia. These could be linked to the rotation of the 1st and 2nd sacral vertebrae in case of their lumbarization. We also clearly established the role of other anomalies of the spine which could induce spinal pain. These included sacralization of L_5, asymmetry of the articular processes in the area of L_5–S_1, clefts in the posterior arches of the lumbosacral vertebrae, and the presence of additional vertebrae and hemivertebrae in the same segment.

10. Osteochondrosis and deformative spondylosis play a significant role in the development of spinal pain. In the initial stages of scoliosis, these conditions are mainly of a compensatory nature, aimed at stabilizing vertebrae in the areas of instability. However, later on, in adults and the elderly, this is followed by the process of decompensation, which is characterized by the destruction of the intervertebral disc and hernial protrusion, and even prolapse of a fragmented nucleus pulposus towards the spinal canal. The growth of osteophytes causes stenosis of the intervertebral foramina and spinal canal, as well as trauma to the anterior and posterior longitudinal ligaments and Lyushka's nerve. This, in essence, is what underlies multifactorial spinal pain syndrome.
11. Despite the fact that the situation is so complex, it is not hopeless. Reduction of the pelvic tilt, as the main factor behind the development of pathological changes, through the use of an insole to compensate for shortening of the limb concerned, gradually normalizes the biomechanics of the musculoskeletal system and eliminates all the mechanisms of spinal pain. Detorsional TPT and local magneto-acoustic therapy also promoted clinical recovery.
12. For patients with spinal pain predominantly in the lumbar area, CT scanning and radiography of the lumbosacral region in two projections, focusing on the L_5–S_1 level, are obligatory. These investigations may reveal signs of dysplasia, which lead to spinal pain. The quality of radiological diagnosis is improved if radiography is complemented by CT scanning and, needless to say, the possibility both of underdiagnosis and overdiagnosis of disc herniation is thus minimized.
13. A huge amount of resources have been spent and great efforts made to treat patients with pathological abnormalities of the spine, joints, internal organs, etc. It would seem that the new generation of children and adolescents is likely to meet the same fate as that of their parents or those adults who are dying prematurely from various diseases. However, the possibility of breaking this 'vicious circle of problems' has become real now. The prevention of diseases is much cheaper and easier and, most importantly, more promising. Orthopaedic surgeons must make a special effort to work on the prophylaxis of different maladies, in close collaboration with other medical specialists, using the information presented in this book.
14. By treating children of all age groups with health problems such as impairments of vision, hearing and speech, allergies, asthma, diabetes and obesity, and by preventing the development of new diseases, we can foster a new generation of healthy people. We do not need huge investments; all we need is the proper organization and provision of preventive and curative services by the health authorities.

Such a programme should include the following.

- Among the measures of foremost importance are systematic examinations of children in pre-school and school for the early detection of spinal deformities. Parents and children should be taught to perform detorsional TPT. Reducing the number of cases of torsion of the spine will improve prospects for a significant decrease in the number of sick children.
- Serial production of orthopaedic insoles must be undertaken as the use of insoles can stop the progression of skeletal deformities in children, adolescents and even adults. In the context of athletes who are training, the use of shoes equipped with the required insole will increase their efficiency and, consequently, help them achieve better results.
- The development and serial production of perambulators and bicycles of the new generation (our construction) are of paramount importance. Their use would create conditions conducive to the formation of the correct posture in early childhood and this, in turn, would in preventing spinal deformities.

We are ready to cooperate with paediatric and adult orthopaedic surgeons and sports physicians. We are also willing to enter into a mutually beneficial collaboration with manufacturers of shoes, perambulators, baby carriages and baby bicycles to supply the market with these vitally important products. Such collaborations may bestow a healthy life on a large number of people, both children and adults!

Epilogue

New conservative method of treatment of scoliosis in children and adults with spinal pain syndrome

ON THE BASIS OF HIS DISCOVERIES, the author has evolved a scheme of non-surgical treatment and prophylactic measures for children with infantile and juvenile forms of scoliosis. This scheme includes exercises of detorsional gymnastics, use of orthopaedic insoles to compensate for relative shortening of one of the legs and magneto-acoustic therapy on the spinal cord. The implementation of this scheme from early childhood to the completion of active growth is directed at restoring the pelvic–spinal balance, physiologically correcting the biomechanics of body muscles and preventing the transformation of functional scoliosis into structural scoliosis. These factors lead to the correct functioning of conductive tracts and spinal nerves, which results in normalization of functioning of various organ systems.

The new non-surgical method of treatment of functional scoliosis is most effective in early childhood. Harmonized development of children ensures a reduction in the number of adult patients in future. The author's suggested scheme has been shown to be effective in more than 8000 patients of Ukraine and Russia.

The following are some clinical examples:

1. Patient E., an 11-year-old boy, presented with S-shaped scoliosis of the thoracic and lumbar parts of the spinal column of the 2nd stage. Relative shortening of the left leg was 3.5 mm. His complaints included headaches, pain in the lower limbs, constant fatigue, progressive myopia and squint. Figures 1A and B show his condition before treatment. At follow-up after 4 months, the spinal axis was correct and the position of the eyes was normal (Figs 1C and D), the length of the legs was identical and the patient had no complaints.

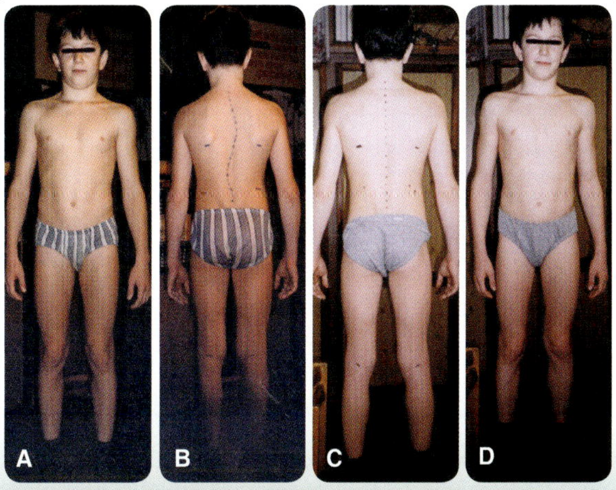

Fig. 1. Patient E., 11 years

2. Patient B., a 12-year-old boy, presented with S-shaped scoliosis of the thoracic and lumbar parts of the spinal column of the 2nd–3rd stages. Relative shortening of the left leg was 15 mm. His complaints included constant headaches, pain in both legs, weakening of sight and vegetovascular dystonia. Two years ago, the patient had undergone treatment elsewhere in connection with cholecystitis, intestinal ulcer, pyelonephritis and cystitis. Figures 2A and B show the condition of the patient before treatment. The results at follow-up 1.5 years later showed that the deformation of the spinal column had reduced (Figs 2C and D), the posture was correct, the position of the eyes was normal and the length of the legs was identical. Though the patient had no complaints, there was a slight asymmetry of the buttocks though the position of the pelvis was correct.

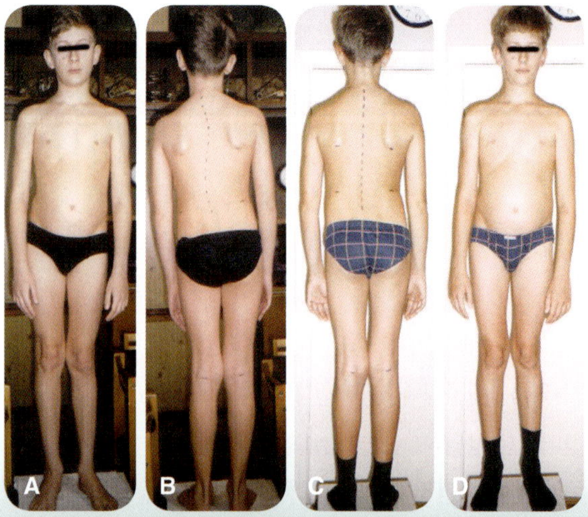

Fig. 2. Patient B., 12 years

3. Patient K., a 12-year-old boy, presented with S-shaped scoliosis of the thoracic and lumbar parts of the spinal column of the 2nd–3rd stages. Relative shortening of the left leg was 10 mm. His complaints included weakening of sight, internal squint, vegetovascular disorders and headaches. Figures 3A and B show the condition of the patient before treatment. The results at follow-up after 5 months showed that the spinal column deformity was removed (Figs 3C and D), the posture was correct, the position of the eyes was normal and the length of the legs was identical. K. had no complaints.

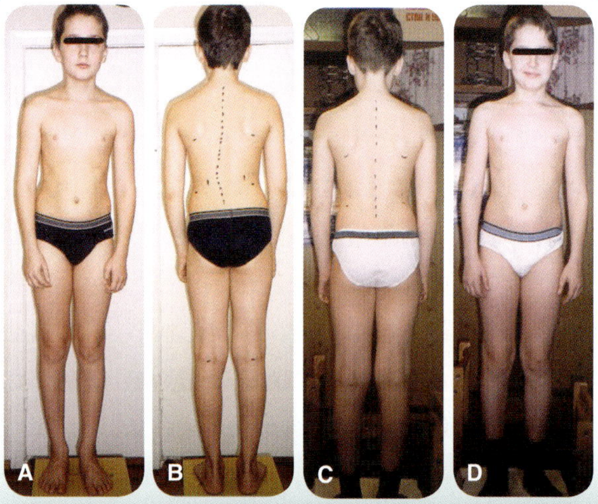

Fig. 3. Patient K., 12 years

4. Patient Z., a 6-year-old boy, presented with kyphoscoliosis deformity of the 2nd–3rd stages. Relative shortening of the left leg was 10 mm. His complaints

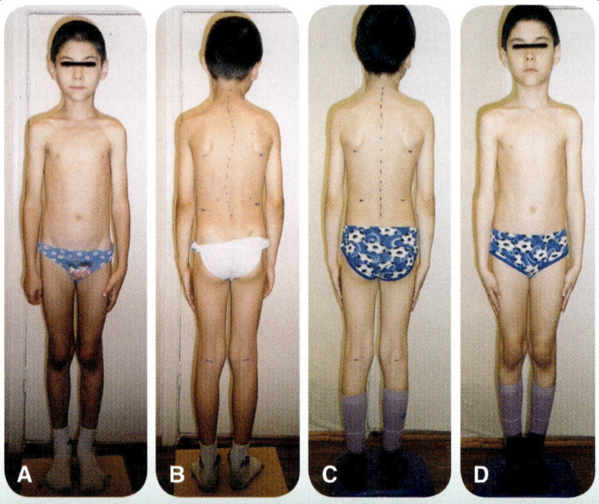

Fig. 4. Patient Z., 6 years

included amblyopia, astigmatism, vegetovascular dystonia and internal squint. He also complained of pain in the arms and lower limbs. Figures 4A and B show the condition of the patient before treatment. The results at follow-up after 6 months showed that the posture was correct, the position of the eyes was normal (Figs 4C and D) and the length of the legs was identical. Z. had no complaints.

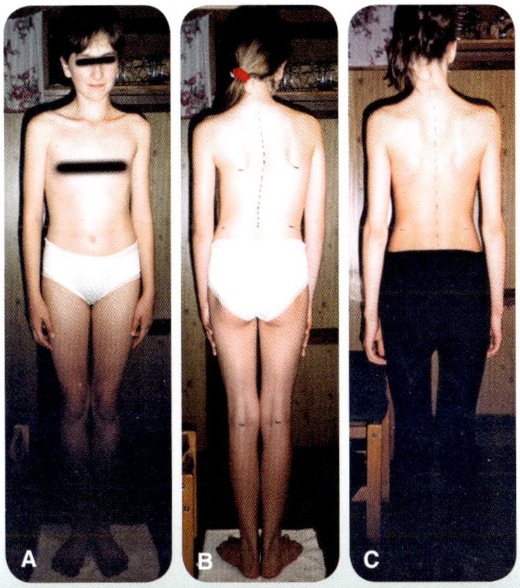

Fig. 5. Patient Ya., 14 years

5. Patient Ya., a 14-year-old girl, presented with S-shaped scoliosis of the thoracic and lumbar parts of the spinal column of the 2nd–3rd stages. Relative shortening of the left leg was 7 mm. Her complaints included marked vegetovascular disorders (emotional instability), headaches, heart pain, and difficulty in breathing. Figures 5A and B show the condition of the patient before treatment. The results at follow-up after 1.5 years showed that the spinal column deformity had been removed (Fig. 5C), her general health had normalized and the length of the legs was identical. Ya. had no complaints.

6. Patient P., an 8.5-year-old girl, presented with increasing S-shaped scoliosis of the thoracic and lumbar parts of the spinal column of the 2nd–3rd stages. Relative shortening of the left leg was 3.5 mm. Her complaints included dyskinesia of the biliary tract, latent internal squint, vegetovascular dystonia, pain in the upper and lower limbs, and recurrent heart pain. Figures 6A and B show the condition of the patient before treatment. The results at follow-up after 8 months showed that there was no deformity of the spinal column (Figs 6C and D), the posture was normal, the vision had normalized and the length of the legs was identical. P. had no complaints.

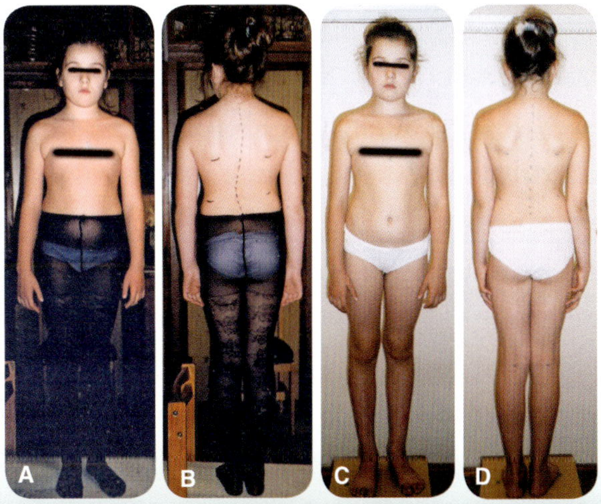

Fig. 6. Patient P., 8.5 years

7. Patient Tch., an 11-year-old girl, presented with progressive S-shaped scoliosis of the thoracic and lumbar parts of the spinal column of the 2nd–3rd stages. Shortening of the left leg was 3.5 mm. Before consulting us, the patient had been under treatment for two years in a special school-sanatorium for children with scoliosis, but with no

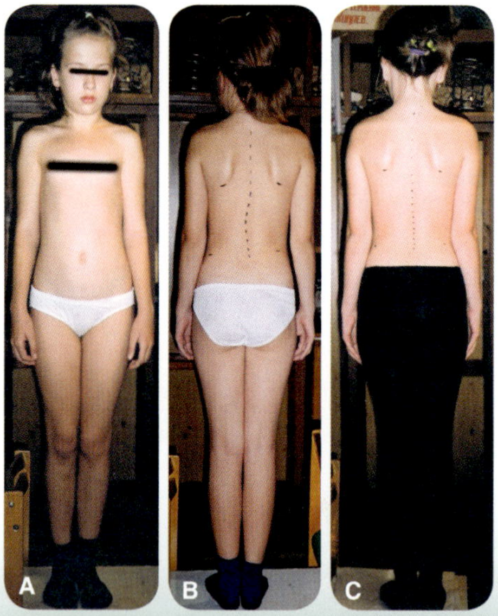

Fig. 7. Patient Tch., 11 years

significant result. Her complaints included pain in the left leg, pain in the heart and undue fatigue. Figures 7A and B show the condition of the patient before treatment. The results of follow-up after 6 months showed that the deformity of the spinal column had been removed (Fig. 7C) and the length of the legs was identical. Tch. had no complaints.

8. Patient K., a 6-year-old girl, presented with S-shaped scoliosis of the thoracic and lumbar parts of the spinal column of the 2nd–3rd stages of dysplastic origin (lumbarization of S_1, spina bifida L_5). Shortening of the left leg was 7 mm. Her complaints included vegetovascular dystonia. During examination at Kiev's surgical hospital, a left ovarian cyst was diagnosed, which was attributed to high levels of oestrogens. She complained of pain in the area of the left ovary and lower limbs. Figures 8A and B show the condition of the patient before treatment. The results at follow-up after 4 months showed that the spinal posture was correct (Figs 8C and D), and the length of the legs was identical. K. had no complaints. An ultrasound showed that the ovarian cyst had disappeared. The level of oestrogens was found to be normal.

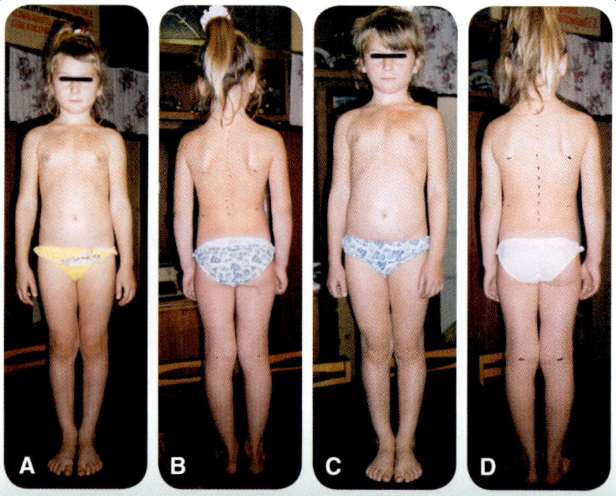

Fig. 8. Patient K., 6 years

9. Patient P., a 6-year-old girl, presented with S-shaped scoliosis of the thoracic and lumbar parts of the spinal column of the 2nd–3rd stages. Relative shortening of the left leg was 7 mm. Her complaints included weakening of sight, squint, vegetovascular disorders, constant headaches and pain in both legs (lumbar ischioneuralgia). Figures 9A

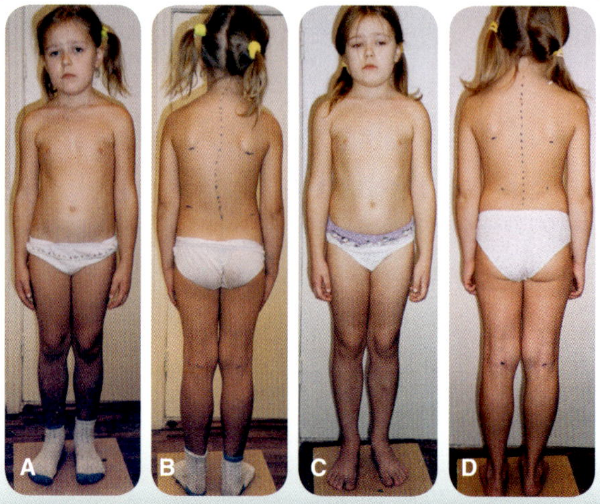

Fig. 9. Patient P., 6 years

and B show the condition of the patient before treatment. The results of follow-up after 4 months showed that the deformity of the spinal column had been reduced, the posture was correct (Figs 9C and D), the length of the legs was identical and the position of the eyes was normal. P. had no complaints.

10. Patient G., a 6-year-old girl, presented with S-shaped scoliosis of the thoracic and lumbar parts of the spinal column of the 2nd–3rd stages. Relative shortening of the left leg was 10 mm. Her mother had noticed increasing deformation of the spine. G.'s complaints included pain in the upper and lower limbs (clinical picture of plexitis and lumbar ischialgia). Figures 10A and B show the condition of the patient before treatment. The results of follow-up after 2 months (Fig. 10C) showed that relative shortening of the left leg had reduced from 10 mm to 7 mm. The results of follow-up after 1.5 years (Fig. 10D) showed that the length of the legs was identical, the spinal posture was correct and she had no symptoms of plexitis and lumbar ischialgia. G. had no complaints.

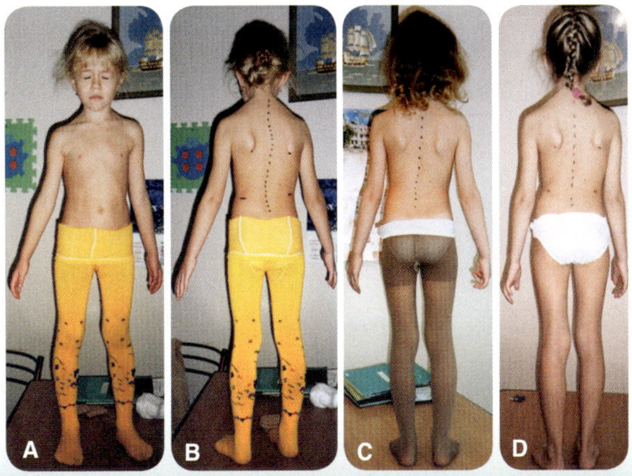

Fig. 10. Patient G., 6 years

On the basis of his investigations and long-term follow-up (more than 12 years) of children with functional scoliosis and spinal pain syndrome, the author makes the following conclusions:

1. As a rule, scoliotic deformity of the spine, even in children, is followed by spinal pain with different localizations.
2. When treatment is provided to children with infantile and juvenile forms of spinal deformity (early-onset scoliosis), the suggested scheme helps in correcting the scoliotic posture (functional scoliosis), which is linked to unilateral spasm of the spinal extensors, muscles of the pelvis and thighs (disturbing the biomechanics of the body). As a result, the lateral curvature can be aligned and the axis of the spine becomes straight.
3. The time it takes to achieve correction of functional scoliosis varies from several months to several years, and depends on the age of the patient, the level of shortening of one of the legs and existence of dysplasia of the lumbar and/or sacral vertebrae.
4. The choice of a correct inlay for the shoe minimizes the possibility of recurrence of spinal deformity. This insole raises the pelvis to the necessary horizontal level.

Information about the changes in the body's position is analysed by the vestibular apparatus. It is then fixed in the cerebellum as a new 'correct' reflex of the vertical position of the body. Thus, correction of functional scoliosis by restoration of the proper biomechanics of the spine and pelvis is the most important stage of treatment.

5. The scoliotic posture (functional scoliosis), if not corrected in young children, transforms later in adults into structural scoliosis, which is characterized by changes in the anatomical features of the bodies of the vertebrae (clinoid shape), underdevelopment of their arches and processes, ligaments, muscles, etc.
6. By treating patients (teenagers and adults) with structural scoliosis, using the author's suggested scheme of treatment, we may achieve correction of the scoliotic posture, a reduction in spinal pain and improvement of general health. But we cannot correct a significantly deformed spine. For this purpose, surgery is recommended to fuse the vertebrae in the maximally correct position, using metal constructions and resecting humpback.
7. Since surgery may be followed by certain complications, many patients and even doctors prefer conservative treatment (which includes swimming, detorsional stretching and flexion muscle exercises, massage, use of insoles, magneto-acoustic therapy, use of brace). Surgery and/or brace are required only for fixation of the spine in the maximally correct position and preventing an increase in deformity. Both methods do not and cannot restore the correct biomechanics of muscles of the spine, pelvis and thighs.
8. The author's scheme of conservative treatment is to be used for at least 2–4 years (or even more), during which the skeleton, vertebrae, muscles, ligaments, etc. get slowly restored to their correct structure without surgical intervention. It is important to note that such self-correction of all structures of the spine proceeds only with the help of continuous correction of the biomechanics of the body. This process is achieved more quickly during childhood because the bones are still growing.
9. This scheme prevents the progression of deformity of the spine in patients of all ages with functional and structural scoliosis.
10. A radical correction of the spine in adults may be achieved only by surgery.

Thus, it becomes clear that correction of scoliotic posture and restoration of the correct biomechanics of the spine, done as early as possible, is the most important element in the treatment of scoliosis; this will prevent the development of structural scoliosis as well as avoid surgical intervention.

Bibliography

1. Abalmasova EA. *To the Etiology of Scoliosis in Children and Adolescents.* Publication of the 1st Congress of Trauma Surgeons of the USSR. M., 1965, pp. 218–20.
2. Arkin A. The Mechanism of Rotation in Combination with Internal Deviation in the Normal Spine. *The Journal of Bone and Joint Surgery* 1950;**32A:**180–8.
3. Babiyak VI, Akimov GA, Bazarov VG, Filimonov VN. *Vestibular and Auditory Disorders in Cervical Osteochondrosis.* K.: Health, 1990, 192 p.
4. Barsov MK. *To the Etiology and Ttreatment of Scoliosis.* M., 1889, 330 p.
5. Belostotski EM—cited after M.M. Zolotareva. *Eye Diseases.* Minsk, Belarus, 1964, 619 p.
6. Bersenev VA. *The Spine and Pain.* K., Avers, 2010, 544 p.
7. Blum F, Leiserson A, Hofstadter L. *Brain, Mind and Behavior,* Verlag, 1988, 248 p.
8. Bobrishchev KV. Back Pain. Poltava: Poltava Literator, 1994, 184 p.
9. Bogdanov FR. *Scolioses. A Surgical Guide,* 4 volumes. M., Medgiz, 1963.
10. Bohart WN. Anatomic Variation and Anomalies of the Spine. *JAMA* 1929;**92:**698.
11. Bohr T. Problems with Myofascial Pain Syndrome and Fibromyalgia Syndrome. *Neurology* 1996;**46:**593–7.
12. Borgesen SE. Herniation of the Lumber Intervertibral Disc on Children and Adolescents. *Acta Orthopaedica Scandinavica* 1974;**45:**540–9.
13. Bragg PS, Maheshvarananda SP, Nordemar R, Preobrazhensky V. *Spine – the key to health.* SPb.: Leila, 1997, 336 pp.
14. Brunk M. *The Importance of Rickets in Childhood as a Cause of Scoliosis in Adult Age.* Copenhagen, 1951, pp. 128–65.
15. Burwell R, Dangerfield P. *A Multifactorial Concept of the Causation of Idiopathic Scoliosis.* 10th International Philip Zorab Symposium: Programme and Abstracts. Oxford, 1998, 48 p.
16. Buryanov A. *Thoracic Osteochondrosis – Methodological Aspects of Restorative Treatment and Rehabilitation.* K.: Health, 1997, 328 p.
17. Chaklin VD. *Pathological Anatomy, Clinical Features and Treatment of Scoliosis.* M.: Medgiz, 1958, 340 p.
18. Cherkeszade DD. *Osteopathic Diagnosis and Treatment of Diseases of the Spine.* M.: Publishing Center Fedorov, 2000, 120 p.
19. Cobb JR. The Problem of the Primary Curve. *The Journal of Bone and Joint Surgery* 1960;**42-A:**1413–25.
20. Dyachenko VA. *Radiographic Osteology (Normal and Variant of Bony System in Radiographic Images).* M.: Medgiz, 1954, 110 pp.
21. Dyadyk AI, Shpilevaya MI, Zdihovskaya II, *et al. Current Approaches to Diagnosis and Treatment of Degenerative Disc Disease: A Method.* Recommendations. Donetsk, 2005, 95 pp.
22. Dzyak A. *Sacral Pain.* Translated from Polish. M.: Medicine, 1981, 220 p.
23. Enneking WF. Pathological Changes in Scoliosis. *The Journal of Bone and Joint Surgery* 1969;**51-A:**165.
24. Evminov V. *How to Overcome Back Pain Forever: The Art of Being Healthy.* K.: SC UKA, 2002, 70 pp.
25. Farkas A. The Pathogenesis of Idiopathic Scoliosis. *The Journal of Bone and Joint Surgery* 1954;**36-A:**617–54.
26. Fishchenko VY, Martynenko GF, Shargorodsky GS, Shvets VA. *Conservative Treatment of Spinal Osteochondrosis.* K.: Health, 1989, 166 pp.

27. Fishchenko VY, Uleschenko VA, Vovk MM, *et al. Conservative Treatment of Scoliosis.* K.: MF-UNITI ATLANT, 1994, 188 p.
28. Fishchenko VY. *Scoliosis: A Scientific Publication.* Makeevka, 2005, 550 pp.
29. Gagman NF. *Causes and Preconditions in the Origin of Scolioses.* M., 1896.
30. Gallie RL, Speight DW, Simon R. *Emergency Orthopedics.* Spine: Translated from English. M.: Medicine, 1995, 432 p.
31. Geel SE. The Fibromyalgia Syndrome: Musculoskeletal Patophysiology. *Seminars in Arthritis and Rheumatism* 1994;**23:**347–53.
32. Gelb H, Siegel P. *Pain Relief Without Drugs*: The Translated from English. Minsk: Polumja, 1990, 143 p.
33. Goryanaya GA. *Get Rid of Osteochondrosis.* K.: Libid, 1991, 80 p.
34. *Great Medical Encyclopedia. Soviet Encyclopedia.* 25 volumes. M., 1962, pp. 593–662.
35. Gruntovsky GH. Results of Manual Therapy in Patients with Acute Spinal Pain. *Orthopaedics, Traumatology and Prosthetics*; 1982;**No.2:**16–19.
36. Grutsa A. *Pathogenesis and Treatment of Idiopathic Scolioses Based on Own Observations.* Jubilee Scientific Session Devoted to the 100th Anniversary of GI Turner: Reports Proc. L., 1959, pp. 273–84.
37. Harrenstein R. Weiteres Uber Fruhskoliose und ihre Behandlung. *Zeitschrift fьr Orthopдdie und Unfallchirurgie* 1933;**No.59:**S.1–S.14.
38. Heine R, Reher H. Die Progredienz der unbehandelten idiopathischen Skoliose bis Wachstumsabschluss. *Zeitschrift fur Orthopedie und Unfallchirurgie* 1975;**Bd. 113:**S.87–S.97.
39. Heuer F. Aetiologie und Mechanik der Scoliose. *Verh Dtsch Orthop Ges* 21 Kongr–Berlin, 1926, S.157.
40. Hildebrandt A. Uber Osteochondrosis im Bereich der Wirbelsaule. *Fortschritte auf dem Gebiete der Rontgenstrahlen* 1933;**47:**551–79.
41. Hubel D. *The Brain.* N.Y.: W.H. Freeman and Company, 1979, 321 p.
42. Hvisyuk NI. *Instability of the Lumbar Spine*: Author's Abstract on Doctoral Thesis for Medical Sciences. H., 1976, 35 pp.
43. Hvisyuk NI, Prodan AI, Puhacheva SS, *et al. Osteochondrosis of the Spine in Children.* K.: Health, 1985, 104 pp.
44. Ilizarov GA, Markhashov AM. *Blood Supply of the Spine and Effect of Trophic Changes and Load on Its Shape: Clinical, Anatomical and Experimental Study.* Chelyabinsk: Urals Book Press, 1981, 224 pp.
45. Isaev A. *Alternative Methods of Treatment for Spinal Osteochondrosis.* K.: S.K.F., 1996, 312 pp.
46. Ivanchenko VA. *Secrets of Vivacity.* M.: Knowledge, 1988, 288 pp.
47. Ivanichev GA. *Manual Medicine (Manual Therapy).* M.: Medpress, 1998, 470 pp.
48. Ivanov GF. *Fundamentals of Normal Human Anatomy* in 2 volumes. M.: Medgiz, 1949, 540 pp.
49. James JIP. *Scoliosis.* Edinburg, London: E.a.S. Livingstone, 1967, 274 p.
50. Jung R (1953) – Citation by Somov EE. *Clinical Anatomy of Human Body.* M.: Medpres-Inform, 2005, 136 p.
51. Kanareikin KF. *Lumbo-sacral pain.* M.: Medicine, 1972, 128 pp.
52. Kasian NA. *Manual Therapy for Osteochondrosis.* M.: Medicine, 1987, 195 pp.
53. Kazmin AI, Kozlov VA. *Some Aspects of Regulation of Water Metabolism of the Intervertebral Disc.* Osteochondrosis of the Spine: Rep. Abstracts. M.: Science, 1972, Part 2, 300 pp.
54. Kazmin AI, Micskevich VA. *Theoretical Aspects of Osteochondrosis.* Medicine and Health Care. M.: Medicine (Surgery Series), 1985, 76 pp.
55. Khodjaev RR. *Familial Forms of Scoliosis (Clinical Features).* Author's Abstract on PhD Thesis for Medical Sciences. M., 1970, 14 pp.
56. Kirillov AI. *Scoliosis. Effective Treatment and Prevention* (Advices of an Experienced Physician). M.: AST, St. Petersburg: Owl, 2007, 128 pp.
57. Kish FM, Santogotai J. *Anatomical Atlas of the Human Body* in 3 volumes. Budapest: Medicine, 1962, Vol. 1, 314 pp.
58. Kleinberg S. *Scoliosis.* Baltimore: Williams & Wilkins, 1951, 256 p.
59. Kondratiev PP. *Congenital Deformations of the Spine.* Proceedings of the Naval Academy, 9 vol. L., 1937, pp. 97–110.

60. Korovessis P, Iliopoulos P, Koureas G, *et al.* Color Doppler Ultrasonography for Evaluation of Anterior Chest Blood Supply: The Possible Role of Anterior Blood Supply by Internal Mammary Artery to the Costosternal Junction in the Etiology of Adolescent Female Right Convex Idiopathic Scoliosis. *European Spine Journal* 2003;**12:**26.
61. Korzh AA, Hvisyuk NI, Sac NN. Some Issues on The Etiology and Pathogenesis of Osteochondrosis of the Lumbar Spine. *Orthopaedics, Traumatology and Prosthetics* 1974;**No.11:**1–10.
62. Korzh AA, Hvisyuk NI, Prodan AI. Manual Therapy for Spinal Osteochondrosis: An Analytical Review of Literature. *Orthopaedics, Traumatology and Prosthetics* 1980;**No.10:**218–21.
63. Kos J. Contribution a l`etude de l`anatomic et de la vascularisation des articulations intervertebrales. *Bulletin de l'Association des anatomiste* 1968;**53:**1088–105.
64. Kozlovsky A. On the Etiology and Treatment of Scoliosis. *Journal of Surgery and Related Specialities* 1927;**9:**253–8.
65. Krapivka I. *Spine – the Core of Health. Notes of Chiropractor.* M.: Gramota, 1997, 119 pp.
66. Krupko IL. *Guidelines for Traumatology and Orthopedics* in 2 volumes. M.: Medicine, 1975.
67. KuznetsovaMA-CitedfromIvanichevGA.*ManualMedicine(ManualTherapy).*M.:MEDpress,1998,470pp.
68. Levitt K, Sachs J, Janda W. *Manual Medicine:* Translated from German. M.: Medicine, 1993, 512 pp.
69. Lindemann K. Aetiologie und Pathogenese der Scoliose. *Handbuch der Orthopadie* 1958;**No.2:**S.160–S.187.
70. Lindenbraten LD. *Variants and Anomalies of Human Organs and Systems in Radiographic Images.* M.: Medgiz, 1954, 92 pp.
71. Lobenko AA, Vasiliev NA, Ignatiev AM. Clinical Manifestations, Diagnosis and Treatment of Degenerative Diseases of the Spine in Water Transport Workers. K.: *Health,* 1991, 96 pp.
72. Long DM. Myofascial Pain and Fibromyalgia Syndrome. *Neurology* 1997;**48:**1740–1.
73. Lovett R. The Mechanism of the Normal Spine and its Relation to Scoliosis. *The Boston Medical and Surgical Journal* 1905;**153:**349–58.
74. Lukacher GY. *Neurologic Manifestations of Spinal Osteochondrosis.* M.: Medicine, 1985, 240 pp.
75. Lyandres ZA *Scolioses Associated with Malformations of the Spine and Surgical Treatment of These Conditions.* Jubilee Scientific Session on the 100th Anniversary of GI Turner: Works. L., 1959, 259–310.
76. Lysenkov NK, Bushkovich VI. *Normal Human Anatomy.* M., L., 1933, 612 pp.
77. Madzhidov NM, Dusmuratov MD. *Thoracic Osteochondrosis and Associated Neurological Syndromes.* Tashkent, 1982, 168 pp.
78. Maheshwari J. *Essential Orthopedics. Scoliosis and Other Spinal Deformities.* New Delhi, 1993, 233–7.
79. Melzack R, Wall PD. Pain Mechanisms. *Science* 1965;**150:**971.
80. Mikhailov MK, Khabibullin IR. *Variants and Anomalies of the Spine on Radiographs.* Kazan, 1986, 32 pp.
81. Mitbreyt IM. *Spondylolisthesis (Pathogenesis, Clinical Features and Treatment).* Author's Abstract on Doctoral Thesis for Medical Sciences. M., 1969, 40 pp.
82. Mitbreyt IM. *Spondylolisthesis.* M.: Medicine, 1978, 271 pp.
83. Mixer WJ, Barr IS. Rupture of the Intervertibral Disk with Involvement of the Spinal Canal. *The New England Journal of Medicine* 1934;**211:**210–14.
84. Movshovich IA. *Scoliosis. Surgical Anatomy and Pathogenesis.* M., Medicine, 1964, 255 pp.
85. Mueller G. *Orthopedics for Practicing Physicians:* Translated from German. SPb., 1913, 191 pp.
86. Nachemson A. L. Low-back pain. It's Etiology and Treatment. *Clinical Medicine* 1971;**No.78:**18–24.
87. Nicoladoni C. *Anatomie und Mechanismus der Scoliose.* Berlin–Wien, 1909, 58 p.
88. Nikitin GD, GP Saldun, NV Kornilov, *et al. Bony and Metal Fixation of The Spine in Diseases, Injuries and Their Consequences.* SPb.: Russian Graphics, 1998, 447 pp.
89. Nordemar R. Back Pain: *Its Causes, Treatment and Prevention* [translated from Swedish]. M.: Medicine, 1991, 144 pp.
90. Novachenko NP. *Fundamentals of Orthopedics and Traumatology.* M.: Medgiz, 1961, 280 pp.
91. Ponseti I, Friedman B. Prognosis in Idiopathic Scoliosis. *The Journal of Bone and Joint Surgery* 1950;**32-A:**381–95.

92. Popelyansky YY, Popelyansky AY. Thoracic Pain Syndromes. *Rheumatology* 1984:**No.4:**65–9.
93. Popelyansky YY. *Orthopedic Neurology* (Vertebro-Neurology): *A Guide for Physicians.* M.: Med. Pres-Inform, 2003, 672 pp.
94. *Popular Medical Encyclopedia.* Section 'The Human'. M., Soviet Encyclopedia, 1961, pp. 1178–85.
95. Puhacheva SS. *Osteochondrosis of the Lumbar Spine in Children, Adolescents and Young Adults.* Author's Abstract on PhD Thesis for Medical Sciences. H., 1979, 26 pp.
96. Rachkov BM. *Osteochondrosis.* St. Petersburg.: Flamingo, 1995, 49 pp.
97. Ratner AY. *Birth Injuries to the Nervous System.* Kazan, 1985, 393 p.
98. Reinberg SA. *Radiologic Diagnosis of Diseases of Bones and Joints,* 2 volumes. M.: Medicine, 1964;**1:**530 pp; **2:**572 pp.
99. Reisman AM, Bagrov FI. *Detorsionnal Exercises in Physiotherapy for Scoliosis.* M.: Medgiz, 1960, 42 pp.
100. Revel MJ. Strabismus. *A History of Orthoptic Techniques.* London: Barrie & Jenkins; 1971, 15 p.
101. Roaf R. Rotation Movements of the Spine with Special Reference to Scoliosis. *The Journal of Bone and Joint Surgery* 1958;**40-B:**312–32.
102. Rogers SP. Mechanism of Scoliosis. *Archives of Surgery* 1933;**No.26:**962–80.
103. Russwurm H, Bjerkeim J, Ronglann E. Intervertibral Disc Herniation in the Young. *Acta Orthopaedica Scandinavica* 1978;**49:**158–63.
104. Samosyuk IZ, Voytanik SA, Popiva TD, Gavata BV. *Manual Therapy, Homeopathy and Acupuncture for Osteochondrosis of the Spine.* K.: Health, 1992, 272 pp.
105. Sampiev MT, Laka AA, Zagorodniy NV. *Scoliosis.* M.: GEOTAR Media, 2008, 144 pp.
106. Sandrigailo LI. *Anatomical and Clinical Atlas of Neurology.* Minsk, 1988, 320 pp.
107. Sapin MR. *Human Anatomy.* M.: Medgiz, 1986, 340 pp.
108. Sapin MR, Bilic GL. *Human Anatomy* in 2 volumes. M.: Alliance-V, 2000, vol 1, 463 pp; vol 2, 432 pp.
109. Schantz AM. *Practical Orthopedics: Translated from German.* M.: Medgiz, 1933, 410 pp.
110. Schapero M. *Amblyopia.* London, 1971, 35–55.
111. Schiano R. *Rosarios 5 Minuten- Gymnastik fur Fitness in Jedem Alter.* Leipzig, 2006, 69 p.
112. Schmidt IR. *Osteochondrosis of the Spine.* Novosibirsk, 1992, 340 pp.
113. Schmidt RF, Thews G. *Human Physiology.* NY: Springer–Verlag, 1983, 797 p.
114. Sechenov IM. *Physiology of the Nervous System.* SPb, 1866, 503 pp.
115. Serdyuk VV, Herzen IG, Faerman DC, Artemenko AP. *The Soviet Union. Device for Magnetotherapy.* Author`s certoficate No.784060. MCI A61N1/42, Odessa Medical Institute. Named after Pirogov N.I. Appl. 18/07/1977, Publ. 01.08.80, 12 p.
116. Serdyuk VV, Ternovoy KS, Apotovsky EL, Roisin VL. *The Soviet Union. Device for magnetotherapy.* Author`s certificate No.1140297, MCI A61N 1/42, Appl. 22/11/1982, Publ. 22.11.82, 10 p.
117. Serdyuk VV, Muhsen SA, Apotovsky EL, Roisin VL. *USSR Patent. Device for Magnetotherapy.* No.32881, Appl. 26.09.1990, 3 pp.
118. Serdyuk VV. *Patent of Ukraine. Device for Magnetotherapy.* No.4119, Appl. 29.06.93, No.94230306, Cl. A 61 N 1/42. *Bulletin* 1994;**No.6:**1–7.
119. Serdyuk VV. Discovery Diploma of Ukraine. *Dependence of Adult Diseases on Deformations of the Spine in Childhood.* Ukrainian Academy of Original Ideas; registered in Academic Registry of Priorities of Intellectual Property, 1995, 2 pp.
120. Serdyuk VV. The Emergence and Development of Spinal Deformities. Medical and Social Aspects. *Theme* 1995;**No. 3/4:**40–41.
121. Serdyuk VV. The Emergence and Development of Spinal Deformities. Medical and Social Aspects. *Theme* 1997;**No. 2:**19–27.
122. Serdyuk VV. Adult Diseases Associated with Spinal Deformities in Childhood. *Inventor of Ukraine* 1998;**No.1:**67–68.
123. Serdyuk VV. On the Nature of Spinal Pain Syndrome. Proceedings of Scientific Conference of Vertebrologists *Relevant Issues of Vertebrology.* H., 1998, pp. 59–61.

124. Serdyuk VV, Komashko OM. Declarative Patent of Ukraine, No. 48,900. *VV Serdyuk's Method for Strabismus Treatment.* Odessa State Medical University, A61F5/00; 2002, Bull. No.8, 8 p.
125. Serdyuk VV. *Magnetothterapy: Past, Present and Future – a reference guide.* K.: Azimuth-Ukraine, 2004, 536 pp.
126. Serdyuk VV, Komashko AM. *Certificate of know-how.* Number HX 025 - Ukraine - Method of Treatment of Inflammation of Trigeminal nerve (Trigeminitis). Ukrainian Academy of Original Ideas; Acad. Rectr from 04/15/05. 3s.
127. Serdyuk VV. *Know-how certificate.* Ukraine - Method of Correction of the Lateral Spinal Curvature. Ukrainian Academy of Original Ideas; Academ. Regist. on 15/04/2005, 3 pp.
128. Serdyuk VV. *Know-how certificate.* Ukraine - Method of Correction of Unequal Length of the Lower Extremities. Academy of Original Ideas; Academic. Registr. on 125/04/2005, 3 pp.
129. Serdyuk VV, Golubov MA. *Ukraine. Device for Correction of Lateral Curvature of the Spine.* Author`s certificate No. 035. Ukrainian Academy of Original Ideas, Registered in Academic registry of priorities of intellectual property. 15.04.05, 3 p.
130. Serdyuk VV. On the Problem of Persistent Lumbosacral Pain Syndrome. In: Serdyuk VV, Wenger WF, Serdyuk EV. *Journal of Naval Medicine* 2006;**No.3:**288–90.
131. Serdyuk VV. Discovery Diploma of Ukraine. *Regularity of Formation of Scoliotic Deformation of the Spine Due to Instability in all its Regions, Which Arise as a Consequence of Unilateral Hypertonus of Spinal Muscles Caused with Asymmetric Functioning of Cerebral Hemispheres.* Ukrainian Academy of Original Ideas; Registered in Academic Registry of Priorities of Intellectual Property; 2008, 2 pp.
132. Serdyuk VV, Svinarev UN. On the Regularity of Formation of Lateral (Scoliotic) Spinal Curvature. *Inventor of Ukraine* 2008;**No.1/2;**109–126.
133. Serdyuk VV. Effect of Spinal Deformities on the Emergence of Various Human Diseases. *Journal of Naval Medicine* 2009;**No.2:**143–9.
134. Serdyuk VV. On the Nature of Various Human Diseases in Relationship to Spinal Deformities. *Inventor of Ukraine* 2009;**No.1:**127–134.
135. Sevastik J. *The Thoracospinal Concept: A New Theory of the Pathogenesis of Idiopathic Scoliosis.* GICD 10th International Congress. Seoul, 1993, pp. 9–13.
136. Severin GS. *Vertebral Artery Syndrome in Cervical Osteochondrosis.* Author's Abstract on PhD Thesis for Medical Sciences. Minsk, 1983, 23 p.
137. Shapiro MN. *The Role of the Intervertebral Disc in Spinal Diseases.* Author's Abstract on Doctoral Thesis for Medical Sciences. Minsk, 1938, 38 pp.
138. Shulutko LI. *Lateral Curvature of the Spine in Children (Scoliosis).* Kazan: Tatknigoizdat, 1968, 134 pp.
139. Simons DG, Travel JG. Myofascial Origin of Low Back Pain. *Postgraduate Medicine* 1983;**73:**66.
140. Sinelnikov RD, Sinelnikov YR. *Atlas of Human Anatomy* in 4 volumes. M.: Medicine, 1967, 1–350 pp.
141. Sitel AB. *Solo for the Spine.* M.: Metaphor, 2006, 223 pp.
142. Sitenko MI. *Lumbar Pain from the Orthopedic Perspective.* 4th Ukrainian Congress of Surgeons: Abstracts of Reports. Kharkov, 1936, 88 pp.
143. Sitenko MI. *Orthopaedics and Traumatology: Selected works.* Kiev: Naukova Dumka, 1991, 136 pp.
144. Somerville E. Rotational Lordosis. The Development of the Single Curve. *The Journal of Bone and Joint Surgery.* 1952;**34-B:**421.
145. Somov EE. *Clinical Anatomy of the Human Eye.* M.: Medpres-Inform, 2005, 136 pp.
146. Sorkin AZ. *Diagnostic Mistakes in Diseases and Malformations of the Osteoarticular Apparatus.* M.: Medicine, 1969, 96 pp.
147. Stillwell D. Structural Deformities of Vertebrae. *The Journal of Bone and Joint Surgery* 1962;**44-A:**611–34.
148. Sutcliffe J. *Forget About Back Pain:* Translated From English. M.: Mahaon, 2002, 112 pp.
149. Tager IL, Kupriyanov WF. *Anomalies of Vertebral Articular Processes – Classification and Significance. Surgery* 1937;**No.4:**88–100.
150. Touzet P, Rigault P. Scoliosis. *La semaine des hapitaux* 1983;**59:**261–6.

151. Travell JG, Simons DG. *Myofascial Pain and Disfunction. The Trigger Point Manual.* Baltimore, London, 1984, 607 p.
152. Tregubov SL. *Fundamentals of Orthopedics.* M.: Medgiz, 1939, 276 pp.
153. Tsivyan YL. *Spinal Injuries.* M.: Medicine, 1971, 312 pp.
154. Tsivyan YL. *Scoliotic Disease and Its Treatment.* Tashkent: Medicine; 1972, 221 pp.
155. Tsivyan YL. *Surgical Treatment of Humps.* M.: Medicine, 1973, 264 pp.
156. Turner GI. Vicious Development of the Spine in the Etiology of its Deformation. *Orthopedics and Traumatology* 1929;**No.1/2:**9–28.
157. Unanov AA, Unanov TA. *Treatment and Prevention of Scoliosis in Children: A Handbook.* Odessa: Astroprint, 2000, 92 pp.
158. Unanov AA. *Essays of Professor Unanov. On the Maternity and Infancy.* Odessa: Astroprint, 2001, 236 pp.
159. Veselovsky VP. *Pathogenesis of Ostheochondrosis of the Spine.* L.: Medgiz, 1984.
160. Veselovsky VP, Samitov OS. *Vertebrogenic Paresthetic Meralgia.* Kazan: Kazan University Publishing, 1988, 136 p.
161. Veselovsky VP, Mikhailov MK, Samitov OS. *Diagnosis of Osteochondrosis Syndromes.* Kazan: Kazan University Publishing, 1990, 136 p.
162. Vorobiev VP. *Human Anatomy* in 2 volumes. M.: Medicine, 1932, Vol. 1, 702 p.
163. Vreden RR. Dysplasias of the Lower Spine, Their Consequences and Treatment. *Orthopedics and Traumatology* 1931;**No.4:**5–10.
164. Vreden RR. *Practical Guide for Orthopedics.* L., 1936, 606 p.
165. Wayne AM, Avrutsky MJ. *Pain and Analgesia.* M.: Medicine, 1997, 280 p.
166. Weisberg J, Shine H. *3 Minutes to a Pain-free Life.* NY: Atria Books, 2005, 301 p.
167. Yamada K., Yamamoto H., Nakagawa Y, *et al.* Etiology of Idiopathic Scoliosis. *Clinical Orthopaedics and Related Research*;1984:**184:**50.
168. Yarom R, Robin G, Gorodetsky R. Yarom R. X-ray Fluorescence Analysis of Muscles in Scoliosis. *Spine* 1978;**3:**142.
169. Yarovoy VK. *Fundamentals of Manual Therapy: A Guide for Physicians and Students.* Sebastopol: NPC 'ecosi-hydrophysics', 1999, 171 pp.
170. Yukina TP, Mikhailova LS. Infantile Scoliosis. *Relevant Issues of Prevention and Treatment of Scoliosis in Children: The All-Union Symposium: Mater.* M., 1984, 21–4.
171. Yumashev GS, Furman ME. *Osteochondroses of the Spine.* M.: Medicine, 1984, 382 pp.
172. Zatsepin TS. *Orthopedics of Childhood and Adolescence.* M.: Medgiz, 1956, 319 pp.
173. Zolotareva MM. *Eye Diseases: Practical Guide for an Ophthalmologist.* Minsk, Belarus, 1964, 619 pp.
174. Zubarev SF. *The Soviet Union. A Method of Treating Strabismus.* Author`s Certificate No. 1641329. 1988, 2 p.